Pharmacokinetics and Drug Metabolism in Canada: The Current Landscape

Special Issue Editors

Neal M. Davies
Kishor M. Wasan

MDPI • Basel • Beijing • Wuhan • Barcelona • Belgrade

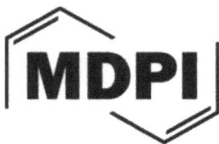

MDPI

Special Issue Editors

Neal M. Davies
University of Alberta
Canada

Kishor M. Wasan
University of British Columbia
Canada

Editorial Office
MDPI AG
St. Alban-Anlage 66
Basel, Switzerland

This edition is a reprint of the Special Issue published online in the open access journal *Pharmaceutics* (ISSN 1999-4923) from 2017–2018 (available at: http://www.mdpi.com/journal/pharmaceutics/special_issues/pkdmcanada).

For citation purposes, cite each article independently as indicated on the article page online and as indicated below:

Lastname, F.M.; Lastname, F.M. Article title. *Journal Name.* **Year**. *Article number*, page range.

First Edition 2018

ISBN 978-3-03842-797-1 (Pbk)
ISBN 978-3-03842-798-8 (PDF)

Table of Contents

About the Special Issue Editors

Neal M. Davies received his undergraduate degree in Pharmacy from the University of Alberta in 1991. In 1996, he completed his Ph.D. in pharmaceutical sciences at the University of Alberta. From 1995 to 1998, he undertook postdoctoral training in pharmacology and toxicology at the University of Calgary. He then joined the University of Sydney as a lecturer in 1998. In 2002, he joined the Washington State University College of Pharmacy as an academic staff member, where he has held the positions of Director of the Pharmaceutical Sciences Graduate Program, Director of Professional and Undergraduate Research, and Director of the Summer Undergraduate Research Fellowship program. From 2011 to 2016 he was Dean of the Faculty of Pharmacy at the University of Manitoba. On September 1, 2016, Dr. Davies commenced his term as Dean and Professor in the Faculty of Pharmacy and Pharmaceutical Sciences at the University of Alberta.

Kishor M. Wasan was appointed Dean of the College of Pharmacy and Nutrition at the University of Saskatchewan in August 2014. He has published over 550 peer-reviewed articles and abstracts in the area of lipid-based drug delivery and lipoprotein–drug interactions. Dr. Wasan completed his undergraduate degree in Pharmacy at the University of Texas at Austin and his Ph.D. in Cellular and Molecular Pharmacology at MD Anderson, University of Texas Medical Center in Houston, Texas . After completing a postdoctoral fellowship in Cell Biology at the Cleveland Clinic, Dr. Wasan joined the Faculty of Pharmaceutical Sciences at the University of British Columbia in 2014. Dr. Wasan has been the recipient of numerous scientific awards, fellowships, and research chairs, including the American Association of Pharmaceutical Scientists New Investigator Award and the Canadian Institutes of Health Research University-Industry Research Chair, and was named a Fellow of the Canadian Academy of Health Sciences.

.

Preface to "Pharmacokinetics and Drug Metabolism in Canada: The Current Landscape"

Canadian Pharmaceutical Scientists have a rich history of groundbreaking research in pharmacokinetics and drug metabolism undertaken primarily throughout its Pharmacy Faculties and within the Pharmaceutical and Biotechnology industry. The principles of drug absorption, distribution, metabolism, and excretion (ADME) is the foundational basis of rationale drug-design, and principled pharmacotherapy. The study of ADME and its descriptive quantitative analysis is the basis of pharmacokinetics. Pharmacokinetics is fundamental in the development of a new chemical entity into a marketable product and is essential in understanding the bioavailability, bioequivalence, and biosimilarities of drugs. Pharmacokinetics and drug metabolism and development studies facilitate an understanding of organ-based functionality. Population pharmacokinetic variability and the modeling of drug concentrations has significant utility in translating individual response in a target patient population underlying advances in precision health.

This book issue serves to highlight and capture the contemporary progress and current landscape of pharmacokinetics and drug metabolism within the prevailing Canadian context and the impact this pharmaceutical sciences research has had on an international scientific community.

This book presents a series of review articles highlighting a summary of the research that investigators from across the country have completed, thus making meaningful and significant contributions to the field. In addition, this special issue has published a series of new leading edge translational research articles demonstrating the continued vibrant collaborative activity of our pharmaceutical sciences community.

Taken together, these papers represent only a fraction of the important and contemporary research in pharmaceutical sciences across Canada and represent the breadth and depth of work carried out in our fine world class institutions by preeminent pharmaceutical scientists in the areas of pharmacokinetics and drug metabolism. Given a recent review of the structure of funding agencies and the recommended improvements to governance and coordination in Canada, strengthening pharmaceutical research and support of early career pharmaceutical scientists is prudent. Canada's future as a knowledge-based economy is strengthened by the pharmaceutical research conducted across the nation and the acquisition of pharmaceutical knowledge, and the success of governments' strategies on technology, innovation, and health sciences could be further enhanced through increased support of leading-edge pharmaceutical investigations highlighted here. Canada, both in research and economically, is more competitive and better positioned on the world stage because of its thriving and vibrant pharmaceutical research community, which this special issue aims to demonstrate.

Neal M. Davies and Kishor M. Wasan

Special Issue Editors

pharmaceutics

MDPI

Editorial

Pharmacokinetics and Drug Metabolism in Canada: The Current Landscape—A Summary of This Indispensable Special Issue

Neal M. Davies [1],* and Kishor M. Wasan [2],*

1   Faculty of Pharmacy and Pharmaceutical Sciences, University of Alberta, Edmonton, AB T6G 2R3, Canada
2   College of Pharmacy and Nutrition, University of Saskatchewan, Saskatoon, SK S7N 2Z4, Canada
*   Correspondence: ndavies@ualberta.ca (N.M.D.); kishor.wasan@usask.ca (K.M.W.);
     Tel.: +1-780-221-0828 (N.M.D.); +1-306-966-3202 (K.M.W.)

Received: 15 January 2018; Accepted: 15 January 2018; Published: 16 January 2018

Canadian Pharmaceutical Scientists have a rich history of groundbreaking research in pharmacokinetics and drug metabolism undertaken primarily throughout its Pharmacy Faculties and within the Pharmaceutical and Biotechnology industry. The principles of drug absorption, distribution, metabolism, and excretion (ADME) is the foundational basis of rationale drug-design, and principled pharmacotherapy. The study of ADME and its descriptive quantitative analysis is the basis of pharmacokinetics. Pharmacokinetics is fundamental in the development of a new chemical entity into a marketable product and is essential in understanding the bioavailability, bioequivalence, and biosimilarities of drugs. Pharmacokinetics and drug metabolism and development studies facilitate an understanding of organ-based functionality. Population pharmacokinetic variability and the modeling of drug concentrations has significant utility in translating individual response in a target patient population underlying advances in precision health.

This special issue serves to highlight and capture the contemporary progress and current landscape of pharmacokinetics and drug metabolism within the prevailing Canadian context and the impact this pharmaceutical sciences research has had on an international scientific community.

This special issue presents a series of review articles highlighting a summary of the research that investigators from across the country have completed, thus making meaningful and significant contributions to the field. El-Kadi and colleagues from the University of Alberta summarized the clinical implications and impact of 20-hydroxyeicosatetraenoic acid in the kidney, liver, lung, and brain as a potential therapeutic target for many diseases [1]. Liu and Coughtrie from the University of British Columbia revised their paper about the latency of uridine diphosphate-glucuronosyltransferases (UGTs) and how the endoplasmic reticulum membrane influences their function [2].

Mahmoud and Shen from the University of Alberta discusses augmented renal clearance (ARC) as a manifestation of enhanced renal function seen in critically ill patients and show that the use of regular unadjusted doses of renally eliminated drugs in patients with ARC might lead to therapy failure [3].

Lin and Wong from the University of British Columbia focus on the development of orally absorbed physiologically based pharmacokinetic (PBPK) models and briefly discuss the major applications of these models in the pharmaceutical industry [4]. Kiang from the University of Alberta and colleagues from University of British Columbia provide a qualitative review on (1) the principles of therapeutic drug monitoring (TDM); (2) alternative matrices for TDM; (3) current evidence supporting the use of interstitial fluid (ISF) for TDM in clinical models; (4) the use of microneedle technologies, which is potentially minimally invasive and pain-free, for the collection of ISF; and (5) future directions [5].

In addition, this special issue has published a series of new leading edge translational research articles demonstrating the continued vibrant collaborative activity of our pharmaceutical sciences community. Edginton with Canadian colleagues from McMaster and Waterloo explored different weight metrics including lean body weight, ideal body weight, and adjusted body weight to determine an alternative dosing strategy that is both safe and resource-efficient in normal and overweight/obese adult patients [6]. Lakowski and colleagues from University of Manitoba and Alberta identified the metabolism, excretion, antioxidant, anti-inflammatory, and anticancer properties of curcuminoids and determined disposition in rodents [7,8]. Simard and colleagues from Université Laval set out to determine if altered protein expression of cardiac and hepatic drug metabolizing enzymes in a mouse model of Type II diabetes lead to the onset and development of cardiovascular disease [9]. Leung, Turgeon, and Michaud from the Université de Montréal presented a study of statin- and loratadine-induced muscle pain mechanisms using human skeletal muscle cells [10]. The same group lead by Michaud and colleagues investigated the specific modulation of cyp2c and cyp3a mRNA levels and activities via diet-induced obesity in mice and the impact of Type II diabetes on drug metabolizing enzymes in liver and extra-hepatic tissues [11].

Davies, Lobenberg, Burczynski, and colleagues from the University of Manitoba and Alberta with international collaborators completed a pharmacokinetic analysis of an oral multicomponent joint dietary supplement in dogs as well as a pharmacokinetic and toxicodynamic characterization of a new doxorubicin derivative with reported lymphatic delivery [12]. Sitar and colleagues from the University of Manitoba and University of Toronto investigated a new theophylline metabolite, theophylline-7β-D-ribofuranoside (theonosine), generated in human and animal lung tissue [13].

Brocks and colleagues from the University of Alberta reported on the development of a selective and sensitive high-performance liquid chromatographic method for the determination of lidocaine in human serum and its application to clinical pharmacokinetics [14]. Foster and colleagues based in Alberta, Canada, and ContraVir Pharmaceuticals Inc., located in Edison, New Jersey, in the United States discussed the in vitro Phase I metabolism of CRV431, a new oral drug candidate for chronic hepatitis B [15].

Piquette-Miller and Gahir from the University of Toronto and Reata Pharmaceuticals, respectively, discussed the role of the PXR genotype and transporter expression in the placental transport of lopinavir in mice [16].

Ellen Wasan and colleagues from the University of Saskatchewan provided an overview of the chitosan-based nanoparticles for various non-parenteral applications and highlighted current research, including sustained release and mucoadhesive chitosan dosage forms that can alter input and pharmacokinetics and targeting [17]. Collier from the University of British Columbia with a cross boarder collaboration with colleagues from Hawaii, USA, unraveled the regulation of hepatic UGT2B15 via methylation in adults of Asian descent [18]. Finally, in a tri-nation international collaboration (Canada, USA, and Qatar) with its roots at the University of Manitoba, Faculty of Pharmacy in Winnipeg, Rachid, Rawas-Qalaji, and Simons extended their investigations towards the development of a novel sublingual epinephrine tablet formulation for anaphylaxis for potential pediatric use in a pre-clinical study [19].

Taken together, these papers represent only a fraction of the important and contemporary research in pharmaceutical sciences across Canada and represent the breadth and depth of work carried out in our fine world class institutions by preeminent pharmaceutical scientists in the areas of pharmacokinetics and drug metabolism. Given a recent review of the structure of funding agencies and the recommended improvements to governance and coordination in Canada, strengthening pharmaceutical research and support of early career pharmaceutical scientists is prudent. Canada's future as a knowledge-based economy is strengthened by the pharmaceutical research conducted across the nation and the acquisition of pharmaceutical knowledge, and the success of governments' strategies on technology, innovation, and health sciences could be further enhanced through increased support of leading-edge pharmaceutical investigations highlighted here. Canada, both in research and economically, is more competitive and better positioned on the world stage because of its thriving and vibrant pharmaceutical research community, which this special issue aims to demonstrate.

Conflicts of Interest: The authors declare no conflict of interest.

References

1. Elshenawy, O.H.; Shoieb, S.M.; Mohamed, A.; El-Kadi, A.O. Clinical Implications of 20-Hydroxyeicosatetraenoic Acid in the Kidney, Liver, Lung and Brain: An Emerging Therapeutic Target. *Pharmaceutics* **2017**, *9*, 9. [CrossRef] [PubMed]
2. Liu, Y.; Coughtrie, M.W.H. Revisiting the Latency of Uridine Diphosphate-Glucuronosyltransferases (UGTs)—How Does the Endoplasmic Reticulum Membrane Influence Their Function? *Pharmaceutics* **2017**, *9*, 32.
3. Mahmoud, S.H.; Shen, C. Augmented Renal Clearance in Critical Illness: An Important Consideration in Drug Dosing. *Pharmaceutics* **2017**, *9*, 36. [CrossRef] [PubMed]
4. Lin, L.; Wong, H. Predicting Oral Drug Absorption: Mini Review on Physiologically-Based Pharmacokinetic Models. *Pharmaceutics* **2017**, *9*, 41. [CrossRef] [PubMed]
5. Kiang, T.K.; Ranamukhaarachchi, S.A.; Ensom, M.H. Revolutionizing Therapeutic Drug Monitoring with the Use of Interstitial Fluid and Microneedles Technology. *Pharmaceutics* **2017**, *9*, 43. [CrossRef] [PubMed]
6. McEneny-King, A.; Chelle, P.; Henrard, S.; Hermans, C.; Iorio, A.; Edginton, A.N. Modeling of Body Weight Metrics for Effective and Cost-Efficient Conventional Factor VIII Dosing in Hemophilia A Prophylaxis. *Pharmaceutics* **2017**, *9*, 47. [CrossRef] [PubMed]
7. Martinez, S.E.; Lillico, R.; Lakowski, T.M.; Martinez, S.A.; Davies, N.M. Pharmacokinetic Analysis of an Oral Multicomponent Joint Dietary Supplement (Phycox®) in Dogs. *Pharmaceutics* **2017**, *9*, 30. [CrossRef] [PubMed]
8. Novaes, J.T.; Lillico, R.; Sayre, C.L.; Nagabushanam, K.; Majeed, M.; Chen, Y.; Ho, E.A.; Oliveira, A.L.P.; Martinez, S.E.; Alrushaid, S.; et al. Disposition, Metabolism and Histone Deacetylase and Acetyltransferase Inhibition Activity of Tetrahydrocurcumin and Other Curcuminoids. *Pharmaceutics* **2017**, *9*, 45. [CrossRef] [PubMed]
9. Drolet, B.; Pilote, S.; Gélinas, C.; Kamaliza, A.-D.; Blais-Boilard, A.; Virgili, J.; Patoine, D.; Simard, C. Altered Protein Expression of Cardiac CYP2J and Hepatic CYP2C, CYP4A, and CYP4F in a Mouse Model of Type II Diabetes—A Link in the Onset and Development of Cardiovascular Disease? *Pharmaceutics* **2017**, *9*, 44. [CrossRef] [PubMed]
10. Leung, Y.H.; Turgeon, J.; Michaud, V. Study of Statin- and Loratadine-Induced Muscle Pain Mechanisms Using Human Skeletal Muscle Cells. *Pharmaceutics* **2017**, *9*, 42. [CrossRef] [PubMed]
11. Maximos, S.; Chamoun, M.; Gravel, S.; Turgeon, J.; Michaud, V. Tissue Specific Modulation of cyp2c and cyp3a mRNA Levels and Activities by Diet-Induced Obesity in Mice: The Impact of Type 2 Diabetes on Drug Metabolizing Enzymes in Liver and Extra-Hepatic Tissues. *Pharmaceutics* **2017**, *9*, 40. [CrossRef] [PubMed]
12. Alrushaid, S.; Sayre, C.L.; Yáñez, J.A.; Forrest, M.L.; Senadheera, S.N.; Burczynski, F.J.; Löbenberg, R.; Davies, N.M. Pharmacokinetic and Toxicodynamic Characterization of a Novel Doxorubicin Derivative. *Pharmaceutics* **2017**, *9*, 35. [CrossRef] [PubMed]
13. Sitar, D.S.; Bowen, J.M.; He, J.; Tesoro, A.; Spino, M. Theophylline-7β-D-Ribofuranoside (Theonosine), a New Theophylline Metabolite Generated in Human and Animal Lung Tissue. *Pharmaceutics* **2017**, *9*, 28. [CrossRef] [PubMed]
14. Al Nebaihi, H.M.; Primrose, M.; Green, J.S.; Brocks, D.R. A High-Performance Liquid Chromatography Assay Method for the Determination of Lidocaine in Human Serum. *Pharmaceutics* **2017**, *9*, 52. [CrossRef] [PubMed]
15. Trepanier, D.J.; Ure, D.R.; Foster, R.T. In Vitro Phase I Metabolism of CRV431, a Novel Oral Drug Candidate for Chronic Hepatitis B. *Pharmaceutics* **2017**, *9*, 51. [CrossRef] [PubMed]
16. Gahir, S.S.; Piquette-Miller, M. The Role of PXR Genotype and Transporter Expression in the Placental Transport of Lopinavir in Mice. *Pharmaceutics* **2017**, *9*, 49. [CrossRef] [PubMed]

17. Mohammed, M.A.; Syeda, J.T.M.; Wasan, K.M.; Wasan, E.K. An Overview of Chitosan Nanoparticles and Its Application in Non-Parenteral Drug Delivery. *Pharmaceutics* **2017**, *9*, 53. [CrossRef] [PubMed]
18. Oeser, S.G.; Bingham, J.P.; Collier, A.C. Regulation of Hepatic UGT2B15 by Methylation in 2 Adults of Asian Descent. *Pharmaceutics* **2018**, *10*, 6. [CrossRef] [PubMed]
19. Rachid, O.; Rawas-Qalaji, M.; Simons, K.J. Epinephrine in anaphylaxis: Preclinical study of pharmacokinetics after sublingual administration of taste-masked tablets for potential pediatric use. *Pharmaceutics* **2017**, accepted.

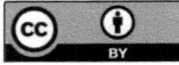

pharmaceutics

MDPI

Review

Clinical Implications of 20-Hydroxyeicosatetraenoic Acid in the Kidney, Liver, Lung and Brain: An Emerging Therapeutic Target

Osama H. Elshenawy [1], Sherif M. Shoieb [1], Anwar Mohamed [1,2] and Ayman O.S. El-Kadi [1,*]

[1]   Faculty of Pharmacy and Pharmaceutical Sciences, University of Alberta, Edmonton T6G 2E1, AB, Canada; oshenawy@ualberta.ca (O.H.E.); shoieb@ualberta.ca (S.M.S.); anwarmoh@ualberta.ca (A.M.)
[2]   Department of Basic Medical Sciences, College of Medicine, Mohammed Bin Rashid University of Medicine and Health Sciences, Dubai, United Arab Emirates
*   Correspondence: aelkadi@ualberta.ca; Tel.: 780-492-3071; Fax: 780-492-1217

Academic Editor: Kishor M. Wasan
Received: 12 January 2017; Accepted: 15 February 2017; Published: 20 February 2017

Abstract: Cytochrome P450-mediated metabolism of arachidonic acid (AA) is an important pathway for the formation of eicosanoids. The ω-hydroxylation of AA generates significant levels of 20-hydroxyeicosatetraenoic acid (20-HETE) in various tissues. In the current review, we discussed the role of 20-HETE in the kidney, liver, lung, and brain during physiological and pathophysiological states. Moreover, we discussed the role of 20-HETE in tumor formation, metabolic syndrome and diabetes. In the kidney, 20-HETE is involved in modulation of preglomerular vascular tone and tubular ion transport. Furthermore, 20-HETE is involved in renal ischemia/reperfusion (I/R) injury and polycystic kidney diseases. The role of 20-HETE in the liver is not clearly understood although it represents 50%–75% of liver CYP-dependent AA metabolism, and it is associated with liver cirrhotic ascites. In the respiratory system, 20-HETE plays a role in pulmonary cell survival, pulmonary vascular tone and tone of the airways. As for the brain, 20-HETE is involved in cerebral I/R injury. Moreover, 20-HETE has angiogenic and mitogenic properties and thus helps in tumor promotion. Several inhibitors and inducers of the synthesis of 20-HETE as well as 20-HETE analogues and antagonists are recently available and could be promising therapeutic options for the treatment of many disease states in the future.

Keywords: 20-hydroxyeicosatetraenoic acid (20-HETE); Cytochrome P450s (CYPs); arachidonic acid (AA); kidney; ischemia/reperfusion (I/R) injury; liver; lung; brain

1. Introduction

Arachidonic acid (AA), which is a major component of cell membrane, is known to be metabolized into different classes of eicosanoids, by cyclooxygenase (COX), lipoxygenase (LOX), and cytochrome P450 (CYP). COX is known to be responsible for production of prostaglandins (PGs); whereas LOX produces mid chain hydroxyeicosatetraenoic acids (HETEs), lipoxins (LXs), and leukotrienes (LTs). CYP enzymes produce epoxyeicosatrienoic acids (EETs) by CYP epoxygenases, and HETEs (terminal, sub-terminal, and mid-chain) by CYP hydroxylases [1–4]. Terminal hydroxylation of AA is known as ω-hydroxylation reaction in which AA is converted to 20-HETE through CYP4A and CYP4F enzymes [5–7]. COX plays an important role in metabolism of 20-HETE providing a diverse range of activities in different organs [8]. 20-HETE is metabolized by COX into hydroxyl analogue of vasoconstrictor prostaglandin H2 (20-OH PGH_2) which is further transformed by isomerases into vasodilator/diuretic metabolites (20-OH PGE_2, 20-OH PGI_2) and vasoconstrictor/antidiuretic metabolites (20-OH Thromboxane A_2. 20-OH PGF_{2a}) [9–11].

A number of selective inhibitors for 20-HETE synthesis have been previously used including 17-octadecynoic acid (17-ODYA), *N*-methylsulfonyl-12,12-dibromododec-11-enamide (DDMS), dibromododec-11-enoic acid (DBDD), *N*-hydroxy-*N'*-(4-butyl-2methylphenyl)formamidine (HET0016), *N*-(3-Chloro-4-morpholin-4-yl)Phenyl-*N'*-hydroxyimido formamide (TS011) and acetylenic fatty acid sodium 10-undecynyl sulfate (10-SUYS) [5,6,12–16]. Nonselective inhibitors of AA metabolism were also used including 1-Aminobenzotriazole (ABT) and Cobalt (II) chloride (CoCl$_2$) [17,18]. Recently, competitive antagonists have been employed including 20-hydroxyeicosa-6(Z),15(Z)-dienoic acid (6,15,20-HEDE; WIT002) and 20-hydroxyeicosa-6(Z),15(Z)-dienoyl]glycine (6,15,20-HEDGE) [5,13–15]. Peroxisome proliferator-activated receptor alpha (PPARα) agonists, such as fenofibrate and clofibrate, or gene therapy were used to upregulate the formation of 20-HETE besides 20-HETE mimetics, 20-hydroxyeicosa-5(Z),14(Z)-dienoic acid (5,14,20-HEDE; WIT003), and *N*-[20-hydroxyeicosa-5(Z),14(Z)-dienoyl]glycine (5,14,20-HEDGE) [13,15] (Figure 1 represents a summarization for 20-HETE modulators commonly used in previous literature).

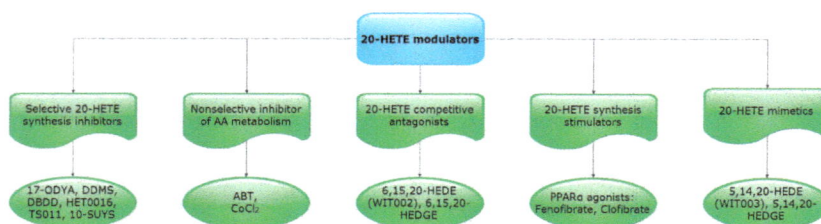

Figure 1. Different 20-hydroxyeicosatetraenoic acid (20-HETE) modulators commonly used to study the role of 20-HETE in vivo and in vitro.

Notably, eicosanoids exert their action through specific receptors called eicosanoid receptors, in addition to non-specific receptors such as PPAR receptors [19]. Recent data demonstrated the identification of a novel G protein-coupled receptor (GPCR) as 20-HETE receptor in the vascular endothelium [20]. The identification of 20-HETE receptor would result in better understanding of molecular mechanisms and clinical implications of 20-HETE in different organs. In this review, 20-HETE role in the kidney, liver, lung and brain during normal physiology, and during pathophysiological disease states will be discussed (summarized in Figure 2).

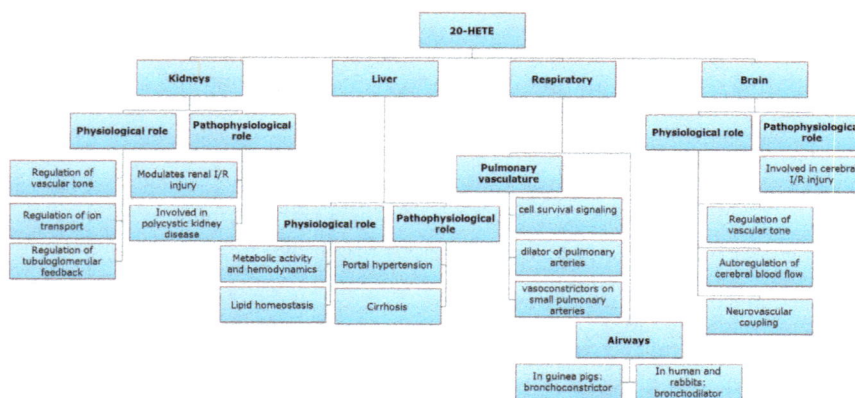

Figure 2. Role of 20-HETE in the kidney, liver, lung and brain during normal physiological and pathophysiological conditions.

Moreover, we will discuss 20-HETE role in mitogenicity. Furthermore, we will discuss the possible therapeutic approaches using 20-HETE mimetics, antagonists as well as synthesis inducers and inhibitors.

2. Role of 20-HETE in the Kidney

The kidney has the highest abundance of CYP among all extrahepatic organs, and the highest level within the kidney was found in the proximal tubules [21,22]. 20-HETE was identified as the major CYP metabolite of AA in the proximal tubule [21] and microsomes of renal cortex [23]. In thick ascending limb of the loop of Henle (TAL), 20-HETE and 20-carboxyeicosatetraenoic acid (20-COOH-AA) are the major AA metabolites of the CYP-dependent pathway [24,25]. 20-HETE is also a major AA metabolite in the renal microvasculature [26–28] and acts as a potent vasoconstrictor; however, its vasoconstrictor actions can be offset by its natriuretic properties [29]. 20-HETE contracts renal microvessels at concentrations of less than 10^{-10} M [30] and sensitizes renal vessels transfected with CYP4A1 cDNA to phenylephrine [31,32]. Also there is a strong evidence that locally produced 20-HETE plays a pivotal role in modulating the myogenic responsiveness of the afferent arteriole and may help explain how deficiencies in the renal production of 20-HETE could foster the initiation of hypertension-induced glomerular injury [33]. Therefore, 20-HETE is the preeminent renal eicosanoid, overshadowing PGE_2 and PGI_2 [8] and plays a role in vascular and tubular abnormalities of renovascular disease states [34]. Interestingly, 20-HETE reduces albumin permeability (P_{alb}), while on the other hand its relatively lowered levels are associated with increased P_{alb}, development of proteinuria and glomerular injury in early hypertension. Pretreatment of Sprague Dawley (SD) rats glomeruli with the 20-HETE mimetic, 5,14,20-HEDE, reduced baseline P_{alb} and opposed the effects of transforming growth factor-beta (TGF-β) to increase P_{alb} [35–37]. Moreover, exogenous 20-HETE or clofibrate treatment protected the glomeruli from increased P_{alb} caused by puromycin aminonucleoside, which is known to be an injurious agent [36].

2.1. Biosynthesis of 20-HETE in the Kidney

20-HETE production in the kidney has been extensively studied in rats, mice, and humans. In this regard, it was found that 20-HETE is formed primarily by CYP4A and CYP4F subfamilies (Figure 3) [5,38].

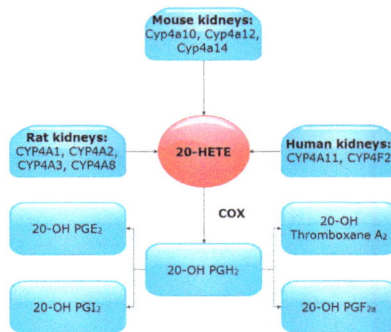

Figure 3. Enzymes responsible for 20-HETE formation and metabolism in different species.

In rat kidney, different CYP4A isoforms were detected, namely CYP4A1, CYP4A2, CYP4A3 and CYP4A8 [26,27,39–41]. Each of these isozymes contribute to a different extent to the basal renal function [42]. For example, CYP4A1 is characterized as a major 20-HETE synthesizing isozyme in the rat kidney [27,43,44]. On the other hand, CYP4A2 is a major contributor to hemodynamic responses, whereas CYP4A3 is a major contributor to tubular responses following nitric oxide (NO) inhibition [42].

CYPA expression and 20-HETE synthesis were the highest in the outer medulla followed by the cortex and lastly the inner medulla/papilla [45]. Also in rats, different CYP4F isoforms have been detected with CYP4F1, CYP4F4, and CYP4F5 being more expressed in the renal cortex than the medulla, while CYP4F6 shows higher medullary expression [46]. In the mouse, however, Cyp4a10, Cyp4a12, and Cyp4a14 are involved in 20-HETE synthesis, of which Cyp4a12a is the predominant 20-HETE synthase [47]. Interestingly, Cyp4a12a expression determines the sex and strain specific differences in 20-HETE generation [48]. Microdissected renal blood vessels and nephron segments from C57BL/6J mice revealed that Cyp4a and Cyp4f isoforms were detected in every segment analyzed [38]. In humans, it was found that microsomes from kidney cortex, converted AA mainly to 20-HETE by CYP4A11 and CYP4F2 [49,50]. Of interest, different human CYP4F2 variants have been identified, of which M433 allele was found to be associated with 56%–66% decrease in 20-HETE production [51].

2.2. Metabolism and Regulation of 20-HETE in the Kidney

Metabolism of 20-HETE by COX (Figure 3) is proposed to represent an important regulatory mechanism in setting preglomerular microvascular tone [52]. Renal vasoconstrictive effect of 20-HETE in response to hyperchloremia was shown to be dependent on COX activity [11]. Also, low-salt intake was found to stimulate the renin-angiotensin system and induces renal vascular expression of CYP4A and COX-2 in arcuate and interlobular arteries while COX-1 was unaffected [52]. It was found that low-salt diet increases 20-HETE levels in the incubate of either arcuate/interlobular or interlobular renal arteries only when COX was inhibited [52]. Thus, the capacity of COX to metabolize 20-HETE to PG analogs, e.g., 20-OH PGF$_{2a}$ and 20-OH PGE$_2$, may be critical to modify the renal vascular and tubular actions of the eicosanoids [53].

With regards to regulation of 20-HETE in the kidney, inhibition of its formation contributes to the cGMP-independent vasodilator response to NO in the renal microcirculation [8,54–58], attenuates myogenic tone and autoregulation of blood flow, and modulates vascular responses to the vasodilators, such as carbon monoxide (CO), and vasoconstrictors such as angiotensin II (AngII) and endothelin (ET) [59]. Interestingly, NO inhibits a variety of heme-containing enzymes, including NO synthase (NOS) and CYP enzymes. For example, it inhibits CYP4A exerting a negative modulatory effect on 20-HETE formation. Inhibition of NOS was found to increase ω-hydroxylase activity, CYP4A expression, and renal efflux of 20-HETE with a concomitant enhanced response to vasoconstrictor agents [8,54–58]. Inhibition of NOS with N(ω)-nitro-L-arginine-methyl ester (L-NAME) greatly increased the expression of ω-hydroxylase protein and induced a 4-fold increase in renal efflux of 20-HETE [55]. In addition, L-NAME increased mean arterial blood pressure and renal vascular resistance (RVR), while reducing renal blood flow and GFR associated with diuresis and natriuresis. Importantly, DBDD, as a 20-HETE synthesis inhibitor, was able to blunt these effects [10]. Sodium nitroprusside, a NO donor, inhibited renal microsomal conversion of AA to 20-HETE and increased vascular diameter in a dose-dependent manner [54,55,57].

Heme and products derived from its metabolism, by heme oxygenase enzymes (HO-1 and HO-2), were found to influence renal function and blood pressure potentially by affecting the expression and activity of hemoproteins, including CYP and COX isoenzymes (COX-1 and COX-2) [45]. HO isoform expression was found to be segmented within the kidney and along the nephron [45]. HO-1 protein in kidney was barely detectable; its contribution to the regulation of hemoproteins became apparent only under pathophysiological conditions that caused HO induction. To the contrast, HO-2 protein was found to be expressed in all kidney structures with higher levels in outer medulla followed by inner medulla/papilla and cortex [45,60]. HO-1 induction was found to suppress microsomal heme, CYP4A and COX-2 protein, and 20 HETE [45,60].

Treatment with clofibrate, a PPAR$_\alpha$ agonist, increased CYP4A protein levels and the subsequent 20-HETE production in microsomes prepared from the renal cortex [61,62]. Moreover, in an in vitro study performed in human renal tubular epithelial cells (HK-2 cell line), Li et al. have demonstrated that cisplatin is a potent inducer of CYP4A11 and it exerts its cytotoxic activity in kidney via increasing production of 20-HETE [63]. In contrast, treatment with pioglitazone, the PPAR$_\gamma$ agonist, neither affected CYP4A nor 20-HETE level [61,62]. Similarly, dexamethasone, an inducer of CYP4A, caused a 2-fold increase in the proximal tubular synthesis of 20-HETE as well as an increase in CYP4A1 mRNA [61]. Another regulator for 20-HETE production is the dietary salt intake which modulates glomerular CYP activity [57]. Hyperchloremia increased 20-HETE release from the rat kidney by 2-fold when compared with low-chloride conditions of renal perfusion [11]. As for AngII, it was found to induce 20-HETE release from preglomerular microvessels [52], whereas vasopressin deficiency elevates the expression of CYP4A protein and renal formation of 20-HETE in the kidney of Brattleboro rats [64].

2.3. Role of 20-HETE in the Kidney

2.3.1. Role of 20-HETE in Preglomerular Vascular Tone Regulation

CYP4A isozymes have the potential to function as an oxygen sensor in mammalian microcirculatory beds and to regulate arteriolar tone by generating 20-HETE in an oxygen-dependent manner [40]. 20-HETE is produced by renal vascular smooth muscle (VSM) cells [65] and participates in the autoregulation of renal blood flow via its effect on vascular tone, ion transport and tubuloglomerular feedback; while excess 20-HETE was found to be excreted in the urine [8,66–69]. Many previous studies have addressed 20-HETE as a second messenger that plays a central role in the regulation of renal vascular tone [38,41,47,48,61,70]. 20-HETE is a potent constrictor produced by the preglomerular vasculature; it contributes to the regulation of tone and myogenic response [40,43,56,71,72]. In addition, 20-HETE contributes to the increase in intracellular calcium in renal micro-VSM cells [73]. The vasoconstrictor response of canine renal arcuate arteries to 20-HETE resembles the myogenic activation of these vessels after elevations in transmural pressure [74].

20-HETE contributes importantly to renal blood flow autoregulation by afferent arterioles [28], and contributes to the development of hypertension by elevating renal vascular resistance [75]. Conversely, in the kidney tubules, 20-HETE suppresses sodium reabsorption and enhances natriuresis, hence, contributing to antihypertensive mechanisms [76]. 20-HETE acts in part by inhibiting the opening of the large-conductance Ca^{2+}-activated K^+ channel, depolarizing VSM cell membrane, and producing sustained increase in intracellular calcium concentration [8,28,59,65,77–81]. Inhibition of 20-HETE formation contributes to the activation of K^+ channels and the vasodilator effects of NO in the renal microcirculation [82]. As for renal medullary perfusion, it seems to be under tonic suppression by 20-HETE, where renal medullary perfusion indices were increased after infusion of HET0016 [83]. Similarly, infusion of 17-ODYA into the renal artery increased cortical and papillary blood flows [66]. In isolated canine renal arcuate arteries, 20-HETE significantly reduced mean open time, the open-state probability, and the frequency of opening a 117-pS K^+ channel recorded from renal VSM cells (Figure 4) [74].

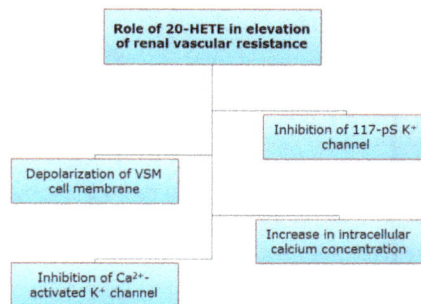

Figure 4. Role of 20-HETE in elevation of renal vascular resistance.

Afferent arteriolar vasoconstriction is partly mediated by the endothelial COX pathway. 20-HETE caused constriction of rabbit afferent arterioles when vascular tone increased with norepinephrine. However, this constriction was significantly attenuated by pretreatment with indomethacin or the thromboxane/endoperoxide receptor antagonist, SQ29548 [75]. 20-HETE metabolites, 20-OH PGE$_2$ and 20-OH PGF$_{2\alpha}$ play significant role in regulating cortical blood flow and medullary blood flow. Renal intra-arterial infusion of 20-HETE was found to decrease cortical blood flow and increase medullary blood flow. These controversial effects were attributable to 20-OH PGF$_{2\alpha}$ that caused vasoconstriction, and 20-OH PGE$_2$ that caused vasodilation in the cortex and medulla [84]. 20-HETE is a second messenger for ET-1 and a mediator for selective renal effects of AngII [8]. ET-1 increased mean arterial blood pressure, renal vascular resistance, while reduced cortical blood flow and renal blood flow, at least in part, by modulating 20-HETE levels via activation of ET receptors [84–87]. However, ET-1 also increased medullary blood flow which seemed to be mediated by the vasodilator prostanoids or by NO via ET receptor activation [85]. As for transgenic animals, KAP-CYP4F2 transgenic mice, predominantly showed renal overexpression of CYP4F2 leading to high 20-HETE in urine and blood, and accounting for the elevation in blood pressure [88]. Cyp4a14 KO mice have prohypertensive status as a result of increased Cyp4a12 expression with associated increased production of 20-HETE and endothelial NOS (eNOS) uncoupling leading to increased oxidative stress, enhanced vasoconstriction as well as a defect in the renal excretory capacity [47]. Recently, it was shown that the dysregulated renal 20-HETE/EET ratio in the hypertensive Cyp4F2 transgenic mice was resulted from the activation of soluble epoxide hydrolase (sEH) and the inhibition of epoxygenase activity suggesting 20-HETE vasoconstrictive activity. Moreover, 20-HETE demonstrated an inverse regulatory effect on the endogenous epoxygenases in the kidney [89].

2.3.2. Role of 20-HETE in Tubular Ion Transport

20-HETE serves as a second messenger that plays a central role in the regulation of sodium reabsorption in the proximal tubule and TAL [21,38,41,47,48,61,70]. 20-HETE inhibits sodium-potassium-chloride (Na$^+$-K$^+$-2Cl$^-$) transporter in the TAL [90]. Moreover, 20-HETE, produced in the proximal tubules, modulates ion transport by regulating Na$^+$-K$^+$-ATPase activity via stimulating protein kinase C (PKC) to phosphorylate the α-subunit of Na$^+$-K$^+$-ATPase [8,28,59,65,91–95]. Additionally, excessive fluid reabsorption in the proximal tubule in the Cyp4a14 knockout mice has led to hypertension which is secondary to 20-HETE-mediated overexpression of sodium-hydrogen exchanger 3 [96–98]. Infusion of 20-HETE at a dose of 100 nmol/kg/min decreased medullary Na$^+$-K$^+$-ATPase activity by 24.2% [99]. 20-HETE serves also as a second messenger for the natriuretic effects of dopamine, parathyroid hormone, and AngII [65,100–102]. In addition, 20-HETE specifically inhibits Na$^+$-Pi co-transporter in proximal tubule-like opossum kidney (OK) cells [103–106]. As for TAL, 20-HETE modulates ion transport by inhibiting the activities of Na$^+$-K$^+$-2Cl$^-$ co-transporter [8,28,65,93,94,107,108]. 20-HETE inhibits Na$^+$-K$^+$-2Cl$^-$ transport, in part, by blocking a 70-pS apical K$^+$ channel, the predominant type of the two apical K$^+$ channels operating under physiological conditions in the TAL of the rat kidney [59,109,110]. DDMS was found to increase the activity of the 70-pS K$^+$ channel significantly [111]. Interestingly, AngII has dual effects on the activity of the apical 70-pS K$^+$ channel in TAL of the rat kidney, where 50 pM AngII has inhibitory effect mediated by 20-HETE, whereas 50–100 nM AngII has stimulatory effect mediated via NO [24]. In addition, 20-HETE was found to be a key mediator in the activation of Na$^+$-independent Mg^{2+} efflux (Figure 5) [112]. Recently, it has been shown that human CYP4A11 transgenic mice have developed a 20-HETE-dependent hypertension associated with 50% increase in sodium chloride cotransporter abundance in the distal tubules [113].

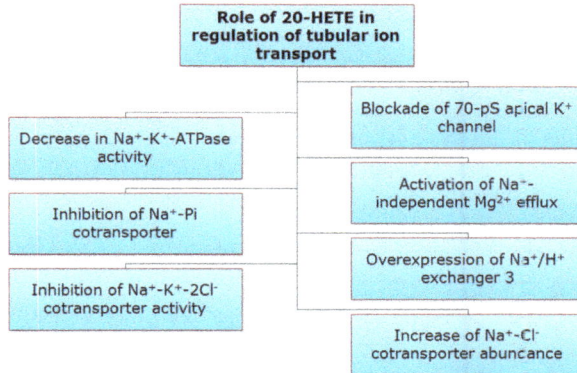

Figure 5. Role of 20-HETE in regulation of tubular ion transport.

2.4. Role of 20-HETE in Pathophysiology of the Kidney

2.4.1. Role of 20-HETE in Renal Ischemia/Reperfusion (I/R) Injury

Acute kidney injury (AKI) is a major consequence following surgery and various medical conditions that significantly increases morbidity and mortality [114–116]. Recent reports suggest that renal I/R injury is the most common cause of AKI [50]. Several reports showed that AA is released from membrane phospholipids in response to ischemia and can be metabolized to 20-HETE that plays an important role in I/R injury which is known to be associated with a patient mortality of up to 50% [117,118]. 20-HETE overexpression in renal I/R injury exacerbates cellular damage by enhancing generation of free radicals and activation of caspase-3 [119]. 20-HETE role in vasoconstriction and inflammation contributes to I/R injury as well [120]. 20-HETE also plays a role in post-ischemic fall in medullary blood flow and its associated long-term decline in renal function [121]. In this regard, the 20-HETE antagonist, 6,15,20-HEDE, accelerated the recovery of medullary perfusion as well as renal medullary and cortical re-oxygenation, during early reperfusion phase, whereas the 20-HETE mimetic, 5,14,20-HEDE, did not improve renal injury and reversed the beneficial effects of 6,15,20-HEDE [120]. Pretreatment of uninephrectomized male Lewis rats with either the HET0016 or 6,15,20-HEDE via the renal artery before exposure to warm ischemia was found to attenuate I/R induced renal dysfunction and to reduce tubular lesion scores, inflammatory cell infiltration, and tubular epithelial cell apoptosis [120]. However contradicting results were obtained in a previous study in which infusion of 5,14-20-HEDE or 5,14-20-HEDGE protected SD rat kidney from I/R injury, whereas HET0016 exacerbated renal injury [15]. Protection provided by 20-HETE analogues was supposed to be due to inhibition of renal tubular sodium transport, increased urine output and sodium excretion, and prevention of post-ischemic fall in medullary blood flow [15]. The contradiction in results could be related to the use of different models and treatment forms. In addition, high systemic HET0016 levels may inhibit not only 20-HETE synthesis, but also the ω-hydroxylation and inactivation of leukotriene B4 resulting in aggravation of ischemic renal damage. Moreover, high doses of 5,14-20-HEDE (mg/kg range) results in high systemic drug levels that acted not only during ischemia but also during reperfusion providing protection for the kidney mainly in reperfusion phase by inhibiting sodium reabsorption, thereby limiting tubular oxygen consumption [120]. In renal transplant patients, the change in dynamics of 20-HETE during early phase of allograft reperfusion was associated with early post-transplant graft function, and extent of 20-HETE release occurring within the first 5 min of allograft reperfusion was found to be a negative predictor of post-transplant allograft function [117,120].

2.4.2. Role of 20-HETE in Polycystic Kidney Diseases

Polycystic kidney diseases are characterized by abnormal proliferation of renal epithelial cells which was found to be mediated by 20-HETE [122–124]. Several pathways known to be involved in polycystic kidney disease have been reported to be activated by 20-HETE such as PKC, Src and EGFR pathways. Expression of CYP4A1, CYP4A2, CYP4A3, and CYP4A8 mRNA was found to be increased in polycystic kidney by 2- to 4-fold as compared to non-cystic SD rat kidney; and daily administration of HET0016 significantly reduced kidney size by 24% [123]. Similarly, Balb/c polycystic kidney mouse, a model of autosomal recessive polycystic kidney disease, treated with HET0016 daily showed significant reduction in kidney size by half and approximately doubled survival rates [122]. Non-cystic Balb/c cells overproducing Cyp4a12 exhibited a 4- to 5-fold increase in cell proliferation compared with control Balb/c cells, however this effect was completely abolished when 20-HETE synthesis was inhibited [122]. These findings suggest that 20-HETE might be a new biomarker and a therapeutic target for polycystic kidney disease [95].

2.5. 20-HETE Mediation of Drug Induced Toxicity in the Kidney

Tian et al. reported that 20-HETE may protect from doxorubicin-induced toxicity of human renal tubular epithelial cells. They found that doxorubicin suppresses CYP4A11 gene expression and protein production in human renal tubular epithelial cells more efficiently than HET0016. This resulted in decreased cell viability and increased lactate dehydrogenase activity when human renal tubular epithelial cells were incubated with doxorubicin for 24h, whereas 20-HETE increased cell survival and decreased lactate dehydrogenase activity in concentration-dependent manner with no reported mechanism. Similar results were obtained when 20-HETE was co-administered with doxorubicin, while, HET0016 was found to exaggerate doxorubicin effect [125]. On the other hand, 20-HETE plays a role in cyclosporin A-induced nephrotoxicity. Rats treated with cyclosporin A suffered from increased renal microsomal conversion of AA to 20-HETE, increased systolic blood pressure, and induced renal damage, whereas pretreatment with HET0016 or ABT attenuated or prevented these effects [126–128]. Interestingly, a recent in vitro study performed in HK-2 cells suggested that cisplatin is a potent inducer of CYP4A11 and 20-HETE biosynthesis and this mechanism of induction is proposed as a novel mechanism of renal tubular toxicity of cisplatin [63].

2.6. Role of 20-HETE in the Renal System during Pregnancy

20-HETE synthesis in the kidney is altered in a time- and site-specific manner during pregnancy suggesting distinct regulatory mechanisms for 20-HETE synthesis in the kidney during pregnancy [129]. In addition, NO interacts with CYP4A proteins in a distinct manner and it interferes with renal microvessels 20-HETE synthesis, emphasizing the important role of 20-HETE in regulating blood pressure and renal function during pregnancy [130,131]. Inhibition of NO synthesis by L-NAME during late pregnancy led to increased production of renal vascular 20-HETE causing significantly higher mean arterial blood pressure and renal vascular resistance, and lower renal blood flow and GFR. Combined treatment with DDMS and L-NAME significantly attenuated these effects [131]. This data suggested that 20-HETE plays a role in hypertension and renal vasoconstriction induced by chronic reduction in uterine perfusion pressure (RUPP) in pregnant rats [132]. ABT decreased mean arterial blood pressure in RUPP rats whereas it had no effect in normal pregnant rats, besides attenuating the differences in renal hemodynamics observed between normal pregnant and RUPP rats [132].

3. Role of 20-HETE in the Liver

3.1. Formation of 20-HETE in the Liver

Interestingly, 50%–75% of CYP-dependent AA metabolites formed by human liver microsomes are 19-HETE and 20-HETE where 20-HETE was found to be the main metabolite formed [93,133]. AA ω-hydroxylation in human liver is catalyzed by CYP4F2, CYP4F3 and CYP4A11 [134];

with CYP4F2 and CYP4F3B, human liver-specific splice variant of CYP4F3, generating most hepatic 20-HETE [134,135]. In human hepatocyte-like HepaRG, hepatoma cell line, induction of CYP4F3B was observed by PGA_1 and by lovastatin leading to increased synthesis of 20-HETE [135,136]. In addition, statins were found to recruit PXR to induce CYP4F3B [136]. On the other hand, isoniazid was found to reduce expression and formation of both CYP4A and 20-HETE, respectively, in the liver [137].

3.2. Role of 20-HETE in the Liver

Very little information is available about the role of 20-HETE in the liver, however it seems that 20-HETE participates in the regulation of liver metabolic activity and hemodynamics [93,138]. 20-HETE is a potent activator of $PPAR_\alpha$ and may exert important functions in lipid homeostasis and in controlling fat-dependent energy supply and metabolism, in addition it is an important inflammatory mediator and may have important role in inflammatory diseases [135,136]. 20-HETE is a weak, COX-dependent, vasoconstrictor of the portal circulation, and it was supposed to be involved in pathophysiology of portal hypertension [93,138]. In addition, 20-HETE was found to be involved in abnormalities related to liver diseases, particularly cirrhosis [93]. While 20-HETE and PGs are excreted at similar rates in normal subjects, it was found that excretory rates of 20-HETE were several-fold higher than those of PGs and TxB_2 in patients with cirrhosis [93,139]. Recently, 20-HETE demonstrated a counter regulatory effect on the endogenous epoxygenases in the liver. Thus the tuning of 20-HETE and EETs formation and degradation may provide therapeutic benefits; given that they have opposite effects in several diseases [89,140]. Interestingly, 20-HETE level in the urine of cirrhotic patients with ascites is much higher than in case of cirrhosis without ascites which in turn is higher than excretion rates in normal individuals [139]. In patients with hepatic cirrhosis, 20-HETE is produced in increased amounts in the preglomerular microcirculation resulting in constriction of renal vasculature, reduction of renal blood flow and depression of renal hemodynamics [93,139]. Of interest, CYP4F2 was found to be exclusively expressed in the liver of CMV-CYP4F2 transgenic mice, driven by cyto-megalovirus (CMV) promoter, with no effect on 20-HETE levels in the urine, kidney, and blood or even on systolic blood pressure. In contrast, KAP-CYP4F2 transgenic mice, driven by kidney androgen-regulated protein (KAP) promoter, were found to overexpress renal CYP4F2 and to have high 20-HETE levels in urine and blood, in addition to elevated blood pressure [88].

4. Role of 20-HETE in the Respiratory System

4.1. Distribution of 20-HETE in Pulmonary Tissues

In the lung, 20-HETE is produced from vascular and non-vascular tissues; it was detected in pulmonary arteries, bronchi, and endothelium [141,142]. 20-HETE modulates many physiological functions such as smooth muscle tone and electrolyte flux [141] and serves as a paracrine factor in the pulmonary circulation when generated from nonvascular tissues [143]. Peripheral lung tissue, small and large pulmonary arteries, airways, and isolated VSM cells from small pulmonary arteries produced 20-HETE when incubated with AA [143]. In adult male rat lung, CYP4A mRNA was detected in pulmonary arterial endothelial and smooth muscle cells, bronchial epithelial and smooth muscle cells, type I epithelial cells, and macrophages. In addition, CYP4A protein was detected in rat pulmonary arteries and bronchi as well as cultured endothelial cells [141]. In rabbit, CYP4A is widely distributed in lung tissues as well [143]. In rats with acute pseudomonas pneumonia, 20-HETE level was depressed in microsomes prepared from lung [144], whereas in cystic fibrosis patients, 20-HETE was detected in freshly obtained sputum suggesting a role in these disease states [145].

4.2. Role of 20-HETE in Pulmonary Cell Survival

20-HETE mediates cell survival signaling in the pulmonary vasculature [146,147], it enhances survival and protects against apoptosis in bovine pulmonary artery endothelial cells (BPAECs) stressed by serum starvation or lipopolysaccharide [148,149]. 20-HETE enhanced survival and protected against apoptosis in mouse pulmonary arteries (PAs) exposed to hypoxia reoxygenation ex vivo [146,148], and similar results obtained with 20-HETE analogs [146]. Protection from apoptosis was found to be dependent on reactive oxygen species (ROS) generation [148]; in addition, ROS is known to modulate vital physiological processes including cell growth, angiogenesis, contraction, and relaxation of VSM [150]. 20-HETE was found to increase both superoxide and NO production in BPAECs resulting in promotion of angiogenesis [148–151]. In addition, 20-HETE maintained the stability of mitochondria membrane and relieved the activation of caspase-9 and caspase-3 [149]. 5,14,20-HEDE and 5,14,20-HEDGE enhanced ROS production in endothelial cell in intact lung ex vivo as well as in cultured pulmonary artery endothelial cells [146].

4.3. Role of 20-HETE in Pulmonary Vascular Tone

20-HETE alters vascular tone signaling in the pulmonary vasculature and plays a role in VSM remodeling [146,147,149,150]. Unlike its constrictor effects on systemic circulation, peripheral arteries, cerebral and renal vessels, 20-HETE is an endothelial-dependent dilator of pulmonary arteries [141,152,153]. 20-HETE relaxed contractile responses to 5-hydroxytryptamine concentration-dependently (0.01–10 microM) in fresh and 1 day culture of pulmonary arteries [154]. 20-HETE was found to induce a dose-dependent vasodilation of isolated human small pulmonary arteries which was inhibited by indomethacin [155], suggesting that 20-HETE could act as a COX-dependent vasodilator for human pulmonary arteries [156]. 20-HETE-dependent pulmonary arteries vasodilation is mediated by increasing intracellular Ca^{2+} concentration and NO release and found to be endothelial-dependent [152,157]. 20-HETE also contributes to vascular endothelial growth factor (VEGF)-stimulated NO release [157,158]; VEGF-induced NO release was attenuated by pretreating the BPAECs with DDMS as well as HET0016 [157]. The potent dilatory response to 20-HETE in human and rabbit pulmonary vascular and bronchiole rings was found to be dependent on an intact endothelium and COX enzyme [93,143]. Human lung microsomes were able to convert 20-HETE into prostanoids suggesting that COX in vascular tissue metabolizes 20-HETE to a vasodilatory compound [155]. Of interest, CYP4 has a unique expression in BPAECs versus systemic arterial endothelial cells suggesting that CYP4 could be an important mediator of endothelial-dependent vasoreactivity in pulmonary arteries [157]. Moreover, a recent study showed that 20-HETE, through gap junctions, appears to modulate smooth muscle myosin heavy chain expression and contribute to the sustained state of hypoxic pulmonary vasoconstriction development [159].

Interestingly, 20-HETE was demonstrated to be more potent vasoconstrictors than phenylephrine and KCl on small pulmonary arteries of rat and did not exhibit any relaxant effects on pulmonary artery rings precontracted with phenylephrine. Potency of 20-HETE as a vasoconstrictor in small pulmonary arteries was attenuated in pulmonary artery rings from lung with pneumonia [156]. It seems that 20-HETE has varied vasoactive effects dependent on the vascular beds studied, where vasoactive effects of 20-HETE can be influenced by the activity of other enzyme systems such as NOS and COX [156]. In sheep pulmonary artery, 20-HETE has a predominant role in the inhibition of vascular Na^+-K^+-ATPase activity, where it significantly attenuated KCl-induced relaxations. In addition, AA caused concentration-dependent inhibition of KCl-induced relaxations and increases basal arterial tone in pulmonary vasculature in sheep, an effect which was completely reversed by 17-ODYA as well as HET0016 [160]. Also in contrast to its action in adult pulmonary circulation, 20-HETE causes constriction in newborn pulmonary resistance-level arteries at resting tone [153] and was found to be released in fetal pulmonary circulation in response to acute increases in pulmonary artery pressure resulting in vasoconstriction [161]. 20-HETE as a vasoconstrictor, causes blockade of Ca^{2+}-activated K^+ (K_{Ca}) channels and inhibits the formation of NO [93]. Inhibition of 20-HETE might have a therapeutic role in neonatal conditions characterized by pulmonary hypertension; DDMS was found to abolish the vasoconstrictor response to ductus arteriosus compression in the presence of nitro-L-arginine (L-NA; to inhibit shear-stress vasodilation) [161].

4.4. Role of 20-HETE in the Airways

In guinea pigs, airway smooth muscle (ASM) cells were found to produce 20-HETE which acted as a bronchoconstrictor and induced concentration-dependent tonic responses [94,162]. However, in human ASM, 20-HETE causes a concentration-dependent relaxation in bronchi precontracted with methacholine or AA [163]. Similarly, 20-HETE produced a concentration-dependent relaxation of rabbit bronchial rings precontracted with KCl or histamine [164]. Differences between observations regarding 20-HETE effect on ASM are likely related to inter-species differences [163]. In rabbit, 20-HETE modulates airway resistance in a COX-dependent manner; 20-HETE-dependent relaxation of bronchial rings was blocked by indomethacin suggesting that epithelial COX converts 20-HETE to a bronchial relaxant which elicited relaxation of bronchial rings [164]. However, in human bronchi, the responses to 20-HETE were not modified by indomethacin pretreatments. Moreover, 20-OH-PGE$_2$ had basically no relaxing effect on bronchi precontracted with methacholine chloride, suggesting that the relaxing effect induced by 20-HETE was not related to prostanoid formation [163]. 20-HETE-dependent hyperpolarization and controlled relaxation of ASM in human distal bronchi depends on activation of large conductance K$_{Ca}$ channels [163]. Interestingly, 20-HETE seems to play an important role in mediating acute ozone-induced airway hyper-responsiveness responsible for increasing morbidity and mortality in patients with obstructive airway diseases and asthma [155]. Interestingly, a recent study performed in Balb/c mice showed that local administration of 20-HETE led to proinflammatory action, associated with airway neutrophilia and macrophage activation, thus contributing to airway hyperresponsiveness [166].

5. Role of 20-HETE in the Brain

5.1. Formation, Metabolism and Regulation of 20-HETE in the Brain

Human CYP2U1 metabolizes AA exclusively to 19-HETE and 20-HETE with abundant transcripts in cerebellum suggesting an important role in fatty acid signaling processes in brain [167]. Brain astrocytes synthesize and release 20-HETE which acts as cerebral arterial myocyte constrictor [168]. In addition, cerebral microvessels convert 20-HETE to 20-COOH-AA which produces vasoconstriction in these vessels, this reaction was found to be catalyzed by alcohol dehydrogenase (ADH), mainly ADH$_4$ [169]. As for regulation, PaCO$_2$ is an important factor in the regulation of cerebral circulation; changes in CO$_2$ concentration could cause changes in cerebral blood flow. CO$_2$ can decrease the expression of brain CYP4A during hypercapnia and increase its expression during hypocapnia, suggesting that 20-HETE plays an important role in CO$_2$-mediated cerebrovascular reactivity [170]. NO was also found to affect 20-HETE synthesis by decreasing its level and inhibiting its formation [171].

5.2. Role of 20-HETE in Regulating Vascular Tone in Brain

Brain does not store glycogen and thus requires a constant supply of glucose and oxygen for the continuous demands of cerebral function [172]; hence, the control of cerebral vessel diameter and cerebral blood flow is of fundamental importance in maintaining healthy brain function [173]. 20-HETE has significant role in the regulation of vascular tone, autoregulation of cerebral blood flow, and the neurovascular coupling (coupling of regional brain blood flow to neuronal activity) [174–176]. 20-HETE was found to be generated in various cell types in the brain and cerebral blood vessels [174,177]. Glial cells, non-neuronal cells, were found to play an important role in mediating neurovascular coupling by inducing the production of EETs and 20-HETE, which dilate and constrict vessels, respectively [178,179]. Recent studies have shown that astrocytes, characteristic star-shaped glial cells, are critical players in the regulation of cerebral blood vessel diameter; astrocytes produce 20-HETE from AA [173]. Furthermore, 20-HETE has been implicated in arteriolar constriction during astrocyte activation in brain slices, and modulates vasodilation in cerebral cortex during sensory activation [171]. 20-HETE synthesis limits the duration of the response to prolonged activation of Group I metabotropic glutamate receptors (mGluR) on astrocytes. Under normal conditions in vivo stimulation of mGluR increases cerebral blood flow [180]. Protein kinase C was found to be an integral part of the signal transduction pathway by which 20-HETE elicits vasoconstriction of cerebral arteries and inhibits the whole cell K^+ current in cat cerebral VSM [181]. 20-HETE also activates L-type calcium current in cerebral arterial smooth muscles [78]. Interestingly, it was found that 20-HETE is an important contributor to cerebral vasoconstriction associated with the onset of ventilation at birth [182]. Recent studies showed that 20-HETE-dependent vasoconstriction in the cerebellum is mediated by metabotropic glutamate receptors [183]. Moreover, 20-HETE induces cerebral parenchymal arteriolar constriction via superoxide production resulting from NADPH oxidase activation, and propofol could prevent this constriction via inhibiting NADPH oxidase [184]. Similarly, 20-HETE inhibitors were found to be associated with a decrease in superoxide production and activation of caspase-3 [185]. Although vasodilation of the brain blood vessels is known to be mediated by prostaglandin E2, nitric oxide production is also needed to suppress 20-HETE formation [186]. Of interest, 20-HETE could dilate mouse basilar artery preconstricted with U-46619, a thromboxane mimetic, in vitro. This action was inhibited by indomethacin suggesting a COX-dependent mechanism. In fact, mouse brain endothelial cells were found to convert 20-HETE to 20-OH-PGE$_2$, which was as potent as PGE$_2$ in dilating the basilar artery [187].

5.3. Role of 20-HETE in Cerebral Ischemia/Reperfusion (I/R) Injury

20-HETE is a potent vasoconstrictor of cerebral microvessels which contributes to I/R injury [188–191] being a mediator of free radical formation and tissue death [119]. 20-HETE plays an important role in the development of neurological and functional deficits, and contributes to infarct size after focal cerebral ischemia [192,193]. It also contributes to neurodegeneration after global cerebral ischemia in immature brain [193]. In rat subarachnoid hemorrhage (SAH) model, 20-HETE formation was found to be substantially elevated in the cerebrospinal fluid (CSF) with a concomitant 30% decrease in cerebral blood flow [189,194,195]. Similar data was obtained in aneurysmal subarachnoid hemorrhage (aSAH) model; 20-HETE was reported to affect cerebral microvascular tone and cerebral blood flow [196]. 20-HETE levels in CSF were also associated with delayed cerebral ischemia, neurological decline, and long-term functional and neuropsychological impairment [196]. GG genotype and G allele of CYP4F2 was associated with ischemic stroke in the male Northern Chinese Han population [197]. Interestingly, 20-HETE was present at physiologically-relevant concentrations in CSF of SAH patients [189].

Inhibitors of 20-HETE synthesis reduced infarct volume and decreased cerebral damage after cerebral ischemia and after I/R in brain without altering blood flow providing direct neuroprotective actions [174,185,198]. In vivo, DDMS and 6,15,20-HEDE were found to attenuate autoregulation of cerebral blood flow to elevation of arterial pressure [175]. HET0016 administration reduced brain damage in a rat model of thromboembolic stroke [199] and it protects blood brain barrier dysfunction after I/R through regulating the expression of MMP-9 and tight junction proteins. Moreover, this protection may be due to inhibition of oxidative stress and JNK pathway [200]. Also, rats treated with HET0016, 90 min prior to temporary middle cerebral artery occlusion, showed 79.6% reduction in 20-HETE in the cortex, pronounced reduction in lesion volume and attenuation of the decrease in cerebral blood flow [191]. 6,15,20-HEDE showed similar effects to HET0016 in reducing infarct size after transient occlusion of the middle cerebral artery [198]. In neonatal piglets, HET0016 administration after hypoxia-ischemia improved early neurological recovery and protected neurons in putamen [193]. Blockade of the synthesis of 20-HETE with TS-011 opposed cerebral vasospasm and reversed the fall in cerebral blood flow following SAH. In addition, it reduced infarct size and improved neurological deficits in ischemic models of stroke [188,201,202]. TS-011 reduced infarct volume in rats after transient occlusion of the middle cerebral artery and reduced neurological deficits as well [198,202]. When given in combination with tissue plasminogen activator, TS-011 improved neurological outcomes in the stroke model in monkey [202]. Thus, TS-011 may provide benefits in patients suffering ischemic stroke [192]. In vitro application of DDMS, or 6,15,20-HEDE eliminated pressure-induced constriction of rat middle cerebral arteries [175]. Organotypic hippocampal slice cultures subjected to oxygen-glucose deprivation (OGD) and reoxygenation showed 2-fold increase in 20-HETE production, however inhibition of 20-HETE synthesis by HET0016 or action by 6,15,20-HEDE reduced the cell death. On the other hand, administration of 5,14,20-HEDE increased injury after OGD [185].

6. Role of 20-HETE in Tumors

Increased generation of 20-HETE was reported to induce mitogenic and angiogenic responses both in vitro and in vivo (summarized in Figure 6) [203,204].

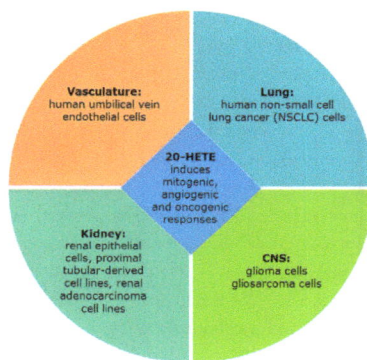

Figure 6. 20-HETE role in carcinogenicity.

In human umbilical vein endothelial cells, administration of 5,14,20-HEDE induced mitogenesis, whereas HET0016 abolished the mitogenic response to VEGF [205]. 20-HETE is also considered a mitogen for smooth muscle cells [43]. 5,14,20-HEDE induced angiogenesis in rat cornea, whereas HET0016 inhibited growth factor-induced angiogenesis by 80%–90% [205]. In lung, 20-HETE was found to promote tumor angiogenesis and metastasis in human non-small cell lung cancer (NSCLC) cells. In vitro, addition of 5,14,20-HEDE or transfection of A549 cells, a human NSCLC cell line, with CYP4A11 expression vector significantly induced invasion, whereas treatment with HET0016 or 6,15,20-HEDE inhibited invasion. In vivo, CYP4A11 transfection significantly increased tumor weight, microvessel density, and lung metastasis, whereas HET0016 or 6,15,20-HEDE administration decreased tumor volume, microvessel density, and spontaneous pulmonary metastasis occurrences [206]. In kidney, 20-HETE has been reported to promote mitogenicity and proliferation in renal epithelial cells [207,208]. In vitro, 20-HETE was found to be a potent mitogen to swine proximal tubular-derived cell lines, LLC-PK1 and opossum kidney (OK) [209]. However no mitogenic effects were observed with 20-HETE in LLCPKcl4, a subclone from the parental LLC-PK1 cells [210]. HET0016 and 6,15,20-HEDE inhibited the proliferation of 786-O and 769-P, human renal adenocarcinoma cell lines, while having little effect on the proliferation of primary cultures of normal human proximal tubule epithelial cells. In vivo, 6,15,20-HEDE administered daily to athymic nude mice implanted subcutaneously with 786-O cells, reduced the growth of the tumors by 84% [207]. In benign prostatic hypertrophy and prostate cancer patients, urinary concentrations of 20-HETE were significantly higher than normal subjects and it was decreased to normal concentrations after removal of prostate gland [211]. Moreover, Vanella et al. showed that ellagic acid (an antioxidant) mediates a new pathway for its chemotherapeutic property, other than its anti-proliferative and pro-differentiation properties, through a mechanism that involves a decrease in 20-HETE synthesis in prostate cancer cells [212]. In human mammary carcinoma, CYP4Z1 which considered a novel CYP4 is over-expressed and was found to be associated with high-grade tumors and poor prognosis, in addition, stable expression of CYP4Z1 in T47D human breast cancer cells lead to higher contents of 20-HETE, whereas HET0016 potently inhibited the tumor-induced angiogenesis with associated changes in the intracellular levels of 20-HETE [213]. Additionally, HET0016 inhibits pro-angiogenic factors and ceases growth of triple negative breast cancer in mice [214].

Similarly, samples from thyroid, breast, colon, and ovarian cancer revealed that expression of CYP4A/4F genes is highly elevated in cancer samples as compared to matched normal tissues [204]. As for CNS, 20-HETE was found to have proto-oncogenic properties in U251 human glioma cells, as pretreatment with exogenous 20-HETE and 5,14,20-HEDE increased U251 cell proliferation [215,216]. Transfection of U251 cells with CYP4A1 cDNA increased the formation of 20-HETE and increased their proliferation rate by 2-fold, whereas HET0016, small interfering RNA (siRNA) against the enzyme, and 6,15,20-HEDE abolished this hyperproliferation [215]. In vivo, implantation of CYP4A1 transfected U251 cells in the brain of nude rats resulted in a 10-fold larger tumor volume after ten days [215]. HET0016 inhibited U251 basal cell proliferation and decreased its induced angiogenesis [216]. Similar results obtained in 9L rat gliosarcoma cells; 5,14,20-HEDE increased its proliferation in vitro, while HET0016 achieved 55% reduction in proliferation after 48 h of incubation. In vivo, chronic administration of HET0016 for two weeks reduced the volume of 9L tumors by 80%, and increased mean survival time of the animals [217]. Interestingly, although both CYP4A mRNA and protein were detected in U251, it did not synthesize 20-HETE in the presence of AA suggesting that HET0016 suppresses U251 proliferation in vitro by mechanisms that may involve activities other than inhibiting 20-HETE synthesis [215,216]. HET0016 is also able to inhibit tumor growth and migration depending on the schedule of drug administration. The addition of HET0016 to vatalanib (a small molecule protein kinase inhibitor that inhibits angiogenesis) may mitigate the undesired effect of vatalanib [218]. Similarly, neither 9L cells grown in vitro nor 9L tumors removed produced 20-HETE when incubated with AA; however, the normal surrounding brain tissue avidly makes 20-HETE. This data suggests that HET0016 may act in vivo by inhibiting the formation of 20-HETE by the surrounding tissue, whereas its antiproliferative effects in vitro seems to be unrelated to its ability to inhibit the formation of 20-HETE [216,217]. In traditional Chinese medicine, Scolopendra subspinipes mutilans L. Koch has been used for cancer treatment for hundreds of years. Scolopendra Polysaccharide-Protein Complex (SPPC) significantly inhibited the growth of S180, mouse sarcoma cell line, transplanted in mice. SPPC prolonged the survival time of H22, mouse hepatoma cell line, bearing mice. SPPC diminished CYP4A and 20-HETE in tumor-associated macrophages [219].

7. Role of 20-HETE in Metabolic Syndrome and Diabetes

Mice fed high-fat diet had significantly higher 20-HETE/(EET+DHET) formation rate ratio in the liver and kidney, suggesting a role in pathogenesis and progression of metabolic syndrome [220]. Moreover, increased levels of 20-HETE significantly disrupt survival and function of endothelial cells in metabolic syndrome leading to impaired coronary collateral growth, hence 20-HETE antagonists could be a potential therapeutic choice in this case [221]. In vitro, 20-HETE has been shown to be involved in adipogenesis. Kim et al. examined the effect of exogenous 20-HETE on mesenchymal stem cell-derived adipocytes and concluded that 20-HETE increased adipogenesis in a concentration-dependent manner [222]. In vivo, 20-HETE contributes to the elevation in vascular reactivity in diabetic animals [223], and was reported to play a role in diabetes-enhanced vasoconstriction of mesenteric and renal vessels [224]. 20-HETE is also involved in the early decrease of retinal hemodynamics in diabetic mice which could be attenuated by HET0016 [224]. Chronic treatment of the diabetic rats with ABT or HET0016 attenuated the responses to vasoconstrictors, norepinephrine, ET-1, and AngII, in mesenteric vascular bed and renal artery segments [223]. Eid et al. suggested that 20-HETE inhibitors could have a pivotal therapeutic potential in the alleviation of diabetic nephropathy [225]. Moreover, hyperglycemia decreases 20-HETE production in the glomeruli suggesting an important role in glomerular damage in the early stage of diabetic nephropathy. Rats treated with streptozotocin for five weeks, to induce diabetes, had a significant decrease in glomerular CYP4A expression; however, when they were treated with clofibrate, glomerular CYP4A expression and 20-HETE production were induced while urinary protein excretion was reduced [37]. Isolated perfused kidney from rats with streptozotocin-induced diabetes show great reduction in 20-HETE release, whereas insulin treatment for two weeks reverses hyperglycemia and renal deficiency in 20-HETE [226].

8. Summary and Conclusions

The formation of 20-HETE has been demonstrated to be through different members of the CYP ω-hydroxylase enzymes, the CYP4A, CYP4F and CYP2U subfamilies. However, the predominant form responsible for 20-HETE formation differs from organ to organ, from species to species and from males to females. For example, Cyp4a12a is the predominant 20-HETE forming enzyme in the mouse kidney and its expression levels dictates the sex and strain specific differences in 20-HETE formation and may explain sex and strain differences in susceptibility to hypertension and target organ damage [48]. In female mice compared to male mice, low AA hydroxylase activity was observed in the kidney and this was associated with very low Cyp4a12a mRNA and protein expression levels, despite high Cyp4a10 and Cyp4a14 expression levels [48]. Thus, these observations highlight the importance of determining the expression of each CYP ω-hydroxylase isoform in different organs.

Although it has been previously reported that 20-HETE plays a negative role in the heart and vasculature [2,3,90,227], it has been demonstrated to have a protective effect in the kidney. 20-HETE plays an anti-hypertensive effect through its regulation of sodium reabsorption in the proximal tubule and TAL [21,38,41,47,48,61,70]. This effect protects the cardiovascular system from salt-retention hypertension, however 20-HETE is a potent constrictor produced by the preglomerular vasculature and could participate in the development of hypertension [40,43,56,71]. Hence it is obvious that a renal 20-HETE level is a double-edged sword, depending on its levels in various locations within the nephron. Moreover, 20-HETE plays a crucial role in renal I/R injury in addition to polycystic kidney diseases. Thus specific targeting of 20-HETE production and/or action might serve as a treatment strategy in renal diseases in the future.

In the liver, the role of 20-HETE is still to be determined although it represents 50%–75% of CYP-dependent AA metabolites in this organ [93,133]. Importantly, it has been demonstrated that 20-HETE is a potent activator of $PPAR_{\alpha}$ and is supposed to exert important functions in lipid homeostasis and in controlling fat-dependent energy supply and metabolism [135,136]. On the other hand, 20-HETE levels have been shown to be elevated in liver pathophysiological disease states such as cirrhotic ascites [139]. Therefore, future studies investigating the physiological and pathophysiological role of hepatic 20-HETE will be of great importance.

The protective effect of 20-HETE is not only limited to the kidney, but it has been also demonstrated in the lung. For example, 20-HETE mediates cell survival signaling in pulmonary vasculature [146,147] and was found to protect against apoptosis in bovine pulmonary artery endothelial cells [148,149]. Moreover, 20-HETE was found to dilate the pulmonary artery in contrast to its vasoconstrictive effect in systemic circulation, peripheral arteries, cerebral and renal vessels [141,152,153]. The controversy between the vasodilator effect of 20-HETE in the lung and its vasoconstrictor effect in other vasculature could be attributed to a COX-dependent transformation of 20-HETE to metabolites possessing vasodilator effects ($20\text{-}OH\text{-}PGI_2$, and $20\text{-}OH\text{-}PGE_2$) [156]. However, this postulation requires further studies to uncover the exact mechanism.

Unlike the other organs, brain metabolizes AA to 20-HETE mainly through CYP2U1 [167], which is abundant in the cerebellum, implicating the importance of this enzyme in 20-HETE mediated fatty acid signaling processes. This is not the only difference between brain and the other organs. That is, brain does not store glycogen [172] as a reservoir of energy and thus requires continuous supply of glucose and oxygen. In this regard, 20-HETE rises as a crucial modulator of brain vascular tone, cerebral blood flow, and neurovascular coupling. Furthermore, 20-HETE is a potent vasoconstrictor for cerebral microvessels contributing to ischemia reperfusion injury [188–191].

Altogether, maintaining homeostatic levels of 20-HETE is pivotal in determining brain functions and altering its levels might contribute to brain pathophysiological disease states.

Of interest, although 20-HETE through its vasoconstrictor effect might appear at the first glance as a tumor suppressor, recent studies have shown that 20-HETE promotes tumor formation through promoting angiogenesis and mitogenesis. Thus targeting its production and/or action might serve as a treatment strategy in carcinogenesis.

Further studies are needed to investigate the exact events and mechanisms associated with different 20-HETE levels in vital organs. Our success in understanding these events would help in rational designing of therapeutic strategies to reduce 20-HETE-mediated disorders.

Acknowledgments: This work was supported by a grant from the Canadian Institutes of Health Research (CIHR) [Grant MOP 106665]. OHE is the recipient of Alberta Innovates-Health Solutions graduate studentship and Alberta Cancer Foundation Scholarship.

Conflicts of Interest: The authors declare no conflict of interest.

Abbreviations

10-SUYS	acetylenic fatty acid sodium 10-undecynyl sulfate
17-ODYA	17-octadecynoic acid
20-COOH-AA	20-carboxyeicosatetraenoic acid
20-HETE	20-hydroxyeicosatetraenoic acid
20-OH PGH2	hydroxyl analogue of vasoconstrictor prostaglandin H2
5,14,20-HEDE; WIT003	20-hydroxyeicosa-5(Z),14(Z)-dienoic acid
5,14,20-HEDGE	N-[20-hydroxyeicosa-5(Z),14(Z)-dienoyl]glycine
6,15,20-HEDE; WIT002	20-hydroxyeicosa-6(Z),15(Z)-dienoic acid
6,15,20-HEDGE	20-hydroxyeicosa-6(Z),15(Z)-dienoyl]glycine
AA	Arachidonic acid
ABT	1-Aminobenzotriazole
ADH	alcohol dehydrogenase
AngII	vasoconstrictors Angiotensin II
aSAH	aneurysmal subarachnoid hemorrhage model
ASM	airway smooth muscle cells
BPAECs	bovine pulmonary artery endothelial cells
CMV	cyto-megalovirus
CO	carbon monoxide
$CoCl_2$	Cobalt(II) chloride
COX	cyclooxygenase
CSF	cerebrospinal fluid
CYP	cytochrome P450
DBDD	dibromododec-11-enoic acid
DDMS	N-methylsulfonyl-12,12-dibromododec-11-enamide
EETs	epoxyeicosatrienoic acids
eNOS	Endothelial NOS
ET	endothelin
EGFR	epidermal growth factor receptor
HET0016	N-hydroxy-N'-(4-butyl-2methylphenyl)formamidine
HETEs	hydroxyeicosatetraenoic acids
HO	heme oxygenase enzymes
I/R	Ischemia/Reperfusion injury
KAP	kidney androgen-regulated protein
K_{Ca}	Ca^{2+}-activated K^+ channels
L-NA	nitro-L-arginine
L-NAME	$N(\omega)$-nitro-L-arginine-methyl ester
LOX	lipoxygenase
LTs	leukotrienes
LXs	lipoxins
mGluR	Group I metabotropic glutamate receptors
NOS	NO synthase
NSCLC	non-small cell lung cancer cells

OGD	oxygen-glucose deprivation
Palb	albumin permeability
PAs	pulmonary arteries
PGs	prostaglandins
PKC	protein kinase C
PPARα	Peroxisome proliferator-activated receptor α
ROS	reactive oxygen species
RUPP	reductions in uterine perfusion pressure
RVR	renal vascular resistance
SAH	subarachnoid hemorrhage model
SD	Sprague Dawley
sEH	soluble epoxide hydrolase
siRNA	small interfering RNA
SPPC	Scolopendra Polysaccharide-Protein Complex
TAL	thick ascending limb of the loop of Henle
TGF-β	transforming growth factor-beta
TS011	*N*-(3-Chloro-4-morpholin-4-yl)Phenyl-*N*′-hydroxyimido formamide
VEGF	vascular endothelial growth factor
VSM	vascular smooth muscle

References

1. Imig, J.D. Epoxides and soluble epoxide hydrolase in cardiovascular physiology. *Physiol. Rev.* **2012**, *92*, 101–130. [CrossRef]

2. Elshenawy, O.H.; Anwar-Mohamed, A.; Abdelhamid, G.; El-Kadi, A.O. Murine atrial hl-1 cell line is a reliable model to study drug metabolizing enzymes in the heart. *Vascul. Pharmacol.* **2012**, *58*, 326–333. [CrossRef] [PubMed]

3. Elshenawy, O.H.; Anwar-Mohamed, A.; El-Kadi, A.O. 20-Hydroxyeicosatetraenoic acid is a potential therapeutic target in cardiovascular diseases. *Curr. Drug Metab.* **2013**, *14*, 706–719. [CrossRef] [PubMed]

4. Maayah, Z.H.; El-Kadi, A.O. The role of mid-chain hydroxyeicosatetraenoic acids in the pathogenesis of hypertension and cardiac hypertrophy. *Arch. Toxicol.* **2016**, *90*, 119–136. [CrossRef] [PubMed]

5. Kroetz, D.L.; Xu, F. Regulation and inhibition of arachidonic acid omega-hydroxylases and 20-hete formation. *Annu. Rev. Pharmacol. Toxicol.* **2005**, *45*, 413–438. [CrossRef] [PubMed]

6. Xu, F.; Falck, J.R.; Ortiz de Montellano, P.R.; Kroetz, D.L. Catalytic activity and isoform-specific inhibition of rat cytochrome P450 4f enzymes. *J. Pharmacol. Exp. Ther.* **2004**, *308*, 887–895. [CrossRef] [PubMed]

7. Fan, F.; Ge, Y.; Lv, W.; Elliott, M.R.; Muroya, Y.; Hirata, T.; Booz, G.W.; Roman. R.J. Molecular mechanisms and cell signaling of 20-hydroxyeicosatetraenoic acid in vascular pathophysiology. *Front Biosci.* **2016**, *21*, 1427–1463.

8. McGiff, J.C.; Quilley, J. 20-HETE and the kidney: Resolution of old problems and new beginnings. *Am. J. Physiol.* **1999**, *277*, 607–623.

9. Carroll, M.A.; McGiff, J.C. A new class of lipid mediators: Cytochrome P450 arachidonate metabolites. *Thorax* **2000**, *55* (Suppl. 2), 13–16. [CrossRef]

10. Oyekan, A.O.; McGiff, J.C. Functional response of the rat kidney to inhibition of nitric oxide synthesis: Role of cytochrome P450-derived arachidonate metabolites. *Br. J. Pharmacol.* **1998**, *125*, 1065–1073. [CrossRef] [PubMed]

11. Askari, B.; Bell-Quilley, C.P.; Fulton, D.; Quilley, J.; McGiff, J.C. Analysis of eicosanoid mediation of the renal functional effects of hyperchloremia. *J. Pharmacol. Exp. Ther.* **1997**, *282*, 101–107. [PubMed]

12. Xu, F.; Straub, W.O.; Pak, W.; Su, P.; Maier, K.G.; Yu, M.; Roman, R.J.; Ortiz De Montellano, P.R.; Kroetz, D.L. Antihypertensive effect of mechanism-based inhibition of renal arachidonic acid omega-hydroxylase activity. *Am. J. Physiol. Regul. Integr. Comp. Physiol.* **2002**, *283*, 710–720. [CrossRef] [PubMed]

13. Williams, J.M.; Murphy, S.; Burke, M.; Roman, R.J. 20-hydroxyeicosatetraeonic acid: A new target for the treatment of hypertension. *J. Cardiovasc. Pharmacol.* **2010**, *56*, 336–344. [CrossRef] [PubMed]

14. Tunctan, B.; Korkmaz, B.; Buharalioglu, C.K.; Firat, S.S.; Anjaiah, S.; Falck, J.; Roman, R.J.; Malik, K.U. A 20-hydroxyeicosatetraenoic acid agonist, n-[20-hydroxyeicosa-5(z),14(z)-dienoyl]glycine, opposes the fall in blood pressure and vascular reactivity in endotoxin-treated rats. *Shock* **2008**, *30*, 329–335. [CrossRef] [PubMed]

15. Regner, K.R.; Zuk, A.; Van Why, S.K.; Shames, B.D.; Ryan, R.P.; Falck, J.R.; Manthati, V.L.; McMullen, M.E.; Ledbetter, S.R.; Roman, R.J. Protective effect of 20-HETE analogues in experimental renal ischemia reperfusion injury. *Kidney Int.* **2009**, *75*, 511–517. [CrossRef] [PubMed]

16. Nakamura, T.; Ishii, T.; Miyata, N.; Taniguchi, K.; Tomishima, Y.; Ueki, T.; Sato, M. Design and synthesis of 1-(4-benzoylphenyl)imidazole derivatives as new potent 20-HETE synthase inhibitors. *Bioorg. Med. Chem. Lett.* **2004**, *14*, 5305–5308. [CrossRef] [PubMed]

17. Yanes, L.L.; Lima, R.; Moulana, M.; Romero, D.G.; Yuan, K.; Ryan, M.J.; Baker, R.; Zhang, H.; Fan, F.; Davis, D.D. Postmenopausal hypertension: Role of 20-HETE. *Am. J. Physiol. Regul. Integr. Comp. Physiol.* **2011**, *300*, 1543–1548. [CrossRef] [PubMed]

18. Chabova, V.C.; Kramer, H.J.; Vaneckova, I.; Vernerova, Z.; Eis, V.; Tesar, V.; Skaroupkova, P.; Thumova, M.; Schejbalova, S.; Huskova, Z. Effects of chronic cytochrome P-450 inhibition on the course of hypertension and end-organ damage in ren-2 transgenic rats. *Vascul. Pharmacol.* **2007**, *47*, 145–159. [CrossRef] [PubMed]

19. Moreno, J.J. Eicosanoid receptors: Targets for the treatment of disrupted intestinal epithelial homeostasis. *Eur. J. Pharmacol.* **2016**, *796*, 7–19. [CrossRef] [PubMed]

20. Garcia, V.; Schwartzman, M.L. Recent developments on the vascular effects of 20-hydroxyeicosatetraenoic acid. *Curr. Opin. Nephrol. Hypertens.* **2017**, *26*, 74–82. [CrossRef] [PubMed]

21. Quigley, R.; Baum, M.; Reddy, K.M.; Griener, J.C.; Falck, J.R. Effects of 20-HETE and 19(s)-HETE on rabbit proximal straight tubule volume transport. *Am. J. Physiol. Renal Physiol.* **2000**, *278*, 949–953.

22. Omata, K.; Abraham, N.G.; Schwartzman, M.L. Renal cytochrome P-450-arachidonic acid metabolism: Localization and hormonal regulation in shr. *Am. J. Physiol.* **1992**, *262*, 591–599.

23. Oliw, E.H. Biosynthesis of 20-hydroxyeicosatetraenoic acid (20-HETE) and 12 (s)-HETE by renal cortical microsomes of the cynomolgus monkey. *Eicosanoids* **1990**, *3*, 161–164. [PubMed]

24. Lu, M.; Zhu, Y.; Balazy, M.; Reddy, K.M.; Falck, J.R.; Wang, W. Effect of angiotensin ii on the apical K$^+$ channel in the thick ascending limb of the rat kidney. *J. Gen. Physiol.* **1996**, *108*, 537–547. [CrossRef]

25. Escalante, B.; Erlij, D.; Falck, J.R.; McGiff, J.C. Cytochrome P450-dependent arachidonate metabolites affect renal transport in the rabbit. *J. Cardiovasc. Pharmacol.* **1993**, *22* (Suppl. 2), 106–108. [CrossRef]

26. Marji, J.S.; Wang, M.H.; Laniado-Schwartzman, M. Cytochrome P-450 4a isoform expression and 20-HETE synthesis in renal preglomerular arteries. *Am. J. Physiol. Renal Physiol.* **2002**, *283*, 60–67. [CrossRef] [PubMed]

27. Wang, M.H.; Guan, H.; Nguyen, X.; Zand, B.A.; Nasjletti, A.; Laniado-Schwartzman, M. Contribution of cytochrome P-450 4a1 and 4a2 to vascular 20-hydroxyeicosatetraenoic acid synthesis in rat kidneys. *Am. J. Physiol.* **1999**, *276*, 246–253.

28. Zhao, X.; Imig, J.D. Kidney cyP450 enzymes: Biological actions beyond drug metabolism. *Curr. Drug Metab.* **2003**, *4*, 73–84. [CrossRef] [PubMed]

29. Ward, N.C.; Tsai, I.J.; Barden, A.; van Bockxmeer, F.M.; Puddey, I.B.; Hodgson, J.M.; Croft, K.D. A single nucleotide polymorphism in the cyp4f2 but not cyp4a11 gene is associated with increased 20-HETE excretion and blood pressure. *Hypertension* **2008**, *51*, 1393–1398. [CrossRef] [PubMed]

30. Harder, D.R.; Campbell, W.B.; Roman, R.J. Role of cytochrome P-450 enzymes and metabolites of arachidonic acid in the control of vascular tone. *J. Vasc. Res.* **1995**, *32*, 79–92. [CrossRef] [PubMed]

31. Wang, J.S.; Zhang, F.; Jiang, M.; Wang, M.H.; Zand, B.A.; Abraham, N.G.; Nasjletti, A.; Laniado-Schwartzman, M. Transfection and functional expression of CYP4A1 and CYP4A2 using bicistronic vectors in vascular cells and tissues. *J. Pharmacol. Exp. Ther.* **2004**, *311*, 913–920. [CrossRef] [PubMed]

32. Kaide, J.; Wang, M.H.; Wang, J.S.; Zhang, F.; Gopal, V.R.; Falck, J.R.; Nasjletti, A.; Laniado-Schwartzman, M. Transfection of CYP4A1 cDNA increases vascular reactivity in renal interlobar arteries. *Am. J. Physiol. Renal Physiol.* **2003**, *284*, 51–56. [CrossRef] [PubMed]

33. Ge, Y.; Murphy, S.R.; Lu, Y.; Falck, J.; Liu, R.; Roman, R.J. Endogenously produced 20-HETE modulates myogenic and TGF response in microperfused afferent arterioles. *Prostaglandin Other Lipid Mediat.* **2013**, *102*, 42–48. [CrossRef] [PubMed]

34. Minuz, P.; Jiang, H.; Fava, C.; Turolo, L.; Tacconelli, S.; Ricci, M.; Patrignani, P.; Morganti, A.; Lechi, A.; McGiff, J.C. Altered release of cytochrome P450 metabolites of arachidonic acid in renovascular disease. *Hypertension* **2008**, *51*, 1379–1385. [CrossRef] [PubMed]

35. Dahly-Vernon, A.J.; Sharma, M.; McCarthy, E.T.; Savin, V.J.; Ledbetter, S.R.; Roman, R.J. Transforming growth factor-β, 20-HETE interaction, and glomerular injury in DAHL salt-sensitive rats. *Hypertension* **2005**, *45*, 643–648. [CrossRef] [PubMed]

36. McCarthy, E.T.; Sharma, R.; Sharma, M. Protective effect of 20-hydroxyeicosatetraenoic acid (20-HETE) on glomerular protein permeability barrier. *Kidney Int.* **2005**, *67*, 152–156. [CrossRef] [PubMed]
37. Luo, P.; Zhou, Y.; Chang, H.H.; Zhang, J.; Seki, T.; Wang, C.Y.; Inscho, E.W.; Wang, M.H. Glomerular 20-HETE, EETs, and TGF-β1 in diabetic nephropathy. *Am. J. Physiol. Renal Physiol.* **2009**, *296*, 556–563. [CrossRef] [PubMed]
38. Stec, D.E.; Flasch, A.; Roman, R.J.; White, J.A. Distribution of cytochrome P-450 4A and 4F isoforms along the nephron in mice. *Am. J. Physiol. Renal Physiol.* **2003**, *284*, 95–102. [CrossRef] [PubMed]
39. Ito, O.; Alonso-Galicia, M.; Hopp, K.A.; Roman, R.J. Localization of cytochrome P-450 4A isoforms along the rat nephron. *Am. J. Physiol.* **1998**, *274*, 395–404.
40. Harder, D.R.; Narayanan, J.; Birks, E.K.; Liard, J.F.; Imig, J.D.; Lombard, J.H.; Lange, A.R.; Roman, R.J. Identification of a putative microvascular oxygen sensor. *Circ. Res.* **1996**, *79*, 54–61. [CrossRef] [PubMed]
41. Yamaguchi, Y.; Kirita, S.; Hasegawa, H.; Aoyama, J.; Imaoka, S.; Minamiyama, S.; Funae, Y.; Baba, T.; Matsubara, T. Contribution of CYP4A8 to the formation of 20-hydroxyeicosatetraenoic acid from arachidonic acid in rat kidney. *Drug Metab. Pharmacokinet.* **2002**, *17*, 109–116. [CrossRef] [PubMed]
42. Hercule, H.C.; Wang, M.H.; Oyekan, A.O. Contribution of cytochrome P450 4a isoforms to renal functional response to inhibition of nitric oxide production in the rat. *J. Physiol.* **2003**, *551*, 971–979. [CrossRef] [PubMed]
43. Jiang, M.; Mezentsev, A.; Kemp, R.; Byun, K.; Falck, J.R.; Miano, J.M.; Nasjletti, A.; Abraham, N.G.; Laniado-Schwartzman, M. Smooth muscle-specific expression of CYP4A1 induces endothelial sprouting in renal arterial microvessels. *Circ. Res.* **2004**, *94*, 167–174. [CrossRef] [PubMed]
44. Nguyen, X.; Wang, M.H.; Reddy, K.M.; Falck, J.R.; Schwartzman, M.L. Kinetic profile of the rat CYP4A isoforms: Arachidonic acid metabolism and isoform-specific inhibitors. *Am. J. Physiol.* **1999**, *276*, 1691–1700.
45. Botros, F.T.; Laniado-Schwartzman, M.; Abraham, N.G. Regulation of cyclooxygenase and cytochrome P450 derived eicosanoids by heme oxygenase in the rat kidney. *Hypertension* **2002**, *39*, 639–644. [CrossRef] [PubMed]
46. Kalsotra, A.; Cui, X.; Anakk, S.; Hinojos, C.A.; Doris, P.A.; Strobel, H.W. Renal localization, expression, and developmental regulation of P450 4f cytochromes in three substrains of spontaneously hypertensive rats. *Biochem. Biophys. Res. Commun.* **2005**, *338*, 423–431. [CrossRef] [PubMed]
47. Fidelis, P.; Wilson, L.; Thomas, K.; Villalobos, M.; Oyekan, A.O. Renal function and vasomotor activity in mice lacking the CYP4A14 gene. *Exp. Biol. Med.* **2010**, *235*, 1365–1374. [CrossRef] [PubMed]
48. Muller, D.N.; Schmidt, C.; Barbosa-Sicard, E.; Wellner, M.; Gross, V.; Hercule, H.; Markovic, M.; Honeck, H.; Luft, F.C.; Schunck, W.H. Mouse CYP4A isoforms: Enzymatic properties, gender- and strain-specific expression, and role in renal 20-hydroxyeicosatetraenoic acid formation. *Biochem. J.* **2007**, *403*, 109–118. [CrossRef] [PubMed]
49. Lasker, J.M.; Chen, W.B.; Wolf, I.; Bloswick, B.P.; Wilson, P.D.; Powell, P.K. Formation of 20-hydroxyeicosatetraenoic acid, a vasoactive and natriuretic eicosanoid, in human kidney. Role of cyp4f2 and cyp4A11. *J. Biol. Chem.* **2000**, *275*, 4118–4126. [CrossRef] [PubMed]
50. Muroya, Y.; Fan, F.; Regner, K.R.; Falck, J.R.; Garrett, M.R.; Juncos, L.A.; Roman, R.J. Deficiency in the formation of 20-hydroxyeicosatetraenoic acid enhances renal ischemia-reperfusion injury. *J. Am. Soc. Nephrol.* **2015**, *26*, 2460–2469. [CrossRef] [PubMed]
51. Stec, D.E.; Roman, R.J.; Flasch, A.; Rieder, M.J. Functional polymorphism in human CYP4F2 decreases 20-HETE production. *Physiol. Genomics* **2007**, *30*, 74–81. [CrossRef] [PubMed]
52. Cheng, M.K.; McGiff, J.C.; Carroll, M.A. Renal arterial 20-hydroxyeicosatetraenoic acid levels: Regulation by cyclooxygenase. *Am. J. Physiol. Renal Physiol.* **2003**, *284*, 474–479. [CrossRef] [PubMed]
53. Carroll, M.A.; Kemp, R.; Cheng, M.K.; McGiff, J.C. Regulation of preglomerular microvascular 20-hydroxyeicosatetraenoic acid levels by salt depletion. *Med. Sci. Monit.* **2001**, *7*, 567–572. [PubMed]
54. Alonso-Galicia, M.; Drummond, H.A.; Reddy, K.K.; Falck, J.R.; Roman, R.J. Inhibition of 20-HETE production contributes to the vascular responses to nitric oxide. *Hypertension* **1997**, *29*, 320–325. [CrossRef] [PubMed]
55. Oyekan, A.O.; Youseff, T.; Fulton, D.; Quilley, J.; McGiff, J.C. Renal cytochrome P450 ω-hydroxylase and epoxygenase activity are differentially modified by nitric oxide and sodium chloride. *J. Clin. Invest.* **1999**, *104*, 1131–1137. [CrossRef] [PubMed]
56. Quilley, J.; Qiu, Y.; Hirt, J. Inhibitors of 20-hydroxyeicosatetraenoic acid reduce renal vasoconstrictor responsiveness. *J. Pharmacol. Exp. Ther.* **2003**, *307*, 223–229. [CrossRef]

57. Ito, O.; Roman, R.J. Regulation of P-450 4a activity in the glomerulus of the rat. *Am. J. Physiol.* **1999**, *276*, 1749–1757.

58. Alonso-Galicia, M.; Sun, C.W.; Falck, J.R.; Harder, D.R.; Roman, R.J. Contribution of 20-HETE to the vasodilator actions of nitric oxide in renal arteries. *Am. J. Physiol.* **1998**, *275*, 370–378.

59. Sarkis, A.; Roman, R.J. Role of cytochrome P450 metabolites of arachidonic acid in hypertension. *Curr. Drug Metab.* **2004**, *5*, 245–256. [CrossRef] [PubMed]

60. Da Silva, J.L.; Zand, B.A.; Yang, L.M.; Sabaawy, H.E.; Lianos, E.; Abraham, N.G. Heme oxygenase isoform-specific expression and distribution in the rat kidney. *Kidney Int.* **2001**, *59*, 1448–1457. [CrossRef] [PubMed]

61. Lin, F.; Abraham, N.G.; Schwartzman, M.L. Cytochrome P450 arachidonic acid omega-hydroxylation in the proximal tubule of the rat kidney. *Ann. N. Y. Acad. Sci.* **1994**, *744*, 11–24. [CrossRef] [PubMed]

62. Ishizuka, T.; Ito, O.; Tan, L.; Ogawa, S.; Kohzuki, M.; Omata, K.; Takeuchi, K.; Ito, S. Regulation of cytochrome P-450 4a activity by peroxisome proliferator-activated receptors in the rat kidney. *Hypertens. Res.* **2003**, *26*, 929–936. [CrossRef] [PubMed]

63. Li, J.; Li, D.; Tie, C.; Wu, J.; Wu, Q.; Li, Q. Cisplatin-mediated cytotoxicity through inducing CYP4A 11 expression in human renal tubular epithelial cells. *J. Toxicol. Sci.* **2015**, *40*, 895–900. [CrossRef] [PubMed]

64. Sarkis, A.; Ito, O.; Mori, T.; Kohzuki, M.; Ito, S.; Verbalis, J.; Cowley, A.W., Jr.; Roman, R.J. Cytochrome P-450-dependent metabolism of arachidonic acid in the kidney of rats with diabetes insipidus. *Am. J. Physiol. Renal Physiol.* **2005**, *289*, 1333–1340. [CrossRef] [PubMed]

65. Maier, K.G.; Roman, R.J. Cytochrome P450 metabolites of arachidonic acid in the control of renal function. *Curr. Opin. Nephrol. Hypertens.* **2001**, *10*, 81–87. [CrossRef] [PubMed]

66. Zou, A.P.; Imig, J.D.; Kaldunski, M.; Ortiz de Montellano, P.R.; Sui, Z.; Roman, R.J. Inhibition of renal vascular 20-HETE production impairs autoregulation of renal blood flow. *Am. J. Physiol.* **1994**, *266*, 275–282.

67. Imaoka, S.; Funae, Y. The physiological role of P450-derived arachidonic acid metabolites. *Nihon Yakurigaku Zasshi* **1998**, *112*, 23–31. [CrossRef] [PubMed]

68. Zou, A.P.; Imig, J.D.; Ortiz de Montellano, P.R.; Sui, Z.; Falck, J.R.; Roman, R.J. Effect of P-450 ω-hydroxylase metabolites of arachidonic acid on tubuloglomerular feedback. *Am. J. Physiol.* **1994**, *266*, 934–941.

69. Schwartzman, M.L.; Omata, K.; Lin, F.M.; Bhatt, R.K.; Falck, J.R.; Abraham, N.G. Detection of 20-hydroxyeicosatetraenoic acid in rat urine. *Biochem. Biophys. Res. Commun.* **1991**, *180*, 445–449. [CrossRef]

70. Roman, R.J.; Alonso-Galicia, M. P-450 eicosanoids: A novel signaling pathway regulating renal function. *News Physiol. Sci.* **1999**, *14*, 238–242. [PubMed]

71. Kauser, K.; Clark, J.E.; Masters, B.S.; Ortiz de Montellano, P.R.; Ma, Y.H.; Harder, D.R.; Roman, R.J. Inhibitors of cytochrome P-450 attenuate the myogenic response of dog renal arcuate arteries. *Circ. Res.* **1991**, *68*, 1154–1163. [CrossRef] [PubMed]

72. Wu, C.C.; Mei, S.; Cheng, J.; Ding, Y.; Weidenhammer, A.; Garcia, V.; Zhang, F.; Gotlinger, K.; Manthati, V.L.; Falck, J.R.; et al. Androgen-sensitive hypertension associates with upregulated vascular CYP4A12-20-HETE synthase. *J. Am. Soc. Nephrol.* **2013**, *24*, 1288–1296. [CrossRef] [PubMed]

73. Zhao, X.; Falck, J.R.; Gopal, V.R.; Inscho, E.W.; Imig, J.D. P2x receptor-stimulated calcium responses in preglomerular vascular smooth muscle cells involves 20-hydroxyeicosatetraenoic acid. *J. Pharmacol. Exp. Ther.* **2004**, *311*, 1211–1217. [CrossRef] [PubMed]

74. Ma, Y.H.; Gebremedhin, D.; Schwartzman, M.L.; Falck, J.R.; Clark, J.E.; Masters, B.S.; Harder, D.R.; Roman, R.J. 20-hydroxyeicosatetraenoic acid is an endogenous vasoconstrictor of canine renal arcuate arteries. *Circ. Res.* **1993**, *72*, 126–136. [CrossRef] [PubMed]

75. Arima, S.; Omata, K.; Ito, S.; Tsunoda, K.; Abe, K. 20-HETE requires increased vascular tone to constrict rabbit afferent arterioles. *Hypertension* **1996**, *27*, 781–785. [CrossRef] [PubMed]

76. Wu, C.C.; Gupta, T.; Garcia, V.; Ding, Y.; Schwartzman, M.L. 20-HETE and blood pressure regulation: Clinical implications. *Cardiol. Rev.* **2014**, *22*, 1–12. [CrossRef] [PubMed]

77. Zou, A.P.; Fleming, J.T.; Falck, J.R.; Jacobs, E.R.; Gebremedhin, D.; Harder, D.R.; Roman, R.J. 20-HETE is an endogenous inhibitor of the large-conductance Ca^{2+}-activated K^{+} channel in renal arterioles. *Am. J. Physiol.* **1996**, *270*, 228–237.

78. Harder, D.R.; Lange, A.R.; Gebremedhin, D.; Birks, E.K.; Roman, R.J. Cytochrome P450 metabolites of arachidonic acid as intracellular signaling molecules in vascular tissue. *J. Vasc. Res.* **1997**, *34*, 237–243. [CrossRef] [PubMed]

79. Roman, R.J.; Harder, D.R. Cellular and ionic signal transduction mechanisms for the mechanical activation of renal arterial vascular smooth muscle. *J. Am. Soc. Nephrol.* **1993**, *4*, 986–996. [PubMed]

80. Imig, J.D.; Zou, A.P.; Stec, D.E.; Harder, D.R.; Falck, J.R.; Roman, R.J. Formation and actions of 20-hydroxyeicosatetraenoic acid in rat renal arterioles. *Am. J. Physiol.* **1996**, *270*, 217–227.

81. Sun, C.W.; Falck, J.R.; Harder, D.R.; Roman, R.J. Role of tyrosine kinase and PKC in the vasoconstrictor response to 20-HETE in renal arterioles. *Hypertension* **1999**, *33*, 414–418. [CrossRef] [PubMed]

82. Sun, C.W.; Alonso-Galicia, M.; Taheri, M.R.; Falck, J.R.; Harder, D.R.; Roman, R.J. Nitric oxide-20-hydroxyeicosatetraenoic acid interaction in the regulation of K$^+$ channel activity and vascular tone in renal arterioles. *Circ. Res.* **1998**, *83*, 1069–1079. [CrossRef] [PubMed]

83. Kuczeriszka, M.; Badzynska, B.; Kompanowska-Jezierska, E. Cytochrome P-450 monooxygenases in control of renal haemodynamics and arterial pressure in anaesthetized rats. *J. Physiol. Pharmacol.* **2006**, *57* (Suppl. 11), 179–185. [PubMed]

84. Oyekan, A.O. Differential effects of 20-hydroxyeicosatetraenoic acid on intrarenal blood flow in the rat. *J. Pharmacol. Exp. Ther.* **2005**, *313*, 1289–1295. [CrossRef] [PubMed]

85. Hercule, H.C.; Oyekan, A.O. Role of no and cytochrome P-450-derived eicosanoids in et-1-induced changes in intrarenal hemodynamics in rats. *Am. J. Physiol. Regul. Integr. Comp. Physiol.* **2000**, *279*, 2132–2141.

86. Hercule, H.C.; Oyekan, A.O. Cytochrome P450 ω/ω-1 hydroxylase-derived eicosanoids contribute to endothelin(a) and endothelin(b) receptor-mediated vasoconstriction to endothelin-1 in the rat preglomerular arteriole. *J. Pharmacol. Exp. Ther.* **2000**, *292*, 1153–1160. [PubMed]

87. Oyekan, A.O.; McAward, K.; McGiff, J.C. Renal functional effects of endothelins: Dependency on cytochrome P450-derived arachidonate metabolites. *Biol. Res.* **1998**, *31*, 209–215. [PubMed]

88. Lai, G.; Liu, X.; Wu, J.; Liu, H.; Zhao, Y. Evaluation of CMV and KAP promoters for driving the expression of human CYP4F2 in transgenic mice. *Int. J. Mol. Med.* **2012**, *29*, 107–112. [PubMed]

89. Zhang, B.; Lai, G.; Liu, X.; Zhao, Y. Alteration of epoxyeicosatrienoic acids in the liver and kidney of cytochrome P450 4f2 transgenic mice. *Mol. Med. Rep.* **2016**, *14*, 5739–5745. [CrossRef] [PubMed]

90. Roman, R.J. P-450 metabolites of arachidonic acid in the control of cardiovascular function. *Physiol. Rev.* **2002**, *82*, 131–185. [CrossRef] [PubMed]

91. Li, D.; Belusa, R.; Nowicki, S.; Aperia, A. Arachidonic acid metabolic pathways regulating activity of renal Na$^+$-K$^+$-atpase are age dependent. *Am. J. Physiol. Renal Physiol.* **2000**, *278*, 823–829.

92. Nowicki, S.; Chen, S.L.; Aizman, O.; Cheng, X.J.; Li, D.; Nowicki, C.; Nairn, A.; Greengard, P.; Aperia, A. 20-hydroxyeicosa-tetraenoic acid (20 HETE) activates protein kinase c: Role in regulation of rat renal Na$^+$-K$^+$-atpase. *J. Clin. Invest.* **1997**, *99*, 1224–1230. [CrossRef] [PubMed]

93. Sacerdoti, D.; Gatta, A.; McGiff, J.C. Role of cytochrome P450-dependent arachidonic acid metabolites in liver physiology and pathophysiology. *Prostaglandins Other Lipid Mediat.* **2003**, *72*, 51–71. [CrossRef]

94. Cloutier, M.; Campbell, S.; Basora, N.; Proteau, S.; Payet, M.D.; Rousseau, E. 20-HETE inotropic effects involve the activation of a nonselective cationic current in airway smooth muscle. *Am. J. Physiol. Lung Cell. Mol. Physiol.* **2003**, *285*, 560–568. [CrossRef] [PubMed]

95. Fan, F.; Muroya, Y.; Roman, R.J. Cytochrome P450 eicosanoids in hypertension and renal disease. *Curr. Opin. Nephrol. Hypertens.* **2015**, *24*, 37–46. [CrossRef] [PubMed]

96. Quigley, R.; Chakravarty, S.; Zhao, X.; Imig, J.D.; Capdevila, J.H. Increased renal proximal convoluted tubule transport contributes to hypertension in CYP4A14 knockout mice. *Nephron Physiol.* **2009**, *113*, 23–28. [CrossRef] [PubMed]

97. Wu, C.C.; Schwartzman, M.L. The role of 20-HETE in androgen-mediated hypertension. *Prostaglandins Other Lipid Mediat.* **2011**, *96*, 45–53. [CrossRef] [PubMed]

98. Holla, V.R.; Adas, F.; Imig, J.D.; Zhao, X.; Price, E., Jr.; Olsen, N.; Kovacs, W.J.; Magnuson, M.A.; Keeney, D.S.; Breyer, M.D. Alterations in the regulation of androgen-sensitive Cyp 4a monooxygenases cause hypertension. *Proc. Natl. Acad. Sci. USA* **2001**, *98*, 5211–5216. [CrossRef] [PubMed]

99. Beltowski, J.; Marciniak, A.; Wojcicka, G.; Gorny, D. The opposite effects of cyclic amp-protein kinase a signal transduction pathway on renal cortical and medullary Na$^+$,K$^+$-atpase activity. *J. Physiol. Pharmacol.* **2002**, *53*, 211–231. [PubMed]

100. Derrickson, B.H.; Mandel, L.J. Parathyroid hormone inhibits Na$^+$-K$^+$-atpase through Gq/G11 and the calcium-independent phospholipase A2. *Am. J. Physiol.* **1997**, *272*, F781–F788. [PubMed]

101. Kirchheimer, C.; Mendez, C.F.; Acquier, A.; Nowicki, S. Role of 20-HETE in D1/D2 dopamine receptor synergism resulting in the inhibition of Na$^+$-K$^+$-ATPase activity in the proximal tubule. *Am. J. Physiol. Renal Physiol.* **2007**, *292*, 1435–1442. [CrossRef] [PubMed]

102. Ominato, M.; Satoh, T.; Katz, A.I. Regulation of Na$^+$-K$^+$-atpase activity in the proximal tubule: Role of the protein kinase c pathway and of eicosanoids. *J. Membr. Biol.* **1996**, *152*, 235–243. [CrossRef] [PubMed]

103. Silverstein, D.M.; Barac-Nieto, M.; Falck, J.R.; Spitzer, A. 20-HETE mediates the effect of parathyroid hormone and protein kinase c on renal phosphate transport. *Prostaglandins Leukot. Essent. Fatty Acids* **1998**, *58*, 209–213. [CrossRef]

104. Silverstein, D.M.; Barac-Nieto, M.; Spitzer, A. Multiple arachidonic acid metabolites inhibit sodium-dependent phosphate transport in ok cells. *Prostaglandins Leukot. Essent. Fatty Acids* **1999**, *61*, 165–169. [CrossRef] [PubMed]

105. Silverstein, D.M.; Spitzer, A.; Barac-Nieto, M. Hormonal regulation of sodium-dependent phosphate transport in opossum kidney cells. *Horm. Res.* **2000**, *54*, 38–43. [CrossRef] [PubMed]

106. Silverstein, D.M.; Spitzer, A.; Barac-Nieto, M. Parathormone sensitivity and responses to protein kinases in subclones of opossum kidney cells. *Pediatr. Nephrol.* **2005**, *20*, 721–724. [CrossRef] [PubMed]

107. Amlal, H.; Legoff, C.; Vernimmen, C.; Paillard, M.; Bichara, M. Na$^+$-K$^+$-Nh^{4+}-2Cl$^-$ cotransport in medullary thick ascending limb: Control by pKa, pKc, and 20-HETE. *Am. J. Physiol.* **1996**, *271*, 455–463.

108. Grider, J.S.; Falcone, J.C.; Kilpatrick, E.L.; Ott, C.E.; Jackson, B.A. P450 arachidonate metabolites mediate bradykinin-dependent inhibition of NACl transport in the rat thick ascending limb. *Can. J. Physiol. Pharmacol.* **1997**, *75*, 91–96. [CrossRef] [PubMed]

109. Wang, W.; Lu, M. Effect of arachidonic acid on activity of the apical K$^+$ channel in the thick ascending limb of the rat kidney. *J. Gen. Physiol.* **1995**, *106*, 727–743. [CrossRef] [PubMed]

110. Gu, R.M.; Wei, Y.; Jiang, H.L.; Lin, D.H.; Sterling, H.; Bloom, P.; Balazy, M.; Wang, W.H. K depletion enhances the extracellular Ca^{2+}-induced inhibition of the apical k channels in the mTAL of rat kidney. *J. Gen. Physiol.* **2002**, *119*, 33–44. [CrossRef] [PubMed]

111. Li, D.; Wei, Y.; Wang, W.H. Dietary K intake regulates the response of apical K channels to adenosine in the thick ascending limb. *Am. J. Physiol. Renal Physiol.* **2004**, *287*, 954–959. [CrossRef] [PubMed]

112. Ikari, A.; Nakajima, K.; Suketa, Y.; Harada, H.; Takagi, K. Activation of Na$^+$-independent Mg^{2+} efflux by 20-hydroxyeicosatetraenoic acid in rat renal epithelial cells. *Jpn. J. Physiol.* **2004**, *54*, 415–419. [CrossRef] [PubMed]

113. Savas, U.; Wei, S.; Hsu, M.H.; Falck, J.R.; Guengerich, F.P.; Capdevila, J.H.; Johnson, E.F. 20-hydroxyeicosatetraenoic acid (HETE)-dependent hypertension in human cytochrome P450 (CYP) 4A11 transgenic mice: Normalization of blood pressure by sodium restriction, hydrochlorothiazide, or blockade of the type 1 angiotensin ii receptor. *J. Biol. Chem.* **2016**, *291*, 16904–16919. [CrossRef] [PubMed]

114. Coca, S.G.; Yusuf, B.; Shlipak, M.G.; Garg, A.X.; Parikh, C.R. Long-term risk of mortality and other adverse outcomes after acute kidney injury: A systematic review and meta-analysis. *Am. J. Kidney Dis.* **2009**, *53*, 961–973. [CrossRef] [PubMed]

115. Bonventre, J.V.; Yang, L. Cellular pathophysiology of ischemic acute kidney injury. *J. Clin. Invest.* **2011**, *121*, 4210–4221. [CrossRef] [PubMed]

116. Siew, E.D.; Davenport, A. The growth of acute kidney injury: A rising tide or just closer attention to detail? *Kidney Int.* **2015**, *87*, 46–61. [CrossRef] [PubMed]

117. Dolegowska, B.; Blogowski, W.; Domanski, L. Is it possible to predict the early post-transplant allograft function using 20-HETE measurements? A preliminary report. *Transpl. Int.* **2009**, *22*, 546–553. [CrossRef] [PubMed]

118. Roman, R.J.; Akbulut, T.; Park, F.; Regner, K.R. 20-HETE in acute kidney injury. *Kidney Int.* **2011**, *79*, 10–13. [CrossRef] [PubMed]

119. Nilakantan, V.; Maenpaa, C.; Jia, G.; Roman, R.J.; Park, F. 20-HETE-mediated cytotoxicity and apoptosis in ischemic kidney epithelial cells. *Am. J. Physiol. Renal Physiol.* **2008**, *294*, 562–570. [CrossRef] [PubMed]

120. Hoff, U.; Lukitsch, I.; Chaykovska, L.; Ladwig, M.; Arnold, C.; Manthati, V.L.; Fuller, T.F.; Schneider, W.; Gollasch, M.; Muller, D.N. Inhibition of 20-HETE synthesis and action protects the kidney from ischemia/reperfusion injury. *Kidney Int.* **2011**, *79*, 57–65. [CrossRef] [PubMed]

121. Regner, K.R.; Roman, R.J. Role of medullary blood flow in the pathogenesis of renal ischemia-reperfusion injury. *Curr. Opin. Nephrol. Hypertens.* **2012**, *21*, 33–38. [CrossRef] [PubMed]

122. Park, F.; Sweeney, W.E.; Jia, G.; Roman, R.J.; Avner, E.D. 20-HETE mediates proliferation of renal epithelial cells in polycystic kidney disease. *J. Am. Soc. Nephrol.* **2008**, *19*, 1929–1939. [CrossRef] [PubMed]

123. Park, F.; Sweeney, W.E., Jr.; Jia, G.; Akbulut, T.; Mueller, B.; Falck, J.R.; Birudaraju, S.; Roman, R.J.; Avner, E.D. Chronic blockade of 20-HETE synthesis reduces polycystic kidney disease in an orthologous rat model of arpkd. *Am. J. Physiol. Renal Physiol.* **2009**, *296*, 575–582. [CrossRef] [PubMed]

124. Klawitter, J.; Klawitter, J.; McFann, K.; Pennington, A.T.; Abebe, K.Z.; Brosnahan, G.; Cadnapaphornchai, M.A.; Chonchol, M.; Gitomer, B.; Christians, U.; et al. Bioactive lipid mediators in polycystic kidney disease. *J. Lipid Res.* **2014**, *55*, 1139–1149. [CrossRef] [PubMed]

125. Tian, T.; Li, J.; Wang, M.Y.; Xie, X.F.; Li, Q.X. Protective effect of 20-hydroxyeicosatetraenoic acid (20-HETE) on adriamycin-induced toxicity of human renal tubular epithelial cell (HK-2). *Eur. J. Pharmacol.* **2012**, *683*, 246–251. [CrossRef] [PubMed]

126. Blanton, A.; Nsaif, R.; Hercule, H.; Oyekan, A. Nitric oxide/cytochrome P450 interactions in cyclosporin a-induced effects in the rat. *J. Hypertens.* **2006**, *24*, 1865–1872. [CrossRef] [PubMed]

127. Seki, T.; Ishimoto, T.; Sakurai, T.; Yasuda, Y.; Taniguchi, K.; Doi, M.; Sato, M.; Roman, R.J.; Miyata, N. Increased excretion of urinary 20-HETE in rats with cyclosporine-induced nephrotoxicity. *J. Pharmacol. Sci.* **2005**, *97*, 132–137. [CrossRef] [PubMed]

128. Vickers, A.E.; Alegret, M.; Meyer, E.; Smiley, S.; Guertler, J. Hydroxyethyl cyclosporin a induces and decreases P4503a and p-glycoprotein levels in rat liver. *Xenobiotica* **1996**, *26*, 27–39. [CrossRef] [PubMed]

129. Wang, M.H.; Zand, B.A.; Nasjletti, A.; Laniado-Schwartzman, M. Renal 20-hydroxyeicosatetraenoic acid synthesis during pregnancy. *Am. J. Physiol. Regul. Integr. Comp. Physiol.* **2002**, *282*, 383–389.

130. Wang, M.H.; Wang, J.; Chang, H.H.; Zand, B.A.; Jiang, M.; Nasjletti, A.; Laniado-Schwartzman, M. Regulation of renal CYP4A expression and 20-HETE synthesis by nitric oxide in pregnant rats. *Am. J. Physiol. Renal Physiol.* **2003**, *285*, 295–302. [CrossRef] [PubMed]

131. Huang, H.; Zhou, Y.; Raju, V.T.; Du, J.; Chang, H.H.; Wang, C.Y.; Brands, M.W.; Falck, J.R.; Wang, M.H. Renal 20-HETE inhibition attenuates changes in renal hemodynamics induced by L-name treatment in pregnant rats. *Am. J. Physiol. Renal Physiol.* **2005**, *289*, 1116–1122. [CrossRef] [PubMed]

132. Llinas, M.T.; Alexander, B.T.; Capparelli, M.F.; Carroll, M.A.; Granger, J.P. Cytochrome P-450 inhibition attenuates hypertension induced by reductions in uterine perfusion pressure in pregnant rats. *Hypertension* **2004**, *43*, 623–628. [CrossRef] [PubMed]

133. Rifkind, A.B.; Lee, C.; Chang, T.K.; Waxman, D.J. Arachidonic acid metabolism by human cytochrome P450s 2c8, 2c9, 2e1, and 1a2: Regioselective oxygenation and evidence for a role for CYP2C enzymes in arachidonic acid epoxygenation in human liver microsomes. *Arch. Biochem. Biophys.* **1995**, *320*, 380–389. [CrossRef]

134. Powell, P.K.; Wolf, I.; Jin, R.; Lasker, J.M. Metabolism of arachidonic acid to 20-hydroxy-5,8,11,14-eicosatetraenoic acid by P450 enzymes in human liver: Involvement of cyp4f2 and CYP4A11. *J. Pharmacol. Exp. Ther.* **1998**, *285*, 1327–1336. [PubMed]

135. Antoun, J.; Goulitquer, S.; Amet, Y.; Dreano, Y.; Salaun, J.P.; Corcos, L.; Plee-Gautier, E. CYP4F3B is induced by PGA1 in human liver cells: A regulation of the 20-HETE synthesis. *J. Lipid Res.* **2008**, *49*, 2135–2141. [CrossRef] [PubMed]

136. Plee-Gautier, E.; Antoun, J.; Goulitquer, S.; Le Jossic-Corcos, C.; Simon, B.; Amet, Y.; Salaun, J.P.; Corcos, L. Statins increase cytochrome P450 4F3-mediated eicosanoids production in human liver cells: A PXR dependent mechanism. *Biochem. Pharmacol.* **2012**, *84*, 571–579. [CrossRef] [PubMed]

137. Poloyac, S.M.; Tortorici, M.A.; Przychodzin, D.I.; Reynolds, R.B.; Xie, W.; Frye, R F.; Zemaitis, M.A. The effect of isoniazid on CYP2E1- and CYP4A-mediated hydroxylation of arachidonic acid in the rat liver and kidney. *Drug Metab. Dispos.* **2004**, *32*, 727–733. [CrossRef] [PubMed]

138. Sacerdoti, D.; Jiang, H.; Gaiani, S.; McGiff, J.C.; Gatta, A.; Bolognesi, M. 11,12-EET increases porto-sinusoidal resistance and may play a role in endothelial dysfunction of portal hypertension. *Prostaglandins Other Lipid Mediat.* **2011**, *96*, 72–75. [CrossRef] [PubMed]

139. Sacerdoti, D.; Balazy, M.; Angeli, P.; Gatta, A.; McGiff, J.C. Eicosanoid excretion in hepatic cirrhosis: Predominance of 20-HETE. *J. Clin. Invest.* **1997**, *100*, 1264–1270. [CrossRef] [PubMed]

140. Imig, J.D.; Hammock, B.D. Soluble epoxide hydrolase as a therapeutic target for cardiovascular diseases. *Nat. Rev. Drug Discov.* **2009**, *8*, 794–805. [CrossRef] [PubMed]

141. Zhu, D.; Zhang, C.; Medhora, M.; Jacobs, E.R. CYP4A mrna, protein, and product in rat lungs: Novel localization in vascular endothelium. *J. Appl. Physiol.* **2002**, *93*, 330–337. [CrossRef] [PubMed]

142. Lakhkar, A.; Dhagia, V.; Joshi, S.R.; Gotlinger, K.; Patel, D.; Sun, D.; Wolin, M.S.; Schwartzman, M.L.; Gupte, S.A. 20-HETE-induced mitochondrial superoxide production and inflammatory phenotype in vascular smooth muscle is prevented by glucose-6-phosphate dehydrogenase inhibition. *Am. J. Physiol. Heart Circ. Physiol.* **2016**, *310*, 1107–1117. [CrossRef] [PubMed]

143. Zhu, D.; Effros, R.M.; Harder, D.R.; Roman, R.J.; Jacobs, E.R. Tissue sources of cytochrome P450 4a and 20-HETE synthesis in rabbit lungs. *Am. J. Respir. Cell Mol. Biol.* **1998**, *19*, 121–128. [CrossRef] [PubMed]

144. Yaghi, A.; Bradbury, J.A.; Zeldin, D.C.; Mehta, S.; Bend, J.R.; McCormack, D.G. Pulmonary cytochrome P-450 2j4 is reduced in a rat model of acute pseudomonas pneumonia. *Am. J. Physiol. Lung Cell. Mol. Physiol.* **2003**, *285*, 1099–1105. [CrossRef] [PubMed]

145. Yang, J.; Eiserich, J.P.; Cross, C.E.; Morrissey, B.M.; Hammock, B.D. Metabolomic profiling of regulatory lipid mediators in sputum from adult cystic fibrosis patients. *Free Radic. Biol. Med.* **2012**, *53*, 160–171. [CrossRef] [PubMed]

146. Jacobs, E.R.; Bodiga, S.; Ali, I.; Falck, A.M.; Falck, J.R.; Medhora, M.; Dhanasekaran, A. Tissue protection and endothelial cell signaling by 20-HETE analogs in intact ex vivo lung slices. *Exp. Cell Res.* **2012**, *16*, 2143–2152. [CrossRef] [PubMed]

147. Zhu, D.; Birks, E.K.; Dawson, C.A.; Patel, M.; Falck, J.R.; Presberg, K.; Roman, R.J.; Jacobs, E.R. Hypoxic pulmonary vasoconstriction is modified by P-450 metabolites. *Am. J. Physiol. Heart Circ. Physiol.* **2000**, *279*, 1526–1533.

148. Dhanasekaran, A.; Bodiga, S.; Gruenloh, S.; Gao, Y.; Dunn, L.; Falck, J.R.; Buonaccorsi, J.N.; Medhora, M.; Jacobs, E.R. 20-HETE increases survival and decreases apoptosis in pulmonary arteries and pulmonary artery endothelial cells. *Am. J. Physiol. Heart Circ. Physiol.* **2009**, *296*, 777–786. [CrossRef] [PubMed]

149. Wang, Z.; Tang, X.; Li, Y.; Leu, C.; Guo, L.; Zheng, X.; Zhu, D. 20-Hydroxyeicosatetraenoic acid inhibits the apoptotic responses in pulmonary artery smooth muscle cells. *Eur. J. Pharmacol.* **2008**, *588*, 9–17. [CrossRef] [PubMed]

150. Medhora, M.; Chen, Y.; Gruenloh, S.; Harland, D.; Bodiga, S.; Zielonka, J.; Gebremedhin, D.; Gao, Y.; Falck, J.R.; Anjaiah, S.; et al. 20-HETE increases superoxide production and activates NAPDH oxidase in pulmonary artery endothelial cells. *Am. J. Physiol. Lung Cell. Mol. Physiol.* **2008**, *294*, 902–911. [CrossRef] [PubMed]

151. Bodiga, S.; Gruenloh, S.K.; Gao, Y.; Manthati, V.L.; Dubasi, N.; Falck, J.R.; Medhora, M.; Jacobs, E.R. 20-HETE-induced nitric oxide production in pulmonary artery endothelial cells is mediated by NADPH oxidase, H_2O_2, and PI3-kinase/Akt. *Am. J. Physiol. Lung Cell. Mol. Physiol.* **2010**, *298*, 564–574. [CrossRef] [PubMed]

152. Yu, M.; McAndrew, R.P.; Al-Saghir, R.; Maier, K.G.; Medhora, M.; Roman, R.J.; Jacobs, E.R. Nitric oxide contributes to 20-HETE-induced relaxation of pulmonary arteries. *J. Appl. Physiol.* **2002**, *93*, 1391–1399. [CrossRef] [PubMed]

153. Fuloria, M.; Eckman, D.M.; Leach, D.A.; Aschner, J.L. 20-hydroxyeicosatetraenoic acid is a vasoconstrictor in the newborn piglet pulmonary microcirculation. *Am. J. Physiol. Lung Cell. Mol. Physiol.* **2004**, *287*, 360–365. [CrossRef] [PubMed]

154. Morin, C.; Guibert, C.; Sirois, M.; Echave, V.; Gomes, M.M.; Rousseau, E. Effects of ω-hydroxylase product on distal human pulmonary arteries. *Am. J. Physiol. Heart Circ. Physiol.* **2008**, *294*, 1435–1443. [CrossRef] [PubMed]

155. Birks, E.K.; Bousamra, M.; Presberg, K.; Marsh, J.A.; Effros, R.M.; Jacobs, E.R. Human pulmonary arteries dilate to 20-HETE, an endogenous eicosanoid of lung tissue. *Am. J. Physiol.* **1997**, *272*, 823–829.

156. Yaghi, A.; Webb, C.D.; Scott, J.A.; Mehta, S.; Bend, J.R.; McCormack, D.G. Cytochrome P450 metabolites of arachidonic acid but not cyclooxygenase-2 metabolites contribute to the pulmonary vascular hyporeactivity in rats with acute pseudomonas pneumonia. *J. Pharmacol. Exp. Ther.* **2001**, *297*, 479–488. [PubMed]

157. Jacobs, E.R.; Zhu, D.; Gruenloh, S.; Lopez, B.; Medhora, M. VEGF-induced relaxation of pulmonary arteries is mediated by endothelial cytochrome P-450 hydroxylase. *Am. J. Physiol. Lung Cell. Mol. Physiol.* **2006**, *291*, 369–377. [CrossRef] [PubMed]

158. Chen, Y.; Medhora, M.; Falck, J.R.; Pritchard, K.A., Jr.; Jacobs, E.R. Mechanisms of activation of eNOS by 20-HETE and VEGF in bovine pulmonary artery endothelial cells. *Am. J. Physiol. Lung Cell. Mol. Physiol.* **2006**, *291*, 378–385. [CrossRef] [PubMed]

159. Kizub, I.V.; Lakhkar, A.; Dhagia, V.; Joshi, S.R.; Jiang, H.; Wolin, M.S.; Falck, J.R.; Koduru, S.R.; Errabelli, R.; Jacobs, E.R. Involvement of gap junctions between smooth muscle cells in sustained hypoxic pulmonary vasoconstriction development: A potential role for 15-HETE and 20-HETE. *Am. J. Physiol. Lung Cell. Mol. Physiol.* **2016**, *310*, 772–783. [CrossRef] [PubMed]

160. Singh, T.U.; Choudhury, S.; Parida, S.; Maruti, B.S.; Mishra, S.K. Arachidonic acid inhibits Na^+-K^+-atpase via cytochrome P-450, lipoxygenase and protein kinase c-dependent pathways in sheep pulmonary artery. *Vascul. Pharmacol.* **2012**, *56*, 84–90. [CrossRef] [PubMed]

161. Parker, T.A.; Grover, T.R.; Kinsella, J.P.; Falck, J.R.; Abman, S.H. Inhibition of 20-HETE abolishes the myogenic response during NOS antagonism in the ovine fetal pulmonary circulation. *Am. J. Physiol. Lung Cell. Mol. Physiol.* **2005**, *289*, 261–267. [CrossRef] [PubMed]

162. Rousseau, E.; Cloutier, M.; Morin, C.; Proteau, S. Capsazepine, a vanilloid antagonist, abolishes tonic responses induced by 20-HETE on guinea pig airway smooth muscle. *Am. J. Physiol. Lung Cell. Mol. Physiol.* **2005**, *288*, 460–470. [CrossRef] [PubMed]

163. Morin, C.; Sirois, M.; Echave, V.; Gomes, M.M.; Rousseau, E. Functional effects of 20-HETE on human bronchi: Hyperpolarization and relaxation due to BKCa channel activation. *Am. J. Physiol. Lung Cell. Mol. Physiol.* **2007**, *293*, 1037–1044. [CrossRef] [PubMed]

164. Jacobs, E.R.; Effros, R.M.; Falck, J.R.; Reddy, K.M.; Campbell, W.B.; Zhu, D. Airway synthesis of 20-hydroxyeicosatetraenoic acid: Metabolism by cyclooxygenase to a bronchodilator. *Am. J. Physiol.* **1999**, *276*, 280–288.

165. Cooper, P.R.; Mesaros, A.C.; Zhang, J.; Christmas, P.; Stark, C.M.; Donaidy, K.; Mittelman, M.A.; Soberman, R.J.; Blair, I.A.; Panettieri, R.A. 20-HETE mediates ozone-induced, neutrophil-independent airway hyper-responsiveness in mice. *PLoS ONE* **2010**, *5*, 10235. [CrossRef] [PubMed]

166. Kokalari, B.; Koziol-White, C.; Jester, W.; Panettieri, R.A.; Haczku, A.; Jiang, Z. 20-hydroxyeicosatetraenoic acid (20-HETE) induces airway inflammation and hyperresponsiveness in mice. In Proceedings of C101. Allergic airway inflammation and hyperresponsiveness: Novel mechanisms and therapy, Washington, DC, USA, 19–24 May 2015; Am Thoracic Soc: New York, NY, USA, 2015; p. 5165.

167. Chuang, S.S.; Helvig, C.; Taimi, M.; Ramshaw, H.A.; Collop, A.H.; Amad, M.; White, J.A.; Petkovich, M.; Jones, G.; Korczak, B. Cyp2u1, a novel human thymus- and brain-specific cytochrome P450, catalyzes ω- and (ω -1)-hydroxylation of fatty acids. *J. Biol. Chem.* **2004**, *279*, 6305–6314. [CrossRef] [PubMed]

168. Gebremedhin, D.; Zhang, D.X.; Carver, K.A.; Rau, N.; Rarick, K.R.; Roman, R.J.; Harder, D.R. Expression of CYP 4A omega-hydroxylase and formation of 20-hydroxyeicosatreanoic acid (20-HETE) in cultured rat brain astrocytes. *Prostaglandins Other Lipid Mediat.* **2016**, *124*, 16–26. [CrossRef] [PubMed]

169. Collins, X.H.; Harmon, S.D.; Kaduce, T.L.; Berst, K.B.; Fang, X.; Moore, S.A.; Raju, T.V.; Falck, J.R.; Weintraub, N.L.; Duester, G.; et al. Omega-oxidation of 20-hydroxyeicosatetraenoic acid (20-HETE) in cerebral microvascular smooth muscle and endothelium by alcohol dehydrogenase 4. *J. Biol. Chem.* **2005**, *280*, 33157–33164. [CrossRef] [PubMed]

170. Qi, L.; Meng, L.; Li, Y.; Qu, Y. Arterial carbon dioxide partial pressure influences CYP4A distribution in the rat brain. *Histol. Histopathol.* **2012**, *27*, 897–903. [PubMed]

171. Liu, X.; Li, C.; Falck, J.R.; Roman, R.J.; Harder, D.R.; Koehler, R.C. Interaction of nitric oxide, 20-HETE, and eets during functional hyperemia in whisker barrel cortex. *Am. J. Physiol. Heart Circ. Physiol.* **2008**, *295*, 619–631. [CrossRef] [PubMed]

172. Pratt, P.F.; Medhora, M.; Harder, D.R. Mechanisms regulating cerebral blood flow as therapeutic targets. *Curr. Opin. Investig. Drugs* **2004**, *5*, 952–956. [PubMed]

173. Gordon, G.R.; Mulligan, S.J.; MacVicar, B.A. Astrocyte control of the cerebrovasculature. *Glia* **2007**, *55*, 1214–1221. [CrossRef] [PubMed]

174. Imig, J.D.; Simpkins, A.N.; Renic, M.; Harder, D.R. Cytochrome P450 eicosanoids and cerebral vascular function. *Expert Rev. Mol. Med.* **2011**, *13*, 7. [CrossRef] [PubMed]

175. Gebremedhin, D.; Lange, A.R.; Lowry, T.F.; Taheri, M.R.; Birks, E.K.; Hudetz, A.G.; Narayanan, J.; Falck, J.R.; Okamoto, H.; Roman, R.J. Production of 20-HETE and its role in autoregulation of cerebral blood flow. *Circ. Res.* **2000**, *87*, 60–65. [CrossRef] [PubMed]

176. Fu, Z.; Nakayama, T.; Sato, N.; Izumi, Y.; Kasamaki, Y.; Shindo, A.; Ohta, M.; Soma, M.; Aoi, N.; Sato, M.; et al. A haplotype of the CYP4F2 gene is associated with cerebral infarction in Japanese men. *Am. J. Hypertens.* **2008**, *21*, 1216–1223. [CrossRef] [PubMed]

177. Berg, R.M. Myogenic and metabolic feedback in cerebral autoregulation: Putative involvement of arachidonic acid-dependent pathways. *Med. Hypotheses* **2016**, *92*, 12–17. [CrossRef] [PubMed]
178. Metea, M.R.; Newman, E.A. Signalling within the neurovascular unit in the mammalian retina. *Exp. Physiol.* **2007**, *92*, 635–640. [CrossRef] [PubMed]
179. Metea, M.R.; Newman, E.A. Glial cells dilate and constrict blood vessels: A mechanism of neurovascular coupling. *J. Neurosci.* **2006**, *26*, 2862–2870. [CrossRef] [PubMed]
180. Liu, X.; Li, C.; Gebremedhin, D.; Hwang, S.H.; Hammock, B.D.; Falck, J.R.; Roman, R.J.; Harder, D.R.; Koehler, R.C. Epoxyeicosatrienoic acid-dependent cerebral vasodilation evoked by metabotropic glutamate receptor activation in vivo. *Am. J. Physiol. Heart Circ. Physiol.* **2011**, *301*, 373–381. [CrossRef] [PubMed]
181. Lange, A.; Gebremedhin, D.; Narayanan, J.; Harder, D. 20-Hydroxyeicosatetraenoic acid-induced vasoconstriction and inhibition of potassium current in cerebral vascular smooth muscle is dependent on activation of protein kinase c. *J. Biol. Chem.* **1997**, *272*, 27345–27352. [CrossRef] [PubMed]
182. Ohata, H.; Gebremedhin, D.; Narayanan, J.; Harder, D.R.; Koehler, R.C. Onset of pulmonary ventilation in fetal sheep produces pial arteriolar constriction dependent on cytochrome P450 omega-hydroxylase activity. *J. Appl. Physiol.* **2010**, *109*, 412–417. [CrossRef] [PubMed]
183. Mapelli, L.; Gagliano, G.; Soda, T.; Laforenza, U.; Moccia, F.; D'Angelo, E.U. Granular layer neurons control cerebellar neurovascular coupling through an NMDA receptor/no-dependent system. *J. Neurosci.* **2017**, *37*, 1340–1351. [CrossRef] [PubMed]
184. Hama-Tomioka, K.; Kinoshita, H.; Azma, T.; Nakahata, K.; Matsuda, N.; Hatakeyama, N.; Kikuchi, H.; Hatano, Y. The role of 20-hydroxyeicosatetraenoic acid in cerebral arteriolar constriction and the inhibitory effect of propofol. *Anesth. Analg.* **2009**, *109*, 1935–1942. [CrossRef] [PubMed]
185. Renic, M.; Kumar, S.N.; Gebremedhin, D.; Florence, M.A.; Gerges, N.Z.; Falck, J.R.; Harder, D.R.; Roman, R.J. Protective effect of 20-HETE inhibition in a model of oxygen-glucose deprivation in hippocampal slice cultures. *Am. J. Physiol. Heart Circ. Physiol.* **2012**, *302*, 1285–1293. [CrossRef] [PubMed]
186. Hall, C.N.; Reynell, C.; Gesslein, B.; Hamilton, N.B.; Mishra, A.; Sutherland, B.A.; O'Farrell, F.M.; Buchan, A.M.; Lauritzen, M.; Attwell, D. Capillary pericytes regulate cerebral blood flow in health and disease. *Nature* **2014**, *508*, 55–60. [CrossRef] [PubMed]
187. Fang, X.; Faraci, F.M.; Kaduce, T.L.; Harmon, S.; Modrick, M.L.; Hu, S.; Moore, S.A.; Falck, J.R.; Weintraub, N.L.; Spector, A.A. 20-Hydroxyeicosatetraenoic acid is a potent dilator of mouse basilar artery: Role of cyclooxygenase. *Am. J. Physiol. Heart Circ. Physiol.* **2006**, *291*, 2301–2307. [CrossRef] [PubMed]
188. Marumo, T.; Eto, K.; Wake, H.; Omura, T.; Nabekura, J. The inhibitor of 20-HETE synthesis, ts-011, improves cerebral microcirculatory autoregulation impaired by middle cerebral artery occlusion in mice. *Br. J. Pharmacol.* **2010**, *161*, 1391–1402. [CrossRef] [PubMed]
189. Poloyac, S.M.; Reynolds, R.B.; Yonas, H.; Kerr, M.E. Identification and quantification of the hydroxyeicosatetraenoic acids, 20-HETE and 12-HETE, in the cerebrospinal fluid after subarachnoid hemorrhage. *J. Neurosci. Methods* **2005**, *144*, 257–263. [CrossRef] [PubMed]
190. Kawasaki, T.; Marumo, T.; Shirakami, K.; Mori, T.; Doi, H.; Suzuki, M.; Watanabe, Y.; Chaki, S.; Nakazato, A.; Ago, Y. Increase of 20-HETE synthase after brain ischemia in rats revealed by pet study with (11)c-labeled 20-HETE synthase-specific inhibitor. *J. Cereb. Blood Flow Metab.* **2012**, *9*, 1737–1746. [CrossRef] [PubMed]
191. Poloyac, S.M.; Zhang, Y.; Bies, R.R.; Kochanek, P.M.; Graham, S.H. Protective effect of the 20-HETE inhibitor het0016 on brain damage after temporary focal ischemia. *J. Cereb. Blood Flow Metab.* **2006**, *26*, 1551–1561. [CrossRef] [PubMed]
192. Tanaka, Y.; Omura, T.; Fukasawa, M.; Horiuchi, N.; Miyata, N.; Minagawa, T.; Yoshida, S.; Nakaike, S. Continuous inhibition of 20-HETE synthesis by ts-011 improves neurological and functional outcomes after transient focal cerebral ischemia in rats. *Neurosci. Res.* **2007**, *59*, 475–480. [CrossRef] [PubMed]
193. Yang, Z.J.; Carter, E.L.; Kibler, K.K.; Kwansa, H.; Crafa, D.A.; Martin, L.J.; Roman, R.J.; Harder, D.R.; Koehler, R.C. Attenuation of neonatal ischemic brain damage using a 20-HETE synthesis inhibitor. *J. Neurochem.* **2012**, *121*, 168–179. [CrossRef] [PubMed]
194. Cambj-Sapunar, L.; Yu, M.; Harder, D.R.; Roman, R.J. Contribution of 5-hydroxytryptamine1b receptors and 20-hydroxyeiscosatetraenoic acid to fall in cerebral blood flow after subarachnoid hemorrhage. *Stroke* **2003**, *34*, 1269–1275. [CrossRef] [PubMed]

195. Takeuchi, K.; Miyata, N.; Renic, M.; Harder, D.R.; Roman, R.J. Hemoglobin, no, and 20-HETE interactions in mediating cerebral vasoconstriction following sah. *Am. J. Physiol. Regul. Integr. Comp. Physiol.* **2006**, *290*, 84–89. [CrossRef] [PubMed]

196. Crago, E.A.; Thampatty, B.P.; Sherwood, P.R.; Kuo, C.W.; Bender, C.; Balzer, J.; Horowitz, M.; Poloyac, S.M. Cerebrospinal fluid 20-HETE is associated with delayed cerebral ischemia and poor outcomes after aneurysmal subarachnoid hemorrhage. *Stroke* **2011**, *42*, 1872–1877. [CrossRef] [PubMed]

197. Deng, S.; Zhu, G.; Liu, F.; Zhang, H.; Qin, X.; Li, L.; Zhiyi, H. CYP4F2 gene V433M polymorphism is associated with ischemic stroke in the male northern chinese han population. *Prog. Neuropsychopharmacol. Biol. Psychiatry* **2010**, *34*, 664–668. [CrossRef] [PubMed]

198. Renic, M.; Klaus, J.A.; Omura, T.; Kawashima, N.; Onishi, M.; Miyata, N.; Koehler, R.C.; Harder, D.R.; Roman, R.J. Effect of 20-HETE inhibition on infarct volume and cerebral blood flow after transient middle cerebral artery occlusion. *J. Cereb. Blood Flow Metab.* **2009**, *29*, 629–639. [CrossRef] [PubMed]

199. Mu, Y.; Klamerus, M.M.; Miller, T.M.; Rohan, L.C.; Graham, S.H.; Poloyac, S.M. Intravenous formulation of n-hydroxy-n'-(4-n-butyl-2-methylphenyl)formamidine (het0016) for inhibition of rat brain 20-hydroxyeicosatetraenoic acid formation. *Drug Metab. Dispos.* **2008**, *36*, 2324–2330. [CrossRef] [PubMed]

200. Liu, Y.; Wang, D.; Wang, H.; Qu, Y.; Xiao, X.; Zhu, Y. The protective effect of HET0016 on brain edema and blood-brain barrier dysfunction after cerebral ischemia/reperfusion. *Brain Res* **2014**, *1544*, 45–53. [CrossRef] [PubMed]

201. Miyata, N.; Seki, T.; Tanaka, Y.; Omura, T.; Taniguchi, K.; Doi, M.; Bandou, K.; Kametani, S.; Sato, M.; Okuyama, S. Beneficial effects of a new 20-hydroxyeicosatetraenoic acid synthesis inhibitor, ts-011 [n-(3-chloro-4-morpholin-4-yl) phenyl-n'-hydroxyimido formamide], on hemorrhagic and ischemic stroke. *J. Pharmacol. Exp. Ther.* **2005**, *314*, 77–85. [CrossRef] [PubMed]

202. Omura, T.; Tanaka, Y.; Miyata, N.; Koizumi, C.; Sakurai, T.; Fukasawa, M.; Hachiuma, K.; Minagawa, T.; Susumu, T.; Yoshida, S.; et al. Effect of a new inhibitor of the synthesis of 20-HETE on cerebral ischemia reperfusion injury. *Stroke* **2006**, *37*, 1307–1313. [CrossRef] [PubMed]

203. Goodman, A.I.; Choudhury, M.; da Silva, J.L.; Schwartzman, M.L.; Abraham, N.G. Overexpression of the heme oxygenase gene in renal cell carcinoma. *Proc. Soc. Exp. Biol. Med.* **1997**, *214*, 54–61. [CrossRef] [PubMed]

204. Alexanian, A.; Miller, B.; Roman, R.J.; Sorokin, A. 20-HETE-producing enzymes are up-regulated in human cancers. *Cancer Genomics Proteomics* **2012**, *9*, 163–169. [PubMed]

205. Chen, P.; Guo, M.; Wygle, D.; Edwards, P.A.; Falck, J.R.; Roman, R.J.; Scicli, A.G. Inhibitors of cytochrome P450 4a suppress angiogenic responses. *Am. J. Pathol.* **2005**, *166*, 615–624. [CrossRef]

206. Yu, W.; Chen, L.; Yang, Y.Q.; Falck, J.R.; Guo, A.M.; Li, Y.; Yang, J. Cytochrome P450 ω-hydroxylase promotes angiogenesis and metastasis by upregulation of vegf and mmp-9 in non-small cell lung cancer. *Cancer Chemother. Pharmacol.* **2011**, *68*, 619–629. [CrossRef] [PubMed]

207. Alexanian, A.; Rufanova, V.A.; Miller, B.; Flasch, A.; Roman, R.J.; Sorokin, A. Down-regulation of 20-HETE synthesis and signaling inhibits renal adenocarcinoma cell proliferation and tumor growth. *Anticancer Res.* **2009**, *29*, 3819–3824. [PubMed]

208. Akbulut, T.; Regner, K.R.; Roman, R.J.; Avner, E.D.; Falck, J.R.; Park, F. 20-HETE activates the RAF/MEK/ERK pathway in renal epithelial cells through an EGFR- and C-SRC-dependent mechanism. *Am. J. Physiol. Renal Physiol.* **2009**, *297*, 662–670. [CrossRef] [PubMed]

209. Lin, F.; Rios, A.; Falck, J.R.; Belosludtsev, Y.; Schwartzman, M.L. 20-Hydroxyeicosatetraenoic acid is formed in response to EGF and is a mitogen in rat proximal tubule. *Am. J. Physiol.* **1995**, *269*, 806–816.

210. Chen, J.K.; Falck, J.R.; Reddy, K.M.; Capdevila, J.; Harris, R.C. Epoxyeicosatrienoic acids and their sulfonimide derivatives stimulate tyrosine phosphorylation and induce mitogenesis in renal epithelial cells. *J. Biol. Chem.* **1998**, *273*, 29254–29261. [CrossRef] [PubMed]

211. Nithipatikom, K.; Isbell, M.A.; See, W.A.; Campbell, W.B. Elevated 12- and 20-hydroxyeicosatetraenoic acid in urine of patients with prostatic diseases. *Cancer Lett.* **2006**, *233*, 219–225. [CrossRef] [PubMed]

212. Vanella, L.; Di Giacomo, C.; Acquaviva, R.; Barbagallo, I.; Li Volti, G.; Cardile, V.; Abraham, N.G.; Sorrenti, V. Effects of ellagic acid on angiogenic factors in prostate cancer cells. *Cancers* **2013**, *5*, 726–738. [CrossRef] [PubMed]

213. Yu, W.; Chai, H.; Li, Y.; Zhao, H.; Xie, X.; Zheng, H.; Wang, C.; Wang, X.; Yang, G.; Cai, X.; et al. Increased expression of CYP4Z1 promotes tumor angiogenesis and growth in human breast cancer. *Toxicol. Appl. Pharmacol.* **2012**. [CrossRef] [PubMed]

214. Borin, T.F.; Zuccari, D.A.; Jardim-Perassi, B.V.; Ferreira, L.C.; Iskander, A.S.; Varma, N.R.; Shankar, A.; Guo, A.M.; Scicli, G.; Arbab, A.S. Het0016, a selective inhibitor of 20-HETE synthesis, decreases pro-angiogenic factors and inhibits growth of triple negative breast cancer in mice. *PLoS ONE* **2014**, *9*, 116247. [CrossRef] [PubMed]

215. Guo, A.M.; Sheng, J.; Scicli, G.M.; Arbab, A.S.; Lehman, N.L.; Edwards, P.A.; Falck, J.R.; Roman, R.J.; Scicli, A.G. Expression of CYP4A1 in U251 human glioma cell induces hyperproliferative phenotype in vitro and rapidly growing tumors in vivo. *J. Pharmacol. Exp. Ther.* **2008**, *327*, 10–19. [CrossRef] [PubMed]

216. Guo, M.; Roman, R.J.; Falck, J.R.; Edwards, P.A.; Scicli, A.G. Human u251 glioma cell proliferation is suppressed by het0016 [*n*-hydroxy-*n'*-(4-butyl-2-methylphenyl)formamidine], a selective inhibitor of CYP4A. *J. Pharmacol. Exp. Ther.* **2005**, *315*, 526–533. [CrossRef] [PubMed]

217. Guo, M.; Roman, R.J.; Fenstermacher, J.D.; Brown, S.L.; Falck, J.R.; Arbab, A.S.; Edwards, P.A.; Scicli, A.G. 9l gliosarcoma cell proliferation and tumor growth in rats are suppressed by *n*-hydroxy-*n'*-(4-butyl-2-methylphenol) formamidine (het0016), a selective inhibitor of CYP4A. *J. Pharmacol. Exp. Ther.* **2006**, *317*, 97–108. [CrossRef] [PubMed]

218. Shankar, A.; Borin, T.F.; Iskander, A.; Varma, N.R.; Achyut, B.R.; Jain, M.; Mikkelsen, T.; Guo, A.M.; Chwang, W.B.; Ewing, J.R. Combination of vatalanib and a 20-HETE synthesis inhibitor results in decreased tumor growth in an animal model of human glioma. *OncoTarget Ther.* **2016**, *9*, 1205–1219.

219. Zhao, H.; Li, Y.; Wang, Y.; Zhang, J.; Ouyang, X.; Peng, R.; Yang, J. Antitumor and immunostimulatory activity of a polysaccharide-protein complex from scolopendra subspinipes mutilans l: Koch in tumor-bearing mice. *Food Chem. Toxicol.* **2012**, *50*, 2648–2655. [CrossRef] [PubMed]

220. Theken, K.N.; Deng, Y.; Schuck, R.N.; Oni-Orisan, A.; Miller, T.M.; Kannon, M.A.; Poloyac, S.M.; Lee, C.R. Enalapril reverses high-fat diet-induced alterations in cytochrome P450-mediated eicosanoid metabolism. *Am. J. Physiol. Endocrinol. Metab.* **2012**, *302*, 500–509. [CrossRef] [PubMed]

221. Joseph, G.; Soler, A.; Hutcheson, R.; Hunter, I.; Bradford, C.; Hutcheson, B.; Gotlinger, K.H.; Jiang, H.; Falck, J.R.; Proctor, S.; et al. Elevated 20-HETE impairs coronary collateral growth in metabolic syndrome via endothelial dysfunction. *Am. J. Physiol. Heart Circ. Physiol.* **2016**. ajpheart 00561. [CrossRef] [PubMed]

222. Kim, D.H.; Puri, N.; Sodhi, K.; Falck, J.R.; Abraham, N.G.; Shapiro, J.; Schwartzman, M.L. Cyclooxygenase-2 dependent metabolism of 20-HETE increases adiposity and adipocyte enlargement in mesenchymal stem cell-derived adipocytes. *J. Lipid Res.* **2013**, *54*, 786–793. [CrossRef] [PubMed]

223. Yousif, M.H.; Benter, I.F.; Dunn, K.M.; Dahly-Vernon, A.J.; Akhtar, S.; Roman, R.J. Role of 20-hydroxyeicosatetraenoic acid in altering vascular reactivity in diabetes. *Auton. Autacoid Pharmacol.* **2009**, *29*, 1–12. [CrossRef] [PubMed]

224. Wang, Z.; Yadav, A.S.; Leskova, W.; Harris, N.R. Inhibition of 20-HETE attenuates diabetes-induced decreases in retinal hemodynamics. *Exp. Eye Res.* **2011**, *93*, 108–113. [CrossRef] [PubMed]

225. Eid, S.; Abou-Kheir, W.; Sabra, R.; Daoud, G.; Jaffa, A.; Ziyadeh, F.N.; Roman, L.; Eid, A.A. Involvement of renal cytochromes P450 and arachidonic acid metabolites in diabetic nephropathy. *J. Biol. Regul. Homeost. Agents* **2013**, *27*, 693–703. [CrossRef] [PubMed]

226. Chen, Y.J.; Li, J.; Quilley, J. Deficient renal 20-HETE release in the diabetic rat is not the result of oxidative stress. *Am. J. Physiol. Heart Circ. Physiol.* **2008**, *294*, 2305–2312. [CrossRef] [PubMed]

227. Tse, M.M.; Aboutabl, M.E.; Althurwi, H.N.; Elshenawy, O.H.; Abdelhamid, G.; El-Kadi, A.O. Cytochrome P450 epoxygenase metabolite, 14,15-eet, protects against isoproterenol-induced cellular hypertrophy in h9c2 rat cell line. *Vascul. Pharmacol.* **2013**, *5*, 363–373. [CrossRef] [PubMed]

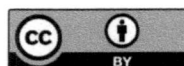

pharmaceutics

MDPI

Review

Revisiting the Latency of Uridine Diphosphate-Glucuronosyltransferases (UGTs)—How Does the Endoplasmic Reticulum Membrane Influence Their Function?

Yuejian Liu and Michael W. H. Coughtrie *

Faculty of Pharmaceutical Sciences, The University of British Columbia, Vancouver, BC V6T 1Z3, Canada; yuejian.liu@alumni.ubc.ca
* Correspondence: michael.coughtrie@ubc.ca; Tel.: +1-604-822-2343

Received: 7 August 2017; Accepted: 28 August 2017; Published: 30 August 2017

Abstract: Uridine diphosphate-glucuronosyltransferases (UGTs) are phase 2 conjugation enzymes mainly located in the endoplasmic reticulum (ER) of the liver and many other tissues, and can be recovered in artificial ER membrane preparations (microsomes). They catalyze glucuronidation reactions in various aglycone substrates, contributing significantly to the body's chemical defense mechanism. There has been controversy over the last 50 years in the UGT field with respect to the explanation for the phenomenon of latency: full UGT activity revealed by chemical or physical disruption of the microsomal membrane. Because latency can lead to inaccurate measurements of UGT activity in vitro, and subsequent underprediction of drug clearance in vivo, it is important to understand the mechanisms behind this phenomenon. Three major hypotheses have been advanced to explain UGT latency: compartmentation, conformation, and adenine nucleotide inhibition. In this review, we discuss the evidence behind each hypothesis in depth, and suggest some additional studies that may reveal more information on this intriguing phenomenon.

Keywords: UDP-glucuronosyltransferase; latency; microsomes; glucuronidation; regulation

1. Introduction

Uridine diphosphate-glucuronosyltransferases (UGTs) comprise a superfamily of phase 2 conjugation enzymes that catalyze the glucuronidation of numerous substrates at functional groups such as –OH, –COOH, –NH$_2$, –SH, and C–C [1]. They are arguably the most important conjugation enzymes facilitating the excretion of various endobiotics such as bilirubin, steroid and thyroid hormones, bile acids, and retinoids, as well as xenobiotics including environmental chemicals, pollutants, and drugs [2]. These substrates are mostly hydrophobic and are conjugated by the UGTs with the glucuronic acid moiety derived from the co-substrate, uridine diphosphate-glucuronic acid (UDPGA). The resulting glucuronide conjugates that are generally more polar and water-soluble are substrates for numerous membrane transporters and thus they can eventually be excreted out of the body in bile and urine (Figure 1).

UGTs are type-I transmembrane glycoproteins mainly located within the smooth endoplasmic reticulum (ER), although some isoforms can be found in the nuclear envelope [3,4]. UGTs demonstrate protein–protein interactions within the superfamily (homo- and hetero-dimers and possibly higher order structures) or with other enzymes such as the cytochromes P450 [5–12], as demonstrated by studies using co-immunoprecipitation, fluorescence microscopy, and Förster resonance energy transfer (FRET), among many other approaches (as summarized in [6]). The interactions have been shown to alter kinetic properties of UGTs [7,9,10].

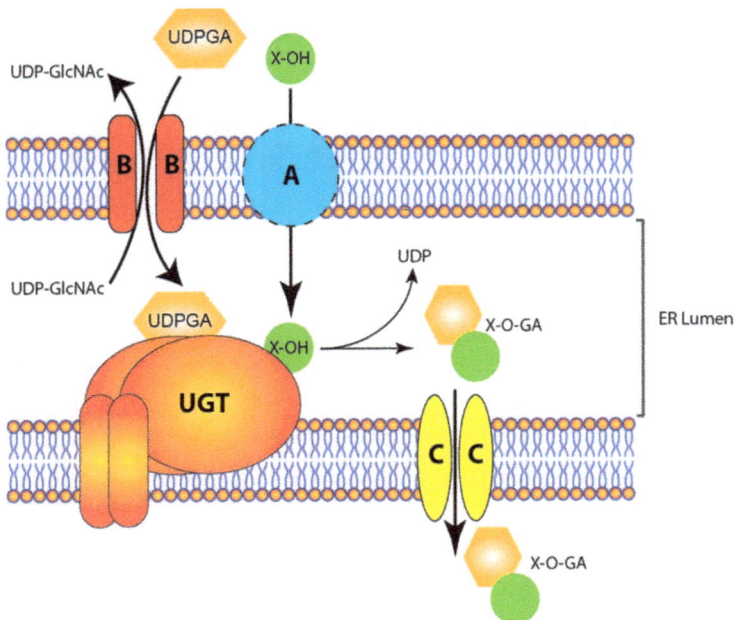

Figure 1. The glucuronidation system in the endoplasmic reticulum. Substrates (X-OH) enter the lumen by diffusion (A), and UDPGA is transported via the UDPGA/UDP-GlcNAc antiporter (UGTrel7, B). Following the conjugation reaction, the glucuronide products (X-O-GA) are removed from the lumen by glucuronide transporter(s) (C). UDPGA: Uridine diphosphate-glucuronic acid; UDP-GLcNAc: UDP-*N*-acetylglucosamine.

Detoxification is divided into two phases [13]. The basic principle is that oxidative metabolism by phase 1 enzymes (such as cytochromes P450, CYP) results in the addition or revealing of a functional group (e.g., –OH, –COOH or –NH$_2$) such that the compounds can be conjugated by phase 2 enzymes such as the UGTs. This necessitates the phase 1 metabolites crossing the ER membrane in order to access the UGT active site. Evidence suggests a functional interaction between the UGT and CYP proteins to facilitate the multistep detoxification process [5,12,14,15].

Besides detoxification, glucuronidation can activate substrates such as certain procarcinogens, as well as morphine that can be converted to morphine 3- and 6-glucuronides, where the latter is a more potent analgesic than the parent drug [16]. Glucuronidation also produces toxic metabolites such as steroid D-ring glucuronides that may be responsible for intrahepatic cholestasis of pregnancy [17]. The human UGT superfamily is divided into five subfamilies: UGT1A, 2A, 2B, 3A, and 8. They are mainly expressed in liver, but are also prevalent in extrahepatic tissues including gastrointestinal tract, kidney, lung, brain, and reproductive tissues [1,18]. The human UGT1A isoforms are generated from a single gene located at chromosome 2q37.1 through alternative splicing. Specifically, there are 13 first exons, including 4 pseudogenes, each of which is controlled by an individual promoter (1A1, 1A2p, 1A3, 1A4, 1A5, 1A6, 1A7, 1A9, 1A13p, 1A10, 1A8, 1A11p, and 1A12p). These 13 exon/promoter pairs are upstream of a second region that consists of 5 common exons under the regulation of a single promoter (exons 2, 3, 4, 5a, and 5b). The mRNA for each UGT1A isoform is generated by splicing one of the first exons with the group of common exons. This mechanism of alternative splicing is conserved in human, mouse, and rat UGTs [19].

2. UGTs and Latency

The majority of the UGT enzyme protein, including its catalytic site, is believed to reside inside the ER lumen (and partially associate with the ER membrane); thus there are physical and physiological barriers to substrates accessing the active site of the enzymes within the ER lumen, as well as to the egress of reaction products from the ER and, subsequently, from the cell. This leads to the phenomenon of latency of UGT activity in preparations of ER (i.e., microsomes). The phenomenon of latency derives from experimental observations that in isolated microsomal preparations, UGTs generally show increased activities after the membranes are physically or chemically disrupted [20–28]. Other enzymes present in the lumen of the ER, such as glucose-6-phosphatase, also display latency [29]. Although the latency of UGTs has been known for more than half a century, the exact mechanism(s) underlying it remain incompletely understood, and this has generated several hypotheses and much heated debate during this time. The phenomenon of latency is an important factor in the consistent underprediction of drug clearance in vivo based on in vitro measurement of UGT activity [30], since it is of particular importance to be able to accurately measure UGT activity in microsomal preparations. Examples of treatments that disrupt microsomal membranes and reveal UGT latency (to different extents) include grinding in sand, sonication, high hydrostatic pressure, detergents, phospholipase A or C, staphylococcal α-toxin, or the pore-forming antibiotic alamethicin [22,23,28,31–39]. It has been postulated that these agents, or physical stressors, act in different ways, for example by allowing unlimited access of substrate and co-substrate to the enzyme's catalytic site; by inducing an alteration in the conformation of the enzyme; by releasing UGT inhibitors from the microsomal lumen; or a combination of these mechanisms which of course are all dependent to some extent on the ER membrane.

Three major hypotheses have been developed over the years to explain latency: compartmentation, conformation, and adenine-nucleotide inhibition. The first two hypotheses mainly address whether the ER membrane limits UGT activity by acting as a barrier blocking access of UDPGA (and potentially aglycone substrate) to the luminal space and thus the UGT active site, or by regulating the conformation of the UGT protein through lipid–protein (or potentially protein–protein) interactions. The last hypothesis was the most recently proposed, based on the inhibitory effects of adenine-containing nucleotides on the UGTs. Under this hypothesis, the membranes might limit UGT activity by sequestering these natural inhibitors in the lumen.

The latency phenomenon makes accurate measurement of UGT activity in microsomal preparations challenging, however it is one of the most important factors to take into consideration in the design of UGT enzyme assays. Different methods of preparation of the microsomal fraction can have major impact on measurable latency, since the level of intactness of the membrane preparation clearly influences the enzyme activity. For example, it has been shown that preparation of microsomal fractions from freshly isolated liver is significantly preferable over frozen tissue, which tends to produce microsomal fractions with much lower levels of intactness [40]. Similarly, microsomes prepared from rat lung tissue exhibited far lower latency levels than those from rat liver, although this may derive from the harsher treatment required to homogenize rat lung tissue [41]. The nature of the disrupting agent also has an impact on the latency—for example some detergents appear to be much harsher than others, resulting in inhibition of UGT activity. In our experience, Lubrol PX has been the most effective detergent for the disruption of the microsomal membrane, and for the solubilization of the UGT protein from the microsomal membrane for purification (e.g., [41,42]). It is generally accepted that the pore-forming antibiotic alamethicin is the membrane disruptor of choice for UGT assays since the UGT enzymes seem less sensitive to variations in its concentration than they are to various detergents [34]. Where liver microsomal preparations are used to generate glucuronide metabolites at a semi-preparative scale, for example for metabolite identification, the issue of latency is also important. For instance, long incubations in the presence of detergents could result in inhibition of the UGT activity, so careful choice of membrane perturbation method would be of particular importance.

Here we review the major hypotheses that have been proposed to explain the phenomenon of latency as it applies to UGTs, and discuss future studies that might be needed to gain a greater understanding of its origins and implications.

3. Compartmentation Hypothesis

This hypothesis is based on the assumption that the highly hydrophilic co-substrate for the glucuronidation reaction, UDPGA, (and possibly certain aglycone substrates) is not able to diffuse across the ER membrane, and therefore that disruption of the membrane integrity is required to reveal the full extent of in vitro UGT activity in microsomal preparations. The discovery of transporters for nucleotide sugars, including UDPGA, has provided very strong evidence in support of this hypothesis.

The barrier function of microsomal membranes was proposed by Winsnes in 1972 [38] and was later elaborated by Berry and Hallinan, who firstly proposed the compartmentation model to explain latency based on previous experimental results [43]. In this model, UGT located on the luminal side of the ER is partially embedded in the membrane, together with a transmembrane UDPGA permease and a lumenal nucleoside diphosphatase (NDPase). This model predicts that UDPGA needs to be transported by the permease into the microsomal lumen where UGT catalyzes glucuronidation reactions, then the NDPase hydrolyzes UDP, a co-product besides the glucuronide conjugate, to facilitate the forward reaction since UDP is an inhibitor of UGTs. Later evidence strongly supports this model, including the prediction of UGT topology and the discovery of UDPGA transporters.

The identification of complete cDNA sequences improved the understanding of many aspects of UGTs such as the ER targeting process and topology [1]. Initial reports on the sequences came from Jackson et al. and Mackenzie et al. for rat liver UGTs [44,45], and allowed researchers to synthesize UGT proteins for studies on post-translational modifications [1,46,47]. In general, UGTs are synthesized as precursors of approximately 530 amino acid residues, and are targeted to the ER by an N-terminal signal sequence. A C-terminal di-lysine motif has been found in several human UGT sequences, and could act as an ER retention signal [48]. Following membrane integration, the N-terminal signal peptide is cleaved and the enzyme is N-glycosylated in the ER lumen. Notably, other internal topological elements within the UGTs might be required to regulate the integration process, as demonstrated for UGT1A6 [49,50]. In this way, the UGTs become mature ER enzymes of just over 500 residues [1]. Although significant portions of the protein may associate with the membrane, approximately 95% of the polypeptide chain is predicted to be luminal, and is connected to the cytosolic C-terminal tail through a 17-residue alpha helix that spans the lipid bilayer.

Although the intimate association between UGT protein and the ER membrane has so far prevented the generation of a complete crystal structure, the predicted topology of UGTs has been well developed. Vanstapel and Blanckaert predicted the catalytic site of bilirubin UGT faces ER lumen [51], which was followed by the development of a more complete topology model by Shepherd et al. [52]. This model was proposed based on the evidence from the authors' own results indicating that the majority of bilirubin UGT (UGT1A1) was not exposed to the cytosol, hydropathy plot analysis [53], and complete cDNA sequences of androsterone UGT [54,55], and rat phenol UGT (UGT1A6) [56]. Site-directed mutagenesis experiments have also confirmed that the UGT proteins are comprised of two domains, one binding the UDPGA (in the conserved C-terminal part of the protein) and one that presumably confers substrate preference located in the less-well conserved N-terminal region [57]. The determination of an X-ray crystal structure (1.8-Å resolution) for the C-terminal domain of human UGT2B7 is another strong piece of evidence confirming the presence of a nucleotide-binding site in the C-terminal half of the UGT proteins [58]. Above all, the sequence information together with recombinant DNA technology have allowed the development of a topology model that is generally accepted today (Figure 1). Compared to the topology proposed by Shepherd et al. [52], the most significant advances include the more specific locations of substrate and co-substrate binding sites, and the presence of transporters for UDPGA and glucuronides. If the binding sites are luminal as predicted, then the rate of glucuronidation might be constrained by the membrane barrier limiting the access of UDPGA, a highly charged molecule synthesized in the cytoplasmic space [59], to the reaction center. Although the complete crystal structure of a UGT protein is unsolved, homology modeling has been used to predict the three-dimensional structure [57]. For example, human UGT1A1 and UGT1A10 were homology-modeled using plant UGT71G1 and UDP-galactose 4-epimerase from *Escherichia coli*, respectively [60,61].

In addition, a transporter (or transporters) might be needed to facilitate the efflux of polar glucuronides out of the ER; this transporting activity has been biochemically demonstrated with a rate comparable to the rate of glucuronide synthesis [62]. Interestingly, the authors suggested that glucuronide efflux could be another rate-limiting step besides UDPGA import, because the rate of glucuronidation is highly variable among intact microsomes and it is unlikely that transport of UDPGA, the universal co-substrate for all glucuronidation reactions, is responsible for all of the variation observed. The identity of glucuronide efflux transporter(s) is still unknown and in contrast to this, UDPGA transporters have been intensively studied and identified, as described below. The role of UDP-*N*-acetylglucosamine (UDP-GlcNAc) has been key to advancing the compartmentation hypothesis.

It is well known that UDP-GlcNAc can activate UGT activity in microsomal preparations in the presence of UDPGA, having been first demonstrated by Pogell and Leloir, who suggested the effect was partly due to inhibition of the breakdown of UDPGA [24]. Later work suggested that UDP-GlcNAc acted as an allosteric effector of UGT [63]. However, it was Berry and Hallinan who proposed the existence of a "UDPGA permease" [43], following on from the suggestion made by Winsnes that UDP-GlcNAc might increase the permeability of the microsomal membrane to UDPGA, thus activating the enzyme [38]. UDP-GlcNAc stimulated UGT activities only when UDPGA was added to preparations of intact microsomes, but not when it was generated in situ by trans-glucuronidation or reverse glucuronidation reactions [64,65], which indicates the stimulation effect of UDP-GlcNAc occurs at the step of UDPGA transport into microsomes. The integrity of microsomal membranes needs to be maintained for UDP-GlcNAc stimulation of UGT activity, because UDP-GlcNAc no longer activated UGTs when microsomal membranes were disrupted by Triton X-100 treatment, sonication, or Lubrol PX treatment [28,31,41]. Interestingly, UGT activity in rat lung microsomes (with 1-naphthol as substrate) was insensitive to UDP-GlcNAc stimulation, unlike in rat liver microsomes [41], although this may be due to excessive mechanical disruption of the membranes during homogenization resulting from the nature of the lung tissue. Taken together, this evidence suggested that UDP-GlcNAc activates UGTs through an indirect mechanism that requires an intact microsomal membrane, presumably by enhancing the transport and access of UDPGA to the catalytic site. Evidence supporting this presumption includes the observation that glucuronidation rate was increased by UDP-GlcNAc when the concentration of UDPGA was high or saturating [24]. Additionally, Berry and Hallinan demonstrated that UDP, UTP, and UDP-glucose showed inhibitory effects on UGT activities only after microsomal membranes were disrupted [43], whereas native UGTs were resistant to the inhibitors, suggesting that these compounds are not transported by the presumptive UDPGA permease [63,66]. Therefore, it was concluded that the presumptive permease has a regulatory role in UGT activities by selectively transporting UDPGA.

Further evidence came from the observations that addition of *N*-ethylmaleimide (NEM) blocked the activation effect of UDP-GlcNAc on native UGT activity within intact microsomes, without a direct inhibition on the enzyme's catalytic site [67]. This piece of evidence suggested the presence of membrane permease-containing thiol groups that are required for the action of UDP-GlcNAc. Indeed, later studies showed that NEM inhibited UDPGA transport into the ER of permeabilized rat hepatocytes, which in turn inhibited glucuronidation of 4-methylumbelliferone (4-MU), a non-selective substrate metabolized by many UGT isoforms [68,69]. However, when microsomal and ER membranes were permeabilized, glucuronidation was not affected by NEM treatment [69].

The discovery of UDPGA transporters was preceded by studies recognizing a carrier-mediated, UDPGA transport activity at the rat liver ER membrane [68–71]. The common question raised by these studies was as to how important UDPGA transport could be to glucuronidation reactions. Bossuyt and Blanckaert carried out a series of studies characterizing the transport activities of UDPGA and UDP-GlcNAc across microsomal membranes [68,72], and were able to connect the two transport systems when UDPGA uptake into the microsomes preloaded with UDP-GlcNAc showed an overshoot effect [69]. Hence, UDP-GlcNAc might be exported by a bidirectional carrier to trans-stimulate the import of UDPGA for UGT catalysis. It turned out that UDPGA transport was both required and necessary for glucuronidation, because the inhibition or stimulation of UDPGA transport by NEM or UDP-GlcNAc, as partly mentioned above, inhibited or stimulated glucuronidation respectively towards 4-MU in microsomes and permeabilized hepatocytes [73]. Indeed, UDPGA transport seemed to be the rate-limiting step of glucuronidation reactions, which formed the basis of the compartmentation hypothesis in that the release of the transport constraint would significantly increase the glucuronidation rate.

A number of nucleotide sugar transporters (NSTs) have now been cloned, expressed and functionally characterized. UDP-galactose transporter-related protein 7 (UGTrel7), a human NST, was shown to transport both UDPGA and UDP-*N*-acetylgalactosamine (UDP-GalNAc) into microsomal vesicles when expressed in *Saccharomyces cerevisiae* [74]. Kobayashi et al. molecularly and functionally characterized four human NSTs, namely UGTrel1, UGTrel7, huYEA4, and huYEA4S, the last two being newly identified human NSTs that are splice variants of each other [75]. These transporters all mediated UDP-GlcNAc-dependent UDPGA uptake into the microsomes isolated from recombinant V79 cells expressing the NST cDNAs, although UGTrel7 was by far the most efficient. These authors also demonstrated that UGTs themselves, at least UGT1 family members, were not significantly involved in the transport of UDPGA. Muraoka et al. subsequently confirmed that UGTrel7 (expressed in *S. cerevisiae*) transported UDPGA in a manner that was much enhanced by UDP-GlcNAc and showed that UGTrel7 was a UDPGA/UDP-GlcNAc antiporter [76]. Therefore, after more than 50 years since the discovery that UDPGA was the co-substrate and glucuronic acid donor for UGTs [77,78], these two papers provided the most direct evidence of how the highly charged co-substrate is delivered to the UGTs in the microsomal lumen, and how UDP-GlcNAc enhances this process. The rapid advance in gene editing technology, such as the CRISPR/Cas9 system, provides an alternate approach to investigating the role of UDPGA transporters in the latency of UGTs. It should be possible, for example, to delete a UDPGA transporter such as UGTrel7 in a cell line (or embryonically in an animal model) to determine the contribution of individual NSTs to UGT latency.

UDPGA transport is a complex process, and probably involves other transport molecules, as described by Rowland et al. who demonstrated that UDPGA uptake into human liver microsomes involves more than one transporter [79]. Other NSTs capable of transporting UDPGA at ER membrane have been identified. For instance, Selva et al. and Goto et al. identified the gene fringe connection (*frc*) that encodes an NST transporting UDPGA, UDP-GlcNAc, and UDP-xylose from the cytoplasm to the lumen of ER/Golgi in *Drosophila* [80,81]. Interestingly, this transporter is important in growth-factor signaling pathways including Wnt/Wingless-, Hedgehog-, fibroblast growth factor-, and Notch-dependent pathways, by transporting UDP-sugars into the Golgi to facilitate the synthesis of heparan sulfate proteoglycan and the glycosylation and maturation of Notch receptor. Lastly, Suda et al. identified the gene *hfrc 1* homologous to *frc* (*Drosophila melanogaster*), *sqv-7* (*Caenorhabditis elegans*), and *UGTrel7* (human) [82]. It encodes an NST that is located at the Golgi and transports UDP-GlcNAc, UDP-glucose, and UDP-mannose.

4. Conformation Hypothesis

The concept that the conformation of the UGT enzyme protein is subject to influence by the hydrophobic lipid environment in the ER membrane, and it is this that controls the activity of enzymes, is the underlying basis of the conformation hypothesis. In contrast to the compartmentation hypothesis, the conformation hypothesis explains latency by assuming that the catalytic site of UGTs is accessible by substrates and UDPGA and the membrane disruption induces the formation of different kinetic forms of the enzyme with increased activity [39].

According to Vessey and Zakim, treatments altering the lipid portion of bovine liver microsomes increased UGT activity at V_{max} towards *p*-nitrophenol, including the addition of phospholipase A or Triton X-100, and sonication [37]. These treatments can alter the lipid composition as well as the integrity of the microsomal membrane. For instance, phospholipase A produces lysophospholipids that can act as detergents when present at high concentrations within the membrane. Therefore, the increase in V_{max} of UGTs could be due to a change in the protein–lipid interaction or greater access of substrates to the catalytic site after the membrane integrity had been lost, or a combination of both. Because Triton treatment only sped up the forward reaction which is the glucuronidation reaction catalyzed by UGTs [37], the activation effect was restricted to the UGTs (not other microsomal components) when the luminal space was fully accessible. Besides, phospholipase A treatment has been shown to alter the binding specificity for UDPGA, allowing for the competitive binding from other UDP-sugars to the UGTs [63,83]. Hence, phospholipase A seems to induce a change in the conformation of the co-substrate binding site that can fit the structures of other UDP-sugars. Overall, these experiments suggested that the effect of membrane perturbants is mainly the alteration of lipid composition which directly affects the enzyme itself, as Zakim and Dannenberg argued [39]. They concluded that the enzyme might exist in different functional states demonstrating different kinetic properties, and the lipid environment controls the enzyme activity by intimately regulating its conformation.

The interaction between substrate and co-substrate binding sites within a single UGT protein was another piece of evidence used to support the existence of multiple conformational forms [84,85]. Vessey and Zakim proposed that *p*-nitrophenol UGTs follow a random order kinetic mechanism after they carried out product inhibition and isotope exchange studies, and so the enzymes can firstly bind substrate or co-substrate and form rapid equilibrium [85]. Interestingly, under high concentrations of *p*-nitrophenol, UGTs showed increased values of V_{max} and $K_{m\ UDPGA}$, which suggested that occupation of the substrate binding site decreased the binding affinity for the co-substrate. The interaction between substrate and co-substrate binding sites was further investigated by Hochman and Zakim who used an enzyme reconstitution system where a delipidated form of purified UGT, called GT_{2p}, was reconstituted into different species of phospholipids to study their influence on the enzyme properties [84]. GT_{2p} represented the second peak of eluted UGT after a hydroxylapatite column purification from pig liver microsomes, and showed a single band of protein following sodium dodecyl sulfate—polyacrylamide (7.5%) gel electrophoresis (SDS-PAGE) [86]. It was shown that the nature of phospholipids used to reconstitute GT_{2p} activity affected the extent to which substrate binding decreased the binding affinity of the co-substrate. In parallel with this result, the α-glucuronidase activity of GT_{2p} was differentially affected by the binding of structural variants of aromatic ethers that only occupy the substrate binding site without being conjugated. Therefore, the binding of a substrate seems to induce a conformational change in the enzyme that possesses an altered co-substrate binding affinity, which is dependent on the surrounding lipid environment.

Further experiments suggested that the physical properties, rather than the chemical structures, of phospholipids surrounding UGTs seemed to play a role in the interaction with the enzymes and regulation of their kinetic patterns. For example, when GT_{2p} was reconstituted into bilayers of 1,2-dimyristoylphosphatidylcholine or 1,2-dipalmitoylphosphatidylcholine lipids in the gel phase, the enzyme displayed non-Michaelis–Menten kinetics, however when the lipids were heated to liquid–crystal phase, the enzyme(s) displayed Michaelis–Menten kinetics [87,88]. The change in enzyme kinetics was solely due to the phase transition of phospholipids independent from a direct effect of increasing temperature. Furthermore, the GT_{2p} demonstrating non-Michaelis–Menten kinetics had two different binding sites for UDPGA per molecule of enzyme, and the appearance of Michaelis–Menten kinetics after phase transition occurred was in parallel with the disappearance of one binding site [87]. These results could be explained by the conformational hypothesis in that the physical state of the phospholipids seems to determine the number of functional binding sites for UDPGA by changing enzyme conformation, although it is possible that the change in membrane fluidity promotes the association/disassembly of UGT monomers by modulating protein–protein interactions. The length and degree of saturation of phospholipid acyl chains are important for regulating membrane fluidity, and have been shown to affect the activity of UGTs [89]. For instance, for the purified pig liver GT_{1p}, the first eluted fraction from a hydroxylapatite column as described by Hochman and Zakim [90], the lysophosphatidylcholine species that had longer acyl chains with more unsaturated bonds led to greater activation at V_{max}. This result further suggested that the interaction between UGTs and phospholipids does not depend on the specific chemical structures of phospholipids. Rather, as Rotenberg and Zakim suggested, the interaction occurs through a non-specific mechanism depending on the physical state of phospholipids [91].

The experiments described above repeatedly emphasize the role of the lipid environment in the regulation of UGT conformation. The change in conformation can in turn alter the rate of glucuronidation presumably by changing the catalytic mechanism, as demonstrated for GT_{2p} reconstituted into different species of lysophosphatidylcholine [86,92]. Specifically, changing the lipids used to reconstitute GT_{2p} from oleoyl lysophosphatidylcholine to stearoyl lysophosphatidylcholine led to changes in the rate of glucuronidation depending on the specific aglycone substrates: a 20-fold decline for *p*-nitrophenol, no change for 1-naphthol and phenol, and a 3-fold decline for *p*-bromophenol. Hence, the specific lipid environment has a selective effect on the glucuronidation rate towards different aglycones. Two mechanisms have been proposed as to how the lipid–protein interaction affects the catalytic rate of UGT (in this case, purified GT_{2p}). Firstly, phospholipids may regulate enzyme–substrate interactions and determine how much inherent binding energy to UDPGA can be shared for catalysis to enhance the reaction rate [92]. Only certain species of lysophosphatidylcholine could influence the enzyme in a way that more inherent binding energy is used for catalysis. Alternatively, phospholipids like oleoyl lysophosphatidylcholine speed up glucuronidation by facilitating the bond breaking between the C1 of glucuronic acid and UDP [86].

Besides kinetic properties and avidity for substrate binding, the lipid environment also regulates the thermal stability of UGTs [91]. Rotenberg and Zakim's data suggest that the GT_{2p} fraction of UGTs existed in three forms through conformational changes: the active form (E), inactive form (E′), and denatured form. The change between E and E′ is controlled by temperature and is reversible, whereas the denatured form is obtained by heating E′ to a certain extent. The specific temperatures required for the occurrence of these conformational changes are dependent on a specific lipid environment. In general, the reconstitution of pure, delipidated GT_{2p} into different species of phosphatidylcholine, such as distearoylphosphatidylcholine, dioleoylphosphatidylcholine, or 1-stearoyl-2-oleoylphosphatidylcholine, stabilized the E form with a greater change in the entropy of the whole system rather than the enthalpy, and slowed down denaturation rate of the E′ form. However, each of these phospholipids affected the thermal stability of GT_{2p} to a different extent depending on the nature of the acyl chains, so the increase in temperature might alter enzyme conformation through modulating the physical state of phospholipids. Using the reconstitution method, Hochman and Zakim showed that only gel-phase phospholipids could reconstitute the sensitivity of the purified GT_{2p} fraction to stimulation by UDP-GlcNAc, a physiological activator of UGTs [90]. Also, GT_{2p} seems to have a favorable interaction with viscous lipids [87]. These data suggest UGTs are restricted by certain forces within a subregion of the ER membrane where the lipids are gel-like, hence it is less likely that the enzymes randomly interact with the bulk phase of lipids within the ER membrane [87,90]. The forces could come from the interactions between UGTs and specific acyl chains in the lipid bilayer, or between different UGT isoforms that preferentially aggregate in the gel-like regions.

Alternatively, the gel-like regions might be formed by lipid rafts, membrane microdomains that are enriched in cholesterol, sphingolipids, and specific proteins such as glycosylphosphatidylinositol (GPI)-anchored proteins and Src-family kinases [93]. These microdomains could be formed by the phase segregation of membrane lipids [93], and/or by anchoring of the lipids to actin filaments [94].

More importantly, the rafts have various functions including endo-, exo-, and transcytosis, polarized intracellular trafficking of specific membrane proteins, and signal transduction [93,95,96]. They can transiently recruit membrane and intracellular proteins to initiate a cellular signaling event [97]. Since the intracellular transport of UGTs to the ER membrane is not fully understood, it is likely that UGTs functionally interact with lipid rafts for the purposes of intracellular transport, ER localization, and/or regulation of the enzyme stability and activity. In vitro and in vivo experiments have demonstrated the effect of cholesterol, a major component of lipid rafts, on the activity of UGTs [98,99]. Specifically, the addition of cholesterol to guinea pig liver microsomes increased UGT activity at V_{max}; diet supplementation that increased the membrane content of cholesterol in guinea pig liver ER showed similar results to that of the in vitro data. In both cases, the activity of UGTs was studied under the native membrane environment. Rotenberg and Zakim reconstituted delipidated GT_{2p} into different phospholipids to study the influence of the lipid environment on the observed cholesterol effect [100]. They showed that the modulation of UGT activity and stability by cholesterol was dependent on specific types of phospholipids surrounding the enzyme. For example, the addition of cholesterol to the bilayers of distearoylphosphatidylcholine decreased enzyme activity but increased stability of the enzyme against thermal denaturation, whereas cholesterol in the bilayers of dioleoylphosphatidylcholine showed little effect on the properties of the enzyme. In order to address the effects of lipid rafts on the activity and stability of UGTs, it is worthwhile to compare the effects of cholesterol in the contexts of raft associated lipids and phospholipids.

Because lipid rafts have been extensively studied with much evidence supporting their existence in living cells, technologies have been developed to monitor raft dynamics such as single molecule tracking together with advanced microscopic analyses [94,97]. These technologies allow researchers to precisely follow the dynamic interactions between raft lipids and raft-associated proteins despite the crowding environment within a cell, and so could be extended to UGTs to follow their interactions with microsomal lipids in real time. A possible experiment would be to use a recombinant system, such as human embryonic kidney 293 (HEK293) cells, where a UGT enzyme and a raft lipid can each be tagged with a Fab-conjugated fluorescent molecule. This would be followed by fluorescence microscopy that records the trajectories of the labeled molecules. The measurement on the time length of co-localization between the enzyme and raft lipid could indicate whether there is a significant interaction between them.

The challenges of using purified membrane protein preparations on the outcome of these experiments has been mentioned several times by Zakim's group [86,87,90]. Integral membrane proteins tend to associate with detergents and other membrane components after they have been isolated, and form mixed micelles with the detergents and phospholipids used to reconstitute the enzymes. Therefore, the properties displayed by the reconstituted GT_{2p} may be artificially affected by other components more than the phosphatidylcholine variants, and may not faithfully reveal UGT–phospholipid interactions. Also, the native structure and function of membrane proteins might be altered during purification before the enzymes are reconstituted into a new lipid environment. Lastly, if UGTs truly have a significant interaction with surrounding phospholipids in the ER membrane, then it is essential that the enzymes are reconstituted into a native lipid environment for functional studies [87]. The studies reported by Zakim and colleagues on the conformational change of UGTs, especially GT_{2p} reconstituted in phosphatidylcholine variants, were mainly carried out on pig liver microsomes, since the activity of *p*-nitrophenol UGTs was greater than that from cow liver microsomes and so was easier to measure [85]. It would be interesting to carry out these studies using liver from other species, particularly humans, to investigate if lipid–protein interaction is a universal mechanism in the regulation of UGT activity, and how much variation among different species that the influence of the lipid environment could have on the enzymes. Nevertheless, Vessey and Zakim observed latency among all the species examined: guinea pigs, mice, rats, cows, rabbits, and humans, using phospholipase A and the detergent *p*-chloromercuribenzoate as the membrane perturbants [101]. The extent of activation by the addition of either reagent varied among the species.

Additionally, most of the kinetic assays were carried out using the substrate *p*-nitrophenol which can be glucuronidated by more than one isoform such as UGT1A6 and 1A1 [102]. This means that the kinetic properties revealed by UGTs could reflect the action of one or multiple isomers. Since protein–protein interactions exist among UGT isoforms, then after altering the lipid phase by changing temperature, the measured kinetic data may not solely represent the regulation from lipid-protein interactions. Above all, the superfamily of UGTs contains many isoforms with overlapping substrate specificity, and these enzymes are widely distributed in the nature from coral and insects to mammals [1]. It is especially important to take these properties into consideration when measuring UGT activity.

It is true that the compartmentation hypothesis is more widely accepted in the field, however the studies by Zakim and colleagues, and others, provide a rich reservoir of data that do indicate that the regulation of UGT activity within the ER membrane environment is complex and may well involve multiple mechanisms.

5. Adenine Nucleotide Inhibition Effect

Recently, the inhibitory effects of adenine and adenine-containing nucleotides on UGT activities have been proposed as another explanation of latency [103–105]. The first report came from Hallinan et al. who demonstrated that activities of UGTs toward *p*-nitrophenol, estradiol, and estrone were suppressed by 4 mM ATP (adenosine triphosphate) in guinea pig liver microsomes [104,106]. Then, Nishimura et al. found that adenine, ATP, NAD^+ (nicotinamide adenine dinucleotide, oxidized), and $NADP^+$ (nicotinamide adenine dinucleotide phosphate, oxidized) inhibited the glucuronidation of 4-MU and estradiol by allosteric binding to UGTs at a site independent from the substrate and co-substrate binding sites, and proposed that membrane perturbations could lead to the release of these inhibitors and hence an increase in glucuronidation activities [105]. AMP (adenosine monophosphate) by itself barely inhibited UGTs, but decreased the potency of inhibitory nucleotides. It is likely that AMP antagonizes the inhibitory nucleotides by competing for the allosteric binding site, as suggested in a later publication [103]. When Nishimura et al. tested 4-MU UGT activity in rat liver microsomes, latency and inhibitory effects of ATP and $NADP^+$ were observed on the UGTs after Brij58 solubilization of the membranes, which suggests the allosteric binding site is luminal [105]. This evidence indirectly supports the compartmentation model since adenine nucleotides must pass the membrane barrier if the UGTs exhibit the native topology, except that the compartmentation model was originally rationalized upon the limited supply of UDPGA for glucuronidation reactions. Lastly, human UGT is also regulated by adenine nucleotides [105]. In microsomes isolated from human embryonic kidney 293 (HEK293) cells that express human UGT1A1, the glucuronidation activity towards estradiol was gradually inhibited by increasing concentrations of ATP, NAD^+, or $NADP^+$.

In 2012, Ishii et al. compared alamethicin- and Brij58-treated microsomes from rat and human livers, and showed the inhibitory potency of adenine nucleotides was lower in the alamethicin-disrupted microsomes [103]. The luminal concentration of ATP in rat liver ER can be as high as 30 μM which is similar to the IC_{50} value measured from Brij58-treated human liver microsomes (33.8 μM), but much lower than that from rat liver microsomes (66.8 μM). Therefore, under physiological conditions, the level of ATP in the ER lumen might be sufficient to suppress UGT activity. These authors also showed that Brij58 and alamethicin treatments could lead to the release of ATP from rat liver microsomes in vitro. Two structural components have been thought to be important for inhibitory nucleotides to bind the allosteric effector site of UGTs [104,105]. The first one is the adenine skeleton. This is because AMP decreased the inhibitory effects of ATP, adenine, NAD^+, and $NADP^+$, and so was thought to compete with the other adenine nucleotides for the common allosteric binding site. The second structural component is a di- or triphosphate moiety attached to the 5′-position of ribose, because neither AMP nor adenosine showed an inhibitory effect on the UGT activity. However, because adenine was able to inhibit UGT and lacks a phosphate group, the significance of the number of phosphates attached to ribose on the inhibitory effect of adenine nucleotides is called into question. Besides adenine-containing nucleotides, GTP and CTP are the only guanine- and cytidine nucleotides that inhibited UGTs, respectively, using 4-MU as the aglycone substrate [104,105]. CTP and ATP had similar IC_{50} values, and so comparable inhibitory effects. GTP, however, was much less potent than ATP.

UDP is a well-known inhibitor of UGTs. However, unlike adenine nucleotides, UDP is believed to compete with the co-substrate UDPGA for binding to UGTs, hence exerting the inhibitory effect on glucuronidation [104,107,108]. The inhibition of UGT by UDP can be prevented by the inclusion of a divalent metal ion in the incubation mixture, for example 10 mM Mg^{2+}.

Despite being a possible explanation of latency, the adenine nucleotides, particularly $NADP^+$, could play a role in the regulation of glucocorticoid levels [105,109]. Specifically, 11 β-hydroxysteroid dehydrogenase reduces $NADP^+$ to produce cortisone from cortisol in hepatic ER lumen. As the level of $NADP^+$ decreases, the inhibitory effect on the UGTs is also decreased, which enables UGTs to glucuronidate excess cortisol. Above all, information on the ER concentrations of adenine nucleotides relative to their cytosolic concentrations and IC_{50} values is needed to further investigate the physiological effects of the nucleotides on glucuronidation and metabolism.

6. Conclusions and Future Direction

The controversy over the underlying mechanisms that explain the latency of UGT activity that is observed in vitro in microsomal preparations has continued for more than half a century. It is clear that disruption of the microsomal membrane by physical and chemical treatments is necessary to reveal full UGT enzyme activity in vitro. Based on the available evidence, it is likely that much of the effect is due to the disruption of the membrane allowing increased access of UDPGA (and potentially also aglycone substrates) to the active site of the enzymes. Critical evidence for this comes from the existence of transporter(s) for UDPGA that presumably regulate access of the co-substrate to the enzyme in vivo. However, it is equally clear that UGT enzyme activity can be regulated by membrane components including phospholipids, cholesterol and indeed other proteins, including other UGTs and CYPs. Some of the effects of membrane disrupting agents such as detergents may well be mediated through their impact on the membrane environment as well as on the UGT proteins themselves.

Readers may ask "why does this matter?", particularly in a time when we know much about the biology, genetics and regulation of UGTs and glucuronidation. One of the main reasons it remains important is that we are still unable to accurately extrapolate in vitro measurements of UGT activity to estimates of in vivo clearance of drugs that are metabolized by glucuronidation. This in vitro–in vivo extrapolation (IVIVE) consistently underpredicts clearance in vivo for such drugs despite significant advances in physiologically-based pharmacokinetic (PBBK) analysis and a far more sophisticated understanding of the physiological factors that influence UGT activity [110,111]. We believe that increasing our understanding of the underlying mechanisms of UGT latency will help to further refine IVIVE for many drugs that are glucuronidated in humans. Advances in analytical tools such as Förster resonance energy transfer, mass spectrometry, etc. provide the technological basis for advancing our knowledge of this important feature of one of the body's key chemical defense mechanisms.

Acknowledgments: Yuejian Liu is supported by the James E. Axelson Outstanding Graduate Scholar Award.

Author Contributions: Yuejian Liu and Michael W. H. Coughtrie reviewed the literature and wrote the paper.

Conflicts of Interest: The authors declare no conflict of interest.

References

1. Radominska-Pandya, A.; Czernik, P.J.; Little, J.M.; Battaglia, E.; Mackenzie, P.I. Structural and functional studies of UDP-glucuronosyltransferases. *Drug Metab. Rev.* **1999**, *31*, 817–899. [CrossRef] [PubMed]
2. Dutton, G.J. *Glucuronidation of drugs and other compounds*; CRC Press: Boca Raton, FL, USA, 1980; ISBN 9780849352959.
3. Fry, D.J.; Wishart, G.J. Apparent induction by phenobarbital of uridine diphosphate glucuronyltransferase activity in nuclear envelopes of embryonic-chick liver. *Biochem. Soc. Trans.* **1976**, *4*, 255–266. [CrossRef] [PubMed]

4. Wishart, G.J.; Fry, D.J. Uridine diphosphate glucuronyltransferase activity in nuclei and nuclear envelopes of rat liver and its apparent induction by phenobarbital. *Biochem. Soc. Trans.* **1977**, *5*, 705–706. [CrossRef]

5. Fremont, J.J.; Wang, R.W.; King, C.D. Coimmunoprecipitation of UDP-glucuronosyltransferase isoforms and cytochrome P450 3A4. *Mol. Pharmacol.* **2005**, *67*, 260–262. [CrossRef] [PubMed]

6. Fujiwara, R.; Nakajima, M.; Oda, S.; Yamanaka, H.; Ikushiro, S.; Sakaki, T.; Yokoi, T. Interactions between human UDP-glucuronosyltransferase (UGT) 2B7 and UGT1A enzymes. *J. Pharm. Sci.* **2010**, *99*, 442–454. [CrossRef] [PubMed]

7. Fujiwara, R.; Nakajima, M.; Yamanaka, H.; Katoh, M.; Yokoi, T. Interactions between human UGT1A1, UGT1A4, and UGT1A6 affect their enzymatic activities. *Drug Metab. Dispos.* **2007**, *35*, 1781–1787. [CrossRef] [PubMed]

8. Ghosh, S.S.; Sappal, B.S.; Kalpana, G.V.; Lee, S.W.; Chowdhury, J.R.; Chowdhury, N.R. Homodimerization of human bilirubin-uridine-diphosphoglucuronate glucuronosyltransferase-1 (UGT1A1) and its functional implications. *J. Biol. Chem.* **2001**, *276*, 42108–42115. [CrossRef] [PubMed]

9. Ikushiro, S.; Emi, Y.; Iyanagi, T. Protein-protein interactions between UDP-glucuronosyltransferase isozymes in rat hepatic microsomes. *Biochemistry* **1997**, *36*, 7154–7161. [CrossRef] [PubMed]

10. Lewis, B.C.; Mackenzie, P.I.; Miners, J.O. Homodimerization of UDP-glucuronosyltransferase 2B7 (UGT2B7) and identification of a putative dimerization domain by protein homology modeling. *Biochem. Pharmacol.* **2011**, *82*, 2016–2023. [CrossRef] [PubMed]

11. Operana, T.N.; Tukey, R.H. Oligomerization of the UDP-glucuronosyltransferase 1A proteins: Homo- and heterodimerization analysis by fluorescence resonance energy transfer and co-immunoprecipitation. *J. Biol. Chem.* **2007**, *282*, 4821–4829. [CrossRef] [PubMed]

12. Taura, K.I.; Yamada, H.; Hagino, Y.; Ishii, Y.; Mori, M.A.; Oguri, K. Interaction between cytochrome P450 and other drug-metabolizing enzymes: Evidence for an association of CYP1A1 with microsomal epoxide hydrolase and UDP-glucuronosyltransferase. *Biochem. Biophys. Res. Commun.* **2000**, *273*, 1048–1052. [CrossRef] [PubMed]

13. Williams, R.T. *Detoxication Mechanisms*, 2nd ed.; Chapman & Hall: London, UK, 1959.

14. Ishii, Y.; Iwanaga, M.; Nishimura, Y.; Takeda, S.; Ikushiro, S.; Nagata, K.; Yamazoe, Y.; Mackenzie, P.I.; Yamada, H. Protein-protein interactions between rat hepatic cytochromes P450 (P450s) and UDP-glucuronosyltransferases (UGTs): Evidence for the functionally active UGT in P450-UGT complex. *Drug Metab. Pharmacokinet.* **2007**, *22*, 367–376. [CrossRef] [PubMed]

15. Takeda, S.; Ishii, Y.; Iwanaga, M.; Mackenzie, P.I.; Nagata, K.; Yamazoe, Y.; Oguri, K.; Yamada, H. Modulation of UDP-glucuronosyltransferase function by cytochrome P450: Evidence for the alteration of UGT2B7-catalyzed glucuronidation of morphine by CYP3A4. *Mol. Pharmacol.* **2005**, *67*, 665–672. [CrossRef] [PubMed]

16. Abbott, F.V.; Palmour, R.M. Morphine-6-glucuronide: Analgesic effects and receptor binding profile in rats. *Life Sci.* **1988**, *43*, 1685–1695. [CrossRef]

17. Vore, M.; Slikker, W. Steroid D-ring glucuronides: A new class of cholestatic agents. *Trends Pharmac. Sci.* **1985**, *6*, 256–259. [CrossRef]

18. Riches, Z.; Collier, A.C. Posttranscriptional regulation of uridine diphosphate glucuronosyltransferases. *Expert. Opin. Drug Metab. Toxicol.* **2015**, *11*, 949–965. [CrossRef] [PubMed]

19. Caspersen, C.S.; Reznik, B.; Weldy, P.L.; Abildskov, K.M.; Stark, R.I.; Garland, M. Molecular cloning of the baboon UDP-glucuronosyltransferase 1A gene family: Evolution of the primate UGT1 locus and relevance for models of human drug metabolism. *Pharmacogenet. Genomics* **2007**, *17*, 11–24. [CrossRef] [PubMed]

20. Halac, E.; Bonevard, E. Solubilization and activation of liver UDP glucuronyltransferase by EDTA. *Biochim. Biophys. Acta* **1963**, *67*, 498–500. [CrossRef]

21. Heirwegh, K.P.; Meuwissen, J.A. Activation in vitro and solubilization of glucuronyltransferase (assayed with bilirubin as acceptor) with digitonin. *Biochem. J.* **1968**, *110*, 31P–32P. [CrossRef] [PubMed]

22. Isselbacher, K.J.; Chrabas, M.F.; Quinn, R.C. The solubilization and partial purification of a glucuronyl transferase from rabbit liver microsomes. *J. Biol. Chem.* **1962**, *237*, 3033–3036. [PubMed]

23. Lueders, K.K.; Kuff, E.L. Spontaneous and detergent activation of a glucuronyltransferase in vitro. *Arch. Biochem. Biophys.* **1967**, *120*, 198–203. [CrossRef]

24. Pogell, B.M.; Leloir, L.F. Nucleotide activation of liver microsomal glucuronidation. *J. Biol. Chem.* **1961**, *236*, 293–298. [PubMed]

25. Stevenson, I.; Greenwood, D.; McEwen, J. Hepatic UDP-glucuronyltransferase in Wistar and Gunn rats - in vitro activation by diethylnitrosamine. *Biochem. Biophys. Res. Commun.* **1968**, *32*, 866–872. [CrossRef]

26. Tomlinson, G.A.; Yaffe, S.J. The formation of bilirubin and p-nitrophenyl glucuronides by rabbit liver. *Biochem. J.* **1966**, *99*, 507–512. [CrossRef] [PubMed]

27. Van Roy, F.P.; Heirwegh, K.P. Determination of bilirubin glucuronide and assay of glucuronyltransferase with bilirubin as acceptor. *Biochem. J.* **1968**, *107*, 507–518. [CrossRef] [PubMed]

28. Winsnes, A. Studies on the activation in vitro of glucuronyltransferase. *Biochim. Biophys. Acta* **1969**, *191*, 279–291. [CrossRef]

29. Burchell, A.; Waddell, I.D. The molecular basis of the hepatic microsomal glucose-6-phosphatase system. *Biochim. Biophys. Acta* **1991**, *1092*, 129–137. [CrossRef]

30. Lin, J.H.; Wong, B.K. Complexities of glucuronidation affecting in vitro in vivo extrapolation. *Curr. Drug Metab.* **2002**, *3*, 623–646. [CrossRef] [PubMed]

31. Berry, C.; Stellon, A.; Hallinan, T. Guinea pig liver microsomal UDP-glucuronyltransferase: Compartmented or phospholipid-constrained? *Biochim. Biophys. Acta* **1975**, *403*, 335–344. [CrossRef]

32. Dannenberg, A.; Wong, T.; Zakim, D. Effect of brief treatment at alkaline pH on the properties of UDP-glucuronosyltransferase. *Arch. Biochem. Biophys.* **1990**, *277*, 312–317. [CrossRef]

33. Dannenberg, A.J.; Kavecansky, J.; Scarlata, S.; Zakim, D. Organization of microsomal UDP-glucuronosyltransferase. Activation by treatment at high pressure. *Biochemistry* **1990**, *29*, 5961–5967. [CrossRef] [PubMed]

34. Fisher, M.B.; Campanale, K.; Ackermann, B.L.; VandenBranden, M.; Wrighton, S.A. In vitro glucuronidation using human liver microsomes and the pore-forming peptide alamethicin. *Drug Metab. Dispos.* **2000**, *28*, 560–566. [PubMed]

35. Graham, A.B.; Wood, G.C. The phospholipid-dependence of UDP-glucuronyltransferase. *Biochem. Biophys. Res. Commun.* **1969**, *37*, 567–575. [CrossRef]

36. Mulder, G.J. The effect of phenobarbital on the submicrosomal distribution of uridine diphosphate glucuronyltransferase from rat liver. *Biochem. J.* **1970**, *117*, 319–324. [CrossRef] [PubMed]

37. Vessey, D.A.; Zakim, D. Regulation of microsomal enzymes by phospholipids. II. Acitvation of hepatic uridine diphosphate-glucuronyltransferase. *J. Biol. Chem.* **1971**, *246*, 4649–4656. [PubMed]

38. Winsnes, A. Kinetic properties of different forms of hepatic UDP glucuronyltransferase. *Biochim. Biophys. Acta* **1972**, *284*, 394–405. [CrossRef]

39. Zakim, D.; Dannenberg, A.J. How does the microsomal membrane regulate UDP-glucuronosyltransferases? *Biochem. Pharmacol.* **1992**, *43*, 1385–1393. [CrossRef]

40. Coughtrie, M.W.H.; Blair, J.N.R.; Hume, R.; Burchell, A. Improved procedure for the preparation of hepatic microsomes to be used in the in vitro diagnosis of inherited disorders of the glucose-6-phosphatase system. *Clin. Chem.* **1991**, *37*, 739–742. [PubMed]

41. Coughtrie, M.W.H. A Molecular Analysis of Biological Variations in UDP-Glucuronosyltransferase Activities. Ph.D. Thesis, University of Dundee, Dundee, UK, 1986.

42. Coughtrie, M.W.H.; Burchell, B.; Bend, J.R. Purification and properties of rat kidney UDP-glucuronosyltransferase. *Biochem. Pharmacol.* **1987**, *36*, 245–251. [CrossRef]

43. Berry, C.; Hallinan, T. Summary of a novel, three-component regulatory model for uridine diphosphate glucuronyltransferase. *Biochem. Soc. Trans.* **1976**, *4*, 650–652. [CrossRef] [PubMed]

44. Jackson, M.R.; McCarthy, L.R.; Corser, R.B.; Barr, G.C.; Burchell, B. Cloning of cDNAs coding for rat hepatic microsomal UDP-glucuronyltransferases. *Gene* **1984**, *34*, 147–153. [CrossRef]

45. Mackenzie, P.I.; Gonzalez, F.J.; Owens, I.S. Cloning and characterization of DNA complementary to rat liver UDP-glucuronosyltransferase mRNA. *J. Biol. Chem.* **1984**, *259*, 12153–12160.

46. Mackenzie, P.I.; Owens, I.S. Cleavage of nascent UDP glucuronosyltransferase from rat liver by dog pancreatic microsomes. *Biochem. Biophys. Res. Commun.* **1984**, *122*, 1441–1449. [CrossRef]

47. Rowland, A.; Miners, J.O.; Mackenzie, P.I. The UDP-glucuronosyltransferases: Their role in drug metabolism and detoxification. *Int. J. Biochem. Cell Biol.* **2013**, *45*, 1121–1132. [CrossRef] [PubMed]

48. Jackson, M.R.; Nilsson, T.; Peterson, P.A. Identification of a consensus motif for retention of transmembrane proteins in the endoplasmic reticulum. *EMBO J.* **1990**, *9*, 3153–3162. [PubMed]

49. Ouzzine, M.; Magdalou, J.; Burchell, B.; Fournel-Gigleux, S. Expression of a functionally active human hepatic UDP-glucuronosyltransferase (UGT1A6) lacking the N-terminal signal sequence in the endoplasmic reticulum. *FEBS Lett.* **1999**, *454*, 187–191. [PubMed]

50. Ouzzine, M.; Magdalou, J.; Burchell, B.; Fournel-Gigleux, S. An internal signal sequence mediates the targeting and retention of the human UDP-glucuronosyltransferase 1A6 to the endoplasmic reticulum. *J. Biol. Chem.* **1999**, *274*, 31401–31409. [CrossRef] [PubMed]

51. Vanstapel, F.; Blanckaert, N. Topology and regulation of bilirubin UDP-glucuronyltransferase in sealed native microsomes from rat liver. *Arch. Biochem. Biophys.* **1988**, *263*, 216–225. [CrossRef]

52. Shepherd, S.R.; Baird, S.J.; Hallinan, T.; Burchell, B. An investigation of the transverse topology of bilirubin UDP-glucuronosyltransferase in rat hepatic endoplasmic reticulum. *Biochem. J.* **1989**, *259*, 617–620. [CrossRef] [PubMed]

53. Kyte, J.; Doolittle, R.F. A simple method for displaying the hydropathic character of a protein. *J. Mol. Biol.* **1982**, *157*, 105–132. [CrossRef]

54. Jackson, M.R.; Burchell, B. The full length coding sequence of rat liver androsterone UDP-glucuronyltransferase cDNA and comparison with other members of this gene family. *Nucleic Acids Res.* **1986**, *14*, 779–795. [CrossRef] [PubMed]

55. Mackenzie, P.I. Rat liver UDP-glucuronosyltransferase. cDNA sequence and expression of a form glucuronidating 3-hydroxyandrogens. *J. Biol. Chem.* **1986**, *261*, 14112–14117. [PubMed]

56. Iyanagi, T.; Haniu, M.; Sogawa, K.; Fujii-Kuriyama, Y.; Watanabe, S.; Shively, J.E.; Anan, K.F. Cloning and characterization of cDNA encoding 3-methylcholanthrene inducible rat mRNA for UDP-glucuronosyltransferase. *J. Biol. Chem.* **1986**, *261*, 15607–15614. [PubMed]

57. Fujiwara, R.; Yokoi, T.; Nakajima, M. Structure and protein-protein interactions of human UDP-glucuronosyltransferases. *Front. Pharmacol.* **2016**, *7*, 388. [CrossRef] [PubMed]

58. Miley, M.J.; Zielinska, A.K.; Keenan, J.E.; Bratton, S.M.; Radominska-Pandya, A.; Redinbo, M.R. Crystal structure of the cofactor-binding domain of the human phase II drug-metabolism enzyme UDP-glucuronosyltransferase 2B7. *J. Mol. Biol.* **2007**, *369*, 498–511. [CrossRef] [PubMed]

59. Axelrod, J.; Kalckar, H.M.; Maxwell, E.S.; Strominger, J.L. Enzymatic formation of uridine diphosphoglucuronic acid. *J. Biol. Chem.* **1957**, *224*, 79–90. [PubMed]

60. Banerjee, R.P.; Pennington, M.W.; Garza, A.; Owens, I.S. Mapping the UDP-glucuronic acid binding site in UDP-glucuronosyltransferase 1A10 by homology-based modeling: Confirmation with biochemical evidence. *Biochemistry* **2008**, *47*, 7385–7392. [CrossRef] [PubMed]

61. Locuson, C.W.; Tracy, T.S. Comparative modelling of the human UDP-glucuronosyltransferases: Insights into structure and mechanism. *Xenobiotica* **2007**, *37*, 155–168. [CrossRef] [PubMed]

62. Revesz, K.; Toth, B.; Staines, A.G.; Coughtrie, M.W.; Mandl, J.; Csala, M. Luminal accumulation of newly synthesized morphine-3-glucuronide in rat liver microsomal vesicles. *Biofactors* **2013**, *39*, 271–278. [CrossRef] [PubMed]

63. Zakim, D.; Vessey, D.A. Membrane dependence of uridine diphosphate glucuronyltransferase: Effect of the membrane on kinetic properties. *Biochem. Soc. Trans.* **1974**, *2*, 1165–1167. [CrossRef]

64. Berry, C.; Hallinan, T. 'Coupled transglucuronidation': A new tool for studying the latency of UDP-glucuronyl transferase. *FEBS Lett.* **1974**, *42*, 73–76. [CrossRef]

65. Vessey, D.A.; Zakim, D. Stimulation of microsomal uridine diphosphate glucuronyltransferase by glucuronic acid derivatives. *Biochem. J.* **1974**, *139*, 243–249. [CrossRef] [PubMed]

66. Winsnes, A. Inhibition of hepatic UDP glucuronyltransferase by nucleotides. *Biochim. Biophys. Acta* **1972**, *289*, 88–96. [CrossRef]

67. Winsnes, A. The effects of sulfhydryl reacting agents on hepatic UDP-glucuronyltransferase in vitro. *Biochim. Biophys. Acta* **1971**, *242*, 549–559. [CrossRef]

68. Bossuyt, X.; Blanckaert, N. Carrier-mediated transport of intact UDP-glucuronic acid into the lumen of endoplasmic-reticulum-derived vesicles from rat liver. *Biochem. J.* **1994**, *302*, 261–269. [CrossRef] [PubMed]

69. Bossuyt, X.; Blanckaert, N. Mechanism of stimulation of microsomal UDP-glucuronosyltransferase by UDP-N-acetylglucosamine. *Biochem J.* **1995**, *305*, 321–328. [CrossRef] [PubMed]

70. Hauser, S.C.; Ziurys, J.C.; Gollan, J.L. A membrane transporter mediates access of uridine 5'-diphosphoglucuronic acid from the cytosol into the endoplasmic reticulum of rat hepatocytes: Implications for glucuronidation reactions. *Biochim. Biophys. Acta* **1988**, *967*, 149–157. [CrossRef]

71. Nuwayhid, N.; Glaser, J.H.; Johnson, J.C.; Conrad, H.E.; Hauser, S.C.; Hirschberg, C.B. Xylosylation and glucuronosylation reactions in rat liver golgi apparatus and endoplasmic reticulum. *J. Biol. Chem.* **1986**, *261*, 12936–12941. [PubMed]

72. Bossuyt, X.; Blanckaert, N. Functional characterization of carrier-mediated transport of uridine diphosphate N-acetylglucosamine across the endoplasmic reticulum membrane. *Eur. J. Biochem.* **1994**, *223*, 981–988. [CrossRef]

73. Bossuyt, X.; Blanckaert, N. Carrier-mediated transport of uridine diphosphoglucuronic acid across the endoplasmic reticulum membrane is a prerequisite for UDP-glucuronosyltransferase activity in rat liver. *Biochem. J.* **1997**, *323*, 645–648. [CrossRef] [PubMed]

74. Muraoka, M.; Kawakita, M.; Ishida, N. Molecular characterization of human UDP-glucuronic acid/UDP-N-acetylgalactosamine transporter, a novel nucleotide sugar transporter with dual substrate specificity. *FEBS Lett.* **2001**, *495*, 87–93. [CrossRef]

75. Kobayashi, T.; Sleeman, J.E.; Coughtrie, M.W.; Burchell, B. Molecular and functional characterization of microsomal UDP-glucuronic acid uptake by members of the nucleotide sugar transporter (NST) family. *Biochem. J.* **2006**, *400*, 281–289. [CrossRef] [PubMed]

76. Muraoka, M.; Miki, T.; Ishida, N.; Hara, T.; Kawakita, M. Variety of nucleotide sugar transporters with respect to the interaction with nucleoside mono- and diphosphates. *J. Biol. Chem.* **2007**, *282*, 24615–24622. [CrossRef] [PubMed]

77. Dutton, G.J.; Storey, I.D.E. The isolation of a compound of uridine diphosphate and glucuronic acid from liver. *Biochem. J.* **1953**, *53*, xxxvii–xxxviii. [PubMed]

78. Storey, I.D.E.; Dutton, G.J. Uridine compounds in glucuronic acid metabolism. 2. The isolation and structure of 'uridine-diphosphate-glucuronic acid'. *Biochem. J.* **1955**, *59*, 279–288. [CrossRef] [PubMed]

79. Rowland, A.; Mackenzie, P.I.; Miners, J.O. Transporter-mediated uptake of UDP-glucuronic acid by human liver microsomes: Assay conditions, kinetics, and inhibition. *Drug Metab. Dispos.* **2015**, *43*, 147–153. [CrossRef] [PubMed]

80. Goto, S.; Taniguchi, M.; Muraoka, M.; Toyoda, H.; Sado, Y.; Kawakita, M.; Hayashi, S. UDP-sugar transporter implicated in glycosylation and processing of notch. *Nat. Cell Biol.* **2001**, *3*, 816–822. [CrossRef] [PubMed]

81. Selva, E.M.; Hong, K.; Baeg, G.H.; Beverley, S.M.; Turco, S.J.; Perrimon, N.; Hacker, U. Dual role of the fringe connection gene in both heparan sulphate and fringe-dependent signalling events. *Nat. Cell Biol.* **2001**, *3*, 809–815. [CrossRef] [PubMed]

82. Suda, T.; Kamiyama, S.; Suzuki, M.; Kikuchi, N.; Nakayama, K.; Narimatsu, H.; Jigami, Y.; Aoki, T.; Nishihara, S. Molecular cloning and characterization of a human multisubstrate specific nucleotide-sugar transporter homologous to drosophila fringe connection. *J. Biol. Chem.* **2004**, *279*, 26469–26474. [CrossRef] [PubMed]

83. Dutton, G.J. Commentary: Control of UDP-glucuronyltransferase activity. *Biochem. Pharmacol.* **1975**, *24*, 1835–1841. [CrossRef]

84. Hochman, Y.; Zakim, D. Studies of the catalytic mechanism of microsomal UDP-glucuronyltransferase. Alpha-glucuronidase activity and its stimulation by phospholipids. *J. Biol. Chem.* **1984**, *259*, 5521–5525. [PubMed]

85. Vessey, D.A.; Zakim, D. Regulation of microsomal enzymes by phospholipids. V. Kinetic studies of hepatic uridine diphosphate-glucuronyltransferase. *J. Biol. Chem.* **1972**, *247*, 3023–3028. [PubMed]

86. Magdalou, J.; Hochman, Y.; Zakim, D. Factors modulating the catalytic specificity of a pure form of UDP-glucuronyltransferase. *J. Biol. Chem.* **1982**, *257*, 13624–13629. [PubMed]

87. Dannenberg, A.; Rotenberg, M.; Zakim, D. Regulation of UDP-glucuronosyltransferase by lipid-protein interactions. Comparison of the thermotropic properties of pure reconstituted enzyme with microsomal enzyme. *J. Biol. Chem.* **1989**, *264*, 238–242. [PubMed]

88. Hochman, Y.; Kelley, M.; Zakim, D. Modulation of the number of ligand binding sites of UDP-glucuronyltransferase by the gel to liquid-crystal phase transition of phosphatidylcholines. *J. Biol. Chem.* **1983**, *258*, 6509–6516. [PubMed]

89. Erickson, R.H.; Zakim, D.; Vessey, D.A. Preparation and properties of a phospholipid-free form of microsomal UDP-glucuronyltransferase. *Biochemistry* **1978**, *17*, 3706–3711. [CrossRef] [PubMed]

90. Hochman, Y.; Zakim, D.A. Comparison of the kinetic properties of two different forms of microsomal UDP-glucuronyltransferase. *J. Biol. Chem.* **1983**, *258*, 4143–4146. [PubMed]

91. Rotenberg, M.; Zakim, D. Effect of phospholipids on the thermal stability of microsomal UDP-glucuronosyltransferase. *Biochemistry* **1989**, *28*, 8577–8582. [CrossRef] [PubMed]

92. Hochman, Y.; Zakim, D.; Vessey, D.A. A kinetic mechanism for modulation of the activity of microsomal UDP-glucuronyltransferase by phospholipids. Effects of lysophosphatidylcholines. *J. Biol. Chem.* **1981**, *256*, 4783–4788. [PubMed]
93. Simons, K.; Ikonen, E. Functional rafts in cell membranes. *Nature* **1997**, *387*, 569–572. [CrossRef] [PubMed]
94. Fujiwara, T.; Ritchie, K.; Murakoshi, H.; Jacobson, K.; Kusumi, A. Phospholipids undergo hop diffusion in compartmentalized cell membrane. *J. Cell Biol.* **2002**, *157*, 1071–1081. [CrossRef] [PubMed]
95. Brown, D.A.; London, E. Functions of lipid rafts in biological membranes. *Annu. Rev. Cell Dev. Biol.* **1998**, *14*, 111–136. [CrossRef] [PubMed]
96. Simons, K.; Toomre, D. Lipid rafts and signal transduction. *Nat. Rev. Mol. Cell Biol.* **2000**, *1*, 31–39. [CrossRef] [PubMed]
97. Suzuki, K.G.; Fujiwara, T.K.; Sanematsu, F.; Iino, R.; Edidin, M.; Kusumi, A. GPI-anchored receptor clusters transiently recruit Lyn and G alpha for temporary cluster immobilization and Lyn activation: Single-molecule tracking study 1. *J. Cell Biol.* **2007**, *177*, 717–730. [CrossRef] [PubMed]
98. Castuma, C.E.; Brenner, R.R. Cholesterol-dependent modification of microsomal dynamics and UDP-glucuronyltransferase kinetics. *Biochemistry* **1986**, *25*, 4733–4738. [CrossRef] [PubMed]
99. Castuma, C.E.; Brenner, R.R. Effect of dietary cholesterol on microsomal membrane composition, dynamics and kinetic properties of UDP-glucuronyltransferase. *Biochim. Biophys. Acta* **1986**, *855*, 231–242. [CrossRef]
100. Rotenberg, M.; Zakim, D. Effects of cholesterol on the function and thermotropic properties of pure UDP-glucuronosyltransferase. *J. Biol. Chem.* **1991**, *266*, 4159–4161. [PubMed]
101. Vessey, D.A.; Zakim, D. Regulation of microsomal enzymes by phospholipids. IV. Species differences in the properties of microsomal UDP-glucuronyltransferase. *Biochim. Biophys. Acta* **1972**, *268*, 61–69. [CrossRef]
102. Peters, W.H.; te Morsche, R.H.; Roelofs, H.M. Combined polymorphisms in UDP-glucuronosyltransferases 1A1 and 1A6: Implications for patients with Gilbert's syndrome. *J. Hepatol.* **2003**, *38*, 3–8. [CrossRef]
103. Ishii, Y.; An, K.; Nishimura, Y.; Yamada, H. ATP serves as an endogenous inhibitor of UDP-glucuronosyltransferase (UGT): A new insight into the latency of UGT. *Drug Metab. Dispos.* **2012**, *40*, 2081–2089. [CrossRef] [PubMed]
104. Ishii, Y.; Nurrochmad, A.; Yamada, H. Modulation of UDP-glucuronosyltransferase activity by endogenous compounds. *Drug Metab. Pharmacokinet* **2010**, *25*, 134–148. [CrossRef] [PubMed]
105. Nishimura, Y.; Maeda, S.; Ikushiro, S.; Mackenzie, P.I.; Ishii, Y.; Yamada, H. Inhibitory effects of adenine nucleotides and related substances on UDP-glucuronosyltransferase: Structure-effect relationships and evidence for an allosteric mechanism. *Biochim. Biophys. Acta* **2007**, *1770*, 1557–1566. [CrossRef] [PubMed]
106. Hallinan, T.; Pohl, K.R.; de Brito, R. Studies on the inhibition of hepatic microsomal glucuronidation by uridine nucleotides or adenosine triphosphate. *Med. Biol.* **1979**, *57*, 269–273. [PubMed]
107. Fujiwara, R.; Nakajima, M.; Yamanaka, H.; Katoh, M.; Yokoi, T. Product inhibition of UDP-glucuronosyltransferase (UGT) enzymes by UDP obfuscates the inhibitory effects of UGT substrates. *Drug Metab. Dispos.* **2008**, *36*, 361–367. [CrossRef] [PubMed]
108. Yokota, H.; Ando, F.; Iwano, H.; Yuasa, A. Inhibitory effects of uridine diphosphate on UDP-glucuronosyltransferase. *Life Sci.* **1998**, *63*, 1693–1699. [CrossRef]
109. Agarwal, A.K.; Monder, C.; Eckstein, B.; White, P.C. Cloning and expression of rat cDNA encoding corticosteroid 11 beta-dehydrogenase. *J. Biol. Chem.* **1989**, *264*, 18939–18943. [PubMed]
110. Rostami-Hodjegan, A. Physiologically based pharmacokinetics joined with in vitro-in vivo extrapolation of ADME: A marriage under the arch of systems pharmacology. *Clin. Pharmacol. Ther.* **2012**, *92*, 50–61. [CrossRef] [PubMed]
111. Gill, K.L.; Houston, J.B.; Galetin, A. Characterization of in vitro glucuronidation clearance of a range of drugs in human kidney microsomes: Comparison with liver and intestinal glucuronidation and impact of albumin. *Drug Metab. Dispos.* **2012**, *40*, 825–835. [CrossRef] [PubMed]

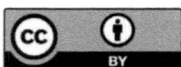

pharmaceutics

MDPI

Review

Augmented Renal Clearance in Critical Illness: An Important Consideration in Drug Dosing

Sherif Hanafy Mahmoud * and Chen Shen

Faculty of Pharmacy and Pharmaceutical Sciences, University of Alberta, Edmonton, AB T6G 1C9, Canada; cshen2@ualberta.ca
* Correspondence: smahmoud@ualberta.ca; Tel.: +1-780-492-5364

Received: 4 August 2017; Accepted: 14 September 2017; Published: 16 September 2017

Abstract: Augmented renal clearance (ARC) is a manifestation of enhanced renal function seen in critically ill patients. The use of regular unadjusted doses of renally eliminated drugs in patients with ARC might lead to therapy failure. The purpose of this scoping review was to provide and up-to-date summary of the available evidence pertaining to the phenomenon of ARC. A literature search of databases of available evidence in humans, with no language restriction, was conducted. Databases searched were MEDLINE (1946 to April 2017), EMBASE (1974 to April 2017) and the Cochrane Library (1999 to April 2017). A total of 57 records were included in the present review: 39 observational studies (25 prospective, 14 retrospective), 6 case reports/series and 12 conference abstracts. ARC has been reported to range from 14 to 80%. ARC is currently defined as an increased creatinine clearance of greater than $130 \text{ mL/min}/1.73 \text{ m}^2$ best measured by 8–24 h urine collection. Patients exhibiting ARC tend to be younger (<50 years old), of male gender, had a recent history of trauma, and had lower critical illness severity scores. Numerous studies have reported antimicrobials treatment failures when using standard dosing regimens in patients with ARC. In conclusion, ARC is an important phenomenon that might have significant impact on outcome in critically ill patients. Identifying patients at risk, using higher doses of renally eliminated drugs or use of non-renally eliminated alternatives might need to be considered in ICU patients with ARC. More research is needed to solidify dosing recommendations of various drugs in patients with ARC.

Keywords: augmented renal clearance; enhanced renal function; critically ill

1. Introduction

Studying the influence of renal dysfunction on the pharmacokinetics of drugs is an important consideration in drug development. In addition, clinicians are vigilant in adjusting the doses of renally eliminated drugs in patients with various degrees of renal impairment to avoid potential toxicities. On the other hand, little attention is given if patients exhibit an augmented renal clearance (ARC). Augmented renal clearance (ARC) is a manifestation of enhanced renal function seen in critically ill patients [1,2]. It is currently defined as an increased creatinine clearance of greater than $130 \text{ mL/min}/1.73 \text{ m}^2$. ARC is a clinical phenomenon rapidly gaining recognition in the world of critical care. Although ARC may have existed long before our current recognition, it wasn't until the early 2010's, that the research group led by Andrew Udy put forth the concept of ARC as an independently existing medical phenomenon [3]. The increased renal clearance of endogenous by-products, various chemicals, toxins, and most importantly medications during ARC manifestation may have a significant impact on patient outcome. The use of regular unadjusted doses of renally eliminated drugs in patients with ARC might lead to therapy failure and worse patient outcome. The purpose of this scoping review was to provide and up-to-date summary of the available evidence pertaining to the phenomenon of ARC including epidemiology, risk factors and pathophysiology of ARC, pharmacokinetic changes of drugs in patients with ARC and suggested assessment and management approach of patients exhibiting ARC.

2. Methods

A literature search of databases of available evidence pertaining to augmented renal clearance (ARC) in humans, with no language restriction, was conducted. Databases searched were MEDLINE (1946 to 12 April 2017), EMBASE (1974 to 12 April 2017) and the Cochrane Library (1999 to 12 April 2017). To ensure that we captured all studies involving augmented renal clearance, we used the following keywords: "augmented renal clearance", "enchanc * renal clear *", "increase * renal clearance", "augmented kidney clearance", "enhance * kidney function *", "ren * ultrafiltrat *", "enhance * creatinine clear *", "increase * kidney function *", and "increase * creatinine clear *". Title and abstract screening were then conducted to identify duplicate studies and studies that were clearly not pertaining to the topic for exclusion. If any doubt arose regarding whether a study was related to ARC, the study was included for full text review. Studies on renal dysfunction (e.g., acute kidney injury, chronic kidney disease, renal dysfunction, etc.) or other clinical phenomena that would alter drug elimination (e.g., cystic fibrosis) were excluded. Non-human studies, non-English studies that could not be easily translated into English using an online translator tool, commentaries, opinion articles, editorials and review articles were excluded. Both authors independently conducted the processes of screening. Then, the full texts of the selected articles were assessed for inclusion in our review. Lastly, a manual search for additional relevant studies was performed by analyzing the reference lists of the selected studies. In case of any discrepancies between the reviewers, further discussion was done to reach a consensus. Data extraction from studies was confirmed by both authors.

3. Results and Discussion

As depicted in Figure 1, databases search resulted in 562 records. After duplicate removal and addition of records from other sources, 322 records remained. After title, abstract and full text screening, a total of 57 records were included in the present review: 39 observational studies (25 prospective, 14 retrospective), 6 case reports/case series and 12 conference abstracts. Because the main body of evidence was derived from observational studies, caution should be exercised while interpreting the results of the included records especially case reports. Table 1 summarizes the studies included in this review.

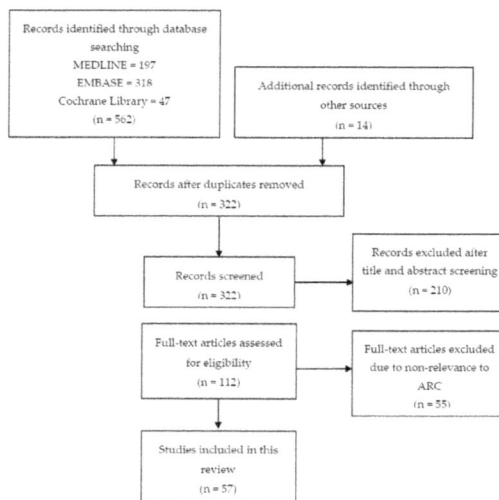

Figure 1. Flow diagram of the literature search for studies addressing augmented renal clearance (ARC).

Table 1. Summary of studies pertaining to ARC.

Author, Year	Study Type	Age (Years) Median (IQR)	Population	N	Sex (% Male)	Measured CrCl (mL/min)—Otherwise Specified	Intervention	Main Results
Barletta et al. [4], 2017	Retrospective observational	48 ± 19	ICU trauma patients where measured SCr available and SCr < 115 µmol/L	133	76	168 ± 65	ARCTIC (Augmented Renal Clearance in Trauma Intensive Care) Scoring system suggested	• 67% of patients identified to have ARC (CrCl > 130 mL/min) • ARC risk factors identified: from multivariate analysis were age < 56 years, age = 56–75 years, SCr < 62 µmol/L, male sex • ARCTIC score > 6 had sensitivity 84% and specificity 68%
Naeem et al. [5], 2017	Prospective observational	ARC: 37 ± 16 Non-ARC: 34 ± 14	ICU patients with SCr < 115 µmol/L	50	ARC: 70 Non-ARC: 60	ARC: 214 ± 46 Non-ARC: 112 ± 11	The effects of ARC on enoxaparin determined; Patients received enoxaparin 40 mg SC daily; Anti-Xa activity measured and compared among patients with and without ARC; measured 24 h CrCl	• 40% of patients identified to have ARC (CrCl > 130 mL/min) • Anti-Xa activity did not differ in both groups at baseline and 4 h after administration • ARC patients had significantly lower anti-Xa activity 12 and 24 h post enoxaparin administration; this implies short duration of action of enoxaparin in patients with ARC.
Udy et al. [6], 2017	Prospective observational (sub-study of BLING II RCT)	ARC: 52 (33–60) Non-ARC: 65 (55–73)	ICU patients with severe sepsis	254	ARC: 73 Non-ARC: 57	ARC: 165 (144–198) Non-ARC: 56 (27–83)	Conducted to determine the effect of ARC on patient outcome; patients randomized to receive beta lactam antibiotics (piperacillin/tazobactam, ticarcillin/clavulanic acid or meropenem) by intermittent or continuous infusion; measured 8 h CrCl	• 18% of patients identified to have ARC (CrCl > 130 mL/min); mainly younger, male and with less organ dysfunction • No outcome differences (ICU-free days or mortality) between ARC and non-ARC • No outcome differences were identified between continuous or intermittent infusion strategy
Udy et al. [7], 2017	Prospective observational	37 (24–49)	ICU (TBI patients with SCr < 120 µmol/L)	11	82	Median (day 1): 201 (76–289)	Measured 8-h CrCl, cardiac output and ANP were determined and correlated	• ARC complicates TBI patients (Measured CrCl generally > 150 mL/min); mainly males and with young age • CrCl was not significantly associated with changes in ANP or cardiac output

Table 1. *Cont.*

Author, Year	Study Type	Age (Years) Median (IQR)	Population	N	Sex (% Male)	Measured CrCl (mL/min)—Otherwise Specified	Intervention	Main Results
Barletta et al. [8], 2016	Retrospective observational	48 ± 18	ICU (trauma)	65	74	169 ± 70	Measured 12-h CrCl compared with CG method, CKD-EPI, and MDRD-4	• 69% of patients identified to have ARC (CrCl > 130 mL/min)—more common in younger patients and patients with SCr < 71 µmol/L • Measured CrCl was significantly higher ($p < 0.001$) than all estimates of CrCl • CG demonstrated lowest amount of bias (38 ± 56 mL/min) compared to CKD-EPI and MDRD-4
Chu et al. [9], 2016	Retrospective observational	Group A: 63 ± 15 Group B: 59 ± 14 Group C: 44 ± 16	Patients treated with vancomycin	148	66	Estimated by CG Group A: 54 ± 17 Group B: 106 ± 15 Group C: 188 ± 50	Vancomycin 1000 mg IV Q12H regimen given; vancomycin levels drawn pre 4th or 5th dose; levels compared across three groups: A (CrCl < 80), B (CrCl 80–129), C (CrCl ≥ 130; ARC)	• Patients with ARC (Group C) had higher percentage of subtherapeutic vancomycin • Vancomycin trough concentrations at steady state: Group A = 25 ± 10, Group B = 15 ± 8, Group C = 9 ± 5 mg/L • Vancomycin trough concentration below 10 mcg/mL: Group A = 0%, Group B = 28%, Group C = 63%
Declercq et al. [10], 2016	Prospective observational	Abdominal Surgery: 63 (51–71) Trauma Surgery: 62 (46–75)	Non-critically ill surgery patients	232	Abdo. Surgery: 74 Trauma Surgery: 58	Abdominal Surgery: 109 (82–135) Trauma Surgery: 109 (85–142)	Aim to assess the prevalence of ARC in non-critically ill surgical patients; Measured 8-h CrCl	• Abdominal surgery patients: 30% of patients identified to have ARC (CrCl > 130 mL/min) • Trauma surgery patients: 35% of patients identified to have ARC (CrCl > 130 mL/min) • The study identified presence of ARC in non-ICU surgery patients especially in younger male patients and undergoing trauma surgery
Hirai et al. [11], 2016	Retrospective observational	4.4 (range 1–15)	Pediatric ICU patients with normal renal function (Japan)	109	59	eGFR estimated by Schwartz formula 160 (range 90–323) mL/min/1.73 m²	Vancomycin 40–60 mg/kg per day given in 2–4 divided doses; vancomycin clearance estimated	• ARC defined as eGFR ≥ 160 mL/min/1.73 m² • Febrile neutropenia is an independent risk factor for ARC • Age and eGFR significantly associated with vancomycin clearance ($p < 0.0001$)

Table 1. *Cont.*

Author, Year	Study Type	Age (Years) Median (IQR)	Population	N	Sex (% Male)	Measured CrCl (mL/min)— Otherwise Specified	Intervention	Main Results
Kawano et al. [12], 2016	Prospective observational	67 (53–77)	ICU (Japan)	111	56	Not reported	Measured 8-h CrCl	• 39% of patients identified to have ARC (CrCl > 130 mL/min/1.73 m²) • Age <63 years was identified as a risk factor for ARC
Roberts et al. [13], 2016	Prospective PK study	61 ± 17	Patients treated with levofloxacin	18	67	Estimated using CG 70 ± 67	Doses of levofloxacin 500 and 750 mg daily have been used; Monte-Carlo simulation conducted to determine PTA in ICU cohort compared to non ICU ones	• For CrCl > 130 and CrCl > 200, levofloxacin 1000 mg Q24H provided the highest target attainment for *S. pneumoniae, P. aeruginosa* and *S. aureus.* • For *H. influenza*, all levofloxacin doses/regimens analyzed were able to achieve >99% attainment
De Cock et al. [14], 2015	Prospective PK study	2.6 (range 0.08–15)	Pediatric ICU	50	60	Not reported	Population PK of amoxicillin/clavulanate in pediatric ICU population; Conventional dosing of 25–35 mg/kg every 6 h was tested.	• In ARC patients; the best dosing is 25 mg/kg over 1 h every 4 h; it produced the best median target attainment by Monte-Carlo Simulation
De Waele et al. [15], 2015	Retrospective observational	62 (50–72)	ICU	1081	63	ARC: 178 (140–243) Non-ARC: 54 (32–82)	Measured 24-h CrCl and ARC risk factors determined	• 56% of patients identified to have ARC (CrCl > 130 mL/min): mainly younger and less likely to be treated with vasopressors • Continuous ARC was present in 33% of patients • ARC incidence 37 per 100 ICU patient-days
Dias et al. [16], 2015	Retrospective observational	Mean 42 (range 20–66)	ICU (TBI patients)	18	89	CG method 199 (Range 62–471)	Cerebrovascular pressure reactivity index (PRx) correlated with CrCl	• A strong negative correlation between CG CrCl and PRX ($r = -0.82$, $p = 0.001$) have been reported • This correlation suggests that reduction in cerebral autoregulation (i.e., after TBI) is associated with an increase in creatinine clearance.

Table 1. *Cont.*

Author, Year	Study Type	Age (Years) Median (IQR)	Population	N	Sex (% Male)	Measured CrCl (mL/min)—Otherwise Specified	Intervention	Main Results
Huttner et al. [17], 2015	Prospective observational	ARC: 41 ± 12 Non-ARC: 51±10	ICU with CrCl ≥ 60 mL/min	100	75	Estimated with CG ARC: 166 (145–200) Non-ARC: 103 (87–113)	They determined the influence of ARC on patient outcome; Standard dose antibiotic regimens given (imipenem/cilastatin 500 mg IV QID; meropenem 2 g IV TID; piperacillin/tazobactam 4.5 g IV TID; cefepime 2 g IV BID)	• 64% of patients identified to have ARC (CrCl > 130 mL/min); mainly younger • ARC predicted undetectable antimicrobials concentrations but was not correlated with clinical failure
Morbitzer et al. [18], 2015	Retrospective observational	CN: 44 (29–52) TH/PI: 48 (40–62)	ICU (TBI)	27	63	Estimated using CG CN: 119 (91–166) TH/PI: 129 (100–156)	Vancomycin pharmacokinetics compared in patients with CN (T = 36–37 C), TH (T=33–34 C) or pentobarbital infusion	• Vancomycin clearance was higher in controlled normothermic patients compared to predicted values based on population parameters
Ruiz et al. [19], 2015	Prospective observational	ARC: 39 ± 16 No ARC: 55 ± 19	ICU (patients with normal SCr)	360	ARC: 75 No ARC: 65	ARC: 173 ± 44 No ARC: 79 ± 30	Measured 24-h CrCl compared with 4 formulas to estimate CrCl/GFR (CG, Robert, MDRD and CKD-EPI methods)	• 33% of patients identified to have ARC (CrCl > 130 mL/min/1.73 m²); mainly trauma patients; younger • Different formulas tended to overestimate CrCl for low eGFR values and underestimate CrCl for normal and high eGFRs • Three factors suggested to identify ARC: Age ≤ 58 years, trauma and eGFR > 108.1 mL/min/1.73 m² as calculated by CKD-EPI
Spadaro et al. [20], 2015	Retrospective observational	Group A: 63 ± 11 Group B: 71 ± 10	ICU	348	Group A: 73 Group B: 69	Group A: 106 ± 41 Group B: 37 ± 16	Vancomycin administration protocol based on measured 24 h CrCl and vancomycin serum measurements; levels compared between two groups: A (CrCl > 50) and B (CrCl ≤ 50) Vancomycin serum trough target: 15–25 mg/L	• 66% of patients had subtherapeutic vancomycin on second determination ARC and increased to 80% on third determination • Patients who had a subtherapeutic vancomycin levels at the first determination had a significant correlation with in-hospital mortality (OR = 2, p = 0.003)

Table 1. *Cont.*

Author, Year	Study Type	Age (Years) Median (IQR)	Population	N	Sex (% Male)	Measured CrCl (mL/min)—Otherwise Specified	Intervention	Main Results
Steinke et al. [21], 2015	Prospective observational	66 (57–74)	ICU	100	61	73 (47–107)	Measured CrCl compared with estimated CrCl using serum cystatin C Hoek formula, CG, and CKD-EPI	• 16% of patients identified to have ARC (CrCl > 130 mL/min/1.73 m²): mainly trauma patients; TBI or SAH • The Hoek formula's precision was higher than CG and CKD-EPI • Authors suggested more studies are needed to identify the rule of Hoek's formula in drug dosing.
Adnan et al. [22], 2014	Prospective observational	34 (24–47)	ICU patients with SCr < 120 μmol/L	49	76	ARC: 173 (141–223) Non-ARC: 91 (64–112)	Measured 24-h CrCl compared with CG method	• 39% of patients identified to have ARC (CrCl > 130 mL/min) • CG method significantly underestimated CrCl in ARC patients
Akers et al. [23], 2014	Prospective observational	45 ± 19	ICU	13	62	Not reported	They determined the ability of the ARC score to predict piperacillin/tazobactam clearance; Piperacillin/tazobactam doses given were (3.375 g IV Q6H or 4.5 g Q6H)	• ARC score had sensitivity 100%, specificity 71% in detecting enhanced clearance of piperacillin/tazobactam
Baptista et al. [24], 2014	Prospective observational	ARC: 49 ± 15 No ARC: 60 ± 18	ICU patients with normal SCr	54	ARC: 64 No ARC: 36	ARC Patients: 161 ± 28 Non-ARC Patients: 105 ± 16	Measured 8-h CrCl compared with CG method, CKD-EPI, and MDRD	• 56% of patients identified to have ARC (CrCl > 130 mL/min) • All formulas underestimated 8h-CrCl for values >120 mL/min/1.73 m² and a overestimated for values <120 mL/min/1.73 m²
Baptista et al. [25], 2014	Prospective observational (Group 1 data were retrospectively collected)	Group 1: 58 ± 16 Group 2: 60 ± 17	ICU	G 1: 79 G 2: 25	Group 1: 66 Group 2: 68	Group 1: 125 ± 67 mL/min/1.73 m² Group 2: 121 ± 54 mL/min/1.73 m²	Continuous infusion Vancomycin dosing nomogram based on 8h measured CrCl was suggested Group 1: retrospective data Group 2: prospective assessment of the nomogram Target vancomycin level: 20–30 mg/L	• 36% and 40% of patients identified to have ARC in groups 1 and 2, respectively (CrCl > 130 mL/min/1.73 m²) • Vancomycin clearance was significantly proportional to measured CrCl

Table 1. *Cont.*

Author, Year	Study Type	Age (Years) Median (IQR)	Population	N	Sex (% Male)	Measured CrCl (mL/min)— Otherwise Specified	Intervention	Main Results
Campassi et al. [26], 2014	Prospective observational	ARC: 48 ± 15 Non-ARC: 65 ± 17	ICU patients with SCr < 115 μmol/L	363	ARC: 48 Non-ARC: 47	ARC: 155 ± 33 Non-ARC: 78 ± 25	CrCl measured by 24 h urine collection; Vancomycin loading dose 15 mg/kg followed by continuous infusion 30 mg/kg/day was given Target trough 15–25 mg/L	• 28% of patients identified to have ARC (CrCl > 120 mL/min/1.73 m²); generally younger; more trauma and obstetric admissions; lower APACHE II scores • 27% of patients who received vancomycin were identified to have ARC and had significantly lower vancomycin levels ($p < 0.05$) than non-ARC patients at 3 days; none of the ARC patients reached target trough despite being administered significantly higher vancomycin doses
Hites et al. [27], 2014	Prospective observational	61 (18–84)	Non-ICU obese (BMI ≥ 30 kg/m²) patients treated with antibiotics	56	50	107 (6–389.0)	They assessed the adequacy of serum concentrations of antimicrobials when given to obese individuals; Standard doses of antibiotics given (Cefepime 2 g TID, Piperacillin/tazobactam 4 g QID, Meropenem 1 g TID); Measured 24-h CrCl determined	• Low levels of antimicrobials were detected following standard doses. • Elevated CrCl was the only predictor of those low concentrations underlining the role of ARC in under-dosing obese individuals.
Udy et al. [28], 2014	Prospective observational	Mean 37 (95% CI 29–44)	ICU patients with SCr < 120 μmol/L and age ≤ 60	20	60	Mean: 168 (95% CI 139–197)	Measured 24-h CrCl determined; various exogenous markers given to detect changes in nephron physiology	• ARC involves increased glomerular filtration, renal tubular secretion of anions and renal tubular reabsorption using various exogenous markers, suggesting that ARC affects many components of the nephron physiology
Udy et al. [29], 2014	Prospective observational	Mean 54 (95% CI 53–56)	ICU patients with SCr < 120 μmol/L	281	63.3	Mean: 108 (95% CI 102–115)	Measured 8-h CrCl determined daily	• 65% of patients identified to have ARC (CrCl > 120 mL/min/1.73 m²); mainly younger, men, multi-trauma victims, and receiving mechanical ventilation • Presence of ICU admission day 1 ARC predicted sustained ARC during ICU stay

Table 1. *Cont.*

Author, Year	Study Type	Age (Years) Median (IQR)	Population	N	Sex (% Male)	Measured CrCl (mL/min)—Otherwise Specified	Intervention	Main Results
Carlier et al. [30], 2013	Prospective observational	56 (48–67)	ICU	61	85	125 (93–175)	Meropenem or piperacillin/tazobactam were given as extended IV infusions; antibiotics concentrations measured; measured 24 h CrCl determined; Meropenem dose: an IV loading of 1 g over 30 min then 1 g Q6H as extended infusion over 3 h; Piperacillin/tazobactam dose: an IV loading of 4.5 g over 30 min then 4.5 g Q6H extended infusion over 3 h.	• 80% of patients identified to have ARC (CrCl > 130 mL/min) • Elevated creatinine clearance is an independent predictor for not achieving meropenem and piperacillin/tazobactam target levels
Claus et al. [31], 2013	Prospective observational	ARC: 54 (44–61) Non-ARC: 66 (57–77)	ICU patients receiving antimicrobial therapies	128	ARC: 73 Non-ARC: 61	98 (57–164) mL/min/1.73 m²	Measured 8 h-CrCl determined; measuring the effect of ARC on antimicrobial therapy failure	• 52% of patients identified to have ARC (CrCl > 130 mL/min/1.73 m²), mainly younger and male • 27% of ARC patients had therapeutic failure (poor clinical response to antimicrobial therapy), more often than non-ARC patients (13%) ($p = 0.04$)
Minkute et al. [32], 2013	Retrospective observational	ARC: 46 (21–66) Non-ARC: 54 (22–86)	Patients treated with vancomycin	36	80	Estimated CG ARC: 151 (131–324) Non-ARC: 103 (90–127)	Vancomycin level comparison between ARC and non-ARC groups	• 50% of patients identified to have ARC (CrCl > 130 mL/min, using CG) • Vancomycin concentrations were lower in ARC group compared to Non-ARC • Vancomycin doses up to 44 mg/kg/day were needed in the ARC group to achieve target trough levels.
Roberts and Lipman [33], 2013	PK study (analysis of Phase III trial data)	58 ± 15	ICU patients with pneumonia	31	93	Estimated by CG 137 ± 71	Population PK of doripenem in critically ill.	• Doripenem clearance correlated with CrCl and was increased compared to non-ICU patients
Shimamoto et al. [34], 2013	Retrospective observational	Non-SIRS: 64 SIRS-2: 54 SIRS-3: 49 SIRS-4: 42	ICU (Septic patients on vancomycin)	105	66	Using CG No-SIRS: 121 ± 51 SIRS-2: 160 ± 65 SIRS-3: 195 ± 70 SIRS-4: 191 ± 77	Identified patients who had SIRS and categorized based on the number of SIRS criteria they had (non-SIRS, SIRS-2, 3 and 4); vancomycin CL and CrCl (CG) determined	• In patients age < 50: higher SIRS score predicted higher vancomycin clearance • In patients age > 50: higher SIRS does not reliably predict higher vancomycin clearance

Table 1. *Cont.*

Author, Year	Study Type	Age (Years) Median (IQR)	Population	N	Sex (% Male)	Measured CrCl (mL/min)— Otherwise Specified	Intervention	Main Results
Udy et al. [35], 2013	Prospective observational	42 ± 17	ICU (trauma, septic; SCr < 110 µmol/L)	71	63	Mean: 135 ± 52	They determined the prevalence and risk factors of ARC	• 58% of patients identified to have ARC; more in trauma patients; generally younger; males, with lower APACHE II, SOFA and higher cardiac index • Three risk factors suggested to predict ARC: age < 50 years, trauma, and SOFA score ≤ 4 (ARC score)
Udy et al. [36], 2013	Prospective observational	51 ± 17	ICU patients with SCr < 121 µmol/L	110	64	Mean: 125 ± 45 mL/min/1.73 m²	Measured 8 h CrCl compared to estimated CrCl (CG and CKD-EPI)	• CKD-EPI and CG underestimated CrCl in patients with ARC • In patients with CKD-EPI eGFR = 60–119 mL/min/1.73 m², 42% had ARC
Baptista et al. [37], 2012	Prospective observational	Non-ARC: 70 (52–79) ARC: 41 (32–56)	ICU septic patients on vancomycin	93	Non-ARC: 71 ARC: 79	Non-ARC: 70 (58–104) ARC: 159 (141–194)	The effect of ARC on vancomycin PK: ARC patients compared to non-ARC patients; measured 24 h CrCl Vancomycin dosing: A loading dose of 1000 mg if wt. < 70 kg or 1500 mg if wt. > 70 kg then 30 mg/kg/day continuous infusion	• Serum vancomycin concentrations in ARC were significantly lower than control group for the 3 days of study
Grootaert et al. [38], 2012	Retrospective observational	59 (48–67)	ICU patients with measured CrCl > 120 mL/min (24-h method)	390	63	148 (132–172) mL/min/1.73 m²	Measured 24-h CrCl compared with CG method (CrCl) and 4-variable MDRD method (eGFR)	• CG and MDRD underestimated measured CrCl in ARC patients
Udy et al. [39], 2012	Prospective observational	53 ± 21	ICU	48	71	134 ± 90	Measured 8 h CrCl; beta lactam antibiotic concentrations measured	• For patients with trough less than MIC and less than 4× MIC: 82 and 72% had CrCl > 130 mL/min/1.73 m², respectively • A 25 mL/min/1.73 m² increase in CrCl is associated with a 60% reduction in the probability of obtaining a trough concentration ≥ 4×MIC

Table 1. *Cont.*

Author, Year	Study Type	Age (Years) Median (IQR)	Population	N	Sex (% Male)	Measured CrCl (mL/min)—Otherwise Specified	Intervention	Main Results
Baptista et al. [40], 2011	Retrospective observational (post hoc analysis)	35 (25–51)	ICU patients with ARC	86	77	162 (145–190) mL/min/1.73 m²	Measured 8-h (Australia) or 24 h (Portugal) CrCl compared with CG, modified CG, 4-variable MDRD and 6-variable MDRD	• All CrCl estimates underestimated measured CrCl • CG estimates had the greatest sensitivity→identified 62% of cohort with ARC; lower sensitivity observed with 4-variable MDRD (47%) and 6-variable MDRD (29%) formulae
Minville et al. [41], 2011	Retrospective observational	NPT: 58 ± 17 PT: 42 ± 18	ICU	284	NPT: 63 PT: 75	NPT: 85 ± 5 PT: 131 ± 5 mL/min/1.73 m²	Measured 24-h CrCl; compared among patients with (NPT) and without polytrauma (PT)	• 37% of patients identified to have ARC (CrCl > 120 mL/min; significantly more trauma patients; younger; had lower SAPS II score; males • Age and trauma independently correlated to CrCl
Spencer et al. [42], 2011	Prospective PK study	54 ± 14	Neuro ICU	12	42	96 ± 32 (estimated, method not reported)	Patients received levetiracetam 500 mg iv every 12 h; levetiracetam levels measured	• Levetiracetam clearance was higher in neurocritical care population compared to healthy volunteers (drug clearance directly proportional to estimated CrCl $r^2 = 0.5$, $p = 0.01$); Higher doses of levetiracetam are recommended in neurocritical care population
Coboova et al. [43], 2015	Case Report	16	ICU (Polytrauma and sepsis)	1	100	Method not reported Day 29: 138 Days 41–51: 340 mL/min/1.73 m²	Vancomycin initiated at doses of 1 g IV every 12 h then titrated up	• A trauma patient who developed ARC later during hospital stay • Vancomycin needed to be increased to up to 6 g per day to achieve therapeutic target trough level • Vancomycin increased to 2 g Q12H, which produced troughs of 15 mg/L and 10 mg/L • Increase in CrCl observed on day 46, vancomycin trough decreased to 5 mg/L, then dose increased to 2 g Q8H (67 mg/kg/day): trough: 19 mg/L.

Table 1. *Cont.*

Author, Year	Study Type	Age (Years) Median (IQR)	Population	N	Sex (% Male)	Measured CrCl (mL/min)— Otherwise Specified	Intervention	Main Results
Abdul-Aziz et al. [44], 2014	Case Report	36	ICU (CNS infection)	1	100	234	Days 1–3: Flucloxacillin 2 g IV Q4H Days 4–16: Flucloxacillin 20 g/day via continuous infusion	• A case report of an ICU patient with CNS infection • Presence of ARC (Measured 8 h) lead to difficulty achieving therapeutic flucloxacillin concentration above MIC with conventional dosing (IV 2 g Q4H) • A continuous infusion of high dose flucloxacillin (20 g/day) was required to achieve clinical cure
Cook et al. [45], 2013	Case Report	22	Neuro ICU (TBI)	1	0	Method not reported 153	They described a case of ARC leading to subtherapeutic vancomycin and levetiracetam levels	• A conventional vancomycin dose 750 mg IV Q12H (17.5 mg/kg/dose) yielded a trough level of 2.2 mg/L (subtherapeutic); dose had to be increased to 1.25 g iv Q8H (29 mg/kg/dose) to achieve a trough of 11 mg/L • Levetiracetam dose was increased from 1000 mg IV BID to 1000 mg Q8H to maintain a trough within reference range (usual dose 0.5–1 g iv Q12H)
Lonsdale et al. [46], 2013	Case Report	44	Neuro ICU (SAH with ventriculitis)	1	100	375 mL/min/1.73 m^2	They described a case of ARC leading to subtherapeutic vancomycin and meropenem levels	• The patient required dose escalation of vancomycin up to 6 g/day (Vancomycin 63 mg/kg/day) in order to achieve therapeutic trough levels (usual dose 45 mg/kg/d for CNS infections) • The patient required dose escalation of meropenem up to 2 g every 6 h in order to achieve therapeutic levels (usual dose 2 g iv Q8H for CNS infections)
Troger et al. [47], 2012	Case Reports	Pt 1: 37 Pt 2: 66	ICU patients with sepsis	2	100	Estimated with CG Pt 1: Initially: 138 Day 5: 276 Pt 2: Initially: 185 Later: 219	Described 2 cases of sepsis patients who required high doses of meropenem secondary to ARC Pt 1: meropenem 1 g IV Q8H then increased to meropenem 2 g IV Q4H Pt 2: meropenem 1 g Q8H then dose increased to1 g Q6H then to 2 g Q6H Meropenem trough target 4–10 mg/L	• Pt 1: meropenem dose was increased to 2 g IV Q4H × 1 week, trough was still <4 mg/L but procalcitonin decreased and clinical improvement was observed • Pt 2: meropenem dose was increased to 2 g Q6H, producing a trough concentration of 8.4 mg/L.

Table 1. *Cont.*

Author, Year	Study Type	Age (Years) Median (IQR)	Population	N	Sex (% Male)	Measured CrCl (mL/min)— Otherwise Specified	Intervention	Main Results
Udy et al. [3], 2010	Case Series	Pt 1: 19 Pt 2: 41 Pt 3: 32	ICU Pt 1 TBI Pt 2 Surgery Pt 3 Burn	3	100	Pt 1: 224 Pt 2: 206 Pt 3: 151 Measured 8 h CrCl	Three case reports of patients with ARC Pt. 1: meropenem Pt 2: vancomycin + meropenem Pt 3: amikacin + ciprofloxacin	• Pt 1: meropenem 1 g Q8H, increased to 2 g Q8H due to undetectable trough serum concentration; pt. still did not have detectable concentration • Pt 2: vancomycin doses were increased up to 4 g (44 mg/kg) continuous infusion over 24-h for clinical cure; Meropenem increased to 1 g Q4H to reach target trough • Pt 3: Amikacin 1 g daily was increased up to 1.2 g Q12H due to undetectable trough levels
Caro et al. [48], 2016 Abstract	Phase I PK study	Range 29–50	ICU patients with ARC (CrCl $\geq$ 180 mL/min estimated by CG)	5	40	Estimated using CG 282 (207–417)	Determined the PK of ceftolozane/tazobactam in patients with ARC	• Study identified higher clearance of ceftolozane/tazobactam in ARC patients compared to non-ARC patients
Goboova et al. [49], 2016 Abstract	Retrospective observational	Mean 42 ± 14	Patients treated with gentamicin	204	78	Method not reported ARC Patients: 166 ± 28 mL/min/1.73 m^2	Identification of the influence of ARC on gentamicin dosing	• 14% of patients identified to have ARC (CrCl > 130 mL/min/1.73 m^2; • 93% of ARC patients were under-dosed (low peak levels) with standard gentamicin regimens
Morbitzer et al. [50], 2016 Abstract	Prospective observational	63 (56–71)	Neuro ICU (Hemorrhagic stroke)	17	27	131 (108–216) mL/min/1.73 m^2	Measured 8-h CrCl compared with CG method; vancomycin trough concentration determined	• CG method underestimated CrCl in ARC patients • Measured vancomycin trough was lower than predicted
Morimoto and Ishikura [51], 2016 Abstract	Prospective observational	Not reported	ICU (Japan)	33	Not reported	Not reported	CrCl measured (method not reported)	• 39% of patients identified to have ARC (CrCl > 130 mL/min/1.73 m^2); mainly younger, less males, had lower APACHE II score and not septic
Dunning and Roberts [52], 2015 Abstract	A survey	N/A	N/A	123	N/A	N/A	A survey of 123 ICU physicians about antibiotic prescribing and renal function assessment	• 15% responded that they would consider modifying the dosage regimen of beta-lactams and vancomycin antimicrobials in patients with ARC This highlights the need for dosing guidance in patients with ARC.

Table 1. *Cont.*

Author, Year	Study Type	Age (Years) Median (IQR)	Population	N	Sex (% Male)	Measured CrCl (mL/min)—Otherwise Specified	Intervention	Main Results
Baptista et al. [53], 2014 Abstract	Retrospective observational	Not reported	ICU	477	Not reported	Not reported	CrCl measured by 8 h urine collection	• 33% of patients identified to have ARC (CrCl > 130 mL/min/1.73 m²) • Urinary creatinine > 45 mg/mL and age < 65 are identified as best predictors of ARC (sensitivity 60%, specificity = 88%); specificity increased to 95% by adding BUN < 7 mmol/L
May et al. [54], 2014 Abstract	Prospective observational	Not reported	Neuro ICU (SAH)	20	Not reported	326 ± 135 mL/min/1.73 m²	Measured 24-h CrCl determined; Monte-Carlo Simulation to achieve levetiracetam doses to achieve trough levels ≥ 6 mg/L	• Estimated CrCl (method not reported) significantly underestimated CrCl • Monte Carlo Simulation suggested that levetiracetam dosing poorly achieved target attainment unless TID was used (as opposed to standard regimen)
Vermis et al. [55], 2014 Abstract	Retrospective observational	Not reported	Patients with hematological malignancies	96	Not reported	CrCl estimated using CG ARC pts: 147 Non-ARC pts: 79	Aimed to determine the prevalence of ARC in a hematological population; Vancomycin continuous infusion: loading 15 mg/kg, maintenance 30 mg/kg given and titrated based on levels Vancomycin trough target: 20 mg/L	• Therapeutic vancomycin trough targets were achieved with dose of 42 mg/kg/day in ARC patients (day 5 post initiation) and with 33 mg/kg/day in non-ARC (day 3 post initiation).
Weigel et al. [56], 2014 Abstract	Retrospective observational	55	ICU patients without renal replacement and receiving vancomycin infusion	287	69	ARC: MDRD eGFR > 130 Non ARC: MDRD eGFR < 130	A vancomycin loading dose of 20 mg/kg was given then adjusted by Therapeutic drug monitoring to target 20–25 mg/L; Vancomycin levels compared in patients with various degrees of eGFR using MDRD	• Subtherapeutic vancomycin levels were more frequent in patients with MDRD > 130 mL/min (55%) i.e., ARC vs. patients with MDRD < 130 mL/min (29%) $p < 0.001$ • Higher than conventional vancomycin dosing is recommended in patients with ARC
Neves et al. [57], 2013 Abstract	Prospective observational	55 ± 13	ICU	54	72	Mean: 138	Measured 8-h CrCl compared with CG method	• ARC identified in 50% of samples • Per subgroup analyses: CrCl > 120 mL/min/1.73 m², CG underestimated measured CrCl; CrCl < 120 mL/min/1.73 m², CG overestimated measured CrCl

Table 1. *Cont.*

Author, Year	Study Type	Age (Years) Median (IQR)	Population	N	Sex (% Male)	Measured CrCl (mL/min)— Otherwise Specified	Intervention	Main Results
Grootaert et al. [58], 2012 Abstract	Retrospective observational	66 (56–75)	ICU patients with measured CrCl available	1317	63	Not reported	Measured 24-h CrCl	• 16% of patients identified to have ARC (CrCl > 120 mL/min): mainly younger, taller, have lower BMI and had longer ICU stay • 30% patients had at least 1 episode of ARC Relative duration of ARC per patient was 5 days in all pts, and 7 days in antimicrobial group
Drust et al. [59], 2011 Abstract	Retrospective observational	Not reported	ICU patients with CrCl > 120 mL/min	15	Not reported	>120	Meropenem plasma concentrations measured	• 27% of patients had appropriate meropenem plasma levels • 67% of patients required higher doses of meropenem (up to 8 g/day) than recommended

ANP = atrial natriuretic peptide; APACHE II = Acute Physiology and Chronic Health Evaluation; ARC = Augmented Renal Clearance; CG = Cockcroft Gault equation; CKD-EPI = Chronic Kidney Disease Epidemiology; CN = controlled normothermia; CrCl = creatinine clearance; GFR = glomerular filtration rate; ICU = intensive care unit; IQR = interquartile range; MDRD = modification of diet in renal disease method; MIC = minimum inhibitory concentration; PK = pharmacokinetic; PT = patient; PTA = probability of target attainment; SAH = subarachnoid hemorrhage; SAPS II = Simplified Acute Physiology Score SCr = serum creatinine; SIRS = systemic inflammatory response syndrome; SOFA = sequential organ failure assessment score; TBI = traumatic brain injury; TH = therapeutic hypothermia. Age and CrCl reported in median (IQR) or mean ± SD.

3.1. ARC Definition and Prevalence

Augmented renal clearance (ARC), also reported as glomerular hyperfiltration or enhanced renal clearance, is an increase in kidney function that results in enhanced clearance of drugs with potential for therapy failure. ARC has been defined using creatinine clearance (CrCl). However, the definition of ARC in relation to CrCl cutoff has varied among studies, thus impeding accurate identification of ARC prevalence among intensive care unit (ICU) patients. Although, many research groups have defined ARC as patients with creatinine clearance > 130 mL/min/1.73 m^2 (Table 1), other creatinine clearance cutoffs have been suggested including ARC cutoff of CrCl > 120 mL/min/m^2 [26,38,41,55,58], and >160 mL/min/1.73 m^2 [11]. The definition of ARC was further complicated with the duration at which CrCl above the suggested cutoff. The majority of the studies have considered one occurrence of CrCl above cutoff is sufficient to acknowledge the presence of ARC. However, both Baptista et al. [24] and DeWaele et al. [15] elected to use the definition of ARC as CrCl > 130 mL/min/1.73 m^2 for more than half of the CrCl measures during a minimum of 72 h of ICU stay. This acknowledges the concern if the current definition of CrCl cutoff (without timeframe specification) truly captures the clinical implication (i.e., the point where changes must be made for renally cleared medications) to patient care. Furthermore, it is not clear if additional cutoffs beyond CrCl of 130 mL/min/1.73 m^2 are needed to stage ARC parallel the categories used to describe renal dysfunction i.e., mild, moderate and severe ARC. However, despite the various definitions observed, based on the large number of studies using the definition CrCl cutoffs of >130 mL/min/1.73 m^2, as well as associated clinical implications at this cut off point, we recommend a unified definition of ARC using CrCl > 130 mL/min/1.73 m^2 as the clinical cut-off in the adult population.

ARC has been reported to range from 14 to 80% (Table 1), suggesting that ARC is a commonly occurring clinical phenomenon. However, these studies may perhaps over- or under-estimate the true prevalence of ARC due to few reasons. First, the most common practice setting where ARC was identified is within the setting of the ICU. Since rigorous patient monitoring is a common practice within the ICU, including daily measures of renal function, it is much easier to identify ARC. In addition, critically ill are exposed to factors that may increase the likelihood of ARC occurrence, such as the use of intravenous fluids, vasopressors and inotropes [60,61]. Second, as discussed above, variations in ARC definitions might impede the true prevalence of ARC. Third, ARC prevalence needs to be interpreted in the context of the study patient selection criteria. For example, exclusion of patients with renal dysfunction will result in higher percentage of patients with ARC and vice versa.

The true onset and duration of ARC in critically ill is not known. In studies that assessed renal function more than one occasion throughout the ICU stay, it appears that the onset of ARC coincides with an acute insult to the body. In a prospective observational study of patients admitted to ICU, Udy et al. have reported that 65% of patients, identified to have ARC, had at least 1 occasion of measured ARC during the first 7 days of admission with 38% of those had ARC on the first day of ICU admission [29]. Occurrence of ARC on day 1 of ICU admission significantly predicted sustained CrCl elevation over the first seven days of the ICU stay (p = 0.019). Similarly, Huttner et al. have reported that 64% of patients had ARC at study enrollment [17]. Duration of ARC has varied among studies owing to difference in monitoring frequency and duration. While many studies have reported persistence of ARC for weeks [17,43,45,46,58], fewer patients exhibited transient ARC lasting for no more than 1 day [31]. Given the current unpredictability of ARC duration, continuous monitoring of patient's renal function is warranted as alteration in drug dosing might be required.

3.2. Pathophysiology

Our current understanding of the ARC pathophysiology remains limited. It has been reported that ARC is associated with increased glomerular filtration, renal tubular secretion of anions, and renal tubular reabsorption using various exogenous markers, suggesting that ARC affects many components of the nephron physiology [28]. It has been suggested that ARC is a hyperdynamic response to insults to the body. In the early study conducted by Ljungberg and Nilsson-Ehle, acute infection has been observed to be associated with enhanced renal clearance [62]. This has been attributed to changes in vascular permeability and increased renal blood flow secondary to elevated body temperature. Similarly, the effect of temperature changes on renal function has been reported in patients exposed to induced hypothermia. In a retrospective study comparing vancomycin pharmacokinetic in patients with controlled normothermia (median temperature = 37.2 °C) to patients with induced hypothermia (median temperature = 34 °C), Morbitzer et al. have demonstrated that vancomycin clearance was higher in controlled normothermic patients [18].

In addition to altered body temperature, insult to the brain could lead to ARC. Dias et al. have identified a possible link between the brain and the kidneys in their retrospective analysis of 18 severe traumatic brain injury (TBI) patients managed with intracranial pressure monitoring in the neurocritical care setting [16]. Analyzing cerebrovascular pressure reactivity index (PRx, a correlation index between intracranial pressure and arterial blood pressure that reflects the capability cerebral arteries to react to changes in blood pressure and is a key element of cerebral autoregulation) in ARC-manifesting patients showed a strong negative correlation ($r = -0.81$, $p < 0.001$) between PRx and creatinine clearance. This correlation suggests that reduction in cerebral autoregulation (i.e., after a TBI) is associated with an increase in creatinine clearance, adding an evidence to the theory that the central autoregulation plays a significant role in the manifestation of ARC. In another study of 11 TBI patients by Udy et al., atrial natriuretic peptide (ANP) levels have been found to be elevated in TBI patients suggesting that ANP following brain may play a role in enhancing glomerular filtration through increased natriuresis and diuresis [7]. The results of the correlation between ANP and CrCl, however, did not reach statistical significance.

Sime et al. have proposed a model of hyperdynamic state to bring forth a pathophysiology model to the occurrence of ARC [63]. It has been suggested that a number of factors consequential to critical illness combine to produce ARC. Systemic inflammatory response syndrome (SIRS) associated with critical illness results in the increase of inflammatory mediators. These mediators produce decrease in vascular resistance in the peripheries and increase in cardiac output. These two responses combine to produce a hyperdynamic state within the body system, resulting in increased renal blood flow, followed by glomerular hyperfiltration that manifest itself as ARC. Additionally, common to the ICU setting, critically ill patients are often subjected to fluid therapy and treatment with vasoactive drugs and inotropes thereby further increasing cardiac output that would more likely to contribute to the already-increased hyperdynamic state. Furthermore, critical illness also may have direct effect on the kidneys, further enhancing renal clearance in ARC. Although this model suggested by Sime et al. provides a logical explanation to the pathophysiology leading to ARC, the exact mechanism to which ARC, as a sequelae of physiological insult, remains uncertain.

3.3. ARC Risk Factors

Various studies (Table 1) have shown that patients exhibiting ARC tend to be younger (<50 years old), of male gender, had a recent history of trauma, and had lower critical illness severity scores such as sequential organ failure assessment score (SOFA) [35], Simplified Acute Physiology Score (SAPS) II [41] or Acute Physiology and Chronic Health Evaluation (APACHE II) [35,51]. Young age appears to be the only risk factor consistently recognized by various epidemiology studies to be able to reliably predict ARC (Table 1). In addition, Hirai et al. have identified febrile neutropenia to be an independent risk factor of ARC the pediatric cancer population [11].

Recognizing the need for a clinical prediction tool to identify patients at risk for manifesting ARC, Baptista et al. [53] have conducted a retrospective study in 447 patients admitted to an ICU at a tertiary hospital over a 1-year period, and assessed patient characteristics on its predictability of ARC occurrence. Urinary creatinine > 45 mg/mL and age < 65 years have been identified as best predictors of ARC (sensitivity 60%, specificity = 88%); specificity increased to 95% by adding BUN < 7 mmol/L. Furthermore, Udy et al. [35]. developed an ARC scoring system based on the risk of factors of age < 50 years old, presence of trauma, and SOFA score $\leq$ 4 (Table 2). This predictive tool was later validated by Akers et al., demonstrating a sensitivity of 100% and specificity of 71% for detecting patients with ARC, based on confirmation data from altered piperacillin/tazobactam pharmacokinetics in ICU patients [23]. Because of the impracticality need to complete a SOFA score in ARC scoring system, Barletta et al. have developed the augmented renal clearance in trauma intensive Care (ARCTIC) scoring system (Table 2) [4]. The ARCTIC scoring system employed the patient factors: serum creatinine, sex and age to identify those with high ARC risk (ARCTIC score > 6). The ARCTIC scoring system produced a sensitivity of 84% and specificity of 68%. Given the need for early recognition of ARC in the ICU setting, the use of the ARC or ARCTIC predictive tools allow for identification of at risk patients, and help direct clinicians to take appropriate interventions (e.g., obtain a measured creatinine clearance, employ more aggressive antibiotic dosing regimen/strategies, etc.).

Table 2. The ARC risk scoring systems.

	ARC Scoring System [23,35]	ARCTIC Scoring System [4]
Criteria	Age 50 or younger = 6 pts Trauma = 3 pts SOFA score ≤ 4 = 1 pt	SCr < 62 μmol/L = 3 pts Male sex = 2 pts Age <56 years = 4 pts Age: 56–75 years = 3 pts
Interpretation	0–6 points→low ARC risk 7–10 points→high ARC risk	>6 points→high ARC risk <6 points→low ARC risk
Sensitivity	100%	84%
Specificity	71%	68%

ARC = augmented renal clearance; ARCTIC = augmented renal clearance in trauma intensive Care (ARCTIC); SOFA = sequential organ failure assessment score; SCr = serum creatinine concentration; pt = point; pts = points.

3.4. Creatinine Clearance: Estimation Methods and ARC

Although risk factors and predictive models offer a method to screen for those at an increased risk for ARC, the actual identification of ARC requires accurate glomerular filtration rate (GFR) determination. While determination of inulin clearance is regarded as the gold standard for measuring GFR because CrCl might overestimate kidney function, affected by muscle mass and physical activity, urinary measurement of creatinine clearance (from 8 to 24 h of urine collection) is currently the most common measurement of renal function in the clinical setting [64]. That's because inulin clearance determination is labor intensive and requires administration of an exogenous substance. Because routine measurement of creatinine clearance is impractical, mathematical estimates of creatinine clearance based on population parameters are often employed to allow for prompt determination. Commonly used mathematical estimates of creatinine clearance/glomerular filtration rate (GFR) include the Cockcroft Gault equation (CG), the Modification of Diet in Renal Diseases (MDRD) formulae, and the Chronic Kidney Disease-Epidemiology (CKD-EPI) equation. These equations all have been validated in various populations, and their respective merits and deficiencies have been described elsewhere [65]. Measured creatinine clearance has been reported in 59% of the included studies. On the other hand creatinine clearance has been estimated only or not reported in 25 and 16% of the included studies, respectively (Table 1). In studies assessing the accuracy of mathematical estimates of creatinine clearance in the ARC population, all the mathematical estimations of creatinine clearance have been found to underestimate the actual measured creatinine clearance in patients with ARC [8,19,21,22,24,36,38,40,50,57].

Comparison of the various mathematical estimates suggest the Cockcroft Gault (CG) formula may be the best method of creatinine clearance estimation in the ARC population. To illustrate, Udy et al. have assessed the accuracy of the CKD-EPI estimation of creatinine clearance in comparison to 8-h measured creatinine clearance in 110 ICU patients [36]. Around 42% of the patients identified by the CKD-EPI equation to have creatinine clearance within the range of 60–119 mL/min/1.73 m^2 exhibited ARC (measured CrCl > 130). In a study conducted by Baptista et al., the CG and MDRD

(4- and 6-variable) estimations of creatinine clearance were compared to measured creatinine clearance using 8-h or 24-h urine sampling [40]. In patients exhibiting ARC, CG estimate was able to detect 62% of the cohort exhibiting ARC, while the MDRD estimations demonstrated lower sensitivity, with the 4-variable MDRD formula detecting 47% of the cohort while the 6-variable MDRD formula was only able to detect 27% of the cohort exhibiting ARC. Similarly, Barletta et al. have found that measured creatinine clearance were significantly higher ($p < 0.001$) than all estimates of creatinine clearance (CG, 4-variable MDRD, and CKD-EPI equation) with the CG method demonstrating the lowest bias [8]. However the CG method may only be used as a screening tool for ARC. Even if a CG estimate show an estimated creatinine clearance within the normal reference range, there is a still a high likelihood that ARC can be present in a patient. Therefore, in the setting of ICU, it would be prudent to assess a patient's measured creatinine clearance at least once, to determine whether a patient is truly experiencing ARC, and to also gauge the level of bias in the estimated creatinine clearance for that patient. Finally, we would like to mention that although serum creatinine used for determination of creatinine clearance is a reliable marker within the general population, consideration must be made when applying this measurement in patients with lower muscle mass, immobility, children or other conditions in which muscle mass are altered. Due to the reduced production of creatinine in these patients, falsely low measures of serum creatinine may inaccurately identify ARC in those populations.

3.5. Drug Therapy in ARC Population

3.5.1. Pharmacokinetic Changes in ARC

In the ICU setting, pharmacokinetic changes to drug therapy in the presence of ARC may have drastic implications on patient outcome. This is especially important to drugs that are renally cleared known to exhibit direct correlation between their renal clearance and creatinine clearance such as aminoglycoside antimicrobials, vancomycin and levetiracetam. Enhanced drug clearance will lead to shorter drug half-life ($t_{\frac{1}{2}}$), lower maximum drug concertation (C_{max}) and lower area under the concentration curve (AUC) which could have direct implication on drugs' pharmacodynamic effects leading to therapy failure. This particularly important for antimicrobials that are time-dependent killers (efficacy depends on the duration of the drug concentration or AUC above the minimum inhibitory concentration (MIC) of the pathogen T > MIC) and concentration-dependent killers (efficacy depends on the Cmax of the drug relative to the MIC of the pathogen). Currently, antimicrobial monograms and various dosing guidelines have not acknowledged the need for alterations to drug dosing regimen in the ARC population. In a survey of ICU physicians in England clarifying their attitudes regarding antibiotic prescribing and assessment of renal function in septic patients, only 15% responded that they would consider modifying the dosage regimen of beta-lactams and vancomycin antimicrobials in patients with ARC [52]. This highlights the need for dosing guidance in patients with ARC.

3.5.2. Vancomycin

Vancomycin, a glycopeptide antibiotic, is one of the antimicrobials of choice for the treatment of serious, life-threatening infections by Gram-positive bacteria. It is a hydrophilic drug that is 80–90% excreted unchanged by the kidneys and its clearance is highly dependent on renal function. Previous pharmacokinetic and pharmacodynamic studies have established that steady state vancomycin trough level is a good surrogate of AUC:MIC which is in turn correlated with treatment success [66].

Currently, there is a growing body of evidence suggesting inadequate therapeutic vancomycin trough levels attained using conventional dosing in patients exhibiting ARC [9,25,26,32,43,45,50,55]. For example, Campassi et al. have reported that 100% of patients with ARC did not have vancomycin trough levels within the target 15–25 mg/L 3 days following vancomycin initiation despite getting high vancomycin doses [26]. Currently, studies on the clinical outcome of subtherapeutic serum concentration of vancomycin in ARC patients are scarce. However, it has been reported that in patients who did not reach therapeutic trough target 15–25 mg/L 48 h post treatment initiation, in-hospital mortality was significantly higher than those who have attained therapeutic target trough (OR = 2.1, $p = 0.003$) [20].

Various vancomycin dosing regimens have been suggested and tested in patients with ARC. In a study by Vermis et al., vancomycin therapeutic drug monitoring (TDM) has been implemented and vancomycin dose adjustment was based on vancomycin trough level 5 days post vancomycin initiation [55]. The average doses successful to achieve trough levels within target were 42 and 33 mg/kg/day in patients with ARC and without ARC, respectively. The authors proposed a loading dose of 25 mg/kg loading dose followed by 40 mg/kg/day for those with CrCl > 130 mL/min. Similarly, Minkute et al. have reported the need for vancomycin doses up to 44 mg/kg/day to achieve trough levels within target [32]. Baptista et al. [25] have suggested a vancomycin dosing strategy using 8 h measured creatinine clearance to achieve a target trough of 25 mg/L. The nomogram suggested has been validated in a second group of patients in the same study and has been found to produce 84% target attainment in patients with ARC.

3.5.3. Beta-Lactam Antimicrobials

Beta-lactams antibiotics are primarily renally eliminated thereby are affected by presence of ARC. Unlike vancomycin or aminoglycosides, therapeutic drug monitoring is not common for beta-lactam antibiotics. Clinicians generally prescribe guideline-recommended regimens without the need to conduct therapeutic drug monitoring. Although following the patients' clinical status after prescribing a beta-lactam is appropriate and acceptable in the general population, dismissal of beta-lactam concentration in the ARC population, where very little evidence exists and no dosing guidelines have been recommended, poses a substantial threat to treatment success and patient outcome. Numerous studies have reported beta-lactam treatment failures (based on sub-therapeutic serum level attainment) when using standard beta-lactam dosing regimens in patients with ARC (discussed below and in Table 1).

Carbapenems

Carbapenems (such as meropenem, imipenem, doripenem and ertapenem) are a family of broad spectrum beta-lactams used for the treatment of multi-drug resistant bacteria. They exhibit time-dependent antibacterial activity and their activity can be best illustrated by the T > MIC pharmacodynamic model [67]. Various studies have reported poor target achievement in ARC patients using conventional regimens. Binder et al. have reported that standard meropenem doses (500–1000 mg every 8 or 12 h) in ICU patients with estimated creatinine >60 mL/min result in lower meropenem AUC secondary to increased clearance suggesting the need for alternate regimen in this population [68]. Similarly, Drust et al. have reported that almost two-thirds of the ICU patents with CrCl > 120 mL/min required higher doses (up to 8 g/day) of meropenem than current recommended therapy to achieve effective plasma meropenem concentrations [59]. In addition, extended infusion have also been suggested for appropriate target T > MIC target attainment and treatment success. Carlier et al. have assessed the efficacy of whether meropenem extended infusion (1 g over 30 min, followed by a maintenance dose of meropenem 1 g infused over a period of 3 h every 8 h) would be a suitable alternative strategy for meropenem dosing in ARC patients [30]. Extended infusion did not improve meropenem plasma concentration by the end of the study, with lower percentage of ARC patients (61%) achieving T > MIC therapeutic target in comparison to non-ARC patients (94%, $p < 0.001$). In addition to meropenem, doripenem pharmacokinetics have been studied in critically ill patients with ARC [33]. Similarly, higher doses of doripenem have been suggested in patients with ARC.

Piperacillin/Tazobactam

Piperacillin/tazobactam is an extended spectrum beta-lactam antibiotic indicated for the treatment of severe multi-drug resistant infections. Like all beta-lactam antibiotics, piperacillin/tazobactam exhibits time-dependent bacterial eradication (T > MIC). Piperacillin/tazobactam is eliminated renally, and dose adjustment of piperacillin/tazobactam has been described for renally impaired population. There are many reports of subtherapeutic target attainment using conventional piperacillin/tazobactam dosing in ICU patients with ARC. Huttner et al. have assessed target attainment of various beta-lactams in the ICU population (ARC observed in 64% of the study cohort) [17]. Subtherapeutic serum concentrations have been reported with intravenous doses of piperacillin/tazobactam 4.5 g every eight hours in 61% of the treated patients. In addition, undetectable piperacillin/tazobactam concentrations were seen in 7% of the patients. To address the issue of subtherapeutic target attainment of piperacillin/tazobactam especially in ICU patients with ARC, various dosage regimens have been tested and suggested [6,23]. A Monte-Carlo simulation conducted by Akers et al. have suggested that doses above the FDA approved doses (up to 36 g per day) might be needed to achieve high probability of target achievement [23]. Unfortunately, the study by Akers et al. was not aimed to assess any of the dosing regimens modelled in their study and these proposed regimens still require validation.

Other Beta-Lactam Antimicrobials

Aside from few other studies [14,48], the evidence of the other members of the beta-lactams is scarce. However, as suggested by the body of evidence on meropenem and piperacillin/tazobactam, it is likely that all beta-lactams that are eliminated renally might be affected by the ARC phenomenon and require further research.

3.5.4. Other Medications

Aminoglycosides are mainly renally eliminated with predictable efficacy based on serum concentrations. Goboova et al. have conducted a retrospective analysis of 204 patients receiving gentamicin, in which 14% of the patients exhibited ARC [49]. The patients in the study were initially treated with conventional gentamicin regimen. Analysis of gentamicin peak concentration at steady state identified 93% of the ARC patients had subtherapeutic steady state concentrations which required dose escalation to attain target peak levels. This highlights the value of therapeutic drug monitoring in the setting of ARC.

Fluoroquinolones are another family of antibiotics affected by altering renal clearance. Due to predictability of current dosing in patients normal or impaired renal function, TDM is not necessary. However, TDM could be of value when using fluoroquinolones in patients with ARC and higher doses may be required. For example, using Monte Carlo simulation, levofloxacin doses of 1 g every 24 h have been suggested for infections caused by *S. pneumoniae*, *P. aeruginosa*, and *S. aureus* in patients with CrCl > 130 mL/min (conventional dosing 0.5–0.75 g every 24 h) [13].

In addition to antimicrobials, other agents have been tested such as levetiracetam and enoxaparin. Levetiracetam is a broad spectrum antiepileptic drug (AED) that has a more favorable side effect profile compared to older AEDs. It displays linear elimination kinetics; therefore dose changes produce relatively predictable changes in serum concentrations. However, it is renally eliminated and its clearance is directly proportional to CrCl and thus could be affected in patients with ARC. There are few reports discussing the enhanced elimination of levetiracetam in TBI and SAH patients with ARC [42,45,54]. Accordingly, Higher initial levetiracetam doses (1 g IV every 8 h) have been suggested in patients with high risk for ARC [42,54]. Enoxaparin, a low molecular weight heparin, also has been reported to be affected by presence of ARC suggested the need for more rigorous monitoring of anti-factor Xa activity in patients with ARC [5].

4. Conclusions

Augmented renal clearance (ARC) is a manifestation of enhanced renal function seen in critically ill patients. The current evidence presented in this review identified the significance of this phenomenon and the need for higher doses of renally eliminated drugs in patients with ARC. More research is needed to solidify dosing recommendations of various drugs in patients with ARC. However, based on the current evidence few recommendations could be put forward to guide clinicians in managing patients presenting with ARC (Figure 2).

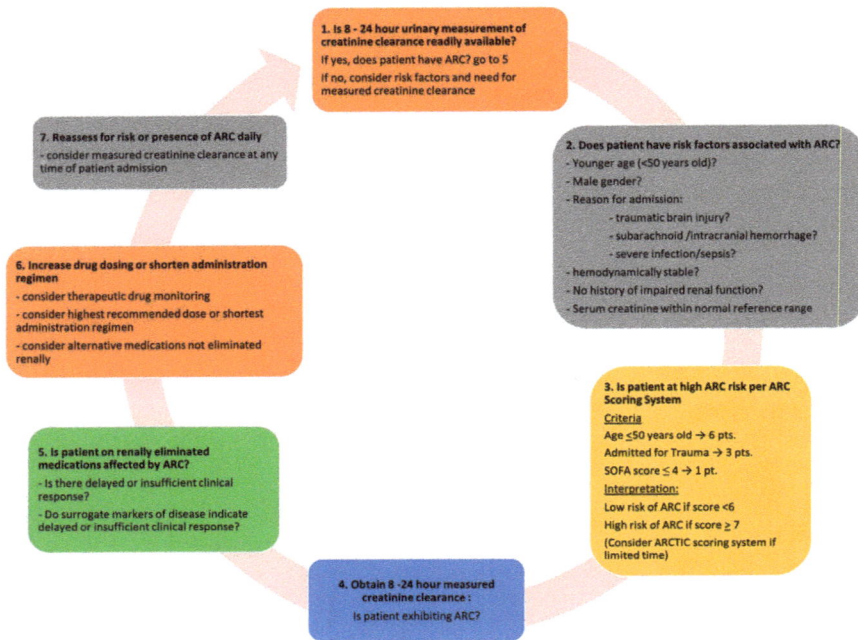

Figure 2. Assessment of ICU patients for augmented renal clearance (ARC).

The recognition of ARC risk factors allows clinicians to screen for at-risk patients. In the ICU setting, the ARC-scoring tool (Table 2) could be used to identify patients suitable for further investigation. If time does not permit the implementation of the ARC-scoring tool, the less time-consuming ARCTIC scoring system (Table 2) could still be considered. Other means of identifying at-risk patients include assessment of patient serum creatinine, estimated creatinine clearance, or delayed clinical response to medication interventions. Upon identification of at-risk patients, a measured 8–24 h creatinine clearance study should be undertaken. Evidence has shown that estimated creatinine clearance carry significant risk of underestimating the renal function of ARC patients in various settings. Therefore, at minimum, determination of a patient's creatinine clearance may be conducted by employing an 8-h urinary measurement, which will aid in the diagnosis of ARC and later-on be used for dosage adjustment of renally cleared medications. We also recommend continued daily monitoring of serum creatinine for those diagnosed with ARC. Due to the unpredictability of ARC manifestation (could be a transient 1-day occurrence or maintained for weeks), we can only determine the manifestation of ARC in an individual through continued measurement of renal function.

Despite many studies seem to suggest that ARC tends to manifest itself during initial ICU admission, any patients, including those with a recent history of acute kidney injury, could exhibit ARC at any time of their hospital admission. For those patients with confirmed ARC, considerations should be made for all renally cleared medications. Therapeutic drug monitoring and dose adjustment could be performed, when possible. Table 3 depicts suggested initial dosing of studied drugs in patients with ARC. For those medications where TDM is not routinely available and there is no sufficient evidence to guide dosage modification in ARC population, the use of the highest approved dose or most frequent administration regimen could be considered with close clinical monitoring. Furthermore, we suggest that consideration be made for alternative therapies that are not affected by altered renal function, such as those medications that are mainly metabolized rather than renally cleared (e.g., use of antiepileptic drugs that are eliminated via metabolism in place of levetiracetam). Finally, although attainment of therapeutic drug levels helps predict efficacy and safety, it is ultimately the patient's clinical status and outcome that should be the anchor for all therapeutic decision making.

Table 3. Suggested dosing recommendations of the studied drugs in adult ARC population.

Drug	Suggested Dosage	Suggestion Basis
Levetiracetam	• Dose: 1000 mg iv Q8H	• Monte-Carlo simulation [42]
Levofloxacin	• Dose: 750–1000 mg iv Q24H	• Monte-Carlo simulation [13] • Levofloxacin 1000 mg Q24H provided the highest target attainment for *S. pneumoniae*, *P. aeruginosa* and *S. aureus*.
Meropenem	• Dose: 2000 mg iv Q8H	• A dose of 1 g iv Q8H reported to be inadequate [27,30] • Doses up to 8 g per day might be required [59]
Piperacillin/Tazobactam	• Dose: 4.5 mg iv Q6H • Extended infusion of the dose over 4 h might be required	• Monte-Carlo simulation [23] • Subtherapeutic serum concentrations have been reported with intravenous doses of piperacillin/tazobactam 4.5 g every eight hours in 61% of the treated patients [17] • Continuous infusion may not improve treatment outcome [6]
Vancomycin	• Initial loading dose: 25–30 mg/kg followed by a maintenance dose of 45 mg/kg/day in divided doses Q8H or continuous infusion • Therapeutic drug monitoring is recommended (target 10–20 mg/L or 15–20 mg/L depending on the indication)	• Doses up to 44 mg/kg/day have been reported to be needed in patients with ARC [32] • Dosage regimens lower than the suggested dosage have resulted in subtherapeutic levels [9,20,37] • A dosing nomogram suggested by Baptista et al. allowed achievement of therapeutic vancomycin levels; average dose was ~47 mg/kg/day in patients with average weight 70 kg and measured CrCl 150 mL/min [25]

ARC = augmented renal clearance; CrCl = creatinine clearance; above recommended doses are based on observational studies and pharmacokinetics simulations. Above doses will need to be tested prospectively to assess its influence on patients' outcome; for antimicrobials, different doses might be needed based on the susceptibility pattern of the microorganisms.

Author Contributions: Sherif Hanafy Mahmoud and Chen Shen conducted literature review and wrote the paper.

Conflicts of Interest: The authors declare no conflict of interest.

References

1. Udy, A.A.; Putt, M.T.; Boots, R.J.; Lipman, J. ARC—Augmented renal clearance. *Curr. Pharm. Biotechnol.* **2011**, *12*, 2020–2029. [CrossRef] [PubMed]
2. Udy, A.A.; Roberts, J.A.; Boots, R.J.; Paterson, D.L.; Lipman, J. Augmented renal clearance: Implications for antibacterial dosing in the critically ill. *Clin. Pharmacokinet.* **2010**, *49*, 1–16. [CrossRef] [PubMed]

3. Udy, A.A.; Putt, M.T.; Shanmugathasan, S.; Roberts, J.A.; Lipman, J. Augmented renal clearance in the intensive care unit: An illustrative case series. *Int. J. Antimicrob. Agents* **2010**, *35*, 606–608. [CrossRef] [PubMed]

4. Barletta, J.F.; Mangram, A.J.; Byrne, M.; Sucher, J.F.; Hollingworth, A.K.; AliOsman, F.R.; Shirah, G.R.; Haley, M.; Dzandu, J.K. Identifying augmented renal clearance in trauma patients: Validation of the augmented renal clearance in trauma intensive care (arctic) scoring system. *J. Trauma Acute Care Surg.* **2017**, *82*, 665–671. [CrossRef] [PubMed]

5. Abdel El Naeem, H.E.M.; Abdelhamid, M.H.E.; Atteya, D.A.M. Impact of augmented renal clearance on enoxaparin therapy in critically ill patients. *Egypt. J. Anaesth.* **2017**, *33*, 113–117. [CrossRef]

6. Udy, A.A.; Dulhunty, J.M.; Roberts, J.A.; Davis, J.S.; Webb, S.A.R.; Bellomo, R.; Gomersall, C.; Shirwadkar, C.; Eastwood, G.M.; Myburgh, J.; et al. Association between augmented renal clearance and clinical outcomes in patients receiving β-lactam antibiotic therapy by continuous or intermittent infusion: A nested cohort study of the BLING-II randomised, placebo-controlled, clinical trial. *Int. J. Antimicrob. Agents* **2017**, *49*, 624–630. [CrossRef] [PubMed]

7. Udy, A.A.; Jarrett, P.; LassigSmith, M.; Stuart, J.; Starr, T.; Dunlop, R.; Deans, R.; Roberts, J.A.; Senthuran, S.; Boots, R.; et al. Augmented renal clearance in traumatic brain injury: A single-center observational study of atrial natriuretic peptide, cardiac output, and creatinine clearance. *J. Neurotrauma* **2017**, *34*, 137–144. [CrossRef] [PubMed]

8. Barletta, J.F.; Mangram, A.J.; Byrne, M.; Hollingworth, A.K.; Sucher, J.F.; AliOsman, F.R.; Shirah, G.R.; Dzandu, J.K. The importance of empiric antibiotic dosing in critically ill trauma patients: Are we under-dosing based on augmented renal clearance and inaccurate renal clearance estimates? *J. Trauma Acute Care Surg.* **2016**, *81*, 1115–1120. [CrossRef] [PubMed]

9. Chu, Y.; Luo, Y.; Qu, L.; Zhao, C.; Jiang, M. Application of vancomycin in patients with varying renal function, especially those with augmented renal clearance. *Pharm. Biol.* **2016**, *54*, 2802–2806. [CrossRef] [PubMed]

10. Declercq, P.; Nijs, S.; D'Hoore, A.; Van Wijngaerden, E.; Wolthuis, A.; De Buck Van Overstraeten, A.; Wauters, J.; Spriet, I. Augmented renal clearance in non-critically ill abdominal and trauma surgery patients is an underestimated phenomenon: A point prevalence study. *J. Trauma Acute Care Surg.* **2016**, *81*, 468–477. [CrossRef] [PubMed]

11. Hirai, K.; Ihara, S.; Kinae, A.; Ikegaya, K.; Suzuki, M.; Hirano, K.; Itoh, K. Augmented renal clearance in pediatric patients with febrile neutropenia associated with vancomycin clearance. *Ther. Drug Monit.* **2016**, *38*, 393–397. [CrossRef] [PubMed]

12. Kawano, Y.; Morimoto, S.; Izutani, Y.; Muranishi, K.; Kaneyama, H.; Hoshino, K.; Nishida, T.; Ishikura, H. Augmented renal clearance in Japanese intensive care unit patients: A prospective study. *J. Intensive Care* **2016**, *4*, 62. [CrossRef] [PubMed]

13. Roberts, J.A.; Cotta, M.O.; Cojutti, P.; Lugano, M.; Rocca, G.D.; Pea, F. Does critical illness change levofloxacin pharmacokinetics? *Antimicrob. Agents Chemother.* **2016**, *60*, 1459–1463. [CrossRef] [PubMed]

14. De Cock, P.A.J.G.; Standing, J.F.; Barker, C.I.S.; de Jaeger, A.; Dhont, E.; Carlier, M.; Verstraete, A.G.; Delanghe, J.R.; Robays, H.; De Paepe, P. Augmented renal clearance implies a need for increased amoxicillin-clavulanic acid dosing in critically ill children. *Antimicrob. Agents Chemother.* **2015**, *59*, 7027–7035. [CrossRef] [PubMed]

15. De Waele, J.J.; Dumoulin, A.; Janssen, A.; Hoste, E.A. Epidemiology of augmented renal clearance in mixed icu patients. *Minerva Anestesiol.* **2015**, *81*, 1079–1085. [PubMed]

16. Dias, C.; Gaio, A.R.; Monteiro, E.; Barbosa, S.; Cerejo, A.; Donnelly, J.; Felgueiras, O.; Smielewski, P.; Paiva, J.A.; Czosnyka, M. Kidney-brain link in traumatic brain injury patients? A preliminary report. *Neurocrit. Care* **2015**, *22*, 192–201. [CrossRef] [PubMed]

17. Huttner, A.; Von Dach, E.; Renzoni, A.; Huttner, B.D.; Affaticati, M.; Pagani, L.; Daali, Y.; Pugin, J.; Karmime, A.; Fathi, M.; et al. Augmented renal clearance, low beta-lactam concentrations and clinical outcomes in the critically ill: An observational prospective cohort study. *Int. J. Antimicrob. Agents* **2015**, *45*, 385–392. [CrossRef] [PubMed]

18. Morbitzer, K.A.; Jordan, J.D.; Rhoney, D.H. Vancomycin pharmacokinetic parameters in patients with acute brain injury undergoing controlled normothermia, therapeutic hypothermia, or pentobarbital infusion. *Neurocrit Care* **2015**, *22*, 258–264. [CrossRef] [PubMed]

19. Ruiz, S.; Minville, V.; Asehnoune, K.; Virtos, M.; Georges, B.; Fourcade, O.; Conil, J.M. Screening of patients with augmented renal clearance in ICU: Taking into account the ckd-epi equation, the age, and the cause of admission. *Ann. Intensiv. Care* **2015**, *5*, 49. [CrossRef] [PubMed]

20. Spadaro, S.; Berselli, A.; Fogagnolo, A.; Capuzzo, M.; Ragazzi, R.; Marangoni, E.; Bertacchini, S.; Volta, C.A. Evaluation of a protocol for vancomycin administration in critically patients with and without kidney dysfunction. *BMC Anesthesiol.* **2015**, *15*, 95. [CrossRef] [PubMed]

21. Steinke, T.; Moritz, S.; Beck, S.; Gnewuch, C.; Kees, M.G. Estimation of creatinine clearance using plasma creatinine or cystatin C: A secondary analysis of two pharmacokinetic studies in surgical ICU patients. *BMC Anesthesiol.* **2015**, *15*, 62. [CrossRef] [PubMed]

22. Adnan, S.; Ratnam, S.; Kumar, S.; Paterson, D.; Lipman, J.; Roberts, J.; Udy, A.A. Select critically ill patients at risk of augmented renal clearance: Experience in a malaysian intensive care unit. *Anaesth. Intensiv. Care* **2014**, *42*, 715–722.

23. Akers, K.S.; Niece, K.L.; Chung, K.K.; Cannon, J.W.; Cota, J.M.; Murray, C.K. Modified augmented renal clearance score predicts rapid piperacillin and tazobactam clearance in critically ill surgery and trauma patients. *J. Trauma Acute Care Surg.* **2014**, *77*, 163. [CrossRef] [PubMed]

24. Baptista, J.P.; Neves, M.; Rodrigues, L.; Teixeira, L.; Pinho, J.; Pimentel, J. Accuracy of the estimation of glomerular filtration rate within a population of critically ill patients. *J. Nephrol.* **2014**, *27*, 403–410. [CrossRef] [PubMed]

25. Baptista, J.P.; Roberts, J.A.; Sousa, E.; Freitas, R.; Deveza, N.; Pimentel, J. Decreasing the time to achieve therapeutic vancomycin concentrations in critically ill patients: Developing and testing of a dosing nomogram. *Crit. Care (Lond. Engl.)* **2014**, *18*, 654. [CrossRef] [PubMed]

26. Campassi, M.L.; Gonzalez, M.C.; Masevicius, F.D.; Vazquez, A.R.; Moseinco, M.; Navarro, N.C.; Previgliano, L.; Rubatto, N.P.; Benites, M.H.; Estenssoro, E.; et al. Augmented renal clearance in critically ill patients: Incidence, associated factors and effects on vancomycin treatment]. *Rev. Bras. Ter. Intensiv.* **2014**, *26*, 13–20. [CrossRef]

27. Hites, M.; Taccone, F.S.; Wolff, F.; Maillart, E.; Beumier, M.; Surin, R.; Cotton, F.; Jacobs, F. Broad-spectrum beta-lactams in obese non-critically ill patients. *Nutr. Diabetes* **2014**, *4*, e119. [CrossRef] [PubMed]

28. Udy, A.A.; Jarrett, P.; Stuart, J.; LassigSmith, M.; Starr, T.; Dunlop, R.; Wallis, S.C.; Roberts, J.A.; Lipman, J. Determining the mechanisms underlying augmented renal drug clearance in the critically ill: Use of exogenous marker compounds. *Crit. Care* **2014**, *18*, 657. [CrossRef] [PubMed]

29. Udy, A.A.; Baptista, J.P.; Lim, N.L.; Joynt, G.M.; Jarrett, P.; Wockner, L.; Boots, R.J.; Lipman, J. Augmented renal clearance in the ICU: Results of a multicenter observational study of renal function in critically ill patients with normal plasma creatinine concentrations. *Crit. Care Med.* **2014**, *42*, 520–527. [CrossRef] [PubMed]

30. Carlier, M.; Carrette, S.; Roberts, J.A.; Stove, V.; Verstraete, A.; Hoste, E.; Depuydt, P.; Decruyenaere, J.; Lipman, J.; Wallis, S.C.; et al. Meropenem and piperacillin/tazobactam prescribing in critically ill patients: Does augmented renal clearance affect pharmacokinetic/pharmacodynamic target attainment when extended infusions are used? *Crit. Care (Lond. Engl.)* **2013**, *17*, R84. [CrossRef] [PubMed]

31. Claus, B.O.M.; Hoste, E.A.; Colpaert, K.; Robays, H.; Decruyenaere, J.; De Waele, J.J. Augmented renal clearance is a common finding with worse clinical outcome in critically ill patients receiving antimicrobial therapy. *J. Crit. Care* **2013**, *28*, 695–700. [CrossRef] [PubMed]

32. Minkute, R.; Briedis, V.; Steponaviciute, R.; Vitkauskiene, A.; Maciulaitis, R. Augmented renal clearance—An evolving risk factor to consider during the treatment with vancomycin. *J. Clin. Parm. Ther.* **2013**, *38*, 462–467. [CrossRef] [PubMed]

33. Roberts, J.A.; Lipman, J. Optimal doripenem dosing simulations in critically ill nosocomial pneumonia patients with obesity, augmented renal clearance, and decreased bacterial susceptibility. *Crit. Care Med.* **2013**, *41*, 489–495. [CrossRef] [PubMed]

34. Shimamoto, Y.; Fukuda, T.; Tanaka, K.; Komori, K.; Sadamitsu, D. Systemic inflammatory response syndrome criteria and vancomycin dose requirement in patients with sepsis. *Intensive Care Med.* **2013**, *39*, 1247–1252. [CrossRef] [PubMed]

35. Udy, A.A.; Roberts, J.A.; Shorr, A.F.; Boots, R.J.; Lipman, J. Augmented renal clearance in septic and traumatized patients with normal plasma creatinine concentrations: Identifying at-risk patients. *Crit. Care (Lond. Engl.)* **2013**, *17*, R35. [CrossRef] [PubMed]

36. Udy, A.A.; Morton, F.J.A.; NguyenPham, S.; Jarrett, P.; LassigSmith, M.; Stuart, J.; Dunlop, R.; Starr, T.; Boots, R.J.; Lipman, J. A comparison of CKD-EPI estimated glomerular filtration rate and measured creatinine clearance in recently admitted critically ill patients with normal plasma creatinine concentrations. *BMC Nephrol.* **2013**, *14*, 250. [CrossRef] [PubMed]

37. Baptista, J.P.; Sousa, E.; Martins, P.J.; Pimentel, J.M. Augmented renal clearance in septic patients and implications for vancomycin optimisation. *Int. J. Antimicrob. Agents* **2012**, *39*, 420–423. [CrossRef] [PubMed]

38. Grootaert, V.; Willems, L.; Debaveye, Y.; Meyfroidt, G.; Spriet, I. Augmented renal clearance in the critically ill: How to assess kidney function. *Ann. Pharmacother.* **2012**, *46*, 952–959. [CrossRef] [PubMed]

39. Udy, A.A.; Varghese, J.M.; Altukroni, M.; Briscoe, S.; McWhinney, B.C.; Ungerer, J.P.; Lipman, J.; Roberts, J.A. Subtherapeutic initial β-lactam concentrations in select critically ill patients: Association between augmented renal clearance and low trough drug concentrations. *Chest* **2012**, *142*, 30–39. [CrossRef] [PubMed]

40. Baptista, J.P.; Udy, A.A.; Sousa, E.; Pimentel, J.; Wang, L.; Roberts, J.A.; Lipman, J. A comparison of estimates of glomerular filtration in critically ill patients with augmented renal clearance. *Crit. Care (Lond. Engl.)* **2011**, *15*, R139. [CrossRef] [PubMed]

41. Minville, V.; Asehnoune, K.; Ruiz, S.; Breden, A.; Georges, B.; Seguin, T.; Tack, I.; Jaafar, A.; Saivin, S.; Fourcade, O.; et al. Increased creatinine clearance in polytrauma patients with normal serum creatinine: A retrospective observational study. *Crit. Care (Lond. Engl.)* **2011**, *15*, R49. [CrossRef] [PubMed]

42. Spencer, D.D.; Jacobi, J.; Juenke, J.M.; Fleck, J.D.; Kays, M.B. Steady-state pharmacokinetics of intravenous levetiracetam in neurocritical care patients. *Pharmacotherapy* **2011**, *31*, 934–941. [CrossRef] [PubMed]

43. Goboova, M.; Kuzelova, M.; Kissova, V.; Bodakova, D.; Martisova, E. An adjustment of vancomycin dosing regimen for a young patient with augmented renal clearance: A case report. *Acta Fac. Pharm. Univ. Comen.* **2015**, *62*, 1–4.

44. Abdul-Aziz, M.; McDonald, C.; McWhinney, B.; Ungerer, J.P.J.; Lipman, J.; Roberts, J.A. Low flucloxacillin concentrations in a patient with central nervous system infection: The need for plasma and cerebrospinal fluid drug monitoring in the ICU. *Ann. Pharmacother.* **2014**, *48*, 1380–1384. [CrossRef] [PubMed]

45. Cook, A.M.; Arora, S.; Davis, J.; Pittman, T. Augmented renal clearance of vancomycin and levetiracetam in a traumatic brain injury patient. *Neurocrit. Care* **2013**, *19*, 210–214. [CrossRef] [PubMed]

46. Lonsdale, D.O.; Udy, A.A.; Roberts, J.A.; Lipman, J. Antibacterial therapeutic drug monitoring in cerebrospinal fluid: Difficulty in achieving adequate drug concentrations. *J. Neurosurg.* **2013**, *118*, 297–301. [CrossRef] [PubMed]

47. Troger, U.; Drust, A.; Martens-Lobenhoffer, J.; Tanev, I.; Braun-Dullaeus, R.; Bode-Boger, S. Decreased meropenem levels in intensive care unit patients with augmented renal clearance: Benefit of therapeutic drug monitoring. *Int. J. Antimicrob. Agents* **2012**, *40*, 370–372. [CrossRef] [PubMed]

48. Caro, L.; Larson, K.; Nicolau, D.; DeWaele, J.; Kuti, J.; Gadzicki, E.; Yu, B.; Rhee, E. PK/PD and safety of 3 g ceftolozane/tazobactam in critically ill augmented renal clearance patients. In Proceedings of the 46th Critical Care Medicine Conference, Honolulu, HI, USA, 21–25 January 2017; p. 661.

49. Goboova, M.; Kuzelova, M.; Fazekas, T.; Kissova, V.; Kakosova, V.; Salkovska, L. The impact of therapeutic drug monitoring (TDM) in optimizing dosage regimens of gentamicin in patients with augmented renal clearance. *Int. J. Clin. Pharm.* **2016**, *38*, 596.

50. Morbitzer, K.; Jordan, D.; Sullivan, K.; Durr, E.; OlmShipman, C.; Rhoney, D. Enhanced renal clearance and impact on vancomycin trough concentration in patients with hemorrhagic stroke. In Proceedings of the Annual Meeting of the American College of Clinical Pharmacy (ACCP), Hollywood, FL, USA, 23–26 October 2016; Volume 36, p. e218.

51. Morimoto, S.; Ishikura, H. An observational prospective study on the onset of augmented renal clearance: The first report. *Crit. Care* **2016**, *20* (Suppl. 2), 182. [CrossRef]

52. Dunning, J.; Roberts, J. Assessment of renal function in dosing antibiotics in septic patients: A survey of current practice within critical care units in england. *Anaesthesia* **2015**, *70*, 21.

53. Baptista, J.P.; Silva, N.; Costa, E.; Fontes, F.; Marques, M.; Ribeiro, G.; Pimentel, J. Identification of the critically ill patient with augmented renal clearance: Make do with what you have! In Proceedings of the 27th Annual Congress of the European Society of Intensive Care Medicine (ESICM), Barcelona, Spain, 27 September–1 October 2014; Volume 40, p. S110.

54. May, C.; Arora, S.; Parli, S.; Bastin, M.T.; Cook, A. Levetiracetam pharmacokinetics in subarachnoid hemorrhage patients with augmented renal clearance: A monte carlo simulation. In Proceedings of the 2014 Annual Meeting of the American College of Clinical Pharmacy (ACCP), Austin, TX, USA, 12–15 October 2014; Volume 34, pp. e261–e262.

55. Vermis, K.; Steel, E.; Vandenbroucke, J. Prevalence of augmented renal clearance in haematological patients and the impact on vancomycin dosing. In Proceedings of the Journal of Oncology Pharmacy Practice. Conference: 14th Symposium of the International Society of Oncology Pharmacy Practitioners, Montreal, QC, Canada, 2–5 April 2014; Volume 20, p. 7.

56. Weigel, J.; Egal, M.; Lima, A.; Koch, B.; Hunfeld, N.G.; Van Gelder, T.; Mouton, J.W.; Groeneveld, A.B.J. Vancomycin is underdosed in patients with high estimated glomerular filtration rate. In Proceedings of the 27th Annual Congress of the European Society of Intensive Care Medicine (ESICM), Barcelona, Spain, 27 September–1 October 2014; p. S252.

57. Neves, M.; Baptista, J.P.; Rodrigues, L.; Pinho, J.; Teixeira, L.; Pimentel, J. Correlation between estimated glomerular filtration rate and measured renal creatinine clearance in critically ill patients with normal serum creatinine. *Nephrol. Dial. Transplant.* **2013**, *28*, 345.

58. Grootaert, V.; Spriet, I.; Decoutere, L.; Debaveye, Y.; Meyfroidt, G.; Willems, L. Augmented renal clearance in the critically ill: Fiction or fact? *Int. J. Clin. Pharm.* **2012**, *34*, 143.

59. Drust, A.; Troger, U.; MartensLobenhoffer, J.; Tanev, I.; BraunDullaeus, R.C.; BodeBoger, S.M. Therapeutic drug monitoring of meropenem is mandatory for critically ill patients with glomerular hyperfiltration. *Br. J. Clin. Pharmacol.* **2011**, *72*, 18.

60. Ichai, C.; Passeron, C.; Carles, M.; Bouregba, M.; Grimaud, D. Prolonged low-dose dopamine infusion induces a transient improvement in renal function in hemodynamically stable, critically ill patients: A single-blind, prospective, controlled study. *Crit. Care Med.* **2000**, *28*, 1329–1335. [CrossRef] [PubMed]

61. Ichai, C.; Soubielle, J.; Carles, M.; Giunti, C.; Grimaud, D. Comparison of the renal effects of low to high doses of dopamine and dobutamine in critically ill patients: A single-blind randomized study. *Crit. Care Med.* **2000**, *28*, 921–928. [CrossRef] [PubMed]

62. Ljungberg, B.; NilssonEhle, I. Advancing age and acute infection influence the kinetics of ceftazidime. *Scand. J. Infect. Dis.* **1989**, *21*, 327–332. [CrossRef] [PubMed]

63. Sime, F.B.; Udy, A.A.; Roberts, J.A. Augmented renal clearance in critically ill patients: Etiology, definition and implications for beta-lactam dose optimization. *Curr. Opin. Pharmacol.* **2015**, *24*, 1–6. [CrossRef] [PubMed]

64. Carlier, M.; Dumoulin, A.; Janssen, A.; Picavet, S.; Vanthuyne, S.; Van Eynde, R.; Vanholder, R.; Delanghe, J.; De Schoenmakere, G.; De Waele, J.J.; et al. Comparison of different equations to assess glomerular filtration in critically ill patients. *Intensive Care Med.* **2015**, *41*, 427–435. [CrossRef] [PubMed]

65. Sunder, S.; Jayaraman, R.; Mahapatra, H.S.; Sathi, S.; Ramanan, V.; Kanchi, P.; Gupta, A.; Daksh, S.K.; Ram, P. Estimation of renal function in the intensive care unit: The covert concepts brought to light. *J. Intensive Care* **2014**, *2*, 31. [CrossRef] [PubMed]

66. Rybak, M.J. The pharmacokinetic and pharmacodynamic properties of vancomycin. *Clin. Infect. Dis.* **2006**, *42* (Suppl. 1), S35–S39. [CrossRef] [PubMed]

67. Mouton, J.W.; Touzw, D.J.; Horrevorts, A.M.; Vinks, A.A. Comparative pharmacokinetics of the carbapenems: Clinical implications. *Clin. Pharmacokinet.* **2000**, *39*, 185–201. [CrossRef] [PubMed]

68. Binder, L.; Schworer, H.; Hoppe, S.; Streit, F.; Neumann, S.; Beckmann, A.; Wachter, R.; Oellerich, M.; Walson, P.D. Pharmacokinetics of meropenem in critically ill patients with severe infections. *Ther. Drug Monit.* **2013**, *35*, 63–70. [CrossRef] [PubMed]

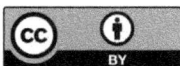

pharmaceutics

MDPI

Review

Predicting Oral Drug Absorption: Mini Review on Physiologically-Based Pharmacokinetic Models

Louis Lin and Harvey Wong *

Faculty of Pharmaceutical Sciences, University of British Columbia, Vancouver, BC V6T 1Z3, Canada;
louis.lin@alumni.ubc.ca
* Correspondence: harvey.wong@ubc.ca; Tel.: +1-604-822-4707

Received: 16 August 2017; Accepted: 22 September 2017; Published: 26 September 2017

Abstract: Most marketed drugs are administered orally, despite the complex process of oral absorption that is difficult to predict. Oral bioavailability is dependent on the interplay between many processes that are dependent on both compound and physiological properties. Because of this complexity, computational oral physiologically-based pharmacokinetic (PBPK) models have emerged as a tool to integrate these factors in an attempt to mechanistically capture the process of oral absorption. These models use inputs from in vitro assays to predict the pharmacokinetic behavior of drugs in the human body. The most common oral PBPK models are compartmental approaches, in which the gastrointestinal tract is characterized as a series of compartments through which the drug transits. The focus of this review is on the development of oral absorption PBPK models, followed by a brief discussion of the major applications of oral PBPK models in the pharmaceutical industry.

Keywords: oral absorption; physiologically-based pharmacokinetic modeling; food-effect; pH effect; formulation simulation

---

1. Introduction

The oral route of drug administration is the most common, as opposed to injections (intravenous, intramuscular, subcutaneous) or inhalation, due to the convenience of administration. However, this route comes with the cost of absorption variability due to the many biological processes involved [1]. For example, variations in oral bioavailability can occur due to individual differences in the pre-systemic metabolism of drugs by the gut and liver. Two fundamental processes describing oral drug absorption include the dissolution of a drug into gastrointestinal (GI) fluid, and the permeation of a dissolved drug through the intestinal wall and into the bloodstream [2]. These processes are complex and are governed by physicochemical properties such as compound solubility and permeability. Other external physiological properties, including the pH environment and metabolic enzymes in the gastrointestinal tract (GIT), also play an important role in influencing oral absorption [3]. Furthermore, the complex interplay between these factors makes the prediction of the oral absorption of drugs difficult.

In the search for new medicines, low oral bioavailability is a common problem faced by scientists in the pharmaceutical industry [4,5]. Therefore, it is valuable to have methodologies that can assess the oral pharmacokinetics (PK) of drug candidates before moving forward with drug development. However, extensive in vivo evaluation in preclinical species can be costly and time consuming. Furthermore, species differences in pharmacokinetics can cause unreliable predictions of oral bioavailability in humans when using in vivo animal data [6,7]. In vitro assays assessing factors such as compound permeability, dissolution, solubility, and metabolic stability offer a more efficient and cost-effective means to evaluate the potential oral bioavailability of large numbers of drug candidates. However, these assays do not fully capture the complex and dynamic nature of the in vivo oral absorption process.

Mathematical models of oral absorption serve as tools to integrate compound data from in vitro assays gathered during the process of drug screening in order to provide in vivo context to these data. The focus of early mathematical models were almost solely on two fundamental compound properties, solubility and permeability. These earlier models were relatively simple and predicted the extent of absorption under more "static" conditions. Examples of these are the Absorption Potential (AP) and the Maximum Absorbable Dose (MAD) equations [8,9]. The AP equation is used to estimate the fraction absorbed of a given dose. The MAD equation estimates the maximum amount of a drug that can be absorbed within a 6-h time frame (meant to simulate small intestinal residence time), assuming drug saturation in the gastrointestinal fluid. Because of their simplicity, they enable rapid assessments of the possible extent of oral bioavailability from smaller information sets [10,11]. However, these models have limited ability to explore more complex phenomenon such as pH-dependent oral absorption and food effects.

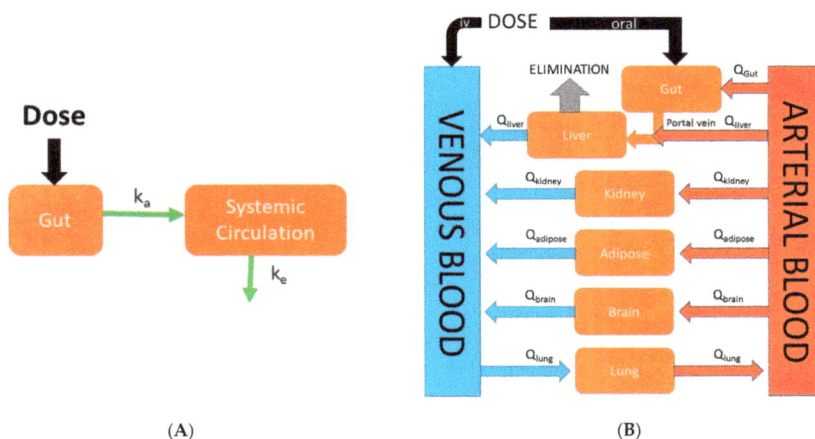

(A)   (B)

Figure 1. Comparison of an empirical classical compartmental model and a mechanistic physiologically-based pharmacokinetic (PBPK) model. (**A**) In the classical compartment model, a drug is inputted into the gut compartment, and absorption into the systemic circulation compartment is governed by the absorption rate constant (k_a). Elimination is described by the elimination rate constant (k_e); (**B**) In the whole-body PBPK model, major organs/tissues are represented by compartments, connected by blood flows (Q). Specific organ blood flows are described by subscripts. Intravenous (IV) dosing inputs drugs directly into venous blood, whereas oral dosing inputs drug into the gut compartment. In this illustration, the liver is the major eliminating organ.

Physiologically-based pharmacokinetic (PBPK) models are mathematical models that describe biological processes in order to mimic biology. They are dynamic in nature and are defined by series of differential equations. While classical compartmental pharmacokinetic models (Figure 1A) simply describe absorption as a single first-order process, PBPK models differ in that they are mechanistic in nature and incorporate physiological processes such as GI transit time and organ blood flows. Although the first PBPK model dates back to 1937, it was not until recently that the use of PBPK models in drug discovery research has rapidly increased in popularity [12]. This increase in popularity of PBPK modeling was largely due to the availability and speed at which ADME (absorption, distribution, metabolism, and excretion) information required as model inputs could be gathered due to advances in in silico and in vitro assays. An example of a generic whole-body PBPK model is shown in Figure 1B. Major tissues/organs are represented by compartments from which blood flows carry a drug into and out of tissue/organ. Specifically, in the case of oral PBPK models the gut is typically described as a series of compartments through which a drug transits (figures in Sections 4 and 5). These models provide a rational means to translate preclinical absorption data to man. For example, one can validate a PBPK model of a particular drug built using rat in vitro data along with in vivo oral pharmacokinetic data in rat. Following the confirmation of a successful prediction of in vivo oral pharmacokinetics using in vitro data in the rat, the physiological parameters and in vitro parameters in the rat PBPK model can be replaced with human parameters in order to predict the human oral pharmacokinetic profile [13]. The use of PBPK modeling in pharmaceutical industry has rapidly expanded in recent times and has been used in sophisticated mechanistic applications such as the prediction of drug-drug interactions, the prediction of pharmacokinetic profiles in special populations, and the assessment of population variability. The specific focus of this review is on the evolution of physiologically-based pharmacokinetic models describing oral absorption. Further, we review the applications of these PBPK models of oral absorption in the current landscape of drug discovery and development.

2. Fundamental Processes for Oral Absorption

The fundamental processes that determine oral absorption include drug or compound dissolution and permeation. Dissolution is the process by which a solid drug dissolves into gastrointestinal fluid. Dissolution is normally described in PBPK models by a form of the Noyes-Whitney equation [14,15]:

$$\frac{dX_{solution}}{dt} = k_{diss} \times \left(S - \frac{X_{solution}}{V} \right) \tag{1}$$

where $X_{solution}$ is the amount of drug in solution at time t, V is the volume of intestinal fluid, and S is the drug solubility. The rate at which the drug dissolves into solution follows first-order kinetics, dependent on the compound specific dissolution constant (k_{diss}), and the concentration gradient surrounding the solid drug ($S - [X_{solution}/V]$).

Following dissolution is permeation, the process by which a dissolved drug crosses the intestinal wall from the GI fluid into the portal vein. A drug is carried from the portal vein to the liver before reaching systemic circulation. Mathematically, permeation is described as a first-order differential equation governed by an absorption constant (k_a) and the amount of drug in solution.

$$\frac{dX_{perm}}{dt} = k_a \times X_{solution} \tag{2}$$

where X_{perm} is the amount of permeated drug. The absorption rate constant (k_a) can be calculated from effective permeability (P_{eff}).

$$k_a = \frac{2P_{eff}}{R} \tag{3}$$

where R refers to the radius of the small intestine. A compound's P_{eff} is calculated from the rate at which it permeates through a membrane (dM_r/dt) using the following equation derived from Fick's Law of Diffusion:

$$P_{eff} = \frac{dM_r/dt}{A \times (C_{GIT} - C_{pv})} \tag{4}$$

where A refers to the area of the membrane, C_{GIT} refers to the concentration in the gastrointestinal tract, and C_{pv} refers to the concentration that has permeated through the intestinal wall and into the portal vein. At the core of both dissolution and permeation equations is the principle of diffusion via a concentration gradient, reflected by ($C_{GIT} - C_{pv}$) for permeation and ($S - [X_{solution}/V]$) for dissolution.

3. Mixing Tank Model

One of the first applications integrating dissolution and permeation processes in an oral PBPK model was the mixing tank model, which treated the GIT as a single well-stirred compartment

(Figure 2) [16]. The amount of drug inputted into the system was assumed to be instantaneously mixed throughout the GIT, and the movement of drug out of this single compartment was assumed to be governed by the intestinal transit time. This model was introduced by Dressman and Fleisher, and was one of the first models to allow for characterization of dissolution rate-limited absorption. Dressman et al. [16] validated this model's ability to estimate the absorption profile for griseofulvin and digoxin using literature data. The model was then used to investigate factors limiting the oral absorption of these two compounds. Increasing dissolution rate and intestinal transit time using the model did not significantly increase bioavailability for griseofulvin, leading to the conclusion that drug solubility was the limiting factor. For digoxin, increasing the dissolution rate by decreasing particle size showed a significant increase in bioavailability, suggesting that the dissolution rate was limiting its absorption. A shortcoming of this early model is that it ignores phenomena such as gut metabolism, hepatic first-pass metabolism, and drug chemical instability. Furthermore, simplifying the entire GIT into a single homogenous compartment assumes that all dissolved drugs are subject to the same absorption rate constant, overlooking heterogeneity along the GIT. Despite the described shortcomings, the mixing tank model served to lay the foundations for the development of later oral PBPK models.

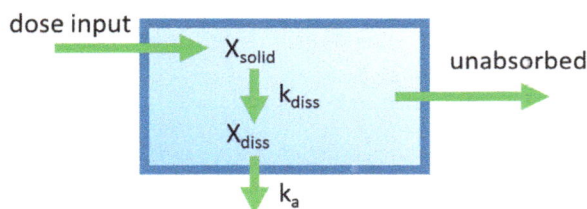

Figure 2. Diagram of the mixing tank model which represents the gastrointestinal (GI) tract as a single well-stirred compartment. k_a is the absorption rate constant, X_{diss} is the amount of drug dissolved in the GI tract. k_{diss} is the dissolution rate constant, and X_{solid} is the dose that has been placed into the GI tract. The oral absorption rate is governed by k_a and X_{diss}. The dissolution rate is governed by X_{solid} and k_{diss}.

4. Compartmental Absorption and Transit Model

A later model of oral absorption that was introduced following the mixing tank model was the compartmental absorption and transit (CAT) model described by Yu et al. [17]. This model characterizes the intestinal tract as a series of compartments as opposed to a single compartment used by the mixing tank model. While a multiple compartment approach has been used prior to describe effects such as gastric emptying, Yu et al. utilized multiple compartments to represent different sections of the small intestine (Figure 3) [18–21]. Specifically, they found that the number of compartments that best fit the small intestine transit time, based on available literature, was seven. The first of the seven compartments represented the duodenum, the next two represented the jejunum, and the final four compartments represented the ileum. The transit of a drug through each small intestine compartment in CAT models is controlled by a transit rate constant (k_t). The movement of drug through the CAT model can be mathematically represented by the following equation:

$$\frac{dY_n}{dt} = k_t \times Y_{n-1} - k_t \times Y_n - k_a \times Y_n \tag{5}$$

where Y_n refers to the amount of a drug in a specific compartment, Y_{n-1} refers to the amount of a drug in the previous compartment, k_t is the transit rate constant, and k_a is the absorption rate constant.

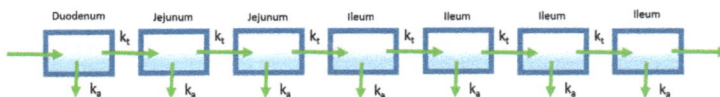

Figure 3. The compartmental absorption and transit (CAT) model extends the mixing tank model to characterize drug transit through the gastrointestinal tract (GIT). Seven well-stirred compartments are used to describe absorption and transit through the small intestine.

An advantage of the CAT model is its mathematic simplicity, as a single rate constant (k_t) is used to describe the transit of a drug through different regions of the small intestine. Yu later added an additional seven compartments such that dissolved and undissolved drugs could be represented [22]. In this model, a rate constant describing dissolution governed the movement of a drug from undissolved compartments into the dissolved drug compartments. This addition allowed the CAT model to capture dissolution rate-limited absorption. The CAT model set the framework for future oral absorption models that incorporated additional features and properties to address its shortcomings.

5. Advanced Compartmental Absorption and Transit Model

Extensions of the early CAT model led to the development of the Advanced Compartment Absorption and Transit (ACAT) model that are implemented in the software GastroPlus® [23]. An early form of the ACAT model adds new compartments describing three different drug states: unreleased drug in formulation, undissolved drug, and dissolved drug (Figure 4). As such, this ACAT model not only allows for investigation of dissolution-rate limited absorption, but also allows exploration of the effect of formulation release rates on oral pharmacokinetics. Like the CAT model, the small intestine is represented by seven compartments in series. In addition, the inclusion of stomach and colon segments allow for incorporation of processes such as gastric emptying and possible colonic absorption. Further, assignment of characteristics such as pH, effective surface area, transporter expression, and GI transit time to each specific compartment accounts for GI heterogeneity [24–28]. Finally, gut and liver metabolism were added to the ACAT model, improving predictions of the extent of oral absorption of drugs that undergo significant gut and liver first-pass metabolism such as propranolol [29].

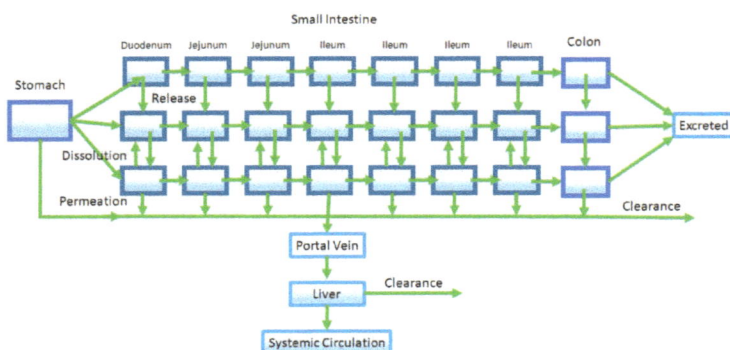

Figure 4. The representative Advanced Compartment Absorption and Transit (ACAT) model pictured here is an extension of the CAT model. Shown in this representative ACAT model, additional compartments are added to characterize features such as stomach and colon absorption, drug release from formulation, and first-pass metabolism from the liver and the gut (shown by the Clearance arrows).

Following the ACAT model, other similar advanced compartmental absorption models have been developed with slight differences in parameters and equations used. The most notable is the Advanced Dissolution Absorption Metabolism (ADAM) model incorporated in the SimCYP® software, which uses the modified Wang and Flanagan method to model dissolution [30,31]. Among the PBPK models of oral absorption, the ACAT and ADAM models remain the most popular.

6. Incorporation of Saturable Processes: Metabolism and Drug Transporters

Metabolism and active transport are two important saturable processes that can have an influence on oral bioavailability [32,33]. As mentioned in the previous section, the incorporation of gut and liver metabolism in the ACAT model helped to correct for over-predictions of the extent of oral absorption for drugs that have significant gut and/or liver first-pass metabolism. A more complex situation is one where both metabolic enzymes and drug transporters are involved in oral absorption of a drug. Metabolic enzymes and drug transporters can have common substrates, which can lead to synergistic effects on oral absorption. Examples of this phenomenon include the impact of the efflux transporter P-glycoprotein and cytochrome P450 3A4 working synergistically to reduce the bioavailability of drugs such as cyclosporin and vinblastine [34–37].

The incorporation of saturable processes such as metabolism and drug transport into PBPK models are accomplished using Michaelis-Menten kinetics, which is described by the following equation:

$$v = \frac{V_{max} \times [s]}{K_m + [s]} \tag{6}$$

where v refers to the rate the particular process being described, V_{max} is the maximum rate of the process, K_m (Michaelis-Menten constant) is the concentration at which the rate is half maximal, and $[s]$ is the compound (substrate) concentration. K_m can also be interpreted as the affinity for the compound to the enzyme or transporter. In cases where the drug concentrations are far below saturation, the equation can be shortened to:

$$v = \frac{V_{max} \times [s]}{K_m} \tag{7}$$

For the case of liver metabolism, these kinetic parameters are commonly estimated in vitro by measuring enzyme activity using liver microsomes or hepatocytes [38–40]. A similar approach can be taken to estimate the kinetics of intestinal metabolism and transport using in vitro methodologies [41]. The success or failure of appropriately capturing the in vivo consequences of these processes on the oral absorption of drugs is highly dependent on the level of understanding how in vitro data generated for these processes translate to an in vivo system. While there is much work performed to understand the in vitro to in vivo translation of metabolic enzyme activity obtained from in vitro experiments, less is known in this regard for drug transport. An example of how saturable processes are incorporated into an oral PBPK model is illustrated in Figure 5. A gut segment is represented in the figure as a GI compartment (representing the lumen) with a separate enterocyte compartment. A drug must pass through the enterocyte compartment prior to being absorbed into the portal vein. Michaelis-Menten kinetics is used to represent both the metabolism and transport processes (Figure 5). Having separate gut segments representing the gastrointestinal tract allows ACAT models to capture the heterogeneity of expression of transporter and enzymes.

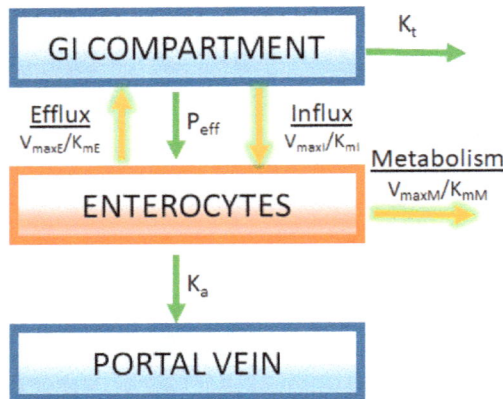

Figure 5. Modeling of transporters and intestinal metabolism is achieved by separately compartmentalizing the enterocytes. Rates of transport and metabolizing enzyme activity are described by Michaelis-Menten kinetics using parameters derived from in vitro enzyme activity assays (V_{maxE}, V_{maxI}, and V_{maxM} are the maximum rate for efflux transporters, influx transporters, and metabolic enzymes respectively; K_{mE}, K_{mI}, and K_{mM} are the Michaelis-Menten constants for efflux transporters, influx transporters, and metabolic enzymes, respectively). In this example, it is assumed that substrate concentrations are far below saturation (Equation (7)).

7. Applications of Oral PBPK Models

PBPK models can have many different applications during the course of drug discovery and development. Simulations using oral PBPK models built using limited drug discovery data can be used to assess the oral absorption of drug candidates by providing in vivo context to all available in vitro data. These early PBPK models have been used to assess oral pharmacokinetics of drug candidates in humans. More detailed simulations can be performed using more refined oral PBPK models at later stages of drug development to inform decisions about drug form selection and formulation optimization. Further, oral PBPK models offer an ideal tool to explore complex dynamic phenomenon such as pH and food effects. The applications of oral PBPK models to guide drug form selection and formulation optimization as well as to investigate pH and food effects are of high value. A more detailed look at these applications is described below.

7.1. Drug Form Selection and Formulation Optimization

Of the various applications of oral PBPK models, one of the applications that has great value is in the area of drug form selection and formulation optimization. The oral absorption of drugs is highly dependent on various drug specific properties such as particle size and drug solubility of different drug forms. Oral PBPK models can be utilized to quantify how changes in these properties influence oral absorption through the use of sensitivity analysis. Sensitivity analysis involves the systematic alteration of a specific drug parameter (e.g., particle size) in an oral PBPK model in order to identify the optimal values required for maximizing oral absorption. Below are descriptions of two studies where sensitivity analysis was used for salt selection and particle size optimization.

7.1.1. Salt Selection

Salt selection for new molecular entities remains a challenge, due to the difficulties in translating in vitro solubility to in vivo bioavailability. For most cases, salt forms with the highest solubility are selected with little regard for other factors (i.e., which salt form has the best solid-state properties for further drug development). In order to assess salt forms with an in vivo context, Chiang and Wong used an oral PBPK model to explore the salt solubility-bioavailability relationship for phenytoin [42]. The exercise identified a solubility of ~0.3 mg/mL that was required in order to produce the maximum bioavailability of phenytoin. Any increase in solubility beyond 0.3 mg/mL was predicted to provide no additional increases in oral bioavailability, as drug solubility would no longer be rate limiting for oral absorption. Phenytoin salts with a wide range of solubility were prepared and administered orally to rats. Despite having a 60-fold difference in solubility, two phenytoin salts—both with solubility >0.3 mg/mL—provided a similar oral bioavailability as predicted by the oral PBPK analysis. This study demonstrates that oral PBPK models can be used to define solubility requirements and provide guidance for salt selection.

7.1.2. Particle Size

A critical factor influencing the oral absorption of poorly soluble drugs is the drug dissolution rate that is dependent on the drug particle size. Particle size of drug product is a characteristic that can be controlled. Therefore, the identification of an optimal particle size is an important consideration in drug development, especially for compounds showing dissolution-rate limited oral absorption. In the Noyes-Whitney equation for dissolution (Equation (1)), particle size is incorporated in the calculation for the dissolution constant.

$$k_{diss} = \frac{3 \times D_{eff} \times S}{r_p^2 \times \rho} \tag{8}$$

where k_{diss} is the dissolution constant, D_{eff} is the effective diffusion coefficient, ρ is the drug density, r_p is the particle size, and S is the solubility. Based on the Noyes-Whitney equation, a smaller particle size (i.e., smaller r_p) translates to more rapid dissolution, due to the increases in the drug particle surface area. However, smaller particle size can require extensive milling of drug products and additional workup.

An example of using PBPK modeling to understand the effect of compound particle size on its in vivo dissolution was reported by Parrott and Lave [43]. As a first step of PBPK model verification, the particle size distribution of a milled and an un-milled compound was characterized. Next, the milled and un-milled compounds were formulated into tablets and administered to monkeys. Particle size distribution data was used as input into a monkey PBPK model, and simulations of the oral monkey plasma concentration-time profiles for the milled and un-milled compounds were performed. PBPK model simulations were compared to in vivo plasma-concentration time profiles from monkey as a means to verify the PBPK model's ability to predict the in vivo dissolution of the milled and un-milled compounds using particle size data. Following model verification, a human PBPK model was used to perform a sensitivity analysis examining the effect of particle size on maximum concentration (C_{max}) and total drug exposure (AUC). The sensitivity analysis suggested that C_{max} was more sensitive to particle changes when compared to AUC. A particle diameter above 24 µm would decrease C_{max} by 20%, whereas a particle diameter above 44 µm would be required for a 20% decrease in AUC. The information from this analysis exemplifies how oral PBPK models can be used to provide guidance on optimal particle size ranges to produce the desired in vivo dissolution profile and resultant oral pharmacokinetic profile.

7.2. Food and pH Effects

A second area of application in which oral PBPK models can serve as a useful tool is in the investigation of pH and food effects on oral bioavailability [44–46]. Of the two phenomena, pH effects are much easier to deal with using PBPK models. As the gastrointestinal tract is represented as a series of compartments in oral PBPK models, a pH effect can be simulated by simply adjusting the pH in the GI compartment of interest. The alteration of pH primarily affects the solubility of the solid drug in the specific compartment, and subsequent simulation with the PBPK model will indicate its effect on oral bioavailability. A more complex phenomenon is food effects on oral absorption. Following food intake, changes in GI transit and gastric pH occur [47]. Further, bile secretions from the gall bladder aid in the dissolution and permeation of lipophilic compounds [48]. Due to the many physiological changes that occur with food intake and the potential for direct food-drug interaction, PBPK modeling of food effects is more challenging. However, as GI physiology can differ between animals and humans, human PBPK models combined with in vitro data may be the most appropriate means to capture and predict how drugs are absorbed in the human fasted and fed states.

7.2.1. Investigating pH Effect

An oral PBPK model was used to investigate the cause of an observed disproportionate increase in drug exposure with increasing dose for ARRY-403 in a single ascending dose study [46]. Findings from the analysis suggested that ARRY-403 dissolved completely in the stomach. The disproportionate increase in ARRY-403 exposure with dose was attributed to dose-limited absorption resulting from ARRY-403's marked pH-dependent solubility. As ARRY-403 had a marked pH-dependent solubility, simulations were performed using the PBPK model to examine the effect of acid-reducing agents on its pharmacokinetics. The PBPK simulations suggested that a clinical study with an acid-reducing agent was warranted. An ARRY-403 clinical study with famotidine co-administration confirmed an acid-reducing agent effect on ARRY-403 exposure that was predicted from model simulations. This example demonstrates the utility of PBPK models for investigation of pH effects on oral absorption.

7.2.2. Investigating Mechanisms of Food Effect

An example of a food effect investigation using PBPK modeling is found in a reported investigation of a decrease in zolpidem drug exposure following administration of a modified release formulation with food [49]. Investigation of the mechanisms of this "negative food effect" was performed using biorelevant dissolution testing and commercially available PBPK modeling software. Based on the analysis, it appeared that the absorption of zolpidem is largely determined by the gastric emptying of the formulation. Because of this, considerable intra- and inter-subject variability in the onset of drug absorption was observed, especially for the immediate release formulation. Further, the release of the zolpidem appeared to be impaired by a high-fat and/or protein environment for both the immediate and modified release formulation.

A second example of using PBPK models to explore the mechanism of an observed food effect was an exploration of a positive food effect of compound X [50]. Compound X is a weak base with pH-dependent solubility that exhibited a significant dose-dependent food effect in humans. As part of the PBPK analysis, a parameter sensitivity analysis was performed to evaluate the effect of particle size on the oral absorption of compound X. It was shown that the oral absorption of compound X can be increased by reducing the particle size (<100 nm) of the active pharmaceutical ingredient under fasted conditions. Therefore, it follows that a reduction of particle size in the formulation of compound X would serve as a mitigation strategy to reduce its food effect.

The two studies described above illustrate the how PBPK models are used in investigations of food effect in humans. Further they illustrate the integration of PBPK models as important tools that can provide an understanding of the mechanisms responsible for observed food effects.

7.3. Predicting Human Oral Pharmacokinetics

A third application of PBPK models of oral absorption includes early attempts to predict human pharmacokinetics following oral dosing of drug candidates. These predictions often occur during the drug discovery phase, and with limited PBPK model verification in humans. An example of this application was described by Liu et al., where the oral pharmacokinetic properties in humans of drug candidate YQA-14, a dopamine D_3 receptor antagonist, was successfully predicted [51]. The authors first verified the PBPK model by comparing the performance of simulations using rat and dog PBPK models with preclinical pharmacokinetic data from rats and dogs, respectively. PBPK models of YQA-14 in rat and dog used in vitro microsomal stability data as model inputs. Both models predicted in vivo PK of the respective species within two-fold of the observed values. Following PBPK model verification, a human PBPK model was built again using in vitro microsomal stability data. This human PBPK model was to simulate the PK behavior of YQA-14 in humans. The resulting human PK simulations were deemed acceptable for further development of the compound. While this study demonstrates some value in using oral PBPK models to predict human oral pharmacokinetics in drug discovery, it does not speak to the performance of such models.

A recent PhRMA (Pharmaceutical Research and Manufacturers of America) initiative assessed the quality of PBPK models in predicting oral human PK profiles of 108 compounds using preclinical data in a blinded manner. The study found that only 23% of oral drug simulations had a medium-high accuracy (up to two-fold error) [52]. Simulations had a general underestimation of oral absorption. Furthermore, inaccuracies mostly occurred in drugs with poorly soluble characteristics, which presents a bigger problem in the context of the current trend of increasing lipophilicity in new chemical entities (NCE) [53]. This study points to the idea that PBPK models using preclinical data perform poorly in predicting oral human pharmacokinetic profiles and highlights a need to continue improving our understanding of oral absorption.

7.4. Performance of Various Applications of PBPK Models of Oral Absorption

Of the three areas of application summarized (Sections 7.1–7.3), evidence in the literature of the poor performance of PBPK models of oral absorption appears largely for the prediction of human oral pharmacokinetics. Typically, the prediction of human oral pharmacokinetics occurs at the transition stage between late drug discovery and early drug development. Less ADME and physicochemical information is available for drug candidate compounds at this transition stage, making it more difficult to build a PBPK model with acceptable performance. Further, human oral PK predictions are made prior to having in vivo human pharmacokinetic data available. In contrast, oral PBPK models used to examine drug form selection and formulation optimization often have the benefit of being more refined. These PBPK models may have been verified using in vivo human PK data available from Phase 1 trials, as much of this work is performed following the initial Phase 1 trial. The same can be said for oral PBPK models used to investigate food and pH effects. The availability of more mechanistic information at later stages of drug development likely provides performance advantages to those PBPK models used to investigate drug form selection, formulation optimization, and food and pH effects when compared to the earlier PBPK models used to predict human oral PK. A challenge will be to improve the performance of PBPK models at earlier stages of drug development where less compound-specific information is available. A better understanding of the in vivo relevance of preclinical data used to build PBPK models may serve to improve predictions of human oral pharmacokinetics of new drug candidates in the long term.

7.5. Model Verification/Validation

Successful application of PBPK models of oral absorption require iterative cycles of model verification/validation involving a comparison of observed pharmacokinetic data to that from PBPK model simulations. The poor performance of the "blinded" PBPK predictions of oral human PK of 108 compounds performed by the PhRMA initiative [51] speaks loudly to the importance of verification and re-verification of PBPK models as new data becomes available.

In the drug discovery phase, only preclinical PK data is available for model verification (Figure 6). At this stage, PBPK model verification consists of a comparison between in vivo PK data typically from rat, dog, or monkey to simulations from PBPK models of rat, dog, or monkey, respectively. At this early phase, the importance of PBPK model verification is to determine if you have identified the important preclinical data inputs (usually in vitro data) to enable your PBPK model to predict the in vivo drug disposition of your compound of interest. If successful predictions are made in preclinical species, human oral PK predictions can be performed with a higher level of confidence. In the drug development phase, both preclinical and human PK data is available for model verification. The availability of human data at this later phase plays a big role in improving the performance of PBPK models developed during clinical development. An advantage of initiating PBPK model-building earlier during drug discovery is that it provides an opportunity for more iterations of model verification and refinement. In a sense, an evolving PBPK model that is initially built during drug discovery can serve as a means to capture in vivo relevant ADME information for compounds of interest. This evolving PBPK model can be passed on to new scientists working on a particular compound as it progresses forward in the drug development process.

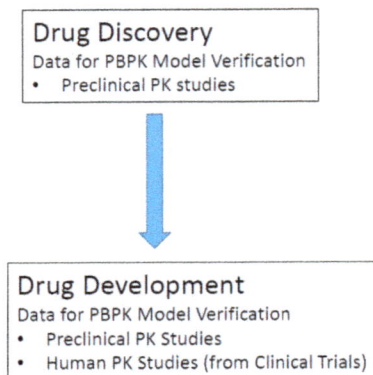

Figure 6. Sources of PK data required for model verification.

8. Conclusions

Computational oral absorption models, in particular PBPK models, provide a powerful tool for researchers and pharmaceutical scientists in drug discovery and development, as they mimic physiologically processes relevant to oral absorption. PBPK models provide in vivo context to in vitro data and allow for a dynamic understanding of in vivo drug disposition that is not typically provided by data from standard in vitro assays. Investigations using oral PBPK models enable informed decision-making, especially with respect to formulation strategies in drug development. PBPK models can also be used to investigate and provide insight into mechanisms responsible for complex phenomena such as food effects.

Ongoing research in the area of oral absorption will increase understanding and allow for the refinement of oral PBPK models. As our understanding of oral absorption improves, the ability of PBPK models to predict oral pharmacokinetics will also improve, providing a better tool for the discovery and development of new medicines in the pharmaceutical industry.

Author Contributions: Louis Lin and Harvey Wong conceived and wrote this paper.

Conflicts of Interest: The authors declare no conflict of interest.

References

1. Sugihara, M.; Takeuchi, S.; Sugita, M.; Higaki, K.; Kataoka, M.; Yamashita, S. Analysis of intra- and intersubject variability in oral drug absorption in human bioequivalence studies of 113 generic products. *Mol. Pharm.* **2015**, *12*, 4405–4413. [CrossRef] [PubMed]
2. Martinez, M.N.; Amidon, G.L. A mechanistic approach to understanding the factors affecting drug absorption: A review of fundamentals. *J. Clin. Pharmacol.* **2002**, *42*, 620–643. [CrossRef] [PubMed]
3. Mudie, D.M.; Amidon, G.L.; Amidon, G.E. Physiological parameters for oral delivery and in vitro testing. *Mol. Pharm.* **2010**, *7*, 1388–1405. [CrossRef] [PubMed]

4. Waring, M.J.; Arrowsmith, J.; Leach, A.R.; Leeson, P.D.; Mandrell, S.; Owen, R.M.; Pairaudeau, G.; Pennie, W.D.; Pickett, S.D.; Wang, J.; et al. An analysis of the attrition of drug candidates from four major pharmaceutical companies. *Nat. Rev. Drug Discov.* **2015**, *14*, 475–486. [CrossRef] [PubMed]

5. Ward, K.W. Optimizing pharmacokinetic properties and attaining candidate selection. In *Reducing Drug Attrition*; Topics in Medicinal Chemistry; Springer: Berlin, Germany, 2012; pp. 73–95. ISBN 978-3-662-43913-5.

6. Chu, X.; Bleasby, K.; Evers, R. Species differences in drug transporters and implications for translating preclinical findings to humans. *Expert Opin. Drug Metab. Toxicol.* **2013**, *9*, 237–252. [CrossRef] [PubMed]

7. Chanteux, H.; Staelens, L.; Mancel, V.; Gerin, B.; Boucaut, D.; Prakash, C.; Nicolas, J.-M. Cross-species differences in the preclinical pharmacokinetics of CT7758, an α4β1/α4β7 integrin antagonist. *Drug Metab. Dispos. Biol. Fate Chem.* **2015**, *43*, 1381–1391. [CrossRef] [PubMed]

8. Dressman, J.B.; Amidon, G.L.; Fleisher, D. Absorption potential: Estimating the fraction absorbed for orally administered compounds. *J. Pharm. Sci.* **1985**, *74*, 588–589. [CrossRef] [PubMed]

9. Johnson, K.C.; Swindell, A.C. Guidance in the setting of drug particle size specifications to minimize variability in absorption. *Pharm. Res.* **1996**, *13*, 1795–1798. [CrossRef] [PubMed]

10. Ding, X.; Rose, J.P.; Van Gelder, J. Developability assessment of clinical drug products with maximum absorbable doses. *Int. J. Pharm.* **2012**, *427*, 260–269. [CrossRef] [PubMed]

11. Sun, D.; Yu, L.X.; Hussain, M.A.; Wall, D.A.; Smith, R.L.; Amidon, G.L. In vitro testing of drug absorption for drug "developability" assessment: Forming an interface between in vitro preclinical data and clinical outcome. *Curr. Opin. Drug Discov. Devel.* **2004**, *7*, 75–85. [PubMed]

12. Torsten, T. Kinetics of distribution of substances administered to the body, I: The extravascular modes of administration. *Arch. Int. Pharmacodyn. Ther.* **1937**, *57*, 205–225.

13. Jones, H.M.; Parrott, N.; Jorga, K.; Lavé, T. A Novel strategy for physiologically based predictions of human pharmacokinetics. *Clin. Pharmacokinet.* **2006**, *45*, 511–542. [CrossRef] [PubMed]

14. Noyes, A.A.; Whitney, W.R. The rate of solution of solid substances in their own solutions. *J. Am. Chem. Soc.* **1897**, *19*, 930–934. [CrossRef]

15. Sugano, K.; Okazaki, A.; Sugimoto, S.; Tavornvipas, S.; Omura, A.; Mano, T. Solubility and dissolution profile assessment in drug discovery. *Drug Metab. Pharmacokinet.* **2007**, *22*, 225–254. [CrossRef] [PubMed]

16. Dressman, J.B.; Fleisher, D. Mixing-tank model for predicting dissolution rate control or oral absorption. *J. Pharm. Sci.* **1986**, *75*, 109–116. [CrossRef] [PubMed]

17. Yu, L.X.; Crison, J.R.; Amidon, G.L. Compartmental transit and dispersion model analysis of small intestinal transit flow in humans. *Int. J. Pharm.* **1996**, *140*, 111–118. [CrossRef]

18. Dressman, J.B.; Fleisher, D.; Amidon, G.L. Physicochemical model for dose-dependent drug absorption. *J. Pharm. Sci.* **1984**, *73*, 1274–1279. [CrossRef] [PubMed]

19. Oberle, R.L.; Amidon, G.L. The influence of variable gastric emptying and intestinal transit rates on the plasma level curve of cimetidine; an explanation for the double peak phenomenon. *J. Pharmacokinet. Biopharm.* **1987**, *15*, 529–544. [CrossRef] [PubMed]

20. Luner, P.E.; Amidon, G.L. Description and simulation of a multiple mixing tank model to predict the effect of bile sequestrants on bile salt excretion. *J. Pharm. Sci.* **1993**, *82*, 311–318. [CrossRef] [PubMed]

21. Bailey, J.M.; Shafer, S.L. A simple analytical solution to the three-compartment pharmacokinetic model suitable for computer-controlled infusion pumps. *IEEE Trans. Biomed. Eng.* **1991**, *38*, 522–525. [CrossRef] [PubMed]

22. Yu, L.X. An integrated model for determining causes of poor oral drug absorption. *Pharm. Res.* **1999**, *16*, 1883–1887. [CrossRef] [PubMed]

23. Agoram, B.; Woltosz, W.S.; Bolger, M.B. Predicting the impact of physiological and biochemical processes on oral drug bioavailability. *Adv. Drug Deliv. Rev.* **2001**, *50* (Suppl. 1), S41–S67. [CrossRef]

24. Jambhekar, S.S.; Breen, P.J. Drug dissolution: Significance of physicochemical properties and physiological conditions. *Drug Discov. Today* **2013**, *18*, 1173–1184. [CrossRef] [PubMed]

25. Dressman, J.B.; Vertzoni, M.; Goumas, K.; Reppas, C. Estimating drug solubility in the gastrointestinal tract. *Adv. Drug Deliv. Rev.* **2007**, *59*, 591–602. [CrossRef] [PubMed]

26. Mouly, S.; Paine, M.F. P-glycoprotein increases from proximal to distal regions of human small intestine. *Pharm. Res.* **2003**, *20*, 1595–1599. [CrossRef] [PubMed]

27. Ungell, A.L.; Nylander, S.; Bergstrand, S.; Sjöberg, A.; Lennernäs, H. Membrane transport of drugs in different regions of the intestinal tract of the rat. *J. Pharm. Sci.* **1998**, *87*, 360–366. [CrossRef] [PubMed]

28. Paine, M.F.; Khalighi, M.; Fisher, J.M.; Shen, D.D.; Kunze, K.L.; Marsh, C.L.; Perkins, J.D.; Thummel, K.E. Characterization of interintestinal and intraintestinal variations in human CYP3A-dependent metabolism. *J. Pharmacol. Exp. Ther.* **1997**, *283*, 1552–1562. [PubMed]

29. Sawamoto, T.; Haruta, S.; Kurosaki, Y.; Higaki, K.; Kimura, T. Prediction of the plasma concentration profiles of orally administered drugs in rats on the basis of gastrointestinal transit kinetics and absorbability. *J. Pharm. Pharmacol.* **1997**, *49*, 450–457. [CrossRef] [PubMed]

30. Jamei, M.Y.J. A Novel Physiologically-Based Mechanistic Model for Predicting Oral Drug Absorption: The Advanced Dissolution, Absorption, and Metabolism (ADAM) Model. Available online: https://www.escholar.manchester.ac.uk/uk-ac-man-scw:108992 (accessed on 12 September 2017).

31. Wang, J.; Flanagan, D.R. General solution for diffusion-controlled dissolution of spherical particles. 1. Theory. *J. Pharm. Sci.* **1999**, *88*, 731–738. [CrossRef] [PubMed]

32. Murakami, T.; Takano, M. Intestinal efflux transporters and drug absorption. *Expert Opin. Drug Metab. Toxicol.* **2008**, *4*, 923–939. [CrossRef] [PubMed]

33. Hurst, S.; Loi, C.-M.; Brodfuehrer, J.; El-Kattan, A. Impact of physiological, physicochemical and biopharmaceutical factors in absorption and metabolism mechanisms on the drug oral bioavailability of rats and humans. *Expert Opin. Drug Metab. Toxicol.* **2007**, *3*, 469–489. [CrossRef] [PubMed]

34. Chan, L.M.S.; Cooper, A.E.; Dudley, A.L.J.; Ford, D.; Hirst, B.H. P-glycoprotein potentiates CYP3A4-mediated drug disappearance during Caco-2 intestinal secretory detoxification. *J. Drug Target.* **2004**, *12*, 405–413. [CrossRef] [PubMed]

35. Wacher, V.J.; Silverman, J.A.; Zhang, Y.; Benet, L.Z. Role of P-glycoprotein and cytochrome P450 3A in limiting oral absorption of peptides and peptidomimetics. *J. Pharm. Sci.* **1998**, *87*, 1322–1330. [CrossRef] [PubMed]

36. Lown, K.S.; Mayo, R.R.; Leichtman, A.B.; Hsiao, H.L.; Turgeon, D.K.; Schmiedlin-Ren, P.; Brown, M.B.; Guo, W.; Rossi, S.J.; Benet, L.Z.; et al. Role of intestinal P-glycoprotein (MDR1) in interpatient variation in the oral bioavailability of cyclosporine. *Clin. Pharmacol. Ther.* **1997**, *62*, 248–260. [CrossRef]

37. Wacher, V.J.; Wu, C.Y.; Benet, L.Z. Overlapping substrate specificities and tissue distribution of cytochrome P450 3A and P-glycoprotein: Implications for drug delivery and activity in cancer chemotherapy. *Mol. Carcinog.* **1995**, *13*, 129–134. [CrossRef] [PubMed]

38. Kumar, S.; Samuel, K.; Subramanian, R.; Braun, M.P.; Stearns, R.A.; Chiu, S.-H.L.; Evans, D.C.; Baillie, T.A. Extrapolation of diclofenac clearance from in vitro microsomal metabolism data: Role of Acyl glucuronidation and sequential oxidative metabolism of the Acyl glucuronide. *J. Pharmacol. Exp. Ther.* **2002**, *303*, 969–978. [CrossRef] [PubMed]

39. Kusuhara, H.; Sugiyama, Y. In vitro-in vivo extrapolation of transporter-mediated clearance in the liver and kidney. *Drug Metab. Pharmacokinet.* **2009**, *24*, 37–52. [CrossRef] [PubMed]

40. Kitamura, S.; Maeda, K.; Sugiyama, Y. Recent progresses in the experimental methods and evaluation strategies of transporter functions for the prediction of the pharmacokinetics in humans. *Naunyn-Schmiedebergs Arch. Pharmacol.* **2008**, *377*, 617. [CrossRef] [PubMed]

41. Gertz, M.; Houston, J.B.; Galetin, A. Physiologically based pharmacokinetic modeling of intestinal first-pass metabolism of CYP3A substrates with high intestinal extraction. *Drug Metab. Dispos.* **2011**, *39*, 1633–1642. [CrossRef] [PubMed]

42. Chiang, P.-C.; Wong, H. Incorporation of physiologically based pharmacokinetic modeling in the evaluation of solubility requirements for the salt selection process: A case study using phenytoin. *AAPS J.* **2013**, *15*, 1109–1118. [CrossRef] [PubMed]

43. Parrott, N.; Lave, T. Applications of physiologically based absorption models in drug discovery and development. *Mol. Pharm.* **2008**, *5*, 760–775. [CrossRef] [PubMed]

44. Abuhelwa, A.Y.; Williams, D.B.; Upton, R.N.; Foster, D.J.R. Food, gastrointestinal pH, and models of oral drug absorption. *Eur. J. Pharm. Biopharm.* **2017**, *112*, 234–248. [CrossRef] [PubMed]

45. Li, X.; Shi, L.; Tang, X.; Wang, Q.; Zhou, L.; Song, W.; Feng, Z.; Ge, J.; Li, J.K.; Yang, L.; et al. Mechanistic prediction of food effects for Compound A tablet using PBPK model. *Saudi J. Biol. Sci.* **2017**, *24*, 603–609. [CrossRef] [PubMed]

46. Chung, J.; Alvarez-Nunez, F.; Chow, V.; Daurio, D.; Davis, J.; Dodds, M.; Emery, M.; Litwiler, K.; Paccaly, A.; Peng, J.; et al. Utilizing physiologically based pharmacokinetic modeling to inform formulation and clinical development for a Compound with pH-dependent solubility. *J. Pharm. Sci.* **2015**, *104*, 1522–1532. [CrossRef] [PubMed]

47. Welling, P.G. Effects of food on drug absorption. *Annu. Rev. Nutr.* **1996**, *16*, 383–415. [CrossRef] [PubMed]

48. Glomme, A.; März, J.; Dressman, J.B. Predicting the intestinal solubility of poorly soluble drugs. In *Pharmacokinetic Profiling in Drug Research*; Testa, B., Krämer, S.D., Wunderli-Allenspach, H., Folkers, G., Eds.; Wiley-VCH: Weinheim, Germany, 2006; pp. 259–280, ISBN 978-3-906390-46-8.

49. Andreas, C.J.; Pepin, X.; Markopoulos, C.; Vertzoni, M.; Reppas, C.; Dressman, J.B. Mechanistic investigation of the negative food effect of modified release zolpidem. *Eur. J. Pharm. Sci.* **2017**, *102*, 284–298. [CrossRef] [PubMed]

50. Zhang, H.; Xia, B.; Sheng, J.; Heimbach, T.; Lin, T.-H.; He, H.; Wang, Y.; Novick, S.; Comfort, A. Application of physiologically based absorption modeling to formulation development of a low solubility, low permeability weak base: Mechanistic investigation of food effect. *AAPS PharmSciTech* **2014**, *15*, 400–406. [CrossRef] [PubMed]

51. Liu, F.; Zhuang, X.; Yang, C.; Li, Z.; Xiong, S.; Zhang, Z.; Li, J.; Lu, C.; Zhang, Z. Characterization of preclinical in vitro and in vivo ADME properties and prediction of human PK using a physiologically based pharmacokinetic model for YQA-14, a new dopamine D3 receptor antagonist candidate for treatment of drug addiction. *Biopharm. Drug Dispos.* **2014**, *35*, 296–307. [CrossRef] [PubMed]

52. Poulin, P.; Jones, R.D.O.; Jones, H.M.; Gibson, C.R.; Rowland, M.; Chien, J.Y.; Ring, B.J.; Adkison, K.K.; Ku, M.S.; He, H.; et al. PHRMA CPCDC initiative on predictive models of human pharmacokinetics, Part 5: Prediction of plasma concentration-time profiles in human by using the physiologically-based pharmacokinetic modeling approach. *J. Pharm. Sci.* **2011**, *100*, 4127–4157. [CrossRef] [PubMed]

53. Williams, H.D.; Trevaskis, N.L.; Charman, S.A.; Shanker, R.M.; Charman, W.N.; Pouton, C.W.; Porter, C.J.H. Strategies to address low drug solubility in discovery and development. *Pharmacol. Rev.* **2013**, *65*, 315–499. [CrossRef] [PubMed]

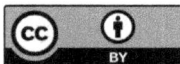

pharmaceutics

MDPI

Review

Revolutionizing Therapeutic Drug Monitoring with the Use of Interstitial Fluid and Microneedles Technology

Tony K.L. Kiang [1], Sahan A. Ranamukhaarachchi [2] and Mary H.H. Ensom [3,*]

[1] Faculty of Pharmacy and Pharmaceutical Sciences, University of Alberta, Edmonton, AB T6G 2E1, Canada; tkiang@ualberta.ca
[2] Department of Electrical and Computer Engineering, University of British Columbia, Vancouver, BC V6T 1Z4, Canada; sahan@microdermics.com
[3] Faculty of Pharmaceutical Sciences, University of British Columbia, Vancouver, BC V6T 1Z3, Canada
*   Correspondence: ensom@mail.ubc.ca; Tel.: +1-604-875-2886

Received: 30 August 2017; Accepted: 7 October 2017; Published: 11 October 2017

Abstract: While therapeutic drug monitoring (TDM) that uses blood as the biological matrix is the traditional gold standard, this practice may be impossible, impractical, or unethical for some patient populations (e.g., elderly, pediatric, anemic) and those with fragile veins. In the context of finding an alternative biological matrix for TDM, this manuscript will provide a qualitative review on: (1) the principles of TDM; (2) alternative matrices for TDM; (3) current evidence supporting the use of interstitial fluid (ISF) for TDM in clinical models; (4) the use of microneedle technologies, which is potentially minimally invasive and pain-free, for the collection of ISF; and (5) future directions. The current state of knowledge on the use of ISF for TDM in humans is still limited. A thorough literature review indicates that only a few drug classes have been investigated (i.e., anti-infectives, anticonvulsants, and miscellaneous other agents). Studies have successfully demonstrated techniques for ISF extraction from the skin but have failed to demonstrate commercial feasibility of ISF extraction followed by analysis of its content outside the ISF-collecting microneedle device. In contrast, microneedle-integrated biosensors built to extract ISF and perform the biomolecule analysis on-device, with a key feature of not needing to transfer ISF to a separate instrument, have yielded promising results that need to be validated in pre-clinical and clinical studies. The most promising applications for microneedle-integrated biosensors is continuous monitoring of biomolecules from the skin's ISF. Conducting TDM using ISF is at the stage where its clinical utility should be investigated. Based on the advancements described in the current review, the immediate future direction for this area of research is to establish the suitability of using ISF for TDM in human models for drugs that have been found suitable in pre-clinical experiments.

Keywords: clinical pharmacokinetics; therapeutic drug monitoring; interstitial fluid; microneedles

1. Introduction

Therapeutic drug monitoring (TDM) is broadly defined as the science or practice of optimizing drug therapy by targeting drug concentrations in biological matrices to the defined therapeutic range in order to increase and decrease the probabilities of efficacy and adverse effects, respectively. Fundamentally, the science of pharmacokinetics (PK) is the underpinning for the practice of TDM; that is, how the absorption, distribution, metabolism, and elimination processes of a drug dictate how TDM is implemented. Not all drugs are subjected to TDM and considerable research is continuing to be conducted on all aspects of TDM today.

From the practical stand point, the traditional gold-standard approach to TDM is to collect blood (hereafter, the term "blood" will be used in this manuscript to infer any biological matrices related to blood, plasma, or serum), because it is relatively easier to obtain compared to other matrices (e.g., organ tissues). Due to the fact that blood remains the gold standard for TDM, the majority of the target range is still being developed in this matrix. However, the primary assumption for using blood for TDM is that drug concentration in the blood compartment is reflective of that attained in the target site, which is not always the case (e.g., concentrations of antibiotics can differ in blood compared to muscle or fat tissues [1]). Moreover, the act of obtaining blood is a relatively invasive procedure which can potentially lead to untoward adverse effects such as iatrogenic infection and psychological unpleasantness [2]. In many patient populations (e.g., elderly, pediatric, anemic) and those with fragile veins, it might be impossible, impractical, or even unethical to obtain this biological fluid for any therapeutic purpose. With the substantial costs associated with collecting and analyzing blood (e.g., salary for nurses, phlebotomists, and lab technicians), it is of great interest for researchers and clinicians to find alternative biological matrices that can be as effective as blood for TDM but without the aforementioned untoward effects.

While many non-blood biological matrices have been investigated in the context of TDM [3], many have limitations that preclude their routine usage in the clinic. One of the few exceptions is interstitial fluid (ISF), which has gained a significant interest and recently fueled the research activities of many laboratories, including ours [1,4–6]. In the context of finding an alternative biological matrix for TDM, this manuscript will provide a qualitative review on: (1) the principles of TDM; (2) alternative matrices for TDM; (3) current evidence supporting the use of ISF for TDM in clinical models; (4) the use of microneedle technologies, which is potentially minimally invasive and pain-free, for the collection of ISF; and (5) future directions.

2. Principles of Therapeutic Drug Monitoring

The term therapeutic drug monitoring is often used interchangeably with clinical pharmacokinetic monitoring. TDM emerged as a clinical discipline in the late 1960s and early 1970s and involves the measurement and interpretation of drug concentrations in order to provide safe and efficacious dosing of drugs. In the past, we applied 4 basic principles to ascertain whether or not to perform routine TDM. These fundamental tenets were: (1) Is there a good relationship between drug concentration and pharmacological response? (2) Does wide interpatient variation exist in drug absorption, distribution, metabolism or excretion? (3) Does the drug have a narrow therapeutic range? and (4) Is the drug's pharmacological response not readily assessable [7,8]?

Given more recent focus on patient-centered care and individualization of dosage regimens as well as judicious use of limited resources, we added to these 4 basic principles and developed a 9-step decision-making algorithm to ascertain whether or not to perform selective TDM for a given patient in a specific scenario. The 9 steps include: (1) Is the patient on the best drug for his/her specific disease state and specific indication? (2) Can the drug be readily measured in the desired biological matrix? (3) Has a good relationship between drug concentration and pharmacologic response been reported in pharmacokinetic studies conducted in humans? (4) Does this relationship still apply to the patient's specific disease state and specific indication? (5) Is the drug's pharmacologic response not readily assessable? (6) Does the drug have a narrow therapeutic range for the specific disease state and indication? (7) Are the pharmacokinetic parameters unpredictable, due to either intrinsic variability or the presence of other confounding factors? (8) Is the duration of drug therapy of a sufficient length for the patient to benefit from clinical pharmacokinetic monitoring? and (9) Will the results of the drug assay make a significant difference in the clinical decision-making process? (i.e., provide more information than sound clinical judgement alone) [7]? If one can answer "yes" to the last question (i.e., quintessential step 9) and "yes" to most of the other questions, then selective TDM is warranted for that particular patient scenario.

From the practical stand point, TDM is usually conducted at steady-state conditions using one or more concentrations. A trough concentration is often used as a surrogate to the area-under-the concentration time curve (AUC), the best marker for drug exposure. Limited sampling strategies (i.e., using 2–4 concentration samples to predict AUC) have become more widely utilized in various disease states as well (e.g., solid organ transplant [9]). Theoretically, once the basic PK characteristics about a drug are known, TDM can be tailored to already-established fundamental PK models (e.g., one, two, three-compartments; oral vs. parenteral; intermittent vs. continuous infusion; linear vs. non-linear (Michaelis-Menten) disposition; well-stirred vs. parallel-tube, etc.). Moreover, a universally accepted idea is that only the free drug is pharmacologically active and subjected to further PK processes (e.g., metabolism or elimination). Because free drug concentrations are not easily accessible, another branch of TDM is the development of static models to "predict" free from total drug concentrations in specific patient populations (e.g., phenytoin [10,11]). Recent advances in physiologically-based PK modeling and population PK modeling [12,13] with Bayesian applications (e.g., so-called "dynamic models" [9]) have further revolutionized the prediction/simulation of drug concentrations for TDM as well.

Since the publication of the decision-making algorithm in 1998, many clinician researchers have used it to critically assess currently available literature and determine the utility of TDM for specific drugs in specific patient scenarios [7]. Examples of papers in various therapeutic classes and special populations are available: central nervous system disorders (e.g., [14,15]), infectious disease (e.g., [16,17]), organ transplant (e.g., [18,19]), pediatric patients (e.g., [20,21]), cancer (e.g., [22]), psychiatric disorders (e.g., [23,24]). This paper will focus on step 2—can the drug be readily measured in the desired biological matrix?

3. Alternative Matrices for Therapeutic Drug Monitoring

Many alternative, less-invasive biological matrices (e.g., ISF, oral fluids, hair, sweat, tears, semen, breast milk, urine) have been investigated for the purpose of TDM [3,25]. In our opinion, with exceptions of a few specific applications where a certain matrix (e.g., tears) is preferred in unique situations (e.g., drug concentrations in eye disorders) [25], only saliva and ISF show the potential to replace blood primarily because drug concentrations can be quantified reliably and consistently in these matrices.

The science and practice of saliva TDM is still undergoing significant evolution [26–29]. Although saliva can be used for the monitoring of illicit drug use (i.e., "doping") [30], the discussion here will focus only on TDM. Saliva is composed of aqueous fluids secreted by three salivary glands [28]. The composition of saliva, with respect to electrolytes and macromolecules, can differ based on intrinsic (e.g., healthy vs. diseased) and extrinsic (e.g., concurrent drugs that modulate the sympathetic or parasympathetic systems; method of saliva simulation) factors [27,28]. A common observation, however, is that protein content is significantly lower in saliva compared to blood [27,28]. There are many advantages and disadvantages of using saliva for diagnostics, which have been extensively reviewed [26–29]. For the purpose of TDM, the primary advantages for using saliva are the non-invasive nature for obtaining this biological fluid and the fact that saliva drug concentration reflects the free (i.e., pharmacologically active) concentration. Because of the latter characteristic, saliva has the distinct benefit over other matrices (e.g., whole tissue, blood) which are protein-rich and require additional analytical techniques to determine free drug concentrations. The primary disadvantages for using saliva for TDM are potential contaminants, drug instability, and lack of phase II metabolites [3,29]. In order for saliva to replace blood for the purpose of TDM, correlations between saliva-blood concentrations also need to be established.

The biochemical properties of xenobiotics (i.e., ionizability, molecular weight, lipophilicity, protein binding) are known to affect the distribution/excretion of drug into saliva [31]. Of these, the ionizability of the drug molecule in saliva appears to play a primary role in the penetration ratio because only unionized drugs can partition into this matrix [29]. Based on these principles, not all drugs are detectable in saliva. The first documented salivary TDM dates back to the 1970s when theophylline [32], digoxin [33], lithium [34], and various anticonvulsant drugs [35] were initially investigated. Since then, the suitability of conducting TDM in saliva for drugs in various therapeutic classes has been reported. While not the primary objective of this paper, the most recent review articles—based on therapeutic classes—on salivary TDM are cited here for the reader's reference: antibiotics [36], anticonvulsants [37], antiretroviral agents [38], and psychotropics [39].

Similar to saliva, ISF has very similar composition as plasma but lower protein content [40]; therefore, drugs are mostly present in ISF in the free (active) form and the matrix is relatively easier to assay compared to blood. Because ISF serves as the connection between vasculature and cells, it acts as a conduit or medium for various signaling molecules and cellular wastes [41], although the exact composition of ISF can differ between organs or locations [40]. In addition to TDM, ISF has been used for other purposes such as diagnostics (e.g., for monitoring the degree of traumatic brain injury) [40] or treatment (e.g., being the primary site for many bacterial infections) [1]. The use of ISF for TDM can have several advantages: potentially pain-free (to be discussed below in the section on sampling techniques, including the use of microneedles), less cumbersome analytical assays (because the matrix is relatively clean and devoid of large macromolecules or cellular debris), and potentially less costly because the collection does not require specially trained personnel. Similar to saliva, however, in order for ISF to replace blood for the purpose of TDM, correlations between ISF-blood concentrations need to be established. On the other hand, unlike saliva, factors influencing the partitioning of drugs between blood and ISF are relatively poorly understood. Although biochemical properties (e.g., ionizability, molecular weight, lipophilicity, protein binding) can theoretically affect drug distribution into ISF, no good correlations have been observed with most of these variables in the currently available literature [1]. Although data are available on drug distribution kinetics (including model-based predictions) into whole tissues (e.g., [42–45]), the ISF compartment would exhibit different physiological properties and warrant an investigation itself. The currently available evidence supporting the use of ISF for TDM in humans is presented in the next section.

4. Current Evidence Supporting the Use of Interstitial Fluid for Therapeutic Drug Monitoring in Clinical Models

For the purpose of this manuscript, data pertaining to cerebral spinal fluid, brain extracellular fluid, tumor ISF, or any internal organ tissue fluid which is not routinely sampled and cannot be characterized non-invasively for the purpose of TDM will be excluded. This approach is similar to exclusion criteria we published previously [1]. Likewise, only studies incorporating microdialysis have been included, because other models (skin blisters, whole tissue) do not adequately reflect the ISF space [1]. Based on our comprehensive investigation in an animal model using an extensive panel of drugs commonly subjected to TDM today [4], a novel scoring algorithm was developed to characterize the suitability of conducting TDM in ISF: directly suitable ("comparable exposure and similar concentration-time profile versus blood"); likely suitable ("different exposure, but similar concentration-time profile versus blood"); unlikely suitable ("detectable in ISF, but different concentration-time profile versus blood"); and not suitable ("not detected in ISF") [4]. We have already used this algorithm to analyze the suitability of using ISF or saliva for TDM in humans for anti-infective drugs [1,36]. The same principles will be employed in this paper to discuss the evidence supporting the use of ISF for TDM of other drug classes. In short, the current state of knowledge on the use of ISF for TDM in humans is still limited. A thorough literature review indicates that only a few drug classes have been investigated (i.e., anti-infectives, anticonvulsants, and miscellaneous other agents). A body of literature is also available on the measurement of drug concentrations in solid tumors [46–52] which is excluded from this paper (i.e., not used routinely for the purpose of TDM) and has been reviewed elsewhere [53,54].

4.1. Anti-Infectives

The majority of the ISF data collected in humans to date is related to anti-infectives because ISF is the primary target compartment of interests for various types of infections [1]. The evidence supporting the use of ISF for TDM for antibiotics has been systematically reviewed by Kiang et al. up to February 2014 [1], which will be summarized briefly. Additional novel data published since this paper will be presented in more detail.

Kiang et al. [1] provided a comprehensive review detailing 87 individual PK comparisons between tissue ISF and blood on various antibiotic classes: penicillins, cephalosporins, fluoroquinolones, carbapenems, oxazolidiones, macrolides, glycopeptides/glycylcycline/lipopeptide and other agents. Overall, different antibiotics exhibited different degrees of penetration into ISF of muscle or adipose tissue [1]. With respect to penicillins, the majority of data were collected on piperacillin, which showed reduced concentration in ISF compared to blood, especially in critically ill (i.e., intensive care) patients. The ability of a specific cephalosporin (i.e., cefaclor, cefixime, cefodizime, cefpirome, cefpodoxime, ceftobiprole, cefuroxime) to penetrate into ISF also appears to be dependent on the type of tissue (i.e., muscle vs. adipose) and the degree of protein binding. In the case of cefpirome, a significant reduction in ISF penetration was observed in critically ill patients, indicating that a potentially more aggressive dosing regimen might be warranted in this patient population [1]. More recently, Roberts et al. [55] compared the pharmacokinetics of cefazolin in subcutaneous ISF and blood in post-trauma critically ill patients ($N = 30$) and found similar exposure (median % penetration ratio of 74%) between the two matrices. Despite the fact that specific pharmacokinetic values were not reported, the concentration-time profiles between the two matrices appear approximately "equivalent", indicating that it is suitable to monitor cefazolin in ISF in this population (albeit cefazolin concentrations are not typically measured in clinical practice). Overall, most of the penicillins and cephalosporins can be categorized as likely suitable drugs for TDM in ISF, due to comparable elimination characteristics but different exposure values in both blood and ISF.

Different degrees of tissue ISF penetration were observed for carbapenems in humans [1]. While doripenem and ertapenem show consistent distribution ratios between different tissues, inconsistent findings were reported for imipenem between muscle and adipose and between studies. The inconsistencies found with imipenem may have been attributed to experimental artifacts, pointing to the potential limitations of comparing findings from multiple sources utilizing different microdialysis calibration techniques. Moreover, imipenem's distribution into ISF in critically ill patients might be dependent on renal function, as evident by contrasting findings shown by Tegeder et al. [56] and Dahyot et al. [57]. More recently, Varghese et al. [58] determined the penetration ratio of meropenem in critically ill patients receiving continuous hemodialysis and noted reduced exposure in subcutaneous ISF (60–74%) compared to blood. Although it was not clear whether the free blood concentration was determined in this study, the concentration-time profiles of meropenem in both matrices exhibited similar characteristics. Overall, the carbapenems can be categorized as likely suitable for TDM in ISF, due to comparable elimination characteristics but different exposure values in both blood and ISF [1].

With respect to the glycopeptides/glycylcycline/lipopeptides, both daptomycin and tigecycline distribute into tissue ISF completely in a manner independent of tissue inflammation or the diagnosis of diabetes [1]. These data suggest that daptomycin and tigecycline could be likely suitable for TDM in ISF (although they are not subjected to routine TDM today). Although vancomycin distributes well into tissues (penetration ratio of 0.8 from comparable exposure in two matrices based on free concentrations) in otherwise healthy subjects with limb infections [59], evidence suggests a reduced penetration in diabetic patients [60,61]. Population modeling also suggests potential suboptimal vancomycin tissue exposure in diabetics which may result in treatment failure [60], but these simulations require further testing in real clinical subjects. The findings for vancomycin in humans of comparable pharmacokinetic characteristics between ISF and blood is consistent with that observed in various animal models, including that published in our own lab [1,62]. Because vancomycin is one of the most frequently monitored drugs in the clinic today, these data suggest that vancomycin could be a potential drug candidate to test the paradigm of using ISF for the purpose of TDM. However, more studies are needed to characterize the effects of intrinsic and extrinsic factors that may affect the disposition characteristics of vancomycin. Further pharmacokinetic modeling is also needed to determine the relationship between ISF and blood concentrations, tailored for the purpose of TDM.

In contrast to the heterogeneity of tissue ISF penetration characteristics observed within many antibiotic classes presented in this manuscript, some consistent class effects of robust tissue distribution could be observed for fluoroquinolones (ciprofloxacin, levofloxacin, moxifloxacin, except for gemifloxacin) and oxazolidinones (linezolid and torezolid) [1], because the distribution ratios appear complete and independent of tissue type (muscle vs. adipose) or disease state (healthy vs. sepsis or diabetes). On the other hand, many macrolide antibiotics (except for telithromycin) penetrate into tissue ISF relatively poorly, resulting in potentially suboptimal drug concentrations at the target site [1]. Based on these characteristics and the available limited data, fluoroquinolones and oxazolidinones in general might be suitable for TDM in ISF whereas the macrolides would not be suitable. While the clinical utility of fluoroquinolone or oxazolidinone TDM still remains to be established, further research is needed to elucidate how drugs in certain classes penetrate into ISF space better than others and careful consideration is needed when selecting and avoiding antibiotic classes for the treatment of tissue infections.

4.2. Anticonvulsants

There is a significant interest regarding TDM for anticonvulsants using alternative body fluids [37,63] and ISF is no exception. The majority of the experiments pertaining to ISF have been conducted with valproic acid [64–67] although preliminary data on other agents (topiramate, carbamazepine, phenytoin, and phenobarbital) are also available [68,69]. Given that patients taking these agents are often monitored on an outpatient basis, having a TDM matrix that is more convenient than blood could potentially improve patient care and quality of life. Although these authors indicated collecting extracellular fluid, their approach (i.e., in vivo microdialysis on subcutaneous tissue) is reflective of free drug concentrations in ISF. The data for valproic acid look promising in that there is a good qualitative correlation between free tissue and blood concentrations in epileptic [64] and healthy subjects [65]. Moreover, the concentration-time profiles of free valproic acid in epileptic patients ($N = 3$) receiving a single dose of valproic acid or in one subject under steady-state conditions were virtually superimposable between ISF and blood [66]. However, a subsequent study using a larger sample size indicated a higher free fraction in plasma under steady-state conditions compared to single-dose conditions [67]. Although specific pharmacokinetic parameters were lacking in these studies to allow a systematic categorization of suitability, these data are suggestive of the general appropriateness of using ISF for TDM for valproic acid. Given that valproic acid is a frequently monitored anticonvulsant drug today, further systematic studies are needed to establish the quantitative relationships between ISF and blood (i.e., using compartmental, population modeling) under various conditions (e.g., single-dose vs. steady-state, healthy vs. various diseased populations requiring valproic acid, mono-therapy vs. polypharmacy, etc.) in order to determine the role of ISF for TDM.

In a single epileptic patient receiving doses of topiramate (not under steady-state conditions) co-administered with phenytoin and dextropropoxifen, the concentration-time profiles of free topiramate in subcutaneous ISF and blood were comparable with a high correlation coefficient (0.99) [69]. Likewise, in single case studies of patients undergoing tapering regimens, carbamazepine and phenobarbital [68] also exhibited similar pharmacokinetic characteristics in subcutaneous ISF and blood up to 70 h post-dose. In Lindberger et al. [68], phenytoin was not detectable in tissue ISF due to extensive binding to the microdialysis tubing. The observation of likely suitable nature with phenobarbital is consistent with our observation in rabbits [4]. Although we noticed the same effects (lack of detection in ISF) with phenytoin in our rabbit experiments, it was not due to recovery, indicating other factors that may prevent phenytoin's distribution into ISF should also be considered. Unfortunately, neither study provided quantitative pharmacokinetic data to allow a systematic determination of suitability of conducting TDM in ISF for these anticonvulsants. Given that topiramate drug concentrations can be used occasionally to guide dosing in refractory, resistant seizure cases, and that phenobarbital and carbamazepine are routinely monitored, more studies in larger patient samples are warranted.

4.3. Miscellaneous Agents

The concentrations of various other drugs have been determined in ISF and compared to blood. Boschmann et al. [70] compared the concentrations of aliskiren in obese hypertensive subjects ($N = 10$)

in adipose ISF, skeletal muscle ISF, and blood under steady-state conditions. Aliskiren appeared to distribute to skeletal muscle ISF (concentration comparable to blood) to a greater extent compared to adipose ISF. Because pharmacokinetic parameters were not characterized in this study, it was not possible to determine the suitability of conducting TDM in ISF for aliskiren. The concentration-time profile of a single healthy subject administered caffeine was illustrated by Stahle et al. [71]. Caffeine presented in the ISF at higher concentrations than blood (i.e., increased exposure), suggesting that additional mechanisms other than simple diffusion might be responsible for its distribution into the tissue compartment. Based on the five individual ISF concentration-time profiles presented in the study, it appeared that the pharmacokinetics of caffeine exhibit large variability in ISF; however, similar information was not provided in blood to draw any correlations. Pharmacokinetic parameters needed for the assessment for suitability of TDM in ISF were not presented for caffeine by Stahle et al. [71]. Stetina et al. [72] characterized the concentration-time profiles of scopolamine (after a single intravenous dose) in adipose tissue ISF and blood in healthy male subjects ($N = 6$) and found similar pharmacokinetic characteristics between the two matrices. Despite reduced maximum concentration and delayed time-to-reach maximum concentration, the overall exposure of scopolamine between the two matrices was essentially the same, as evident by a distribution ratio approaching unity. These characteristics suggest that scopolamine can potentially be a suitable agent to be monitored in ISF, although TDM for scopolamine is not currently clinically indicated.

5. Microneedle Technologies for Interstitial Fluid Collection for Therapeutic Drug Monitoring

Microneedle technologies have been used in non-clinical and clinical settings for their TDM, diagnostics, and physiological health monitoring using ISF rather than blood, as described here. ISF is trapped in its extracellular matrices of skin [73] leading to difficulties in extracting in biosensing applications. Considering limited availability of ISF in the skin (~20 nL mm^{-2} in the epidermis and ~800 nL mm^{-2} in the dermis [73]), extracting large volumes of ISF for bioanalysis is a major hurdle in developing sensors that rely on ISF extraction. Development of microneedle-integrated biosensors can potentially provide commercially feasible solutions to TDM and diagnostics [74]. A summary of microneedle strategies used for ISF collection and TDM is presented in Table 1.

Table 1. Summary of microneedle strategies used for interstitial fluid (ISF) collection and therapeutic drug monitoring.

Microneedle Device Strategy	Description	Indication	Testing Model	ISF Volume Collected/Required
ISF extraction and off-device analysis	Glass hollow microneedle (0.7–1.5 mm long) and vacuum-assisted ISF collection [75]	Glucose	Tail vein of rats, finger tips of humans	1–10 μL
	Dissolving microneedle "poke" followed by vacuum suction [62]	Vancomycin	Male Wistar rats	2 μL
	Solid microneedle arrays "poked" the skin, and hydrogel "patch" collected ISF [76]	Glucose and sodium ion concentration	Human subjects	<10 μL
	Hydrogel forming microneedle array [77–79]	Theophylline, caffeine, glucose	Pigs, rats, and human subjects	-
ISF extraction and on-device analysis	Hollow microneedles with integrated ISF collection reservoir [80]	Glucose	Human subject	-
	Hollow microneedle array integrated with screen-printed enzyme sensor [81]	Glucose	In vitro bench testing	10 μL
	Hollow microneedle integrated with optofluidic sensor [6]	Vancomycin	In vitro bench testing	0.6 nL
Continuous ISF monitoring	Hollow microneedle integrated with buffer-filled glucose sensor [82]	Glucose	Human subjects	-

5.1. Interstitial Fluid Extraction Devices for Off-Device Analysis

Several studies have successfully demonstrated techniques for ISF extraction from the skin, followed by analysis of its content outside the ISF-collecting microneedle device (hereafter termed "off-device analysis"). For example, Wang et al. [75] used a glass microneedle device to penetrate 0.7–1.5 mm into the skin in hairless rats and healthy adults, and collect 1–10 µL of ISF using a 200–500 mm Hg vacuum for 2 to 10 min for glucose measurement. Sakaguchi et al. [76] overcame vacuum-assisted extraction by applying a solid microneedle array to create micropores on the skin surface followed by a hydrogel patch to collect ISF by swelling action for glucose and sodium ion concentration measurement. Donnelly et al. [77] developed a hydrogel-forming microneedle array, using blends of hydrolyzed poly(methyl-vinylether-*co*-maleic anhydride) and polyethylene glycol crosslinked by esterification, which increased its mass when applied to skin, due to ISF uptake by the hydrogel. Caffarrel-Salvador et al. [78], Romanyuk et al. [79], and Chang et al. [83] showed that extremely small volumes of ISF (<20 µL) can be extracted by similar hydrogel-forming swellable microneedle-arrays over 1 to 2 h in porcine, human (Figure 1) [78], rat [79]. and mice [83] skins.

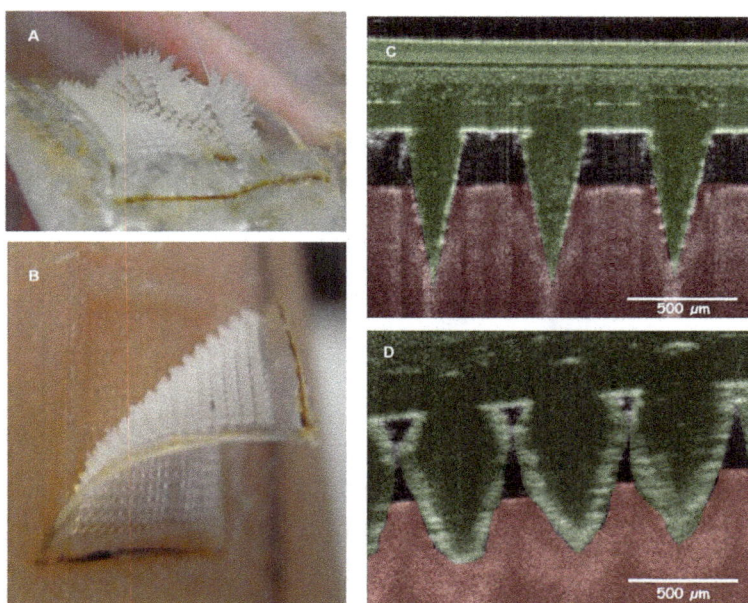

Figure 1. Hydrogel-forming microneedles for extraction of analytes from ISF Figure obtained from Caffarel-Salvador et al. with permission [78]. A hydrogel forming microneedle array (**A**) before application into the skin and (**B**) after application where microneedles are swollen. Optical coherent tomography images show the microneedle arrays after skin insertion (**C**) before swelling, and (**D**) after swelling.

Research conducted to date have failed to demonstrate commercial feasibility of ISF extraction followed by off-device analysis for various reasons. These include prolonged ISF extraction time, need for multiple steps between sample extraction and bioanalysis, need to further extract and/or transfer the fluid from the collection apparatus to a separate site for analysis, extremely low volume of ISF collected, and evaporation of ISF leading to measurement variability and error [74].

5.2. Interstitial Fluid Extraction for On-Device Analysis

Microneedle-integrated biosensors were built to extract ISF and perform the biomolecule analysis on-device, with a key feature of not needing to transfer ISF to a separate instrument. Mukerjee et al. [80] devised a hollow silicone microneedle-integrated system to collect water, glycerol, ISF, and whole blood. ISF was extracted in vivo from human earlobe skin over a 15 to 20-min period, and analyzed qualitatively for glucose [80]. Zimmerman et al. [84] developed a hollow silicon microneedle array integrated into an enzymatic glucose sensor with a porous dialysis membrane, and showed a significant sensor response after exposure to ISF ex vivo. Strambini et al. [81] developed a similar glucose sensor with hollow silicon-dioxide microneedle arrays (1×10^6 needles cm^{-2}) connected to chip consisting screen-printed enzymatic glucose sensor integrated to the backside of the microneedle array for ISF collection and bioanalysis. Ex vivo evaluation showed rapid detection of glucose [81]. Although more commercially feasible than ISF collection devices for off-device analysis, devices with integrated on-device analytical capabilities consist of some challenges, including the need for microliter-level volumes of ISF for analysis, prolonged time to collect ISF, and transfer of ISF to the backside of the microneedle for bioanalysis.

Ranamukhaarachchi et al. [6] developed a point-of-care TDM device by integrating a gold-coated hollow microneedle with an optofluidic sensing system to detect vancomycin in sub-nanoliter volumes of fluid in vitro. Vancomycin receptors were immobilized inside the microneedle lumen (Figure 2), which collected 0.6 nL of sample (i.e., ISF) within seconds, and caused vancomycin to bind to the microneedle lumen for quantification.

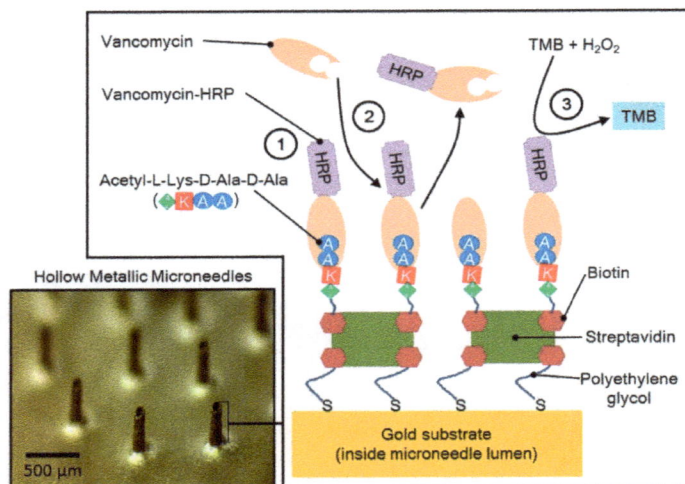

Figure 2. Functionalization of gold-coated hollow microneedle lumens for fluid collection, drug binding, and detection. Figure obtained from Ranamukhaarachchi et al. with permission [6].

The extremely small sample volume, capability to detect low concentration TDM drugs, rapid operation from collection to analysis (altogether less than 5 min TDM time), and lack of need for sample transfer from the collection site to analytical site were key advantages of this system. However, this system needs to be validated in pre-clinical and clinical studies [74].

5.3. Continuous Monitoring Microneedle Devices

The most promising applications for microneedle-integrated biosensors is continuous monitoring of biomolecules from the skin's ISF. Jina et al. [82] developed a hollow microneedle-integrated continuous glucose monitoring (CGM) biosensor, and demonstrated accurate and continuous glucose measurements in humans using ISF up to 72 h. The sensing chamber (Figure 3), located behind the microneedle array, was filled with a buffer solution to transfer glucose passively from ISF to sensor, eliminating the need for removal of ISF from the skin [82]. The main advantages of this system are lack of volume requirement for ISF extraction, real-time bioanalysis, and limited number of steps to obtain bioanalytical results [74].

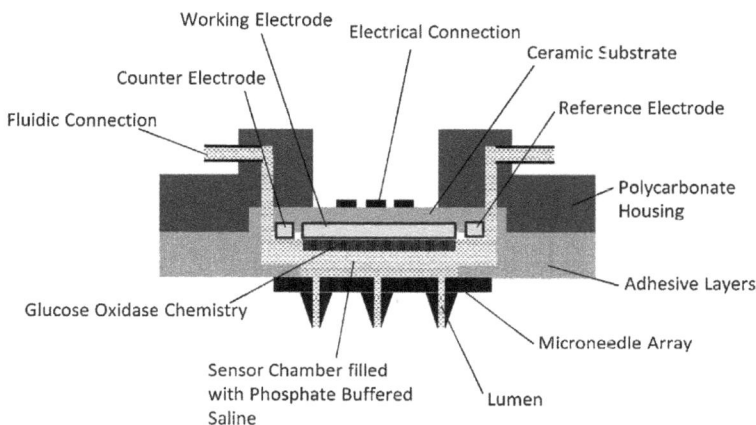

Figure 3. Continuous glucose monitoring biosensor. Figure obtained from Chua et al. with permission [85].

5.4. Other Methods for ISF Extraction

Microdialysis catheters can be implanted in or under the skin and used to extract biomolecules, such as glucose, from ISF [86]. Other systems such as ultrafiltration [87], reverse iontophoresis [88], and sonophoresis [89] have all been used previously to extract ISF as well, but their potential is limited compared to more minimally-invasive technologies such as microneedle-based systems.

6. Future Directions

The conventional paradigm of monitoring drug concentrations in blood might be impractical, costly, and sometimes unethical in certain patient populations (e.g., pediatric, elderly, or those with "bad" veins). A new way of conducting TDM using ISF is gaining momentum in the research community and, in our opinion, is at the stage where its clinical utility should be investigated. In this review paper, we have presented (1) the principles of TDM; (2) alternative matrices for TDM; (3) current evidence supporting the use of ISF for TDM in clinical models; and (4) the use of microneedle technologies, which is potentially minimally invasive and pain-free, for the collection of ISF. Based on these advancements, the immediate future direction for this area of research is to establish the suitability of using ISF for TDM in human models for drugs that have been found "suitable" in pre-clinical experiments. In order to do this, a systematic approach involving compartmental modeling, physiologically-based modeling, and population pharmacokinetic modeling would have to be utilized. The effects of intrinsic and extrinsic factors that can potentially affect the pharmacokinetics of particular drugs in ISF should be incorporated into these clinical studies to fully capture the covariates and variabilities associated with this approach. In the more distant future, microneedle devices, such as those described in this review, that are minimally invasive and potentially pain-free should be tested on humans to determine their utility in the collection of ISF. Ultimately, we envision point-of-care devices where pain-free ISF collection (via a microneedle-like device), drug concentration assessment, and dosing can be done in real time, at the bedside.

Acknowledgments: No sources of funding were received for the preparation of this manuscript. The authors would like to acknowledge Urs O. Häfeli, for his invaluable input and guidance.

Conflicts of Interest: The authors declare no conflict of interest.

References

1. Kiang, T.K.; Hafeli, U.O.; Ensom, M.H. A Comprehensive Review on the Pharmacokinetics of Antibiotics in Interstitial Fluid Spaces in Humans: Implications on Dosing and Clinical Pharmacokinetic Monitoring. *Clin. Pharmacokinet.* **2014**, *53*, 695–730. [CrossRef] [PubMed]
2. Koka, S.; Beebe, T.J.; Merry, S.P.; DeJesus, R.S.; Berlanga, L.D.; Weaver, A.L.; Montori, V.M.; Wong, D.T. The Preferences of Adult Outpatients in Medical or Dental Care Settings for Giving Saliva, Urine or Blood for Clinical Testing. *J. Am. Dent. Assoc.* **2008**, *139*, 735–740. [CrossRef] [PubMed]
3. Pichini, S.; Altieri, I.; Zuccaro, P.; Pacifici, R. Drug Monitoring in Nonconventional Biological Fluids and Matrices. *Clin. Pharmacokinet.* **1996**, *30*, 211–228. [CrossRef] [PubMed]
4. Kiang, T.K.; Schmitt, V.; Ensom, M.H.; Chua, B.; Hafeli, U.O. Therapeutic Drug Monitoring in Interstitial Fluid: A Feasibility Study using a Comprehensive Panel of Drugs. *J. Pharm. Sci.* **2012**, *101*, 4642–4652. [CrossRef] [PubMed]
5. Hafeli, U.O.; Ensom, M.H.; Kiang, T.K.; Stoeber, B.; Chua, B.A.; Pudek, M.; Schmitt, V. Comparison of Vancomycin Concentrations in Blood and Interstitial Fluid: A Possible Model for Less Invasive Therapeutic Drug Monitoring. *Clin. Chem. Lab. Med.* **2011**, *49*, 2123–2125. [CrossRef] [PubMed]
6. Ranamukhaarachchi, S.A.; Padeste, C.; Dubner, M.; Hafeli, U.O.; Stoeber, B.; Cadarso, V.J. Integrated Hollow Microneedle-Optofluidic Biosensor for Therapeutic Drug Monitoring in Sub-Nanoliter Volumes. *Sci. Rep.* **2016**, *6*, 29075. [CrossRef] [PubMed]
7. Ensom, M.H.; Davis, G.A.; Cropp, C.D.; Ensom, R.J. Clinical Pharmacokinetics in the 21st Century. Does the Evidence Support Definitive Outcomes? *Clin. Pharmacokinet.* **1998**, *34*, 265–279. [CrossRef] [PubMed]
8. DiPiro, J.; Blouin, R.; Pruemer, J.; Spruill, W. *Concepts in Clinical Pharmacokinetics: A Self-Instructional Course*, 2nd ed.; American Society of Health-System Pharmacists Inc.: Bethesda, MD, USA, 1996; p. 200.
9. Kiang, T.K.; Ensom, M.H. Therapeutic Drug Monitoring of Mycophenolate in Adult Solid Organ Transplant Patients: An Update. *Expert Opin. Drug Metab. Toxicol.* **2016**, *12*, 545–553. [CrossRef] [PubMed]
10. Kiang, T.K.; Ensom, M.H. A Comprehensive Review on the Predictive Performance of the Sheiner-Tozer and Derivative Equations for the Correction of Phenytoin Concentrations. *Ann. Pharmacother.* **2016**, *50*, 311–325. [CrossRef] [PubMed]
11. Cheng, W.; Kiang, T.K.; Bring, P.; Ensom, M.H. Predictive Performance of the Winter-Tozer and Derivative Equations for Estimating Free Phenytoin Concentration. *Can. J. Hosp. Pharm.* **2016**, *69*, 269–279. [CrossRef] [PubMed]
12. Kiang, T.K.; Sherwin, C.M.; Spigarelli, M.G.; Ensom, M.H. Fundamentals of Population Pharmacokinetic Modelling: Modelling and Software. *Clin. Pharmacokinet.* **2012**, *51*, 515–525. [CrossRef] [PubMed]
13. Sherwin, C.M.; Kiang, T.K.; Spigarelli, M.G.; Ensom, M.H. Fundamentals of Population Pharmacokinetic Modelling: Validation Methods. *Clin. Pharmacokinet.* **2012**, *51*, 573–590. [CrossRef] [PubMed]
14. Bring, P.; Ensom, M.H. Does Oxcarbazepine Warrant Therapeutic Drug Monitoring? A Critical Review. *Clin. Pharmacokinet.* **2008**, *47*, 767–778. [CrossRef] [PubMed]
15. Tan, J.; Paquette, V.; Levine, M.; Ensom, M.H. Levetiracetam Clinical Pharmacokinetic Monitoring in Pediatric Patients with Epilepsy. *Clin. Pharmacokinet.* **2017**. [CrossRef] [PubMed]
16. Kuo, I.F.; Ensom, M.H. Role of Therapeutic Drug Monitoring of Voriconazole in the Treatment of Invasive Fungal Infections. *Can. J. Hosp. Pharm.* **2009**, *62*, 469–482. [CrossRef] [PubMed]
17. Ng, K.; Mabasa, V.H.; Chow, I.; Ensom, M.H. Systematic Review of Efficacy, Pharmacokinetics, and Administration of Intraventricular Vancomycin in Adults. *Neurocrit. Care* **2014**, *20*, 158–171. [CrossRef] [PubMed]
18. Stenton, S.B.; Partovi, N.; Ensom, M.H. Sirolimus: The Evidence for Clinical Pharmacokinetic Monitoring. *Clin. Pharmacokinet.* **2005**, *44*, 769–786. [CrossRef] [PubMed]

19. Ng, J.C.; Leung, M.; Wright, A.J.; Ensom, M.H. Clinical Pharmacokinetic Monitoring of Leflunomide in Renal Transplant Recipients with BK Virus Reactivation: A Review of the Literature. *Clin. Pharmacokinet.* **2017**, *56*, 1015–1031. [CrossRef] [PubMed]

20. Kendrick, J.G.; Carr, R.R.; Ensom, M.H. Pharmacokinetics and Drug Dosing in Obese Children. *J. Pediatr. Pharmacol. Ther.* **2010**, *15*, 94–109. [PubMed]

21. Strong, D.K.; Lai, A.; Primmett, D.; White, C.T.; Lirenman, D.S.; Carter, J.E.; Hurley, R.M.; Virji, M.; Ensom, M.H. Limited Sampling Strategy for Cyclosporine (Neoral) Area under the Curve Monitoring in Pediatric Kidney Transplant Recipients. *Pediatr. Transplant.* **2005**, *9*, 566–573. [CrossRef] [PubMed]

22. Teng, J.F.; Mabasa, V.H.; Ensom, M.H. The Role of Therapeutic Drug Monitoring of Imatinib in Patients with Chronic Myeloid Leukemia and Metastatic or Unresectable Gastrointestinal Stromal Tumors. *Ther. Drug Monit.* **2012**, *34*, 85–97. [CrossRef] [PubMed]

23. Schwenger, E.; Dumontet, J.; Ensom, M.H. Does Olanzapine Warrant Clinical Pharmacokinetic Monitoring in Schizophrenia? *Clin. Pharmacokinet.* **2011**, *50*, 415–428. [CrossRef] [PubMed]

24. Seto, K.; Dumontet, J.; Ensom, M.H. Risperidone in Schizophrenia: Is there a Role for Therapeutic Drug Monitoring? *Ther. Drug Monit.* **2011**, *33*, 275–283. [CrossRef] [PubMed]

25. Raju, K.S.; Taneja, I.; Singh, S.P.; Wahajuddin. Utility of Noninvasive Biomatrices in Pharmacokinetic Studies. *Biomed. Chromatogr.* **2013**, *27*, 1354–1366. [CrossRef] [PubMed]

26. Haeckel, R.; Hanecke, P. The Application of Saliva, Sweat and Tear Fluid for Diagnostic Purposes. *Ann. Biol. Clin.* **1993**, *51*, 903–910.

27. Aps, J.K.; Martens, L.C. Review: The Physiology of Saliva and Transfer of Drugs into Saliva. *Forensic Sci. Int.* **2005**, *150*, 119–131. [CrossRef] [PubMed]

28. Nunes, L.A.; Mussavira, S.; Bindhu, O.S. Clinical and Diagnostic Utility of Saliva as a Non-Invasive Diagnostic Fluid: A Systematic Review. *Biochem. Med.* **2015**, *25*, 177–192. [CrossRef] [PubMed]

29. Mullangi, R.; Agrawal, S.; Srinivas, N.R. Measurement of Xenobiotics in Saliva: Is Saliva an Attractive Alternative Matrix? Case Studies and Analytical Perspectives. *Biomed. Chromatogr.* **2009**, *23*, 3–25. [CrossRef] [PubMed]

30. Anizan, S.; Huestis, M.A. The Potential Role of Oral Fluid in Antidoping Testing. *Clin. Chem.* **2014**, *60*, 307–322. [CrossRef] [PubMed]

31. Haeckel, R. Factors Influencing the saliva/plasma Ratio of Drugs. *Ann. N. Y. Acad. Sci.* **1993**, *694*, 128–142. [CrossRef] [PubMed]

32. Levy, G.; Ellis, E.F.; Koysooko, R. Indirect Plasma-Theophylline Monitoring in Asthmatic Children by Determination of Theophylline Concentration in Saliva. *Pediatrics* **1974**, *53*, 873–876. [PubMed]

33. Jusko, W.J.; Gerbracht, L.; Golden, L.H.; Koup, J.R. Digoxin Concentrations in Serum and Saliva. *Res. Commun. Chem. Pathol. Pharmacol.* **1975**, *10*, 189–192. [PubMed]

34. Neu, C.; DiMascio, A.; Williams, D. Saliva Lithium Levels: Clinical Applications. *Am. J. Psychiatry* **1975**, *132*, 66–68. [PubMed]

35. McAuliffe, J.J.; Sherwin, A.L.; Leppik, I.E.; Fayle, S.A.; Pippenger, C.E. Salivary Levels of Anticonvulsants: A Practical Approach to Drug Monitoring. *Neurology* **1977**, *27*, 409–413. [CrossRef] [PubMed]

36. Kiang, T.K.; Ensom, M.H. A Qualitative Review on the Pharmacokinetics of Antibiotics in Saliva: Implications on Clinical Pharmacokinetic Monitoring in Humans. *Clin. Pharmacokinet.* **2016**, *55*, 313–358. [CrossRef] [PubMed]

37. Patsalos, P.N.; Berry, D.J. Therapeutic Drug Monitoring of Antiepileptic Drugs by use of Saliva. *Ther. Drug Monit.* **2013**, *35*, 4–29. [CrossRef] [PubMed]

38. Ter Heine, R.; Beijnen, J.H.; Huitema, A.D. Bioanalytical Issues in Patient-Friendly Sampling Methods for Therapeutic Drug Monitoring: Focus on Antiretroviral Drugs. *Bioanalysis* **2009**, *1*, 1329–1338. [CrossRef] [PubMed]

39. Pichini, S.; Papaseit, E.; Joya, X.; Vall, O.; Farre, M.; Garcia-Algar, O.; de laTorre, R. Pharmacokinetics and Therapeutic Drug Monitoring of Psychotropic Drugs in Pediatrics. *Ther. Drug Monit.* **2009**, *31*, 283–318. [CrossRef] [PubMed]

40. Venkatesh, B.; Morgan, T.J.; Cohen, J. Interstitium: The Next Diagnostic and Therapeutic Platform in Critical Illness. *Crit. Care Med.* **2010**, *38*, S630–S636. [CrossRef] [PubMed]

41. Wiig, H.; Swartz, M.A. Interstitial Fluid and Lymph Formation and Transport: Physiological Regulation and Roles in Inflammation and Cancer. *Physiol. Rev.* **2012**, *92*, 1005–1060. [CrossRef] [PubMed]

42. Poulin, P. Drug Distribution to Human Tissues: Prediction and Examination of the Basic Assumption in in Vivo Pharmacokinetics-Pharmacodynamics (PK/PD) Research. *J. Pharm. Sci.* **2015**, *104*, 2110–2118. [CrossRef] [PubMed]

43. Poulin, P. A Paradigm Shift in Pharmacokinetic-Pharmacodynamic (PKPD) Modeling: Rule of Thumb for Estimating Free Drug Level in Tissue Compared with Plasma to Guide Drug Design. *J. Pharm. Sci.* **2015**, *104*, 2359–2368. [CrossRef] [PubMed]

44. Poulin, P.; Haddad, S. Advancing Prediction of Tissue Distribution and Volume of Distribution of Highly Lipophilic Compounds from a Simplified Tissue-Composition-Based Model as a Mechanistic Animal Alternative Method. *J. Pharm. Sci.* **2012**, *101*, 2250–2261. [CrossRef] [PubMed]

45. Poulin, P.; Schoenlein, K.; Theil, F.P. Prediction of Adipose Tissue: Plasma Partition Coefficients for Structurally Unrelated Drugs. *J. Pharm. Sci.* **2001**, *90*, 436–447. [CrossRef]

46. Konings, I.R.; Sleijfer, S.; Mathijssen, R.H.; de Bruijn, P.; Ghobadi Moghaddam-Helmantel, I.M.; van Dam, L.M.; Wiemer, E.A.; Verweij, J.; Loos, W.J. Increasing Tumoral 5-Fluorouracil Concentrations during a 5-Day Continuous Infusion: A Microdialysis Study. *Cancer Chemother. Pharmacol.* **2011**, *67*, 1055–1062. [CrossRef] [PubMed]

47. Konings, I.R.; Engels, F.K.; Sleijfer, S.; Verweij, J.; Wiemer, E.A.; Loos, W.J. Application of Prolonged Microdialysis Sampling in Carboplatin-Treated Cancer Patients. *Cancer Chemother. Pharmacol.* **2009**, *64*, 509–516. [CrossRef] [PubMed]

48. Muller, M.; Mader, R.M.; Steiner, B.; Steger, G.G.; Jansen, B.; Gnant, M.; Helbich, T.; Jakesz, R.; Eichler, H.G.; Blochl-Daum, B. 5-Fluorouracil Kinetics in the Interstitial Tumor Space: Clinical Response in Breast Cancer Patients. *Cancer Res.* **1997**, *57*, 2598–2601. [PubMed]

49. Muller, M.; Brunner, M.; Schmid, R.; Mader, R.M.; Bockenheimer, J.; Steger, G.G.; Steiner, B.; Eichler, H.G.; Blochl-Daum, B. Interstitial Methotrexate Kinetics in Primary Breast Cancer Lesions. *Cancer Res.* **1998**, *58*, 2982–2985. [PubMed]

50. Blochl-Daum, B.; Muller, M.; Meisinger, V.; Eichler, H.G.; Fassolt, A.; Pehamberger, H. Measurement of Extracellular Fluid Carboplatin Kinetics in Melanoma Metastases with Microdialysis. *Br. J. Cancer* **1996**, *73*, 920–924. [CrossRef] [PubMed]

51. Thompson, J.F.; Siebert, G.A.; Anissimov, Y.G.; Smithers, B.M.; Doubrovsky, A.; Anderson, C.D.; Roberts, M.S. Microdialysis and Response during Regional Chemotherapy by Isolated Limb Infusion of Melphalan for Limb Malignancies. *Br. J. Cancer* **2001**, *85*, 157–165. [CrossRef] [PubMed]

52. Quist, S.R.; Quist, J.; Birkenmaier, J.; Stauch, T.; Gollnick, H.P. Pharmacokinetic Profile of Methotrexate in Psoriatic Skin Via the Oral Or Subcutaneous Route using Dermal Microdialysis Showing Higher Methotrexate Bioavailability in Psoriasis Plaques than in Non-Lesional Skin. *J. Eur. Acad. Dermatol. Venereol.* **2016**, *30*, 1537–1543. [CrossRef] [PubMed]

53. Zhou, Q.; Gallo, J.M. In Vivo Microdialysis for PK and PD Studies of Anticancer Drugs. *AAPS J.* **2005**, *7*, E659–E667. [CrossRef] [PubMed]

54. Chu, J.; Gallo, J.M. Application of Microdialysis to Characterize Drug Disposition in Tumors. *Adv. Drug Deliv. Rev.* **2000**, *45*, 243–253. [CrossRef]

55. Roberts, J.A.; Udy, A.A.; Jarrett, P.; Wallis, S.C.; Hope, W.W.; Sharma, R.; Kirkpatrick, C.M.; Kruger, P.S.; Roberts, M.S.; Lipman, J. Plasma and Target-Site Subcutaneous Tissue Population Pharmacokinetics and Dosing Simulations of Cefazolin in Post-Trauma Critically Ill Patients. *J. Antimicrob. Chemother.* **2015**, *70*, 1495–1502. [CrossRef] [PubMed]

56. Tegeder, I.; Schmidtko, A.; Brautigam, L.; Kirschbaum, A.; Geisslinger, G.; Lotsch, J. Tissue Distribution of Imipenem in Critically Ill Patients. *Clin. Pharmacol. Ther.* **2002**, *71*, 325–333. [CrossRef] [PubMed]

57. Dahyot, C.; Marchand, S.; Bodin, M.; Debeane, B.; Mimoz, O.; Couet, W. Application of Basic Pharmacokinetic Concepts to Analysis of Microdialysis Data: Illustration with Imipenem Muscle Distribution. *Clin. Pharmacokinet.* **2008**, *47*, 181–189. [CrossRef] [PubMed]

58. Varghese, J.M.; Jarrett, P.; Wallis, S.C.; Boots, R.J.; Kirkpatrick, C.M.; Lipman, J.; Roberts, J.A. Are Interstitial Fluid Concentrations of Meropenem Equivalent to Plasma Concentrations in Critically Ill Patients Receiving Continuous Renal Replacement Therapy? *J. Antimicrob. Chemother.* **2015**, *70*, 528–533. [CrossRef] [PubMed]

59. Housman, S.T.; Bhalodi, A.A.; Shepard, A.; Nugent, J.; Nicolau, D.P. Vancomycin Tissue Pharmacokinetics in Patients with Lower-Limb Infections Via in Vivo Microdialysis. *J. Am. Podiatr. Med. Assoc.* **2015**, *105*, 381–388. [CrossRef] [PubMed]

60. Hamada, Y.; Kuti, J.L.; Nicolau, D.P. Vancomycin Serum Concentrations do Not Adequately Predict Tissue Exposure in Diabetic Patients with Mild to Moderate Limb Infections. *J. Antimicrob. Chemother.* **2015**, *70*, 2064–2067. [CrossRef] [PubMed]

61. Skhirtladze, K.; Hutschala, D.; Fleck, T.; Thalhammer, F.; Ehrlich, M.; Vukovich, T.; Muller, M.; Tschernko, E.M. Impaired Target Site Penetration of Vancomycin in Diabetic Patients Following Cardiac Surgery. *Antimicrob. Agents Chemother.* **2006**, *50*, 1372–1375. [CrossRef] [PubMed]

62. Ito, Y.; Inagaki, Y.; Kobuchi, S.; Takada, K.; Sakaeda, T. Therapeutic Drug Monitoring of Vancomycin in Dermal Interstitial Fluid using Dissolving Microneedles. *Int. J. Med. Sci.* **2016**, *13*, 271–276. [CrossRef] [PubMed]

63. Linder, C.; Andersson, M.; Wide, K.; Beck, O.; Pohanka, A. A LC–MS/MS Method for Therapeutic Drug Monitoring of Carbamazepine, Lamotrigine and Valproic Acid in DBS. *Bioanalysis* **2015**, *7*, 2031–2039. [CrossRef] [PubMed]

64. Stahle, L.; Alm, C.; Ekquist, B.; Lundquist, B.; Tomson, T. Monitoring Free Extracellular Valproic Acid by Microdialysis in Epileptic Patients. *Ther. Drug Monit.* **1996**, *18*, 14–18. [CrossRef] [PubMed]

65. Lindberger, M.; Tomson, T.; Stahle, L. Validation of Microdialysis Sampling for Subcutaneous Extracellular Valproic Acid in Humans. *Ther. Drug Monit.* **1998**, *20*, 358–362. [CrossRef] [PubMed]

66. Lindberger, M.; Tomson, T.; Wallstedt, L.; Stahle, L. Distribution of Valproate to Subdural Cerebrospinal Fluid, Subcutaneous Extracellular Fluid, and Plasma in Humans: A Microdialysis Study. *Epilepsia* **2001**, *42*, 256–261. [PubMed]

67. Lindberger, M.; Tomson, T.; Stahle, L. Unbound Valproate Fraction in Plasma and Subcutaneous Microdialysate in Steady State and After a Single Dose in Humans. *Ther. Drug Monit.* **2003**, *25*, 378–383. [CrossRef] [PubMed]

68. Lindberger, M.; Tomson, T.; Lars, S. Microdialysis Sampling of Carbamazepine, Phenytoin and Phenobarbital in Subcutaneous Extracellular Fluid and Subdural Cerebrospinal Fluid in Humans: An In Vitro and In Vivo Study of Adsorption to the Sampling Device. *Pharmacol. Toxicol.* **2002**, *91*, 158–165. [CrossRef] [PubMed]

69. Lindberger, M.; Tomson, T.; Ohman, I.; Wallstedt, L.; Stahle, L. Estimation of Topiramate in Subdural Cerebrospinal Fluid, Subcutaneous Extracellular Fluid, and Plasma: A Single Case Microdialysis Study. *Epilepsia* **1999**, *40*, 800–802. [CrossRef] [PubMed]

70. Boschmann, M.; Nussberger, J.; Engeli, S.; Danser, A.H.; Yeh, C.M.; Prescott, M.F.; Dahlke, M.; Jordan, J. Aliskiren Penetrates Adipose and Skeletal Muscle Tissue and Reduces Renin-Angiotensin System Activity in Obese Hypertensive Patients. *J. Hypertens.* **2012**, *30*, 561–566. [CrossRef] [PubMed]

71. Stahle, L.; Arner, P.; Ungerstedt, U. Drug Distribution Studies with Microdialysis. III: Extracellular Concentration of Caffeine in Adipose Tissue in Man. *Life Sci.* **1991**, *49*, 1853–1858. [CrossRef]

72. Stetina, P.M.; Madai, B.; Kulemann, V.; Kirch, W.; Joukhadar, C. Pharmacokinetics of Scopolamine in Serum and Subcutaneous Adipose Tissue in Healthy Volunteers. *Int. J. Clin. Pharmacol. Ther.* **2005**, *43*, 134–139. [CrossRef] [PubMed]

73. Groenendaal, W.; von Basum, G.; Schmidt, K.A.; Hilbers, P.A.; van Riel, N.A. Quantifying the Composition of Human Skin for Glucose Sensor Development. *J. Diabetes Sci. Technol.* **2010**, *4*, 1032–1040. [CrossRef] [PubMed]

74. Ranamukhaarachchi, S. Skin Mechanics, Intradermal Delivery and Biosensing with Hollow Metallic Microneedles. Ph.D. Thesis, University of British Columbia, Vancouver, BC, Canada, December 2016.

75. Wang, P.M.; Cornwell, M.; Prausnitz, M.R. Minimally Invasive Extraction of Dermal Interstitial Fluid for Glucose Monitoring using Microneedles. *Diabetes Technol. Ther.* **2005**, *7*, 131–141. [CrossRef] [PubMed]

76. Sakaguchi, K.; Hirota, Y.; Hashimoto, N.; Ogawa, W.; Sato, T.; Okada, S.; Hagino, K.; Asakura, Y.; Kikkawa, Y.; Kojima, J.; et al. A Minimally Invasive System for Glucose Area Under the Curve Measurement using Interstitial Fluid Extraction Technology: Evaluation of the Accuracy and Usefulness with Oral Glucose Tolerance Tests in Subjects with and without Diabetes. *Diabetes Technol. Ther.* **2012**, *14*, 485–491. [CrossRef] [PubMed]

77. Donnelly, R.F.; Mooney, K.; Caffarel-Salvador, E.; Torrisi, B.M.; Eltayib, E.; McElnay, J.C. Microneedle-Mediated Minimally Invasive Patient Monitoring. *Ther. Drug Monit.* **2014**, *36*, 10–17. [CrossRef] [PubMed]

78. Caffarel-Salvador, E.; Brady, A.J.; Eltayib, E.; Meng, T.; Alonso-Vicente, A.; Gonzalez-Vazquez, P.; Torrisi, B.M.; Vicente-Perez, E.M.; Mooney, K.; Jones, D.S.; et al. Hydrogel-Forming Microneedle Arrays Allow Detection of Drugs and Glucose in Vivo: Potential for use in Diagnosis and Therapeutic Drug Monitoring. *PLoS ONE* **2015**, *10*, e0145644. [CrossRef] [PubMed]

79. Romanyuk, A.V.; Zvezdin, V.N.; Samant, P.; Grenader, M.I.; Zemlyanova, M.; Prausnitz, M.R. Collection of Analytes from Microneedle Patches. *Anal. Chem.* **2014**, *86*, 10520–10523. [CrossRef] [PubMed]

80. Mukerjee, E.V.; Collins, S.D.; Isseroff, R.R.; Smith, R.L. Microneedle Array for Transdermal Biological Fluid Extraction and in Situ Analysis. *Sens. Actuators A Phys.* **2004**, *114*, 267–275. [CrossRef]

81. Strambini, L.M.; Longo, A.; Scarano, S.; Prescimone, T.; Palchetti, I.; Minunni, M.; Giannessi, D.; Barillaro, G. Self-Powered Microneedle-Based Biosensors for Pain-Free High-Accuracy Measurement of Glycaemia in Interstitial Fluid. *Biosens. Bioelectron.* **2015**, *66*, 162–168. [CrossRef] [PubMed]

82. Jina, A.; Tierney, M.J.; Tamada, J.A.; McGill, S.; Desai, S.; Chua, B.; Chang, A.; Christiansen, M. Design, Development, and Evaluation of a Novel Microneedle Array-Based Continuous Glucose Monitor. *J. Diabetes Sci. Technol.* **2014**, *8*, 483–487. [CrossRef] [PubMed]

83. Chang, H.; Zheng, M.; Yu, X.; Than, A.; Seeni, R.Z.; Kang, R.; Tian, J.; Khanh, D.P.; Liu, L.; Chen, P.; et al. A Swellable Microneedle Patch to Rapidly Extract Skin Interstitial Fluid for Timely Metabolic Analysis. *Adv. Mater.* **2017**, *37*. [CrossRef] [PubMed]

84. Zimmermann, S.; Fienbork, D.; Flounders, A.W.; Liepmann, D. In-Device Enzyme Immobilization: Wafer-Level Fabrication of an Integrated Glucose Sensor. *Sens. Actuators B Chem.* **2004**, *99*, 163–173. [CrossRef]

85. Chua, B.; Desai, S.P.; Tierney, M.J.; Tamada, J.A.; Jina, A.N. Effect of Microneedles Shape on Skin Penetration and Minimally Invasive Continuous Glucose Monitoring In Vivo. *Sens. Actuators A Phys.* **2013**, *203*, 373–381. [CrossRef]

86. Heinemann, L.; Glucose Monitoring Study Group. Continuous Glucose Monitoring by Means of the Microdialysis Technique: Underlying Fundamental Aspects. *Diabetes Technol. Ther.* **2003**, *5*, 545–561. [CrossRef] [PubMed]

87. Tiessena, R.G.; Kapteinab, W.A.; Venemaa, K.; Korf, J. Slow Ultrafiltration for Continuous In Vivo Sampling: Application for Glucose and Lactate in Man. *Anal. Chim. Acta* **1999**, *379*, 327–335. [CrossRef]

88. Tamada, J.A.; Bohannon, N.J.; Potts, R.O. Measurement of Glucose in Diabetic Subjects using Noninvasive Transdermal Extraction. *Nat. Med.* **1995**, *1*, 1198–1201. [CrossRef] [PubMed]

89. Kost, J.; Mitragotri, S.; Gabbay, R.A.; Pishko, M.; Langer, R. Transdermal Monitoring of Glucose and Other Analytes using Ultrasound. *Nat. Med.* **2000**, *6*, 347–350. [CrossRef] [PubMed]

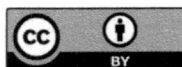

pharmaceutics

MDPI

Article

Modeling of Body Weight Metrics for Effective and Cost-Efficient Conventional Factor VIII Dosing in Hemophilia A Prophylaxis

Alanna McEneny-King [1], Pierre Chelle [1], Severine Henrard [2], Cedric Hermans [3], Alfonso Iorio [4,5] and Andrea N. Edginton [1,*]

[1] School of Pharmacy, University of Waterloo, Waterloo, ON N2L 3G1, Canada; amceneny@uwaterloo.ca (A.M.-K.); pierre.chelle@uwaterloo.ca (P.C.)
[2] Louvain Drug Research Institute, Clinical Pharmacy Research Group and Institute of Health and Society (IRSS), Université catholique de Louvain, 1348 Brussels, Belgium; severine.henrard@uclouvain.be
[3] Haemostasis and Thrombosis Unit, Division of Haematology, Cliniques universitaires Saint-Luc, Université catholique de Louvain, 1348 Brussels, Belgium; cedric.hermans@uclouvain.be
[4] Department of Health Evidence, Research Methods and Impact, McMaster University, Hamilton, ON L8S 4L8, Canada; io002a@mcmaster.ca
[5] Department of Medicine, McMaster University, Hamilton, ON L8S 4L8, Canada
* Correspondence: aedginto@uwaterloo.ca; Tel.: +1-519-888-4567 (ext. 21315)

Received: 9 September 2017; Accepted: 12 October 2017; Published: 17 October 2017

Abstract: The total body weight-based dosing strategy currently used in the prophylactic treatment of hemophilia A may not be appropriate for all populations. The assumptions that guide weight-based dosing are not valid in overweight and obese populations, resulting in overdosing and ineffective resource utilization. We explored different weight metrics including lean body weight, ideal body weight, and adjusted body weight to determine an alternative dosing strategy that is both safe and resource-efficient in normal and overweight/obese adult patients. Using a validated population pharmacokinetic model, we simulated a variety of dosing regimens using different doses, weight metrics, and frequencies; we also investigated the implications of assuming various levels of endogenous factor production. Ideal body weight performed the best across all of the regimens explored, maintaining safety while moderating resource consumption for overweight and obese patients.

Keywords: hemophilia A; conventional factor VIII; dose metrics; obesity; population pharmacokinetics

1. Introduction

Hemophilia A is an inherited bleeding disorder resulting from a deficiency in clotting factor VIII (FVIII), causing spontaneous and recurring joint bleeds, eventually leading to arthropathy and premature death if left untreated. The mainstay of severe hemophilia treatment is prophylactic replacement of the missing factor. The typical aim of prophylaxis is to maintain a clotting factor level of at least 1 IU dL^{-1}, based on the observation that patients with moderate hemophilia (i.e., those with baseline factor levels >1 IU dL^{-1}) are less prone to the spontaneous bleeds and subsequent arthropathy seen in more severe cases [1]. In a study of 65 boys with severe hemophilia A, only regular prophylactic infusions were shown to prevent joint damage as compared to on-demand treatment [2]. While there is global unanimity that prophylaxis should be initiated before joint disease is sustained [3,4], the implementation of this approach is quite variable [5]. No optimal dosing regimen has been identified; instead, an individualized approach that accounts for the patient's physical activity, current (and accepted future) musculoskeletal condition, and the availability of resources has been suggested [6,7]. Ideally, the patient's pharmacokinetic (PK) profile is taken into account to define a truly individualized regimen that optimizes both safety and resource utilization [8]. To facilitate the adoption of PK-based dosing regimens, tools such as the Web Accessible Population Pharmacokinetics Service—Hemophilia (WAPPS-Hemo [9,10]) provide estimates of individual PK parameters from a minimal number of samples by leveraging population PK data. Despite the development of these platforms, the majority of hemophilia patients are still dosed according to total body weight, as initially proposed by Ingram in 1981 [11]. For instance, hemophilic children in Canada are started on a once-weekly regimen (50 IU kg^{-1}), then step up to either twice weekly (30 IU kg^{-1}) or every 48 h (25 IU kg^{-1}) as required; prophylaxis regimens in the Netherlands (Utrecht protocol: 15–30 IU kg^{-1} three times per week) and Sweden (Malmö protocol: 25–40 IU kg^{-1} three times per week), though proposing different intensities and targeting different levels, are based on the same principle [12].

The normalization of life expectancy of individuals with hemophilia brings new challenges to hemophilia care. Overweight and obesity rates amongst hemophiliacs now match the epidemic proportions that are seen in the general population [13]. A 2011 study conducted in Ontario found 28.8% of enrolled hemophiliacs were overweight or obese, compared to 26% of healthy controls [14]. Obesity also comes with a higher risk for hemophilic arthropathy; joint range of motion has been shown to negatively correlate with body mass index (BMI) [15]. Furthermore, the total body weight-based dosing regimen currently used in hemophilia treatment may not be appropriate for overweight and obese populations. Calculations for weight-adjusted dosing are based on the following formula:

$$\text{Dose (IU)} = \frac{\text{total body weight (kg)} \times \text{desired increase in FVIII level (\%)}}{\text{IVR}} \tag{1}$$

In vivo recovery (IVR) is a parameter used to describe clotting factor pharmacokinetics, and reflects the rise in factor activity (in this case, FVIII) after a dose is administered. Although it has been suggested that an individual IVR value be determined for each patient [16], typically an IVR of 2 IU dL^{-1}/IU kg^{-1} is assumed. For example, a desired increase to normal FVIII levels (100%) would lead to a 50 IU kg^{-1} dose being administered. However, the assumption that IVR equals 2 for all is not always valid. A study by Henrard et al. found that overweight patients (BMI > 29.6 kg·m^{-2}) had a median IVR of 2.70, while underweight patients (BMI < 20.3 kg·m^{-2}) had a median IVR of 1.60 [17].

The emerging proportion of overweight and obesity in the general population has prompted research efforts aimed at identifying pharmacokinetic differences (and the corresponding dose adjustments) in this population. The relationship between body size and clearance is well established; a 2012 systematic review of this topic found that more than half of all identified models for clearance included a covariate for body size, most commonly as a power function [18]. Obesity specifically influences several factors affecting drug disposition, including body composition, metabolism by CYP450 enzymes, and plasma protein levels [19]. The most striking differences are observed for highly lipophilic drugs, where volume of distribution changes dramatically in the obese population [20]. However, this is not the case for clotting factor concentrates. FVIII concentrates are typically confined to the vascular space, with volumes of distribution approximating plasma volume (48 mL·kg^{-1}) [21]. Since vasculature represents a very small fraction (0.005–0.010) of adipose tissue volume [22], an excess (or scarcity) of fat does not significantly alter the volume of distribution of FVIII. As a result, overweight and obese patients are likely overdosed when dose is calculated using total body weight [23]. A similar issue has been noted for dosing of unfractionated heparin, another compound whose volume of distribution is approximately equal to the plasma volume; obese children achieved comparable anticoagulation at a lower weight-based dose [24]. Hemophilia treatment is expensive, with annual costs in the hundreds of thousands for those on prophylaxis [2], and while prophylaxis does achieve better health outcomes, these come at a significant cost that is not automatically offset by prevention of other expenses [25]. As the clotting factor itself represents the majority of the cost of prophylaxis [26], overdosing can introduce a significant waste of resources [27]. This study will explore alternative dosing regimens that optimize both safety and resource utilization in overweight and obese hemophiliacs.

2. Methods

Population generation, simulation, and data analysis were all conducted in Matlab R2009.

2.1. Population Generation

The generated population of virtual individuals consists of two equal sized bins classified by BMI using the cut-offs defined by Henrard et al. [17] The first group consists of average weight subjects (BMI between 20.3 and 29.6 kg·m^{-2}); the second group represents an overweight and obese population with BMI between 29.6 kg·m^{-2} and 40.0 kg·m^{-2}. These cut-off values for BMI were found to be the strongest predictors of FVIII IVR. Each group contains 1000 simulated subjects with a uniform BMI distribution. Heights were derived from the distribution provided by the NHANES database [28]. A uniform distribution of BMI's was simulated and the total body weights were calculated as the product of BMI and the square of height.

2.2. Definitions of Weight Metrics

The following weight metrics were defined for each virtual patient from their simulated total body weight (TBW, kg), height (HT, cm) and BMI (kg·m^{-2}):

1. Lean body weight (LBW) [29]

$$LBW = \frac{9270 \times TBW}{6680 + 216 \times BMI},$$

(2)

2. Ideal body weight (IBW—Lorentz formula)

$$IBW = HT - 100 - \left(\frac{HT - 150}{4}\right),$$

(3)

3. Adjusted body weight (ABW)

$$ABW_{25} = IBW + 0.25 \times (TBW - BW),$$

(4)

$$ABW_{40} = IBW + 0.4 \times (TBW - IBW).$$

(5)

We used the semi-mechanistic model for LBW developed by Janmahasatian et al. [30] as it has been found to better describe the full range of adult heights and weights [20]. IBW was calculated using Lorentz's formula, which takes into account the patient's height and sex but not total body weight. ABW was the first weight metric intended for use in pharmacokinetic studies; it involves adding a proportion of the excess weight above IBW [30]. This proportion is variable, ranging from 25–50%, with 40% being used most commonly; in this study, we examined both 25% (ABW$_{25}$) and 40% (ABW$_{40}$) correction factors. Correlation plots for all body size metrics are presented in Supplementary Figures S1 and S2 for normal and overweight/obese individuals, respectively.

2.3. Population Pharmacokinetic Model

Simulations were performed using the 2-compartment structure described by Garmann et al. [31] for BAY 81-8973 (Kovaltry®, Bayer, Leverkusen, Germany), built on 183 subjects. Of the 109 patients above 18 years of age, the BMI range was 15.0–38.3 kg·m^{-2}. The details of the model structure are presented in Table 1. For each simulated individual, PK parameters were calculated. Each virtual individual was then dosed based on various weight metrics and their PK was simulated.

Table 1. Details of the model developed by Garmann et al. [31]. CL: clearance; Q: intercompartmental clearance; V_1: volume of the central compartment; V_2: volume of the peripheral compartment; RUV: residual unexplained variability; BSV: between subject variability; LBW: lean body weight.

Parameter	Estimate	Covariate Effect	BSV (%CV)
CL (dL·h^{-1})	1.88	$\theta_{CL}\left(\frac{LBW}{51.1}\right)^{0.610}$	37.0
Q (dL·h^{-1})	1.90		
V_1 (dL)	30.0	$\theta_{V_1}\left(\frac{LBW}{51.1}\right)^{0.950}$	11.2
V_2 (dL)	6.37		
Proportional RUV (%CV)	26.7		
Additive RUV (IU dL^{-1})	1.10		

2.4. Simulation and Assessment of Treatment Regimens

For each virtual individual, FVIII levels and individual PK parameters were simulated assuming a baseline factor level of 0.5 IU dL^{-1}. FVIII levels were simulated using time steps of 0.2 h following dosing regimens for four weeks to ensure that steady state was reached, and results from the 5th week were used in subsequent analysis steps. In a first instance, we analyzed a typical dosing strategy (20 IU kg^{-1} TBW every 48 h) to evaluate its appropriateness.

We then simulated various regimens wherein equal doses were given at regular intervals (i.e., 48 h). Each patient was dosed from 10 IU kg^{-1} for each weight metric (10 IU kg^{-1} of TBW, 10 IU kg^{-1} of LBW, etc.) up to 210 IU kg^{-1}. Initially, the dose step was 2 IU kg^{-1} for doses up to 100 IU kg^{-1} and 10 IU kg^{-1} for doses between 100 and 210 IU kg^{-1}. After reviewing the results, the dose step was reduced to 0.1 IU kg^{-1} between 20 and 30 IU kg^{-1}, as this was the range of most interest. A regimen was considered to be safe for a BMI group if 95% of the simulated population within that group had factor levels above 1 IU dL^{-1} at all times ($C_{min} \geq 1$ IU dL^{-1}). The lowest dose per weight metric that met this safety criterion was identified and considered to be the optimal regimen for that particular metric and BMI group. A secondary measure of safety was the 95th quantile for time spent below 1 IU dL^{-1}; in other words, the amount of time per week spent below trough for the 5% of the population not meeting the safety criteria. To evaluate economic differences between regimens, we calculated the mean weekly consumption on each optimal regimen to determine which dosing regimen met safety requirements while minimizing resource expenditure. This process was then repeated for a Monday-Wednesday-Friday (M-W-F) dosing schedule. For these simulations, the optimal dose for each metric (determined in the previous simulations) was administered on Monday and Wednesday, and the Friday dose was increased until the safety criterion was reached. To evaluate the importance of the earlier assumption of 0.5 IU dL^{-1} baseline, we repeated the above simulations assuming a baseline of 0 IU dL^{-1} to observe if similar trends emerged.

3. Results

Simulations of the typical regimen of 20 IU kg^{-1} TBW every 48 h were completed and the results are summarized in Table 2. We then investigated the hypothesis that a TBW-based dosing regimen results in overdosing in overweight and obese patients by determining the TBW-based dose required to meet the 1 IU dL^{-1} safety criterion in 95% of these patients. At a dose of 20 IU kg^{-1} TBW, the median minimum concentration (C_{min}) throughout the week for these patients was 5.4 IU dL^{-1}; the average consumption associated with this dosing regimen was 7.25×10^3 IU per person per week. However, this population requires only 14 IU kg^{-1} TBW to meet the 95% safety criterion, which corresponds to an average weekly consumption of 5.07×10^3 IU per person.

Table 2. Comparison of the typical 20 IU kg^{-1} total body weight (TBW) dose and the lowest dose meeting the safety threshold (i.e., 14 IU kg^{-1} TBW) in overweight and obese patients. Results are presented as median (90% confidence interval).

Measure	Regimen	
	20 IU kg^{-1} TBW, Q48 h	14 IU kg^{-1} TBW, Q48 h
C_{min} (IU dL^{-1})	5.4 (1.2–17.3)	3.9 (1.0–12.3)
Consumption (IU per person per week)	7260 (5730–8780)	5080 (4010–6140)

Following this initial investigation, we explored dosing regimens using alternative weight metrics. The correlation between each weight metric and BMI is shown in Figure 1. We began by administering a dose of 10 IU kg^{-1} of each weight metric on a Q48 h dosing schedule. Once steady state was reached, the percentage of patients with $C_{min} \geq 1.0$ IU dL^{-1} was calculated. If this percentage was below 95%, the dose was incrementally increased until this threshold was reached. We then calculated the mean weekly consumption associated with the minimum dose required to reach the safety criterion for each metric to assess cost-effectiveness. Since a Monday-Wednesday-Friday dosing schedule is commonly used in hemophilia A prophylaxis, we performed analogous simulations using this schedule instead of a regular 48 h interval. We used the optimal doses found in the previous study on Monday and Wednesday, and then increased the dose on Fridays to compensate for the longer interval until the safety criterion was met.

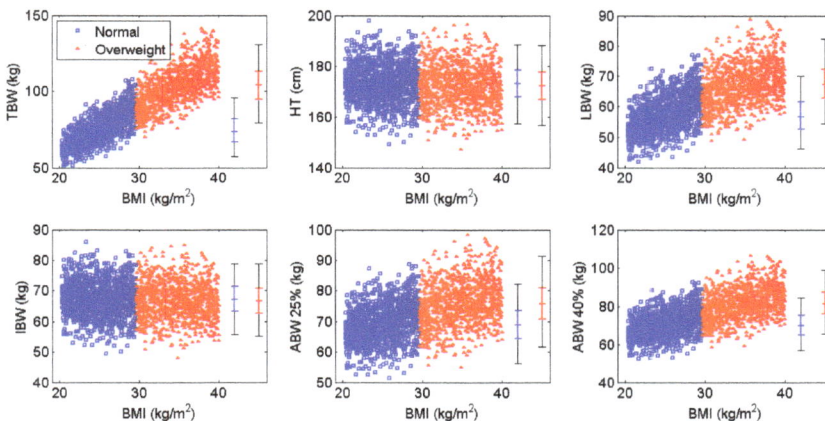

Figure 1. Correlation of body weight metrics with body mass index (BMI) for each BMI subgroup (blue = normal weight, red = overweight and obese). TBW: total body weight; HT: height; LBW: lean body weight; IBW: ideal body weight; ABW: adjusted body weight.

Tables 3 and 4 summarize the doses per kg of each weight metric required to reach the 95% safety criterion (when infused every 48 h or Monday-Wednesday-Friday, respectively) and the associated weekly consumption in each of the BMI categories and in the merged population, assuming a baseline factor level of 0.5 IU dL^{-1}. The most appropriate regimen is the one that meets the safety requirements while consuming the least amount of factor concentrate. For patients within the normal BMI range, LBW produced the optimal regimen for both dosing schedules; for the overweight and obese cohort, an IBW-based dosing regimen was found to be most cost-effective. Furthermore, the range of mean weekly consumption across the various weight metrics was much tighter for the normal BMI subgroup (125 IU per person per week) as compared to the overweight/obese subgroup (483 IU per person per week). When the two subgroups were combined, ABW with a 25% correction factor proved to be ideal for the Q48 h regimen, with IBW a very close second with a difference of just 5 IU per person per week. Both ABW_{25} and IBW perform almost identically in terms of safety for both BMI subgroups for the Q48 h regimen (Figure 2). However, IBW performed better than all other weight metrics when a Monday-Wednesday-Friday schedule was adopted, with a difference in consumption of over 100 IU per person per week when compared to the next best metric (LBW). Nevertheless, the amount of time spent below 1 IU dL^{-1} is significantly greater when following a Monday-Wednesday-Friday regimen as compared to the Q48 h dosing schedule (Figure 3b); additionally, an extremely high Friday dose (>125 IU kg^{-1} TBW) is required to meet the 95% safety requirement, whereas a dose of 18 IU kg^{-1} TBW is successful for the Q48 h regimen (Figure 3a).

Table 3. Summary of safety and economic evaluations of different weight metrics used in a Q48 h regimen across BMI subgroups, assuming a baseline factor level of 0.5 IU dL^{-1}. Dose is the dose required to have 95% of patients with a steady state C_{min} over 1 IU dL^{-1}. Optimal regimens for each subgroup and the overall population are bolded. IBW: ideal body weight, ABW: adjusted body weight.

Metric	Normal		Overweight and Obese		All BMI Categories		
	Dose (IU kg^{-1})	Mean Consumption (IU per Person per Week)	Dose (IU kg^{-1})	Consumption (IU per Person per Week)	Dose (IU kg^{-1})	Mean Consumption (IU per Person per Week)	Difference in Consumption from TBW
TBW	20.0	5202	14.0	5074	18.0	5603	-
LBW	**25.6**	**5114**	21.3	5028	23.8	5186	−417
IBW	22.2	5222	**20.7**	**4828**	22.1	5176	−427
ABW_{25}	21.7	5239	20.0	5311	**20.4**	**5171**	−432
ABW_{40}	21.1	5173	18.0	5129	20.0	5301	−302

Table 4. Summary of safety and economic evaluations of different weight metrics used in a Monday-Wednesday-Friday regimen across BMI subgroups, assuming a baseline factor level of 0.5 IU dL^{-1}. Dose is the Friday dose required to have 90% of patients with a weekly $C_{min} \geq 1$ IU dL^{-1}. Optimal regimens for each subgroup and the overall population are bolded.

Metric	Normal		Overweight and Obese		All BMI Categories		
	Dose (IU kg^{-1})	Consumption (IU per Person per Week)	Dose (IU kg^{-1})	Consumption (IU per Person per Week)	Dose (IU kg^{-1})	Consumption (IU per Person per Week)	Difference in Consumption from TBW
TBW	74	8174	54	9320	62	8716	-
LBW	**94**	**8082**	82	8740	88	8442	−274
IBW	78	8213	**84**	**8543**	**80**	**8312**	−404
ABW_{25}	78	8195	72	8558	76	8459	−258
ABW_{40}	76	8126	68	8792	72	8481	−235

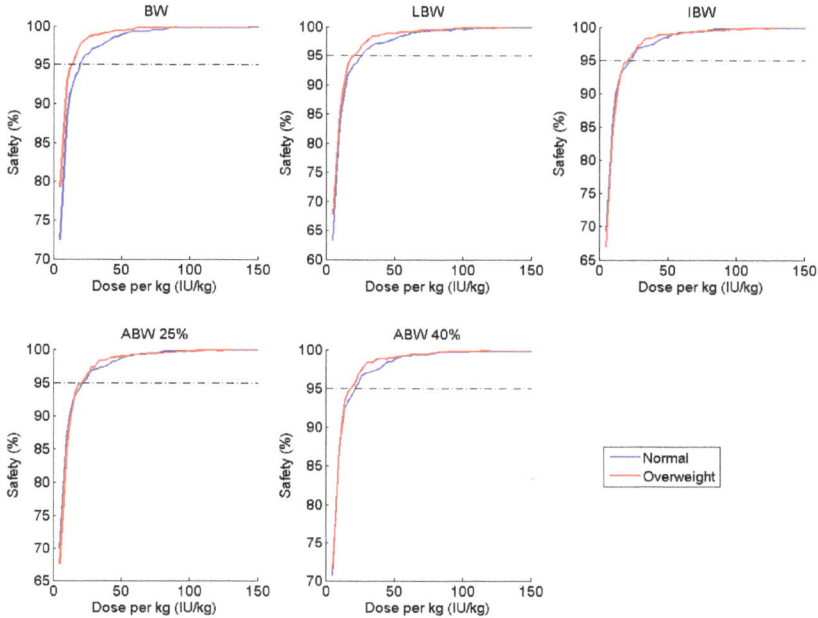

Figure 2. Percentage of patients with $C_{min} \geq 1$ IU dL^{-1} (safety) at various doses per kg of various weight metrics, stratified by BMI subgroup, administered at 48-h intervals.

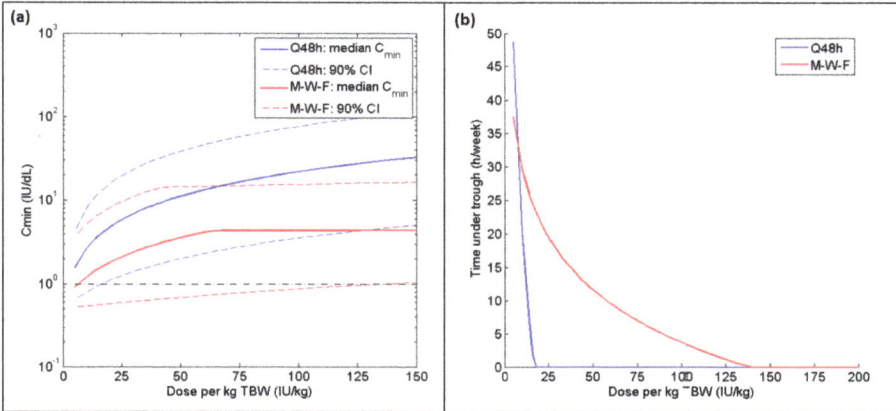

Figure 3. (**a**) Median and 90% confidence intervals for C_{min} and (**b**) 95th quantile for time spent below 1 IU dL^{-1} (hours per week) for TBW-based dosing regimen administered at different intervals for the combined group (normal + overweight/obese) for both Q48 h (blue) and Monday-Wednesday-Friday (red) dosing schedules. For the Q48 h regimen, all doses are increasing along the *X*-axis; for the Monday-Wednesday-Friday schedule, only the Friday dose is changing (Monday and Wednesday doses are fixed at 20 IU per kg TBW).

Ideal body weight continued to perform well in simulations with an assumed baseline of 0 IU dL^{-1}. The safety ratio versus dose curves are once again nearly identical for both BMI subgroups (Figure 4), although consumption was approximately doubled as compared to the Q48 h regimen.

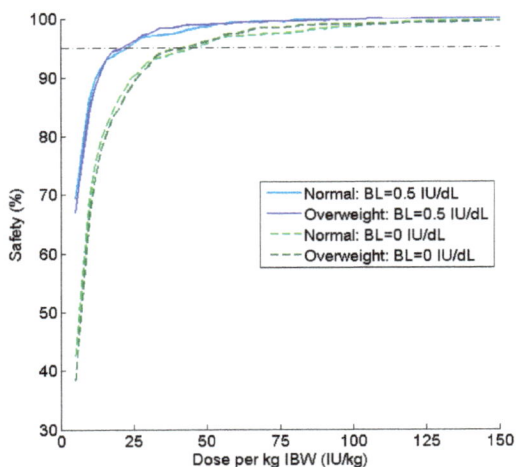

Figure 4. Comparison of safety profiles for patients simulated with baseline 0.5 IU dL^{-1} and 0 IU dL^{-1} for a Q48 h regimen. Safety (%) is the percentage of patients with $C_{min} \geq 1$ IU dL^{-1} at various doses per kg of IBW.

4. Discussion

We began by assessing the safety and cost-effectiveness of a typical 20 IU kg^{-1} TBW, Q48 h regimen in an overweight and obese patient population. For comparison, we determined the TBW-based dose required to meet the safety criterion. At a dose of 14 IU kg^{-1} TBW, 95% of patients had FVIII levels of at least 1 IU dL^{-1} at all times; the median C_{min} was 3.9 IU dL^{-1} and the mean consumption was just over 5000 IU per person per week. By contrast, the 20 IU kg^{-1} TBW regimen produced a median C_{min} of 5.4 IU dL^{-1} with a mean consumption of 7250 IU per person per week. Hence, the standard TBW-based dosing protocol results in over 40% higher consumption than required in the overweight and obese population; assuming a cost of $1 US per unit of concentrate, this amounts to over $100,000 US in excess spending per person annually. From this evaluation, it is clear that TBW does not represent the optimal body weight metric to guide FVIII dosing.

Simulations using dosing regimens based on alternative weight metrics (LBW, IBW, ABW$_{25}$, and ABW$_{40}$) were carried out using the two most common dosing schedules in hemophilia A prophylaxis: a regular 48 h regimen and a Monday-Wednesday-Friday regimen. Adapting a Monday-Wednesday-Friday timetable made it extremely difficult to meet the safety requirement, regardless of which weight metric was used to define the dose. While patients are often advised to increase their FVIII dose on Friday, a simple doubling of the dose is not sufficient. A potentially harmful Friday dose of 140 IU kg^{-1} TBW was required for 95% of patients to have a $C_{min} \geq 1$ IU dL^{-1}, compared to 18 IU kg^{-1} TBW to meet this safety minimum when infused every 48 h. Furthermore, the time spent below 1 IU dL^{-1} (and, consequently, the risk of bleeding events [32]) is significantly greater when following a Monday-Wednesday-Friday regimen, even if the Friday dose is twice or three times greater than the Monday and Wednesday doses (Figure 3b). In fact, a 2010 study in which FVIII was administered three times per week found that over 80% of bleeds occurred 48–72 h post-infusion [33]. The Monday-Wednesday-Friday treatment schedule, while more convenient, is no longer considered to be optimal therapy due to this increased vulnerability to bleeds during the weekend, with alternate day dosing representing the ideal regimen [34,35].

Due to analytical limitations, it can be difficult to obtain an exact measure of a patient's baseline factor level. Many assays have a lower limit of quantification of 1 IU dL^{-1} [36,37], which is greater than endogenous levels for severe hemophilia patients. To balance both safety and resource utilization, we ran initial simulations with an assumed baseline of 0.5 IU dL^{-1}. However, it is known that many severe hemophilia patients possess a genetic mutation such that no functional FVIII is produced endogenously. For this reason, the simulations were performed again using a baseline of 0 IU dL^{-1} to ensure similar trends were observed within this sub-population. Notably, a 95% safe ratio can be achieved in a population with no endogenous FVIII production at a reasonable dose (34 IU kg^{-1} TBW) if administered every 48 h. However, it is not possible to meet that safety threshold in this population if a Monday-Wednesday-Friday dosing schedule is employed. If the safety criteria is lowered to 90%, it can be met, but only with extremely high Friday doses (between 130 and 180 IU kg^{-1} for the various weight metrics) and associated weekly consumption (>16,000 IU per person per week); a study by Collins et al. found similarly high doses (>100 IU kg^{-1} for patients with average half-lives, and up to 400 IU kg^{-1} in extreme cases) were required to maintain FVIII levels above 1 IU dL^{-1} throughout the week when following this dosing schedule [38]. These results suggest that a regular dosing interval of 48 h offers significant advantages over the weekly Monday-Wednesday-Friday schedule in terms of both safety and cost-effectiveness.

After exploring all combinations of dosing schedule and baseline factor level, we determined that IBW-based dosing provides a safe and cost-effective regimen in the majority of scenarios, with ABW$_{25}$ producing fairly similar results. Ideal body weight performed almost exactly the same in terms of safety between the normal and overweight groups across all of the doses and regardless of baseline, as evidenced by the closeness of the curves shown in Figures 2 and 4. Further, IBW was the most cost-effective in three out of four simulations; in the fourth, it differed by only 5 IU per person per week from the optimal regimen (ABW$_{25}$). If we compare the optimal regimen for a Q48 h schedule with a baseline of 0.5 IU dL^{-1} (i.e., 20.7 IU kg^{-1} IBW) to a 20 IU kg^{-1} TBW, this alterative regimen offers a savings of over 2000 IU per person per week (or nearly \$110,000 US annually) for overweight and obese patients. Thus, IBW-based dosing offers a similar safety profile to the currently used TBW strategy while moderating the economic burden of clotting factor prophylaxis.

This exercise was limited by the constraints of the data. The model used herein was built on PK data from a specific brand of FVIII concentrate, although brand has not generally been found to significantly influence PK. A second limitation to the applicability of this approach is that the source data is largely from older (10+ years of age) patients, and the opinions on use of prophylaxis in adults are varied [39–41]. Obesity rates are also increasing rapidly amongst pediatric patients and similar dosing adjustments are likely appropriate in this population, but cannot be confirmed in this study. Further study of pediatric populations (and validated pediatric population PK models) is required in order to determine a dosing regimen that applies not only to all BMI's but also to all ages.

As the prevalence of obesity has risen in the general population, a number of studies have been conducted to investigate the frequency of overweight and obesity among hemophilia patients, complications such as co-morbidities and decreased quality of life, and recommendations for management strategies. Many pharmacokinetic studies exploring the relationship between excess body weight and plasma volume (and, by extension, in vivo recovery) have postulated that dosing according to body weight results in overdosing and an ineffective use of resources, suggesting instead that dosing be guided by LBW or IBW [42,43]. This study compared several weight metrics and confirmed that an IBW-based regimen is both safe and cost-effective across a range of BMI's. Ideal body weight produced slightly better results than other weight metrics because it is calculated based solely on height; as shown in Figure 1, there is no correlation between IBW and BMI as observed with the other metrics investigated.

Although we were able to identify a weight metric that is more suitable for a variable population, the high inter-individual variability in PK handling of factor concentrates precludes the definition of a single, "one dose fits all" strategy. In order to optimize prophylaxis, regimens should be tailored to the individual PK profile. This process has been facilitated by the development of the WAPPS-Hemo service (www.wapps-hemo.org), a Canadian-based user-friendly and industry-independent platform that produces estimates of individual PK parameters through a Bayesian iterative approach.

The WAPPS-Hemo service also includes a module for dosing regimen development, wherein clinicians can predict the effects of changing dose, frequency, or targeted trough for a specific patient before implementing these changes in practice. While PK-tailored dosing regimens may offer the best results, weight-based strategies are still the norm, but these can be optimized by adapting a different weight metric (i.e., IBW) to guide safe and cost-effective dosing at a population level.

5. Conclusions

In summary, we conducted simulations based on a previously published model of a conventional FVIII to explore the appropriateness of different weight metric-based dosing regimens for hemophilia A prophylaxis for overweight and obese patients. Regimens were required to produce a $C_{min} \geq 1$ IU dL^{-1} in 95% of the population, and then the average consumption for each regimen was calculated to evaluate resource-effectiveness. From this study, we conclude that ideal body weight performs the best, maintaining safety while tempering factor consumption for overweight and obese patients.

Supplementary Materials: The following are available online at www.mdpi.com/1999-4923/9/4/47/s1, Figure S1: Correlation plots for all body size metrics used in simulations for the normal BMI subgroup. Diagonal elements contain histograms. Figure S2: Correlation plots for all body size metrics used in simulations for the overweight/obese subgroup. Diagonal elements contain histograms.

Acknowledgments: We thank Dirk Garmann for helpful comments. This work was funded by the Canadian Institute of Health Research (CIHR) as a doctoral award to AMK.

Author Contributions: Severine Henrard, Alanna McEneny-King, Andrea N. Edginton and Cedric Hermans conceived of the project. Alanna McEneny-King and Pierre Chelle completed the data analysis and all authors participated in manuscript preparation.

Conflicts of Interest: The authors declare no conflict of interest.

References

1. Den Uijl, I.E.; Mauser Bunschoten, E.P.; Roosendaal, G.; Schutgens, R.E.; Biesma, D.H.; Grobbee, D.E.; Fischer, K. Clinical severity of haemophilia A: Does the classification of the 1950s still stand? *Haemophilia* **2011**, *17*, 849–853. [CrossRef] [PubMed]
2. Manco-Johnson, M.J.; Abshire, T.C.; Shapiro, A.D.; Riske, B.; Hacker, M.R.; Kilcoyne, R.; Ingram, J.D.; Manco-Johnson, M.L.; Funk, S.; Jacobson, L.; et al. Prophylaxis versus episodic treatment to prevent joint disease in boys with severe hemophilia. *N. Engl. J. Med.* **2007**, *357*, 535–544. [CrossRef] [PubMed]
3. Fischer, K.; Collins, P.W.; Ozelo, M.C.; Srivastava, A.; Young, G.; Blanchette, V.S. When and how to start prophylaxis in boys with severe hemophilia without inhibitors: Communication from the SSC of the ISTH. *J. Thromb. Haemost.* **2016**, *14*, 1105–1109. [CrossRef] [PubMed]
4. Berntorp, E.; Spotts, G.; Patrone, L.; Ewenstein, B.M. Advancing personalized care in hemophilia A: Ten years' experience with an advanced category antihemophilic factor prepared using a plasma/albumin-free method. *Biologics* **2014**, *8*, 115–127. [CrossRef] [PubMed]
5. Petrini, P. Identifying and overcoming barriers to prophylaxis in the management of haemophilia. *Haemophilia* **2007**, *13* (Suppl. 2), 16–22. [CrossRef] [PubMed]
6. Oldenburg, J. Optimal treatment strategies for hemophilia: Achievements and limitations of current prophylactic regimens. *Blood* **2015**, *125*, 2038–2044. [CrossRef] [PubMed]
7. Bjorkman, S.; Folkesson, A.; Jonsson, S. Pharmacokinetics and dose requirements of factor VIII over the age range 3–74 years: A population analysis based on 50 patients with long-term prophylactic treatment for haemophilia A. *Eur. J. Clin. Pharmacol.* **2009**, *65*, 989–998. [CrossRef] [PubMed]
8. Carlsson, M.; Berntorp, E.; Bjorkman, S.; Lethagen, S.; Ljung, R. Improved cost-effectiveness by pharmacokinetic dosing of factor VIII in prophylactic treatment of haemophilia A. *Haemophilia* **1997**, *3*, 96–101. [CrossRef] [PubMed]
9. Iorio, A.; Keepanasseril, A.; Foster, G.; Navarro-Ruan, T.; McEneny-King, A.; Edginton, A.N.; Thabane, L. WAPPS-Hemo co-investigator network Development of a Web-Accessible Population Pharmacokinetic Service-Hemophilia (WAPPS-Hemo): Study Protocol. *JMIR Res. Protoc.* **2016**, *5*, e239. [CrossRef] [PubMed]

10. McEneny-King, A.; Foster, G.; Iorio, A.; Edginton, A.N. Data Analysis Protocol for the Development and Evaluation of Population Pharmacokinetic Models for Incorporation into the Web-Accessible Population Pharmacokinetic Service—Hemophilia (WAPPS-Hemo). *JMIR Res. Protoc.* **2016**, *5*, e232. [CrossRef] [PubMed]

11. Ingram, G.I. Calculating the dose of factor VIII in the management of haemophilia. *Br. J. Haematol.* **1981**, *48*, 351–354. [CrossRef] [PubMed]

12. Poon, M.C.; Lee, A. Individualized prophylaxis for optimizing hemophilia care: Can we apply this to both developed and developing nations? *Thromb. J.* **2016**, *14*, 32. [CrossRef] [PubMed]

13. Ullman, M.; Zhang, Q.C.; Brown, D.; Grant, A.; Soucie, J.M. Hemophilia Treatment Center Network Investigators Association of overweight and obesity with the use of self and home-based infusion therapy among haemophilic men. *Haemophilia* **2014**, *20*, 340–348. [CrossRef] [PubMed]

14. Revel-Vilk, S.; Komvilaisak, P.; Blanchette, V.; Stain, A.M.; Floros, G.; Cochrane, A.; Blanchette, C.; Hang, M.; Roberts, E.A.; Ling, S.C. The changing face of hepatitis in boys with haemophilia associated with increased prevalence of obesity. *Haemophilia* **2011**, *17*, 689–694. [CrossRef] [PubMed]

15. Young, G. New challenges in hemophilia: Long-term outcomes and complications. *Hematol. Am. Soc. Hematol. Educ. Program.* **2012**, *2012*, 362–368.

16. Shapiro, A.D.; Korth-Bradley, J.; Poon, M.C. Use of pharmacokinetics in the coagulation factor treatment of patients with haemophilia. *Haemophilia* **2005**, *11*, 571–582. [CrossRef] [PubMed]

17. Henrard, S.; Speybroeck, N.; Hermans, C. Impact of being underweight or overweight on factor VIII dosing in hemophilia A patients. *Haematologica* **2013**, *98*, 1481–1486. [CrossRef] [PubMed]

18. McLeay, S.C.; Morrish, G.A.; Kirkpatrick, C.M.; Green, B. The relationship between drug clearance and body size: Systematic review and meta-analysis of the literature published from 2000 to 2007. *Clin. Pharmacokinet.* **2012**, *51*, 319–330. [CrossRef] [PubMed]

19. Cheymol, G. Effects of obesity on pharmacokinetics implications for drug therapy. *Clin. Pharmacokinet.* **2000**, *39*, 215–231. [CrossRef] [PubMed]

20. Hanley, M.J.; Abernethy, D.R.; Greenblatt, D.J. Effect of obesity on the pharmacokinetics of drugs in humans. *Clin. Pharmacokinet.* **2010**, *49*, 71–87. [CrossRef] [PubMed]

21. Bjorkman, S.; Oh, M.; Spotts, G.; Schroth, P.; Fritsch, S.; Ewenstein, B.M.; Casey, K.; Fischer, K.; Blanchette, V.S.; Collins, P.W. Population pharmacokinetics of recombinant factor VIII: The relationships of pharmacokinetics to age and body weight. *Blood* **2012**, *119*, 612–618. [CrossRef] [PubMed]

22. Kawai, R.; Lemaire, M.; Steimer, J.L.; Bruelisauer, A.; Niederberger, W.; Rowland, M. Physiologically based pharmacokinetic study on a cyclosporin derivative, SDZ IMM 125. *J. Pharmacokinet. Biopharm.* **1994**, *22*, 327–365. [CrossRef] [PubMed]

23. Tuinenburg, A.; Biere-Rafi, S.; Peters, M.; Verhamme, P.; Peerlinck, K.; Kruip, M.J.; Laros-Van Gorkom, B.A.; Roest, M.; Meijers, J.C.; Kamphuisen, P.W.; et al. Obesity in haemophilia patients: Effect on bleeding frequency, clotting factor concentrate usage, and haemostatic and fibrinolytic parameters. *Haemophilia* **2013**, *19*, 744–752. [CrossRef] [PubMed]

24. Taylor, B.N.; Bork, S.J.; Kim, S.; Moffett, B.S.; Yee, D.L. Evaluation of weight-based dosing of unfractionated heparin in obese children. *J. Pediatr.* **2013**, *163*, 150–153. [CrossRef] [PubMed]

25. Risebrough, N.; Oh, P.; Blanchette, V.; Curtin, J.; Hitzler, J.; Feldman, B.M. Cost-utility analysis of Canadian tailored prophylaxis, primary prophylaxis and on-demand therapy in young children with severe haemophilia A. *Haemophilia* **2008**, *14*, 743–752. [CrossRef] [PubMed]

26. Johnson, K.A.; Zhou, Z.Y. Costs of Care in Hemophilia and Possible Implications of Health Care Reform. *Hematol. Am. Soc. Hematol. Educ. Program.* **2011**, *1*, 413. [CrossRef] [PubMed]

27. Majumdar, S.; Ostrenga, A.; Latzman, R.D.; Payne, C.; Hunt, Q.; Morris, A.; Iyer, R. Pharmacoeconomic impact of obesity in severe haemophilia children on clotting factor prophylaxis in a single institution. *Haemophilia* **2011**, *17*, 717–718. [CrossRef] [PubMed]

28. Fryar, C.D.; Gu, Q.; Ogden, C.L.; Flegal, K.M. Anthropometric Reference Data for Children and Adults: United States, 2011–2014. *Vital Health Stat. 3* **2016**, *39*, 1–46.

29. Janmahasatian, S.; Duffull, S.B.; Ash, S.; Ward, L.C.; Byrne, N.M.; Green, B. Quantification of lean bodyweight. *Clin. Pharmacokinet.* **2005**, *44*, 1051–1065. [CrossRef] [PubMed]

30. Green, B.; Duffull, S.B. What is the best size descriptor to use for pharmacokinetic studies in the obese? *Br. J. Clin. Pharmacol.* **2004**, *58*, 119–133. [CrossRef] [PubMed]

31. Garmann, D.; McLeay, S.; Shah, A.; Vis, P.; Maas Enriquez, M.; Ploeger, B.A. Population pharmacokinetic characterization of BAY 81–8973, a full-length recombinant factor VIII: Lessons learned—Importance of including samples with factor VIII levels below the quantitation limit. *Haemophilia* **2017**, *23*, 528–537. [CrossRef] [PubMed]

32. Collins, P.W.; Blanchette, V.S.; Fischer, K.; Bjorkman, S.; Oh, M.; Fritsch, S.; Schroth, P.; Spotts, G.; Astermark, J.; Ewenstein, B. Break-through bleeding in relation to predicted factor VIII levels in patients receiving prophylactic treatment for severe hemophilia A. *J. Thromb. Haemost.* **2009**, *7*, 413–420. [CrossRef] [PubMed]

33. Collins, P.; Faradji, A.; Morfini, M.; Enriquez, M.M.; Schwartz, L. Efficacy and safety of secondary prophylactic vs. on-demand sucrose-formulated recombinant factor VIII treatment in adults with severe hemophilia A: Results from a 13-month crossover study. *J. Thromb. Haemost.* **2010**, *8*, 83–89. [CrossRef] [PubMed]

34. Collins, P.W.; Fischer, K.; Morfini, M.; Blanchette, V.S.; Bjorkman, S.; International Prophylaxis Study Group Pharmacokinetics Expert Working Group. Implications of coagulation factor VIII and IX pharmacokinetics in the prophylactic treatment of haemophilia. *Haemophilia* **2011**, *17*, 2–10. [CrossRef] [PubMed]

35. Richards, M.; Williams, M.; Chalmers, E.; Liesner, R.; Collins, P.; Vidler, V.; Hanley, J. Paediatric Working Party of the United Kingdom Haemophilia Doctors' Organisation A United Kingdom Haemophilia Centre Doctors' Organization guideline approved by the British Committee for Standards in Haematology: Guideline on the use of prophylactic factor VIII concentrate in children and adults with severe haemophilia A. *Br. J. Haematol.* **2010**, *149*, 498–507. [PubMed]

36. Shapiro, A.D. Long-lasting recombinant factor VIII proteins for hemophilia A. *Hematol. Am. Soc. Hematol. Educ. Program.* **2013**, *2013*, 37–43. [CrossRef] [PubMed]

37. Barrowcliffe, T.W. Monitoring haemophilia severity and treatment: New or old laboratory tests? *Haemophilia* **2004**, *10* (Suppl. 4), 109–114. [CrossRef] [PubMed]

38. Collins, P.W.; Bjorkman, S.; Fischer, K.; Blanchette, V.; Oh, M.; Schroth, P.; Fritsch, S.; Casey, K.; Spotts, G.; Ewenstein, B.M. Factor VIII requirement to maintain a target plasma level in the prophylactic treatment of severe hemophilia A: Influences of variance in pharmacokinetics and treatment regimens. *J. Thromb. Haemost.* **2010**, *8*, 269–275. [CrossRef] [PubMed]

39. Ljung, R. Aspects of prophylactic treatment of hemophilia. *Thromb. J.* **2016**, *14*, 30. [CrossRef] [PubMed]

40. Jackson, S.C.; Yang, M.; Minuk, L.; Sholzberg, M.; St-Louis, J.; Iorio, A.; Card, R.; Poon, M.C. Prophylaxis in older Canadian adults with hemophilia A: Lessons and more questions. *BMC Hematol.* **2015**, *15*. [CrossRef] [PubMed]

41. Oldenburg, J.; Brackmann, H.H. Prophylaxis in adult patients with severe haemophilia A. *Thromb. Res.* **2014**, *134* (Suppl. 1), S33–S37. [CrossRef] [PubMed]

42. Graham, A.; Jaworski, K. Pharmacokinetic analysis of anti-hemophilic factor in the obese patient. *Haemophilia* **2014**, *20*, 226–229. [CrossRef] [PubMed]

43. Komwilaisak, P.; Blanchette, V. Pharmacokinetic studies of coagulation factors: Relevance of plasma and extracellular volume and body weight. *Haemophilia* **2006**, *12* (Suppl. 4), 33. [CrossRef]

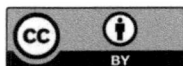

pharmaceutics

MDPI

Article

Pharmacokinetic Analysis of an Oral Multicomponent Joint Dietary Supplement (Phycox®) in Dogs

Stephanie E. Martinez [1,2], Ryan Lillico [2], Ted M. Lakowski [2], Steven A. Martinez [3] and Neal M. Davies [2,4,*]

[1] Department of Veterinary Clinical Sciences, College of Veterinary Medicine, Washington State University, Pullman, WA 99164, USA; smartinez@vetmed.wsu.edu

[2] College of Pharmacy, Rady Faculty of Health Sciences, University of Manitoba, Winnipeg, MB R3E 0T5, Canada; umlillic@myumanitoba.ca (R.L.); ted.lakowski@umanitoba.ca (T.M.L.)

[3] Comparative Orthopedic Research Laboratory, Department of Veterinary Clinical Sciences, College of Veterinary Medicine, Washington State University, Pullman, WA 99164, USA; martinez@vetmed.wsu.edu

[4] Faculty of Pharmacy and Pharmaceutical Sciences, University of Alberta, Edmonton, AB T6G 2H7, Canada

[*] Correspondence: ndavies@ualberta.ca; Tel.: +1-780-221-0828

Received: 19 July 2017; Accepted: 13 August 2017; Published: 18 August 2017

Abstract: Despite the lack of safety, efficacy and pharmacokinetic (PK) studies, multicomponent dietary supplements (nutraceuticals) have become increasingly popular as primary or adjunct therapies for clinical osteoarthritis in veterinary medicine. Phycox® is a line of multicomponent joint support supplements marketed for joint health in dogs and horses. Many of the active constituents are recognized anti-inflammatory and antioxidant agents. Due to a lack of PK studies in the literature for the product, a pilot PK study of select constituents in Phycox® was performed in healthy dogs. Two novel methods of analysis were developed and validated for quantification of glucosamine and select polyphenols using liquid chromatography-tandem mass spectrometry. After a single oral (PO) administrated dose of Phycox®, a series of blood samples from dogs were collected for 24 h post-dose and analyzed for concentrations of glucosamine HCl, hesperetin, resveratrol and naringenin. Non-compartmental PK analyses were carried out. Glucosamine was detected up to 8 h post-dose with a T_{max} of 2 h and C_{max} of 9.69 µg/mL. The polyphenols were not found at detectable concentrations in serum samples. Co-administration of glucosamine in the Phycox® formulation may enhance the absorption of glucosamine as determined by comparison of glucosamine PK data in the literature.

Keywords: glucosamine; nutraceutical; osteoarthritis; pharmacokinetics; polyphenols; veterinary medicine

---

1. Introduction

Osteoarthritis (OA) continues to present significant therapeutic problems in humans, equines, canines and other companion animals despite its clinical prevalence. Non-steroidal anti-inflammatory agents (NSAIDs) remain the most common therapies across species for attenuation of clinical signs of OA [1–3]. NSAIDs act by inhibiting cyclooxygenases, which are involved in the production of prostaglandins resulting in analgesic, anti-inflammatory and antipyretic effects [4,5]. Chronic use of NSAIDs is associated with adverse effects including gastrointestinal ulcers, liver toxicity, hemorrhaging and negative effects on chondrocytes and cartilage-matrix formation [1,4–7]. Due to the possible adverse effects of NSAIDs, there has been an interest in human and veterinary medicine to identify dietary supplements (nutraceuticals) that may serve as safer, efficacious alternatives or adjuncts to NSAIDs for the management of OA [8].

Presently, multicomponent formulations are a trend in dietary supplements and nutraceuticals with the notion that several chemical constituents may interact with multiple targets to evoke interdependent pharmacological activities to achieve optimal and potentially synergistic effects [9]. In regards to pharmacological and pharmacokinetic (PK) evaluations, multicomponent dietary supplements pose increased difficulty in comparison to a supplement containing a single chemical constituent; not only due to the increase in the amount of chemical constituents to monitor but also the increased potential for xenobiotic–xenobiotic interaction. Clearly, PK analysis is required on the major constituents present in these formulations; however, the reports of polyPK analyses of dietary supplements are lacking in the literature [9]. A comprehensive understanding of the absorption, distribution, metabolism and excretion of dietary supplements and natural health products is important for sustaining effective concentrations of active compounds at the sites of action but, unfortunately, many dietary supplements for both human and veterinary health do not undergo PK evaluation and are sold with dosing instructions without any scientific rationale [10]. The lack of PK evaluation for commercial dietary supplements is particularly evident in veterinary medicine as no federal testing requirements are in place despite the increased clinical use of these dietary supplements [11–13].

Joint health products such as glucosamine hydrochloride and chondroitin sulfate represent the largest category of dietary supplements in veterinary medicine. A novel product that falls into this category is the multicomponent Phycox® product line produced by Dechra Veterinary Products (Overland Park, KS, USA). The Phycox® line produces products formulated for dogs and horses marketed as a joint health supplement that supports joint mobility and healthy bone structure [14]. Table 1 contains the extensive list of active ingredients of Phycox® soft chews for dogs. Many of the ingredients are not single chemical constituents but complex matrices, such as the Phycox® active ingredient consisting of a proprietary blue-green algae extract containing biliprotein, c-phycocyanin, citrus bioflavonoids, grape seed extract and turmeric; all of which have been reported to possess anti-inflammatory and/or antioxidant properties in vitro, and, in some cases, in vivo [15–23]. Furthermore, flaxseed is a source of fatty acid omega-3, as alpha-linoleic acid (ALA) is a precursor to eicosapentaenoic acid (EPA) and docosahexaenoic acid (DHA), each of which could also have potential bioactivity and therapeutic properties. Additionally, a recent study from our group demonstrated that many Phycox® constituents as well as the whole preparation possess cyclooxygenase-2 inhibitory activities and, in an in vitro model of canine OA, no significant difference between the Phycox® preparation and the NSAID, carprofen, were found in the reduction of most OA biomarkers warranting further clinical investigations of Phycox® [11]. It is entirely possible that the major components of the formulation including glucosamine, MSM, creatine, ALA, etc. may have a peripheral role.

Table 1. Phycox® soft chew formula for canines (Pieloch 2006) (Phycox® active ingredient is a proprietary blue-green algae extract).

Active Ingredients Per Soft Chew	
Glucosamine hydrochloride	450 mg
Methylsulfonylmethane	400 mg
Creatine monohydrate	250 mg
Alpha-linolenic acid	200 mg
Proprietary blend of citrus bioflavonoids, calcium phosphate, manganese sulfate, ascorbic acid (vitamin C), zinc sulfate, alpha lipoic acid, and grape seed extract	132 mg
Turmeric	50 mg
Phycox active	30 mg
Eicosapentaenoic acid (EPA)	9 mg
Docosahexaenoic acid (DHA)	6 mg
Boron	100 µg
Selenium	10 µg
Alpha tocopheryl acetate (vitamin E)	25 IU
Inactive ingredients	
Flaxseed oil, hydrolyzed vegetable protein, magnesium stearate, marine lipid concentrates, natural liver flavor, and sucrose	

To our knowledge, there are no studies published evaluating the PK disposition or the in vivo metabolism of the constituents of Phycox® when administered via the Phycox® soft chew in the dog. Individual PK studies in dogs exist for the following Phycox® constituents: glucosamine [1,13], resveratrol (found in grape seed extract) [24] and naringenin (found in citrus bioflavonoids) [25,26]. The objectives of this study were to develop and validate the methods of analysis using liquid chromatography-tandem mass spectometry (LC-MS/MS) for glucosamine (Figure 1A), *trans*-resveratrol (Figure 1B), ±naringenin (Figure 1B) and ±hesperetin (component of citrus bioflavonoids) (Figure 1B), to quantify *trans*-resveratrol, ±naringenin and ±hesperetin in Phycox® soft chews and to describe the pharmacokinetics of glucosamine, *trans*-resveratrol, ±naringenin, and ±hesperetin following administration of a single Phycox® soft chew to female Beagle dogs in a pilot study.

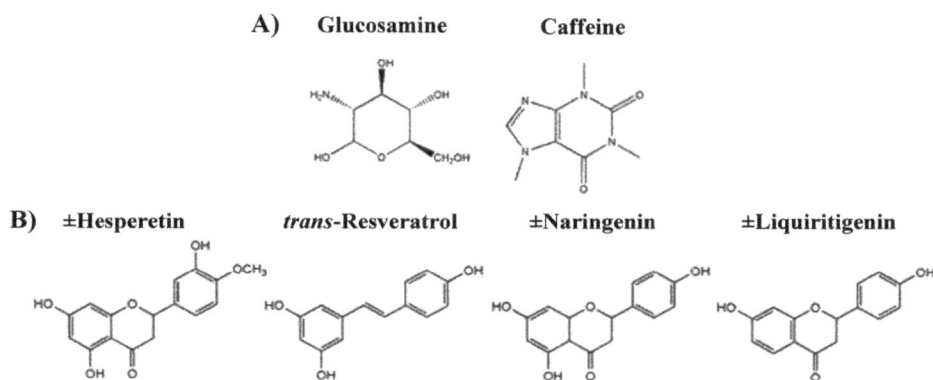

Figure 1. (**A**) Chemical structures of glucosamine and the internal standard caffeine; (**B**) chemical structures of ±hesperetin, ±naringenin, *trans*-resveratrol and the internal standard ±liquiritigenin.

2. Materials and Methods

2.1. Chemicals and Reagents

Phycox® canine chewable whole tablets and the individual components, glucosamine hydrochloride, grape seed extract, citrus bioflavonoids, and Phycox® premix were provided by Dechra Veterinary Products. ±Naringenin, ±hesperidin, ±liquiritigenin. caffeine, *trans*-resveratrol, β-glucuronidase type IX A (β-glucuronidase), were purchased from Sigma-Aldrich (St. Louis, MO, USA). β-Glucosidase from almonds was purchased from Tokyo Chemical Industry Co., Ltd. (Tokyo, Japan). Formic acid was purchased from Acros Organics (Geel, Belgium). HPLC-grade acetonitrile and methanol were purchased from EMD Millipore (Gibbstown, NJ, USA). Ultrapure water from a Milli-Q water system was used (Millipore, Billerica, MA, USA).

2.2. Analytical System and Conditions

The LC-MS/MS system used (Shimadzu, Kyoto, Japan) was connected to the liquid chromatography portion consisting of two Nexera™ LC-30AD pumps, a Nexera™ SIL-30AC auto injector, a CMB-2-A Prominence system controller, a DGU-20A5R degassing unit and a CT0-20A Prominence column oven. Data analysis was accomplished using Shimadzu LabSolutions (Version 5.3) software.

The LC-MS/MS was operated in DUIS mode (electrospray ionization and atmospheric pressure chemical ionization) using multiple reaction monitoring (MRM). The LC-MS/MS conditions consisted of a curved desolvation line temperature of 250 °C and heating block temperature of 400 °C. Nebulizing gas we delivered at 2 L/min and drying gas was delivered at 15 L/min.

2.3. Glucosamine

The analytical system described above was used for serum glucsamine concentration analysis. The analytical column used was a Primesep 200 (3.0 μm, 2.1 × 100 mm) (SIELC Technologies, Wheeling, IL, USA) mixed function cation exchange column. The mobile phase consisted of a pH gradient with mobile phases A (0.05% aqueous formic acid) and B (1% formic acid) in 50% aqueous acetonitrile. The gradient was as follows: 0% B for 3 min, linear gradient from 0% to 80% B in 2.5 min, linear gradient from 80% to 100% B in 0.1 min, and from 100% to 0% B in 1 min. The column equilibrated for 3 min at 0% B prior to the next injection. Separation was carried out at 35 ± 0.5 °C with a flow rate of 0.4 mL/min. Both glucosamine and the internal standard, caffeine, were monitored in positive mode. Table 2 describes the parent and daughter ion mass to charge ratios (*m/z*) used along with the collision energy of each compound.

Table 2. Mass spectral multiple reaction monitoring data for glucosamine, ±hesperetin, ±naringenin, *trans*-resveratrol and the internal standards caffeine and ±liquiritigenin.

Compound	Parent Ion *m/z*	Daughter Ion *m/z*	Collision Energy (eV)
Glucosamine	180.20	162.10	10
Caffeine (internal standard)	194.90	138.00 42.00 110.15	19 36 24
±Hesperetin	302.80	153.10	24.0
±Naringenin	273.90	153.10	24.0
trans-Resveratrol	228.80	135.10 107.20	13.0 23.0
±Liquiritigenin (internal standard)	257.90	137.0	−22.0

2.4. Polyphenols

The analytical system described above was used for serum polyphenol analysis. The analytical column used was a Waters ACQUITY UPLC® BEH C_{18} column (3.0 μm, 2.1 × 100 mm) (Waters Corporation, Milford, MA, USA). An isocratic mobile phase consisting of 50% aqueous methanol with 0.1% formic acid was employed. Separation was carried out at 40 ± 0.5 °C with a flow rate of 0.4 mL/min. ±Liquiritigenin was used as the internal standard. All compounds were monitored in positive mode. Table 2 describes the parent and daughter ion mass to charge ratios (*m/z*) used along with the collision energy of each compound.

2.5. Stock and Working Standard Solutions

Methanolic stock solutions of glucosamine, caffeine, ±hesperetin, ±naringenin, *trans*-resveratrol and ±liquiritigenin were prepared at 100 μg/mL concentrations. These solutions were protected from light and stored at −20 °C between uses for no longer than 3 months. Calibration standards in serum and methanol were prepared from stock solutions by sequential dilution, yielding a series of concentrations; 0.005, 0.01, 0.05, 0.1, 0.5, 1.0, 5.0, 10 and 20 μg/mL for glucosamine, ±hesperetin, ±naringenin and *trans*-resveratrol. Quality control (QC) samples were prepared from stock solutions by dilution to yield target concentration of 0.075, 1.5, and 15 μg/mL.

2.6. Sample Preparation for Standard Curves

2.6.1. Glucosamine

The working standards of glucosamine were added to blank dog serum (100 μL) in microcentrifuge tubes to achieve the desired final concentration previously described along with 40 μL of internal standard, caffeine (diluted to a concentration of 0.1 μg/mL from stock solution). One milliliter of cold acetonitrile (−20 °C) was added to the samples to precipitate proteins. The samples were vortexed and centrifuged at 20,160× *g* for 5 min. The supernatant was transferred to new microcentrifuge tubes and evaporated to dryness using a Savant SPD1010 SpeedVac Concentrator (Thermo Fisher Scientific, Inc., Asheville, NC, USA). The residues were reconstituted with 50 μL of starting mobile phase (0.05% aqueous formic acid), vortexed for 30 seconds and centrifuged at 20,160× *g* for 5 min. The supernatants were transferred to 30 kDa centrifugal filter tubes and centrifuged for 30 min at 9000× *g*. The filtrate was transferred to HPLC vials and 5 μL were injected into the LC-MS/MS system.

2.6.2. Polyphenols

The working standards of ±hesperetin, ±naringenin and *trans*-resveratrol were added to blank dog serum (100 μL) in microcentrifuge tubes to achieve the desired final concentration previously described along with 20 μL of internal standard, ±liquiritigenin (diluted to a concentration of 10 μg/mL from stock solution). One milliliter of cold acetonitrile (−20 °C) was added to the samples to precipitate proteins. The samples were vortexed and centrifuged at 20,160× *g* for 5 min. The supernatant was transferred to new microcentrifuge tubes and evaporated to dryness using a Savant SPD1010 SpeedVac Concentrator. The residues were reconstituted with 50 μL of mobile phase (50% aqueous methanol with 0.1% formic acid), vortexed for 30 seconds and centrifuged at 20,160× *g* for 5 min. The supernatants were transferred to 30 kDa centrifugal filter tubes and centrifuged for 30 min at 9000× *g*. The filtrate was transferred to HPLC vials and 5 μL were injected into the LC-MS/MS system.

2.7. Precision, Accuracy and Recovery

The inter-day precision and accuracy of the two assays were determined from the results of three replicate assays on three different days during a one-week period. Three standard curves (0.001–20 μg/mL) with the inclusion of the 3 QC sample concentrations (0.075, 1.5, and 15 μg/mL) for each assay were used. The precision of the assays was evaluated by the coefficient of variations (CV) of the QC samples. The accuracies were determined by the mean percentage error of measured concentrations to the expected concentrations (percent bias) of the QC samples using the constructed standard curves.

Recoveries of glucosamine and the polyphenols at the QC sample concentrations were determined. Recovery was assessed by the comparing the measured values of QC samples in methanol to theoretical values of QC samples.

2.8. Content Analysis of Polyphenols in Phycox®

The amount of glucosamine in each Phycox® soft chew is known and listed under the active ingredients on the packaging. However, specific amounts of ±hesperetin, ±naringenin and *trans*-resveratrol contained in the citrus bioflavonoids and grape seed extract ingredients, respectively, are unknown. To determine the amount of ±hesperetin, ±naringenin and *trans*-resveratrol in one Phycox® soft chew, content analyses of the whole soft chew, the premix and individual ingredient constituents of grape seed extract and citrus bioflavonoids were undertaken. The polyphenol extraction procedure from dietary supplements has previously been described [27]. Briefly, three samples of soft chews from different lots were weighed and then pulverized. The premix, grape seed extract and citrus bioflavonoids were already in powdered form. One gram of each product was weighted and placed in 15 mL tubes. Methanolic extractions were performed by adding 4 mL of methanol to each tube and then placing them on a rocking platform shaker at room temperature ($23 \pm 1\,°C$) for 3 h. Tubes were centrifuged for 10 min at $5000\times g$. The supernatants were collected in duplicate 100 μL aliquots (aglycone and total). The total samples were dried to completion using a Savant SPD1010 SpeedVac Concentrator and then reconstituted with phosphate-buffered saline (200 μL at pH 7.4). Twenty microliters of β-glucosidase (750 U/mL in phosphate buffered saline at pH 7.4) was added and samples were incubated for 48 h at $37\,°C$ in a shaking incubator. β-Glucosidase acts by cleaving the glycosidic sugar moieties frequently present in plant extracts as previously described [28]. Cold acetonitrile (1 mL, $23 \pm 1\,°C$) was added to stop the enzymatic reaction. To both sets of samples, the internal standard, 20 μL of 10 μg/mL ±liquiritigenin in methanol, was added. Samples were centrifuged at $20,160\times g$ for 5 min. The supernatants were collected and dried to completion using a Savant SPD1010 SpeedVac Concentrator. Samples were reconstituted in mobile phase (50 μL of 50% aqueous methanol with 0.1% formic acid), vortexed and centrifuged at $20,160\times g$ for 5 min. The supernatants were transferred to 30 kDa centrifugal filter tubes and centrifuged for 30 min at $9000\times g$. The filtrate was transferred to HPLC vials and 5 μL were injected into the LC-MS/MS system.

2.9. Animals and Compliance with Ethical Standards

The animal research protocol used in this study was reviewed and approved by the Institutional Animal Care and Use Committee at Washington State University (protocol #04224-011, approved 21 December 2014). Four commercially available purpose-bred intact female research Beagles from an Association for Assessment and Accreditation of Laboratory Animal Care (AALAC) certified source were used for the study. All dogs were 2 years of age at the onset of the study with a weight of 9.25 ± 0.81 kg (mean $\pm$ SD; range 8.4–10.2 kg). Animals were housed in AALAC approved facilities for animal research for 80 days acclimating to their environment prior to the initiation of the study. All dogs were fed a standard canine formulation (Proactive Health™ Adult Minichunks, IAMS, Mason, OH, USA) ration twice daily and housed in a temperature and humidity controlled room; $21\,°C$ and 30%, respectively, while under 12 h light cycle conditions. The dogs underwent daily examinations and weekly body weight assessments. All animals were also given daily enrichment activities before, during, and after the study. At study termination all animals were transferred to an unrelated study.

2.10. Pharmacokinetic Studies

Dogs were fasted 12 h prior to the study but provided free access to water. Each subject was administered a single Phycox® soft chew and a series of blood samples (3 mL) were collected at 0, 1, 2, 4, 6, 8, 12 and 24 h post-dose via saphenous or cephalic vein depending on the temperament of the animals. Animals were fed after 2 h post-dose. Following centrifugation of the blood samples, serum was removed and stored at $-80\,°C$ until analyzed.

2.11. Treatment of Pharmacokinetic Samples

2.11.1. Glucosamine

One hundred microliters of serum from each PK sample was placed into a microcentrifuge tube. To all samples, except 0 h, 40 μL of 0.1 μg/mL internal standard stock solution (caffeine) was added along with 1.0 mL of cold acetonitrile ($-20\,°C$) to precipitate proteins. The samples were vortexed and centrifuged at $20,160\times g$ for 5 min. The supernatant was transferred to new microcentrifuge tubes and evaporated to dryness using a Savant SPD1010 SpeedVac Concentrator. The residues were reconstituted with 50 μL of starting mobile phase (0.05% aqueous formic acid), vortexed and centrifuged at $20,160\times g$ for 5 min. The supernatants were transferred to 30 kDa centrifugal filter tubes and centrifuged for 30 min at $9000\times g$. The filtrate was transferred to HPLC vials and 5 μL were injected into the LC-MS/MS system.

2.11.2. Polyphenols

The PK serum samples were separated into two sets of microcentrifuge tubes (total and aglycone) with 100 μL of serum in each. To the total samples, 20 μL β-glucuronidase (500 U/mL in 6.8 pH phosphate buffer) was added and incubated for 2 h at 37 °C [28]. To all samples except 0 h, 20 μL of 10 μg/mL internal standard stock solution (±liquiritigenin) was added along with 1.0 mL of cold acetonitrile (−20 °C) to precipitate proteins. The supernatant was transferred to new microcentrifuge tubes and evaporated to dryness using a Savant SPD1010 SpeedVac Concentrator. The residues were reconstituted with 50 μL of mobile phase (50% aqueous methanol with 0.1% formic acid), vortexed and centrifuged at 20,160× *g* for 5 min. The supernatants were transferred to 30 kDa centrifugal filter tubes and centrifuged for 30 min at 9000× *g*. The filtrate was transferred to HPLC vials and 5 μL were injected into the LC-MS/MS system.

2.12. Pharmacokinetic Analysis

PK samples were analyzed using Phoenix WinNonlin software (ver. 6.3; Certara, St. Louis, MO, USA) to derive the pharmacokinetic parameters for each individual dog and expressed as mean ± SEM. A non-compartmental analysis was used to calculate the PK parameters including area under the curve ($AUC_{0-\infty}$), the peak serum concentration (C_{max}), time to reach peak serum concentration (T_{max}), the apparent volume of distribution (Vd/F), the elimination half-life ($t_{1/2}$), and the apparent clearance (CL/F). The elimination rate constant (KE), was estimated by log-linear regression of the serum concentrations. The $AUC_{0-\infty}$ was calculated using the long-linear trapezoidal rule for data from time of dosing to the last measured concentration plus the quotient of the last measured concentration divided by KE/2.303. The concentration time points of the animals were subjected to non-compartmental modeling. The aglycone concentrations of ±hesperetin, ±naringenin and *trans*-resveratrol were used for modeling.

2.13. Data Analysis

Compiled data were presented as mean and standard error of the mean (mean ± SEM). Where possible, the data were analyzed for statistical significance using SigmaPlot software (v. 13.0, SystatSoftware, Inc., San Jose, CA, USA). Student's t-test was employed for unpaired samples to compare means between two groups, with a value of $p < 0.05$ considered statistically significant. The quantifications of concentrations were based on calibration curves constructed using the peak area ratio (PAR) of glucosamine and the polyphenols to internal standards, against the concentrations of glucosamine and the polyphenols using unweighted least squares linear regression.

3. Results

3.1. LC-MS/MS Analyses

3.1.1. Glucosamine

Various compositions of mobile phase and columns were tested to achieve the best resolution of glucosamine. Optimal separation was achieved with the combination of a Primesep 200 mixed function cation exchange column and pH gradient mobile phase consisting of: (A) 0.05% aqueous formic acid; and (B) 1% formic acid, in 50% aqueous acetonitrile with the following gradient: 0% B for 3 min, linear gradient from 0% to 80% B in 2.5 min, linear gradient from 80% to 100% B in 0.1 min, and from 100% to 0% B in 1 min. Following the gradient, the column was equilibrated for 3 min at 0% B prior to the next injection. Separation was best achieved using a flow rate of 0.4 mL/min and maintaining the column 35 ± 0.5 °C. Caffeine was selected as the internal standard owing to its similar chromatographic behavior and ionization efficiency to glucosamine. No interfering peaks co-eluted with the peaks of interest (Figure 2A). The retention times for glucosamine and caffeine were 2.7 min and 4.9 min, respectively, in serum (Figure 2B,C).

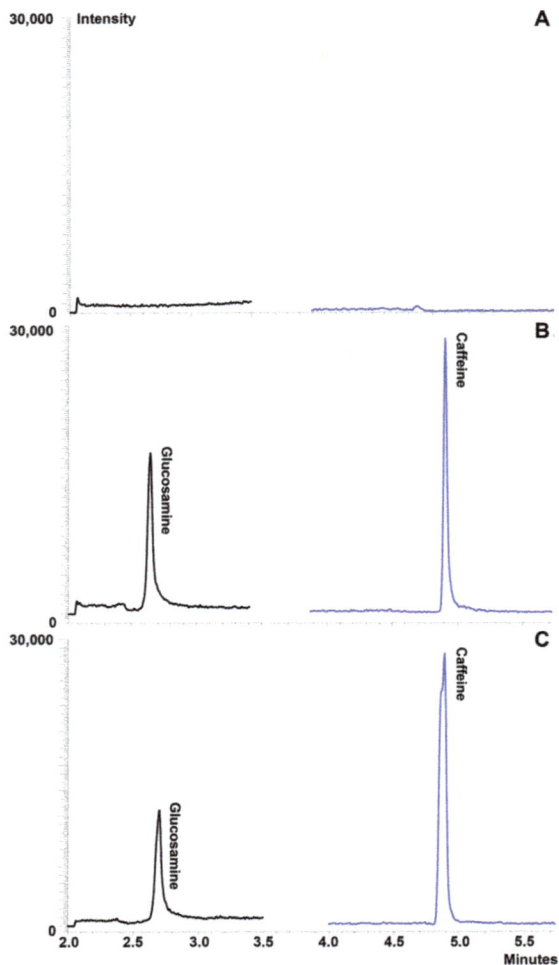

Figure 2. Representative chromatograms of glucosamine in serum: (**A**) blank serum demonstrating no interfering peaks co-eluted with the compounds of interest; (**B**) serum containing glucosamine and the internal standard at glucosamine at 10 µg/mL; and (**C**) pharmacokinetic sample at 2 h post-dose (450 mg glucosamine HCl via administration of one Phycox® soft chew).

3.1.2. Polyphenols

As with glucosamine, various compositions of mobile phases and columns were investigated to achieve the best resolution of the compounds. Optimal separation was achieved using a simple, reverse-phase isocratic mobile phase consisting of 50% aqueous methanol with 0.1% formic acid with a flow rate of 0.4 mL/min. Separation of the compounds was achieved using a Waters ACQUITY UPLC® BEH C$_{18}$ column at 40 ± 0.5 °C. ±Liquiritigenin was used as the internal standard due to its structural similarity to the compounds of interest. No interfering peaks co-eluted with the peaks of interest (Figure 3A). The retention times for ±hesperetin, *trans*-resveratrol, ±naringenin and ±liquiritigenin were 2.3 min, 1.6 min, 2.1 min and 1.4 min, respectively (Figure 3B).

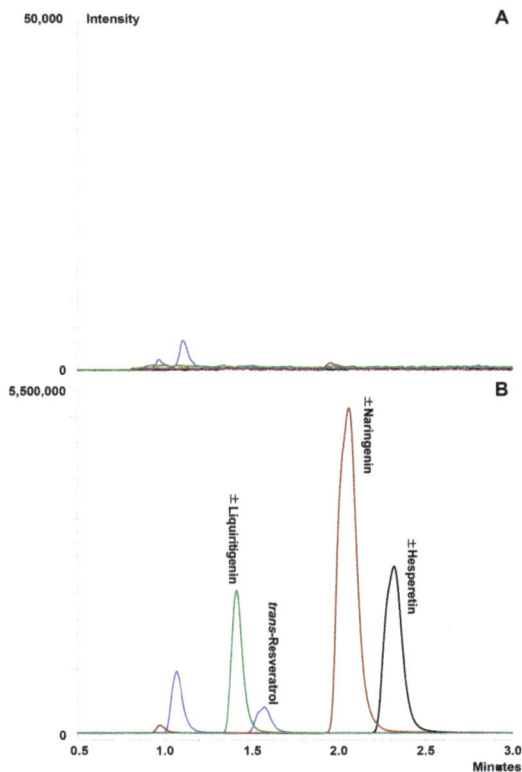

Figure 3. Representative chromatograms of ±hesperetin, trans-resveratrol and ±naringenin in serum: (**A**) blank serum demonstrating no interfering peaks co-eluted with the compounds of interest; and (**B**) serum containing polyphenols (20 μg/mL) and the internal standard.

3.2. Linearity and Limit of Quantification

3.2.1. Glucosamine

Calibration curves for glucosamine were linear from 5 ng/mL to 20 μg/mL in serum. The calibration curves showed good coefficient of determination (R^2) > 0.95. The limit of quantitation for the method was 5 ng/mL. The limit of detection for the method was calculated by measuring the average background noise in blank samples at the retention time of the peaks of interest. Limit of detection was taken to be five times the background response and determined to be 1 ng/mL.

3.2.2. Polyphenols

Calibration curves for ±hesperetin, *trans*-resveratrol and ±naringenin were linear from 5 ng/mL to 20 μg/mL in serum. The calibration curves for each compound showed good coefficient of determination (R^2) > 0.99, (R^2) > 0.97 and (R^2) > 0.99 for ±hesperetin, *trans*-resveratrol and ±naringenin, respectively. The limits of detection for all three compounds were 5 ng/mL. The limits of detection for the method were calculated by measuring the average background noise in blank samples at the retention times of the peaks of interest and then limit of detection were taken to be five times the background response. Limit of detection for all compounds was found to be 1 ng/mL.

3.3. Precision, Accuracy and Recovery

3.3.1. Glucosamine

The LC-MS/MS assay showed excellent accuracy and interday precision with a bias < 20% for the low QC sample (0.075 µg/mL) and < 3% for the medium (1.5 µg/mL) and high (15 µg/mL) QC samples along with CVs between 2.93 and 12.2% for the QC sample evaluated (Table 3). The recovery (extraction efficiency) of the assay was determined to be 34% in serum. These data indicate that the developed LC-MS/MS method for glucosamine quantitation is accurate, precise and reproducible.

Table 3. Accuracy and precision of the LCMS quantitative analysis of glucosamine, ±hesperetin, *trans*-resveratrol and ±naringenin (*n* = 3).

Analyte	Nominal Value (µg/mL)	Measured Value (µg/mL) (Mean ± SEM)	CV (%)	Bias (%)
Glucosamine				
Low	0.075	0.063 ± 0.000	2.93	−16.4
Medium	1.5	1.46 ± 0.102	12.2	−2.91
High	15	14.6 ± 0.989	11.7	−2.45
±Hesperetin				
Low	0.075	0.087 ± 0.000	0.662	14.2
Medium	1.5	1.44 ± 0.062	7.40	−3.64
High	15	13.7 ± 0.155	1.97	−9.87
trans-Resveratrol				
Low	0.075	0.088 ± 0.000	0.267	17.7
Medium	1.5	1.47 ± 0.063	7.49	−2.87
High	15	14.6 ± 0.219	2.57	−1.50
±Naringenin				
Low	0.075	0.083 ± 0.004	7.98	10.1
Medium	1.5	1.55 ± 0.102	11.4	3.30
High	15	14.3 ± 0.219	2.78	−2.28

3.3.2. Polyphenols

The LC-MS/MS assay showed excellent accuracy and inter-day precision for all three compounds. The bias for ±hesperetin was < 15% for all QC concentrations and the CV was between 0.662 and 7.40% (Table 3). The bias for *trans*-resveratrol was < 18% for the low QC sample (0.075 µg/mL) and < 3% for the medium (1.5 µg/mL) and high (15 µg/mL) QC samples. The CVs for resveratrol were between 0.267% and 7.49%. The recovery (extraction efficiency) of the assay was determined to be 54.8%, 62.1% and 54.3% in serum for ±hesperetin, *trans*-resveratrol and ±naringenin, respectively. Bias for ±naringenin was < 12% for all QC samples and the CVs were between 2.78% and 11.4%. These data (Table 3) indicate that the developed LC-MS/MS method is accurate, precise and reproducible for all three compounds.

3.3.3. Content Analysis of Polyphenols in Phycox®

The LC-MS/MS method of analysis for ±hesperitin, *trans*-resveratrol and ±naringenin was successfully applied to the determination and quantification of the compounds in Phycox® soft chews, premix as well as the constituents; citrus bioflavonoids and grape seed extract. It was determined that ±hesperitin, *trans*-resveratrol and ±naringenin are present as the aglycones and not a mixture of aglycones and glycosides as determined by the lack of differences in concentrations between aglycone and total (incubated with β-glucosidase to cleave sugar moieties) samples. ±Hesperitin was determined to be the most prevalent of the three polyphenols in the premix, citrus bioflavonoids and Phycox® soft chews. The concentration of ±hesperidin in the citrus bioflavonoids constituent was determined to be 362 µg/g and 80.8 µg/g in the Phycox® premix. It was determined that a single Phycox® soft chew contains 36.1 ± 5.39 µg of ±hesperetin. ±Naringenin was found at much lower concentrations than ±hesperetin in all of the samples. ±Naringenin was found to contain 68.6 µg/g and the Phycox® premix was found to contain 6.77 µg/g ±naringenin. A single Phycox® soft chew was determined to contain 2.88 ± 0.280 µg of naringenin. *Trans*-resveratrol was found at the lowest concentration in all samples of the three polyphenols measured. It was determined that the grape seed extract ingredient contains 0.681 µg/g of *trans*-resveratrol and the Phycox® premix contains 0.482 µg/g. A single Phycox® soft chew was found to contain 0.554 ± 0.177 µg of *trans*-resveratrol. The amount of grape seed extract and citrus bioflavonoids in each Phycox® soft chew is proprietary information and not disclosed on the label claims.

3.4. Glucosamine

The LC-MS/MS method of analysis for glucosamine was successfully applied to the determination and quantification of glucosamine in canines following administration of a single Phycox® soft chew containing 450 mg of glucosamine hydrochloride. At time zero, no detectable concentrations of glucosamine were found. The mean serum concentration over time profile for glucosamine is shown in Figure 4. The pharmacokinetic parameters for glucosamine were calculated using non-compartmental analysis and are summarized in Table 4. These data indicate following PO administration of the Phycox® soft chew, glucosamine was absorbed slowly into the systemic circulation with an average T_{max} of 2 h and an average C_{max} of 9.69 µg/mL, followed by elimination during the next 8 h, after which serum concentrations were below quantifiable concentrations (5 ng/mL). The apparent $t_{1/2}$ of glucosamine after PO administration of the Phycox® soft chew was approximately 35 min.

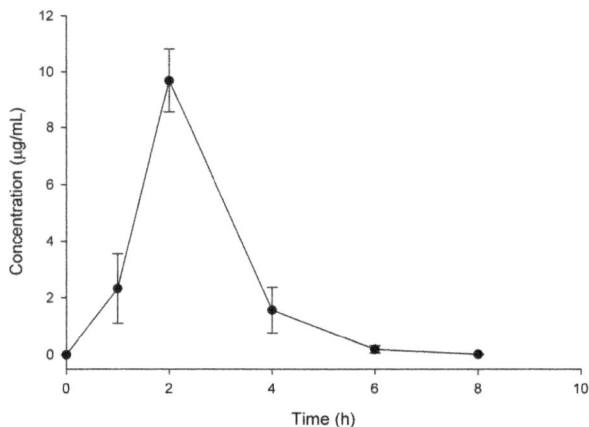

Figure 4. Glucosamine disposition in serum following oral administration of one Phycox® soft chew containing 450 mg of glucosamine hydrochloride (n = 4, mean ± SEM).

Table 4. Pharmacokinetic parameters of glucosamine (450 mg) administered in one Phycox® soft chew in the dog (n = 4).

Pharmacokinetic Parameter	Mean ± SEM
$AUC_{0-\infty}$ (µg·h/mL)	20.4 ± 2.34
Vd/F (L/kg)	2.10 ± 0.254
CL/F (L/h/kg)	2.56 ± 0.446
$t_{1/2}$ (h)	0.584 ± 0.034
T_{max} (h)	2.00 ± 0.000
C_{max} (µg/mL)	9.69 ± 1.14

3.5. Polyphenols

±Hesperetin, *trans*-resveratrol and ±naringenin were not detected at quantifiable concentrations as either the aglycone or glucuronidated metabolite. Therefore, no pharmacokinetic parameters could be derived.

4. Discussion

Although the developed LC-MS/MS method for the quantification of ±hesperetin, *trans*-resveratrol and ±naringenin with a limit of quantification of 5 ng /mL proved to be sensitive, accurate and reproducible, when applied to the quantification of the compounds in canines following PO administration of a single Phycox® soft chew containing 36.1 ± 5.39 µg of ±hesperetin, 0.554 ± 0.177 µg of *trans*-resveratrol and 2.88 ± 0.280 µg of ±naringenin, no compounds were detected at quantifiable concentrations as either the aglycone or glucuronidated metabolite. This is not unexpected given the extremely small quantities of these compounds administered via one Phycox® soft chew and the generally low bioavailability of polyphenols in mammals [29,30]. Presently, there is no information on the bioavailability ±naringenin, ±hesperetin or *trans*-resveratrol in the literature in dogs. As the amounts of racemic flavonoids were so small no attempts were made to examine stereochemistry although we possess validated methods to do so in follow up studies if quantifiable in serum or urine [31–33].

Two previous studies have evaluated the oral pharmacokinetics of glucosamine HCl in Beagle dogs. Adebowale et al. [1] administered 1500–2000 mg of glucosamine HCl to eight dogs and used non-compartmental modeling to derive PK parameters. They report T_{max} values of glucosamine between 1.1 and 1.6 h and C_{max} values between 7.1 and 12.1 µg/mL [1]. The serum-concentration time curve reported in Adebowale et al. [1] was similar in shape to the curve reported in this study but the half-lives were reported to be between 1.52–2.4 h, which is 3–5 times longer than the half-live reported in this study [1]. After 4 h post-dose, Adebowale et al. [1] was not able to detect glucosamine [1]. The method employed by the study utilized a validated HPLC method with a limit of quantification of 1.25 µg/mL and involved pre-column derivatization [1]. The amount of glucosamine administered in the present study was 3.3 to 4.4 less than those administered in the study by Adebowale et al. [1] but the method employed in this study was 250 times more sensitive allowing for detection of much smaller concentrations of glucosamine. Various LC-MS-MS assays are validated in the literature across various fluids and species [33–35]. The current assay performance using 100 µL of serum is analytically comparable and robust. The second report of glucosamine HCl PK in dogs administered 1000 mg of glucosamine HCl to four male dogs using two commercially available chewable tablet formulations [12]. T_{max} and C_{max} values were reported to range 4.2–5.0 h and 1.8–2.6 µg/mL, respectively. The serum-concentration time curves reported by Maxwell et al. [12] were formulation dependent. The time curves generated by Maxwell et al. featured clear secondary peaks for two tablet products but not for the solution administered. A secondary peak has previously been reported in PO glucosamine HCl disposition in rats [32]. $t_{1/2}$ was not reported by Maxwell et al. [12] At 12 h post-dose, Maxwell et al. was not able to detect glucosamine [12]. The method employed by the study used a modified HPLC method with a limit of quantification of 0.05 µg/mL (10 fold higher limit of quantitation than the method presented in this study) and involved pre-column derivatization [12]. To our knowledge, this is the first report of glucosamine PK in fasted dogs following PO administration of a multicomponent dietary supplement.

Administering glucosamine via a Phycox® soft chew may enhance the absorption of glucosamine compared to previous studies where glucosamine HCl was administered alone or in conjunction with chondroitin sulfate [1,12]; however, this is not the first observation in the literature of a change in glucosamine disposition when co-administered with another compound besides chondroitin sulfate to dogs. Quian et al. [34] found that when glucosamine was co-administered with chitosan to Beagle dogs, absorption of glucosamine was increased compared to absorption of glucosamine administered alone likely due to chitosan's ability to reversibly act on the epithelial tight junction to increase the paracellular permeability of glucosamine across the mucosal epithelial [34]. While chitosan is not present in Phycox®, it may be possible that other components of Phycox® are able to increase glucosamine transcellular or paracellular permeability across the mucosal epithelial thereby enhancing absorption; however, it is also common that the pharmacokinetics of a given compound in a multi-component mixture may be significantly different from that of the single compound due to drug-drug interactions [9,36,37] With the plethora of chemical constituents in Phycox® it is feasible that several constituents are interacting with multiple targets to increase absorption of glucosamine. The importance of fasting and gender on the pharmacokinetics of glucosamine remains to be further delineated.

5. Conclusions

Two method of analysis to detect glucosamine, ±hesperetin, *trans*-resveratrol and ±naringenin in dog serum were developed using a LC-MS/MS. These methods were found to be sensitive, reproducible and accurate. The methods were applied to a single-dose PK study of the multicomponent dietary supplement, Phycox®. Additionally, the method for quantification of ±hesperetin, *trans*-resveratrol and ±naringenin was employed to determine the amount of each compound in a single dose of Phycox® as it is not disclosed on the label claim. No polyphenols at quantifiable concentrations were found as aglycones or glucuronide metabolites in the PK samples; however, glucosamine was successfully quantified using a novel method which requires no pre-column derivatization allowing PK parameters to be derived. The PK disposition of glucosamine was characterized by a slow absorption and a rapid terminal $t_{1/2}$ of almost 35 min. While our PK parameters were at variance from previously reported PK parameters of glucosamine in fed Beagle dogs, the analytical method employed in this current study possessed greater sensitivity than previous studies. Future studies to determine the influence of gender and fasting and the mechanism whereby glucosamine absorption is increased by Phycox® constituents as low glucosamine bioavailability may be considered a limiting factor for its therapeutic utility and improved absorption may result in increased efficacy for the clinical management of OA. Additionally, future studies should investigate the multiple-dosing PK of the constituents of Phycox® as well as the PK of other bioactive constituents of the dietary supplement in both canines and equines since oral bioavailability and PK play an important role in the optimization of OA therapeutics for the management of clinical OA in people and other animals.

Acknowledgments: The authors acknowledge the University of Manitoba Graduate Fellowship, Manitoba Graduate Scholarship and Pfizer Canada Centennial Pharmacy Research Award given to SEM during her graduate studies. The authors also acknowledge the Leslie F. Buggey Graduate Scholarship and the Maurice Faiman Graduate Scholarship awarded to Ryan Lillico and the Natural Sciences and Engineering Research Council (NSERC) Canada (RGPIN-2015-06543, 2015–2020) awarded to Theodore M. Lakowski. The authors also acknowledge the valuable assistance provided by the staff of the Comparative Orthopedic Research Laboratory at Washington State University for this study and Dechra Veterinary Products for their funding support of this project.

Author Contributions: Steven A. Martinez, Neal M. Davies, Stephanie E. Martinez, Ryan Lillico and Theodore M. Lakowski conceived and designed the experiments; Steven A. Martinez, Stephanie E. Martinez, and Ryan Lillico performed the experiments; Stephanie E. Martinez, Neal M. Davies, Ryan Lillico, Theodore M. Lakowski and Steven A. Martinez analyzed the data; Neal M. Davies, Ryan Lillico, Stephanie E. Martinez, Steven A. Martinez and Theodore M. Lakowski contributed reagents/materials/analysis tools; and Stephanie E. Martinez, Steven A. Martinez, Neal M. Davies, Theodore M. Lakowski and Ryan Lillico wrote the paper.

Conflicts of Interest: The authors declare no conflict of interest. The University of Manitoba (Neal M. Davies) was academically subcontracted by Washington State University (Steven A. Martinez) in collaboration to carry out these analyses and studies. Dechra Veterinary Products provided funding to Washington State University but was not involved in the study design, collection, analysis and interpretation of the data, the writing of the manuscript, or the decision to submit the manuscript for publication. The authors had full access to all data in this study and take complete responsibility for the integrity of the data and accuracy of the data analysis, and have no conflicts of interest with the sponsoring company to declare.

References

1. Adebowale, A.; Du, J.; Liang, Z.; Leslie, J.L.; Eddington, N.D. The bioavailability and pharmacokinetics of glucosamine hydrochloride and low molecular weight chondroitin sulfate after single and multiple doses to beagle dogs. *Biopharm. Drug Dispos.* **2002**, *23*, 217–225. [CrossRef] [PubMed]

2. Henrotin, Y.; Sanchez, C.; Balligand, M. Pharmaceutical and nutraceutical management of canine osteoarthritis: present and future perspectives. *Vet. J.* **2005**, *170*, 113–123. [CrossRef] [PubMed]

3. Rychel, J.K. Diagnosis and treatment of osteoarthritis. *Top. Companion Anim. Med.* **2010**, *25*, 20–25. [CrossRef] [PubMed]

4. Hulse, D. Treatment methods for pain in the osteoarthritic patient. *Vet. Clin. North. Am. Small Anim. Pract.* **1998**, *28*, 361–375. [CrossRef]

5. Day, R.O.; Graham, G.G. Non-steroidal anti-inflammatory drugs (NSAIDs). *Br. Med. J.* **2013**, *3195*, 1–7.

6. Dingle, J.T. The effect of nonsteroidal antiinflammatory drugs on human articular cartilage glycosaminoglycan synthesis. *Osteoarthr. Cartil.* **1999**, *7*, 313–314. [CrossRef] [PubMed]

7. Wolfe, M.M.; Lichtenstein, D.R.; Singh, G. Gastrointestinal toxicity of nonsteroidal antiinflammatory drugs. *N. Engl. J. Med.* **1999**, *340*, 1888–1899. [CrossRef] [PubMed]

8. Vandeweerd, J.M.; Coisnon, C.; Clegg, P.; Cambier, C.; Pierson, A.; Hontoir, F.; Saegerman, C.; Gustin, P.; Buczinski, S. Systematic review of efficacy of nutraceuticals to alleviate clinical signs of osteoarthritis. *J. Vet. Intern. Med.* **2012**, *26*, 448–456. [CrossRef] [PubMed]

9. Lan, K.; Zie, G.; Jia, W. Towards polypharmacokinetics: pharmacokinetics of multicomponent drugs and herbal medicines using a metabolomics approach. *Evid. Based Complement. Alternat. Med.* **2013**, *2013*, 819147. [CrossRef] [PubMed]

10. He, S.-M.; Chan, E.; Zhou, S.F. Properties of herbal medicines in humans: evidence, challenges andstrategies. *Curr. Pharm. Des.* **2011**, *17*, 357–407. [CrossRef] [PubMed]

11. Martinez, S.E.; Chen, Y.; Ho, E.A.; Martinez, S.A.; Davies, N.M. Pharmacological effects of a C-phycocyanin-based multicomponent nutraceutical in an in vitro canine chondrocyte model of osteoarthritis. *Can. J. Vet. Res.* **2015**, *79*, 241–249. [PubMed]

12. Comblain, F.; Serisier, S.; Barthelemy, N.; Balligand, M.; Henrotin, Y. Review of dietary supplements for the management of osteoarthritis in dogs in studies from 2004 to 2014. *J. Vet. Pharmacol. Ther.* **2016**, *39*, 1–15. [CrossRef] [PubMed]

13. Maxwell, L.K.; Regier, P.; Satyanarayana, A. Comparison of glucosamine absorption after administration of oral liquid, chewable, and tablet formulations to dogs. *J. Am. Anim. Hosp. Assoc.* **2016**, *52*, 90–94. [CrossRef] [PubMed]

14. Pieloch, M.J. Method of use and dosage composition of bluegreen algae extract for inflammation in animals. US Patent 7025965 B1, 11 April 2006.

15. Reddy, C.M.; Bhat, V.B.; Kiranmai, G.; Reddy, M.N.; Reddanna, P.; Madyastha, K.M. Selective inhibition of cyclooxygenase-2 by C-phycocyanin, a biliprotein from Spirulina platensis. *Biochem. Biophys. Res. Commun.* **2000**, *277*, 599–603. [CrossRef] [PubMed]

16. Neil, K.M.; John, P.; Orth, M.W. The role of glucosamine and chondroitin sulfate in treatment for and prevention of osteoarthritis in animals. *J. Am. Vet. Med. Assoc.* **2005**, *226*, 1079–1088. [CrossRef] [PubMed]

17. Debbi, E.M.; Agar, G.; Fichman, G.; Ziv, Y.B.; Kardosh, R.; Halperin, N.; Elbaz, A.; Beer, Y.; Debi, R. Efficacy of methylsulfonylmethane supplementation on osteoarthritis of the knee: a randomized controlled study. *BMC Complement. Altern. Med.* **2011**, *11*, 50. [CrossRef] [PubMed]

18. Woo, Y.J.; Joo, Y.B.; Jung, Y.O.; Ju, J.H.; Cho, M.L.; Oh, H.J.; Jhun, J.Y.; Park, M.K.; Park, J.S.; Kang, C.M.; et al. Grape seed proanthocyanidin extract ameliorates monosodium iodoacetate-induced osteoarthritis. *Exp. Mol. Med.* **2011**, *43*, 561–570. [CrossRef] [PubMed]

19. Mahmoud, A.M.; Ashour, M.B.; Abdel-Moneim, A.; Ahmed, O.M. Hesperidin and naringin attenuate hyperglycemia-mediated oxidative stress and proinflammatory cytokine production in high fat fed/streptozotocin-induced type 2 diabetic rats. *J. Diabetes Complicat.* **2012**, *26*, 483–490. [CrossRef] [PubMed]

20. Mohammadi, S.; Najafi, M.; Hamzeiy, H.; Maleki-Dizaji, N.; Pezeshkian, M.; Sadeghi-Bazargani, H.; Darabi, M.; Mostafalou, S.; Bohlooli, S.; Garjani, A. Protective effects of methylsulfonylmethane on hemodynamics and oxidative stress in monocrotaline-induced pulmonary hypertensive rats. *Adv. Pharmacol. Sci.* **2012**, 507278. [CrossRef] [PubMed]

21. Aggarwal, B.B.; Gupta, S.C.; Sung, B. Curcumin: an orally bioavailable blocker of TNF and other pro-inflammatory biomarkers. *Br. J. Pharmacol.* **2013**, *169*, 1672–1692. [CrossRef] [PubMed]
22. Al-Rejaie, S.S.; Abuohashish, H.M.; Al-Enazi, M.M.; Ahmed, M.M.; Al-Rejaie, S.S. Protective effect of naringenin on acetic acid-induced ulcerative colitis in rats. *World J. Gastroenterol.* **2013**, *19*, 5633–5644. [CrossRef] [PubMed]
23. Asher, G.N.; Spelman, K. Clinical utility of curcumin extract. *Altern. Ther. Health Med.* **2013**, *19*, 20–22.
24. Muzzio, M.; Huang, Z.; Hu, S.; Johnson, W.D.; McCormick, D.L.; Kapetanovic, I.M. Determination of resveratrol and its sulfate and glucuronide metbaolites in plasma by LC-MS/MS and their pharmaockinetics in dogs. *J. Pharm. Biomed. Anal.* **2012**, *59*, 201–208. [CrossRef] [PubMed]
25. Mata-Bilbao; Mde, L.; Andres-Lacueva, C.; Roura, E.; Jáuregui, O.; Escribano, E.; Torre, C.; Lamuela-Raventós, R.M. Absorption and pharmacokinetics of grapefruit flavanones in beagles. *Br. J. Nutr.* **2007**, *98*, 86–92. [CrossRef] [PubMed]
26. Yang, C.P.; Liu, M.H.; Zou, W.; Guan, X.L.; Lai, L.; Su, W.W. Toxicokinetics of naringin and its metabolite naringenin after 180-day repeated oral administration in beagle dogs assayed by rapid resolution liquid chromatogrpahy/tandem mass spectrometric method. *J. Asian Nat. Prod. Res.* **2012**, *14*, 68–75. [CrossRef] [PubMed]
27. Remsberg, C.M.; Good, R.L.; Davies, N.M. Ingredient consistency of commercially available polyphenol and tocopherol nutraceuticals. *Pharmaceutics* **2010**, *2*, 50–60. [CrossRef] [PubMed]
28. Roupe, K.A.; Yáñez, J.A.; Teng, X.W.; Davies, N.M. Pharmacokinetics of selected stilbenes: Rhapontigenin, piceatannol and pinosylvin in rats. *J. Pharm. Pharmacol.* **2006**, *58*, 1443–1450. [CrossRef] [PubMed]
29. Yang, C.; Tsai, S.; Chao, P.L.; Yen, H.; Chien, T.; Hsiu, S. Determination of hesperetin and its conjugate metabolites in serum and urine. *J. Food Drug Anal.* **2002**, *10*, 143–148. [CrossRef]
30. Scheepens, A.; Tan, K.; Paxton, J.W. Improving the oral bioavailability of beneficial polyphenols through designed synergies. *Genes Nutr.* **2010**, *5*, 75–87. [CrossRef] [PubMed]
31. Yáñez, J.; Davies, N.M. Stereospecific high-performance liquid chromatographic analysis of naringenin in urine. *J. Pharm. Biomed. Anal.* **2005**, *39*, 164–169. [CrossRef] [PubMed]
32. Yáñez, J.; Teng, X.W.; Roupe, K.; Davies, N.M. Stereospecific high-performance liquid chromatographic analysis of hesperetin in biological matrices. *J. Pharm. Biomed. Anal.* **2005**, *37*, 591–595. [CrossRef] [PubMed]
33. Roda, A.; Sabatini, L.; Barbieri, A.; Guardigli, M.; Locatelli, M.; Violante, F.S.; Rovati, L.C.; Persiani, S. Development and validation of a sensitive HPLC-ESI-MS/MS method for the direct determination of glucosamine in human plasma. *J. Chromatogr. B* **2006**, *844*, 119–126. [CrossRef] [PubMed]
34. Pastorini, E.; Rotini, R.; Guardigli, M.; Vecchiotti, S.; Persiani, S.; Trisolino, G.; Antonioli, D.; Rovati, L.C.; Roda, A. Development and validation of a HPLC-ES-MS/MS method for the determination of glucosamine in human synovial fluid. *J. Pharm. Biomed. Anal.* **2009**, *50*, 1009–1014. [CrossRef] [PubMed]
35. Zhong, S.; Zhong, D.; Chen, X. Improved and simplified liquid chromatography/electrospray ionization mass spectrometry method for the analysis of underivatized glucosamine in human plasma. *J. Chromatogr. B* **2007**, *854*, 291–298. [CrossRef] [PubMed]
36. Ibrahim, A.; Gilzad-kohan, M.H.; Aghazadeh-Habashi, A.; Jamali, F. Absorption and Bioavailability of Glucosamine in the Rat. *J. Pharm. Sci.* **2012**, *101*, 2574–2583. [CrossRef] [PubMed]
37. Qian, S.; Zhang, Q.; Wang, Y.; Lee, B.; Betageri, G.V.; Chow, M.S.; Huang, M.; Zuo, Z. Bioavailability enhancement of glucosamine hydrochloride by chitosan. *Int. J. Pharm.* **2013**, *455*, 365–373. [CrossRef] [PubMed]

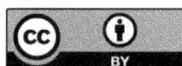

pharmaceutics

MDPI

Article

Disposition, Metabolism and Histone Deacetylase and Acetyltransferase Inhibition Activity of Tetrahydrocurcumin and Other Curcuminoids

Júlia T. Novaes [1,†], Ryan Lillico [1,†], Casey L. Sayre [2], Kalyanam Nagabhushanam [3],
Muhammed Majeed [3], Yufei Chen [1], Emmanuel A. Ho [4], Ana Luísa de P. Oliveira [1],
Stephanie E. Martinez [5], Samaa Alrushaid [1], Neal M. Davies [6,*] and Ted M. Lakowski [1,*]

[1] The Rady Faculty of Health Sciences, College of Pharmacy, Pharmaceutical Analysis Laboratory, University of Manitoba, Winnipeg, MB R3E 0T5, Canada; juliatnovaes@gmail.com (J.T.N.); umLillic@myumanitoba.ca (R.L.); umche355@myumanitoba.ca (Y.C.); analuisapoliv@gmail.com (A.L.d.P.O.); umalrush@myumanitoba.ca (S.A.)
[2] College of Pharmacy, Roseman University of Health Sciences, South Jordan, UT 84096, USA; csayre@roseman.edu
[3] Sabinsa Corporation, 20 Lake Drive, East Windsor, NJ 08520, USA; kalyanam@sabinsa.com (K.N.); mmjd52@hotmail.com (M.M.)
[4] Faculty of Science, School of Pharmacy, University of Waterloo, Kitchener, ON N2G 1C5, Canada; emmanuel.ho@uwaterloo.ca
[5] Department of Veterinary Clinical Sciences, College of Veterinary Medicine, Washington State University, Pullman, WA 99164-6610, USA; smartinez@vetmed.wsu.edu
[6] Faculty of Pharmacy and Pharmaceutical Sciences, University of Alberta, Edmonton, AB T6G 2R3, Canada
* Correspondence: ndavies@ualberta.ca (N.M.D.); ted.lakowski@umanitoba.ca (T.M.L.);
  Tel.: +1-780-492-2429 (N.M.D.); +1-204-272-3173 (T.M.L.)
† These Authors contributed equally to this work.

Received: 21 August 2017; Accepted: 11 October 2017; Published: 12 October 2017

Abstract: Tetrahydrocurcumin (THC), curcumin and calebin-A are curcuminoids found in turmeric (*Curcuma longa*). Curcuminoids have been established to have a variety of pharmacological activities and are used as natural health supplements. The purpose of this study was to identify the metabolism, excretion, antioxidant, anti-inflammatory and anticancer properties of these curcuminoids and to determine disposition of THC in rats after oral administration. We developed a UHPLC–MS/MS assay for THC in rat serum and urine. THC shows multiple redistribution phases with corresponding increases in urinary excretion rate. In-vitro antioxidant activity, histone deacetylase (HDAC) activity, histone acetyltransferase (HAT) activity and anti-inflammatory inhibitory activity were examined using commercial assay kits. Anticancer activity was determined in Sup-T1 lymphoma cells. Our results indicate THC was poorly absorbed after oral administration and primarily excreted via non-renal routes. All curcuminoids exhibited multiple pharmacological effects in vitro, including potent antioxidant activity as well as inhibition of CYP2C9, CYP3A4 and lipoxygenase activity without affecting the release of TNF-α. Unlike curcumin and calebin-A, THC did not inhibit HDAC1 and PCAF and displayed a weaker growth inhibition activity against Sup-T1 cells. We show evidence for the first time that curcumin and calebin-A inhibit HAT and PCAF, possibly through a Michael-addition mechanism.

Keywords: curcumin; tetrahydrocurcumin; calebin-A; UHPLC–MS/MS; pharmacokinetics; antioxidant; anti-inflammatory; anticancer; HDAC; HAT

1. Introduction

Turmeric from *Curcuma longa* is a popular spice known to contain curcuminoids and has been used traditionally as a natural health product [1]. There are many compounds of the curcuminoid family that are thought to produce its effects, the most studied being curcumin (**1**) (Figure 1) [2]. Curcumin is a deep yellow, poorly water-soluble substance that has been claimed to exhibit a variety of effects including antioxidant, anti-inflammatory, antiviral, antifungal, antibacterial, anticancer, antidiabetic and neuroprotective properties [3]. The effects elicited by curcumin are thought to be partly a result of its activity inhibiting the histone lysine acetyltransferases (HATs) p300/CBP [4] as well as histone deacetylases (HDACs) such as HDAC1 [5]. Inhibition of enzymes that catalyze lysine acetylation are known to have a variety of effects on gene expression and such activity confers a potential epigenetic mechanism to curcumin that has led to its exploration as an anticancer medication. Indeed, several HDAC inhibitors are already in use alone or in combination for the treatment of cancer and several groups have thought to exploit curcumin for its HDAC inhibition activity. This activity has been shown to suppress some DNA damage repair pathways and may be used to increase the effectiveness of existing cancer treatments [6]. Despite its poor bioavailability, curcumin has even been shown to suppress medulloblastoma growth in vivo through its HDAC inhibition activity [7]. Inhibition of HAT is currently being explored as a new class of cancer treatment, but despite promising results, no HAT inhibitors are currently approved; therefore, the anticancer potential of the HAT inhibition of curcumin has not been explored as much as its HDAC inhibition activity [8]. Curcumin is thought to exhibit its HAT inhibition activity by a Michael-addition reaction, alkylating the active-site cysteines of HAT [9].

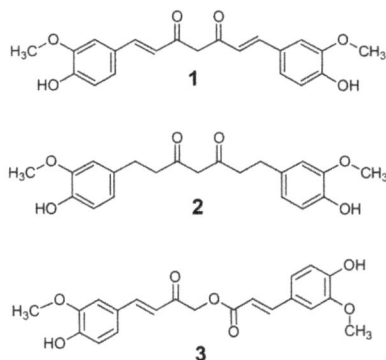

Figure 1. The structures of curcuminoids curcumin (**1**), tetrahydrocurcumin (THC) (**2**) and calebin-A (**3**). Both THC and curcumin are shown in the keto tautomer.

Another important consequence of inhibiting HAT activity is the repression of genes important in the inflammatory response. For example, some HAT inhibitors have been shown to inhibit the NF-κB pathway [10,11]. Recently, HAT inhibitors having a similar mechanism of inhibition to curcumin [9] have been shown to reduce expression of COX2, yielding anti-inflammatory and analgesic effects [12]. Although a great deal of attention has been paid to curcumin, there are many other curcuminoid-type compounds in turmeric that have potential pharmacological activities, such as tetrahydrocurcumin (THC) (**2**) and calebin-A (**3**) (Figure 1) [2].

Calebin-A has been studied for its antioxidant, anti-inflammatory and anticancer effects that have been demonstrated in vitro by inhibition of cyclooxygenase and lipoxygenase; it may also have cytochrome P450 inhibitory activity, as it appears to interact with CYP2D6 and CYP1A2 [2]. It has also been shown to inhibit dipeptidyl peptidase-4 (DPP-4), which is a membrane glycoprotein and serine exopeptidase that is implicated in type 2 diabetes mellitus through its activity inhibiting incretin release, including GLP-1 [13]. Inhibitors of DPP-4, such as gliptins, are currently used clinically as hypoglycemic agents. Calebin-A has potential as an adjuvant for cancer therapy, increasing the effectiveness of currently used cancer treatments, as it has been shown to directly inhibit P-glycoprotein and has been co-administered with vincristine to treat multidrug-resistant human gastric cancer cells. Furthermore, calebin-A also appears to modulate the mitogen-activated protein-kinase pathway. These data suggest the calebin-A may be an effective cancer treatment [1], however, a major drawback is that it has an extremely low oral bioavailability, much like curcumin [2].

THC is another curcuminoid found in turmeric that is produced by the reduction of curcumin [14]. It can be synthesized in the laboratory by hydrogenation of curcumin, yielding a colorless substance. THC can also be produced in vivo through Phase I metabolism in the liver by hepatic reductases, and as a result, after oral administration it is found as free THC and conjugated as glucuronides. Like curcumin and calebin-A, THC is also thought to have several biological activities; among the most studied are its antioxidant properties. In fact, the antioxidant role of THC has been studied as a potential preventative treatment for cardiovascular disease by reducing the formation of atherosclerotic lesions. THC has also been studied for its anti-inflammatory activity, both as a treatment for arthritis and cancer [14]. Like calebin-A and curcumin, THC is an inhibitor of P-glycoprotein, and because of this, THC has been explored as a potential way to overcome multidrug resistance in cancer [15].

THC has a number of attractive properties not shared with curcumin that may make it superior. For example, THC is significantly more stable under physiological pH and temperature conditions than curcumin [16]. Moreover, it is slightly more soluble in water, making it much easier to formulate into an acceptable dosage form than curcumin which, as stated above, has had longstanding issues with its near-insolubility in water and a number of other common solvents.

Currently, there are few studies in the literature about curcuminoids, apart from curcumin. Considering the depth of study of curcumin as a treatment for cancer among other diseases, the fact that curcumin is metabolized to THC, and the fact that THC has therapeutic potential in its own right, it is necessary to describe the pharmacological effects and pharmacokinetic characteristics of THC. In this study we developed a bioanalytical assay to quantify THC in urine and serum using ultra-high-performance liquid chromatography–mass spectrometry (UHPLC–MS/MS) to characterize its pharmacokinetics in rats after oral (PO) administration. We also identify the HDAC and HAT activities, as well as the antioxidant, anti-inflammatory and cell viability activities of THC compared to curcumin and calebin-A. As far as we know, this is the first study to dose rats with THC and measure serum and urine concentrations of THC.

2. Materials and Methods

2.1. Chemicals and Reagents

Tetrahydrocurcumin, curcumin and calebin-A were provided by Sabinsa Corporation® (Piscataway, NJ, USA). Sulfaphenazole, ketoconazole, α-naphthoflavone, quinidine, DMSO, PEG-400 and β-glucuronidase type IX A (β-glucuronidase) were purchased from Sigma-Aldrich (St. Louis, MO, USA). Analytical-grade formic acid and HPLC-grade acetonitrile were purchased from Fisher Scientific. Ultrapure water from a Milli-Q® system (Millipore, Billerica, MA, USA) was used for mobile phase. The antioxidant activity kit, cyclooxygenase-1 and -2 inhibitor screening kits, lipoxygenase inhibitor screening kit, HDAC1 and PCAF inhibitor screening kits were purchased from Cayman Chemical Company (Ann Arbor, MI, USA). Vivid® CYP2C9 green screening kit, Vivid® CYP3A4 green screening kit, Vivid® CYP1A2 blue screening kit and Vivid® CYP2D6 blue screening kit were bought from Life Technologies™ (Carlsbad, CA, USA). Human CXCL9/MIG, Human TNF-α, Human IFN-γ and Human CXCL10/IP-10 DuoSet® ELISA kits, solutions and reagents were purchased from R & D Systems® (Minneapolis, MN, USA). CellTiter 96® AQueous One Solution Cell Proliferation Assay (MTS) was purchased from Promega (Madison, WI, USA). Heat-inactivated fetal bovine serum was purchased from Gibco® by Life Technologies™ and Roswell Park Memorial Institute (RPMI) 1640 medium and Penicillin Streptomycin solution were purchased from Corning.

2.2. UHPLC–MS/MS Analysis and Conditions

THC was analyzed using the Shimadzu Nexera UHPLC coupled to a Shimadzu LCMS 8040 triple quadrupole mass spectrometer (Shimadzu, Kyoto, Japan). Chromatography was performed using a Waters Acquity UPLC BEH C18 column under isocratic conditions with 45% aqueous acetonitrile in 0.1% formic acid at a flow rate of 0.4 mL/min. THC and the internal standard (curcumin) were measured using Multiple Reaction Monitoring (MRM) in positive mode using the transitions m/z 373.3 > 137.1 and m/z 369.3 > 177.1, respectively. Data analysis was performed with the LabSolutions software version 5.72 (Shimadzu, Kyoto, Japan).

2.3. Animals

Surgically-modified, exposed jugular vein-catheterized (polyurethane-silastic blended catheter), adult male CD Sprague-Dawley rats (250–300 g) were purchased from Charles River Laboratories (St. Constant, QC, Canada). Rats received free access to food (Purina Rat Chow 5001) and water in the animal facility for at least 3 days before use. Rats were housed in temperature-controlled rooms with a 12 h light/dark cycle. Animal ethics approval was obtained from University of Manitoba Office of Research Ethics and Compliance (protocol 11-064) and a minimal number of rats were utilized to answer the hypothesis tested.

2.4. Pharmacokinetic Study

THC was provided as a dry powder from Sabinsa Corporation® and this was dissolved in a mixture of DMSO 2% and 98% PEG-400. Each rat was placed in a separate metabolic cage and fasted for 12 h prior to dosing with free access to water. On the day of experiment, the animals ($N = 3$) received a single dose of THC by oral gavage (500 mg/kg) in a volume not exceeding 1 mL. Animals had free access to water pre- and post-dosing, and food (Purina Rat Chow 5001) was provided 2 hours post-dosing. A series of blood samples (0.3 mL) were collected at 0, 15 and 30 min, and 1, 2, 4, 6, 12, 24, 48 and 72 h post-dose. At 72 h after administration, the animals were euthanized and exsanguinated. Immediately after each blood collection time point (except the terminal point), the cannula was flushed with 0.3 mL of 0.9% saline to replenish the collected blood volume. The dead volume of the cannula was replaced with sterile heparin/50% dextrose catheter lock solution (SAI Infusion Technologies, Strategic Applications, Lake Villa, IL, USA) to maintain the patency of the cannula as advised in the technical sheet supplied with the animals from Charles River. Following centrifugation of blood samples at 15,000 rpm for 5 min, serum was collected and placed into 2 mL tubes at −20 °C until further analysis. Urine samples were collected at 0, 2, 6, 12, 24, 48 and 72 h post-dose and placed in 15 mL tubes. The exact urine volume of each sample was recorded then stored at −20 °C until further analysis.

2.5. Standard Solutions and Standard Curve Preparation

Stock solutions of THC and curcumin were prepared in acetonitrile and calibration standards were prepared from these stocks in blank urine and serum into a series of concentrations: 0.005, 0.01, 0.05, 0.1, 0.5, 1.0, 5.0 and 10.0 μg/mL. Briefly, 100 μL of serum or urine, 50 μL of internal standard (curcumin 1 μg/mL) and the corresponding concentration of THC stock solution were combined and vortexed in a 2 mL microtube. Ice-cold acetonitrile (1 mL) was added to precipitate serum proteins from solution and the same was done in urine for consistency. These solutions were vortexed, centrifuged and the supernatants were collected and evaporated to dryness by a stream of nitrogen gas. The pellet was reconstituted with 50 μL of 45% aqueous acetonitrile (ACN) with 0.1% formic acid (F.A.) and injected into the UHPLC–MS/MS. The accuracy was measured from three standard curves on three separate days and precision measured with 4 quality control (QC) samples at the low, mid and high range of the curve. The accuracy and precision of the assay were 89.2 ± 10% and 95.1 ± 4.9%, respectively.

2.6. Serum and Urine Sample Preparation

Serum and urine samples (100 μL) were treated with 20 μL of 500 U/mL β-glucuronidase, vortexed and incubated at 37 °C for 2 h to release any glucuronide conjugates. 50 μL of internal standard (curcumin 1 μg/mL) was added, vortexed and rapidly, 1 mL of cold acetonitrile was added to precipitate the proteins present in both samples. Urine and serum samples were vortexed and centrifuged at 15,000 rpm for 5 min. The supernatants were collected and evaporated to dryness by nitrogen gas. Samples were reconstituted with 50 μL of mobile phase (45% ACN, 0.1% F.A.) and vortexed. The samples were transferred to HPLC vials and 10 μL was injected into the UHPLC system for each sample.

2.7. Cytochrome P450 Inhibition Determination

CYP2C9, CYP3A4, CYP1A2 and CYP2D6 assays were performed to assess metabolism and inhibition of human P450 isozymes involved using Vivid® CYP450 screening kits and CYP450 BACULOSOMES® Plus Reagents. CYP450 BACULOSOMES® Plus Reagents express only one CYP450 enzyme, preventing metabolism by other CYP450s. For CYP2C9, the substrate was BOMF and the positive control inhibitor sulfaphenazole; for CYP3A4, DBOMF was the substrate and ketoconazole the positive control inhibitor; for CYP1A2, the substrate was EOMCC and the positive control inhibitor naphthoflavone; for CYP2D6, the substrate was EOMCC and the positive control inhibitor quinidine. The assays were performed using the excitation and emission wavelengths recommended by the manufacturer. To run the assay, 50 μL of Master Pre-Mix was added with 40 μL of THC, curcumin and calebin-A, at 0.01, 0.1, 1.0, 10.0, 50.0 and 100.0 μM dissolved in DMSO. The plate was incubated for 10 min at room temperature (25 ± 1 °C) on a plate shaker. Then, 10 μL of Vivid® Substrate was added to each well to start the reaction. Less than 2 min after the reaction had started, the measurement of fluorescence was performed using the Synergy HT multi-well plate reader and Gen5 data analysis software (Biotek Instruments Inc., Winooski, VT, USA). The assay was done in triplicate. The reading was performed at 1 min intervals for 60 min. Inhibition was calculated as $(1 - (X - B/A - B)) \times 100\%$, where X was the average of compound fluorescence, A was the average of solvent control and B was the average of inhibition in the presence of positive inhibitor control. The percent inhibition was calculated relative to a fixed concentration of the positive control. For more information of assay protocols, please refer to the instructions for the kits (Vivid® CYP2C9 Green Screening Kit—Cat. no. P2860; Vivid® CYP3A4 Green Screening Kit—Cat. No. P2857; Vivid® CYP1A2 Blue Screening Kit—Cat. No. P2863 and Vivid® CYP2D6 Blue Screening Kit—Cat. No. P2972 from Life Technologies).

2.8. Antioxidant Capacity Determination

Total antioxidant capacity of THC, curcumin and calebin-A was measured using the antioxidant assay kit (Cayman Chemical, Ann Arbor, MI, USA) following the standard protocol from the manufacturer. The assay measures the inhibition of oxidation of 2,2′-azino-bis(3-ethylbenzothiazoline-6-sulphonic acid) (ABTS) by metmyoglobin. THC, curcumin and calebin-A were prepared in DMSO for concentrations of 1, 5, 10, 50 and 100 μg/mL. The antioxidant capacity of each curcuminoid was expressed as Trolox equivalents. The assay was performed in triplicate and absorbance at 750 nm was measured using the Synergy HT plate reader (Biotek Instruments Inc., Winooski, VT, USA). For more information regarding the assay protocol, please refer to the instructions for the kit (Antioxidant Assay kit from Cayman Chemical—Cat. No. 709091).

2.9. Cyclooxygenase Inhibition Determination

Cyclooxygenase is a bifunctional enzyme exhibiting both COX and peroxidase activities. This assay was used to measure the inhibition of COX-1 and -2 of THC, curcumin and calebin-A. Concentrations of 1, 10 and 250 μg/mL of THC, curcumin and calebin-A were prepared using DMSO. The assay was performed in quadruplet using a COX Inhibitor Screening Assay Kit from Cayman

Chemical (Cat. No. 560131) according to the manufacturer's instructions. The measurement of absorbance was performed at 415 nm within 10 min at room temperature using the Synergy HT multi-well plate reader and Gen5 data analysis software (Biotek Instruments Inc., Winooski, VT, USA).

2.10. Lipoxygenase Inhibition

We detected the lipoxygenase activity of the curcuminoids using a Lipoxygenase Inhibitor Screening Assay Kit from Cayman Chemical (Ann Arbor, MI, USA, Cat. No. 760700a) using linoleic acid as the substrate according to the manufacturer's recommended instructions. Briefly, concentrations of 1, 10 and 250 µg/mL of THC, curcumin and calebin-A were prepared in DMSO and 10 µL of each were combined with 90 µL of 15-lipoxygenase derived from soybean. 10 µL of linoleic acid was added to start the reaction. The plate was covered and placed on a shaker for 5 min. Then, 100 µL of chromogen was added. The plate was covered and placed on a shaker for 5 min again. The assay was performed in triplicate. The absorbance was measured at 500 nm using the Synergy HT multi-well plate reader and Gen5 data analysis software (Biotek Instruments Inc., Winooski, VT, USA). For additional information of assay protocol, please refer to the instructions for the kit.

2.11. Cellular Growth Inhibition Assay (MTS)

The CellTiter 96® AQueous One Solution Cell Proliferation Assay (MTS, Promega, Madison, WI, USA) was used to measure proliferation inhibition of cultured cells. Briefly, Sup-T1 cells were cultured in RPMI 1640 supplemented with 10% FBS and 1% penicillin/streptomycin at 37 °C and 5% CO_2. 2×10^5 cells/mL were seeded in each well and THC, curcumin and calebin-A, at 0.1, 0.5, 1.0, 5.0, 10.0, 50.0 and 100.0 µM dissolved in DMSO, were added to their respective wells and incubated for 24, 48 and 72 h. The MTS reagent was added and incubated for 4 h. Absorbance was recorded at 490 nm in Synergy HT multi-well plate reader and Gen5 data analysis software (Biotek Instruments Inc., Winooski, VT, USA). Sup-T1 cells were used in this study because curcuminoids are thought in part to work via an HDAC inhibitor mechanism and as some HDACs are approved for some T-cell lymphomas, we used Sup-T1 cells because they are a T-cell lymphoma cell line that is established. To the best of our knowledge no other study has measured the effects of THC on Sup-T1 cells.

2.12. Cellular Inflammatory Cytokine Release Assay (TNF-α)

Sup-T1 cells were prepared and seeded as above and separately treated with THC, curcumin and calebin-A at 5, 10, 50 and 100 µM. Cell culture supernatant was collected and used to determine released TNF-α using the Human TNF-alpha DuoSet ELISA kit (DY210, R & D systems, Minneapolis, MN, USA) following the standard manufacturer's protocol, optimized using recombinant TNF-α. The optical density was determined in Synergy HT multi-well plate reader and Gen5 data analysis software (Biotek Instruments Inc., Winooski, VT, USA). The data were analyzed using SigmaPlot 12.2 (Systat Software Inc., San Jose, CA, USA).

2.13. HDAC1 and PCAF Inhibition Assays

Curcuminoids were tested for direct HDAC1 and PCAF inhibitory activity using the fluorescent-based HDAC1 or PCAF inhibitor screening assay kit ((HDAC1) 10011564, (PCAF) 10006515, Cayman, Ann Arbor, MI, USA) according to manufacturer's instructions. THC, curcumin and calebin-A, at 0.1, 1.0, 10.0, 50.0, 100.0 and 250.0 µg/mL dissolved in DMSO, were prepared and screened. Fluorescence was measured for both assays using excitation/emission wavelengths of 340/460 nm using Synergy HT multi-well plate reader and Gen5 data analysis software (Biotek Instruments Inc., Winooski, VT, USA).

Data for the PCAF and HDAC1 inhibition and viability assays were used to derive percent changes based on no treatment controls. Each of three data sets were then fit to a 4-parameter logistic regression using SigmaPlot 12.2 to derive IC_{50} values, which were then used to determine the mean and SD.

3. Results

3.1. Chromatography

The central 3,5-dione structure of THC and curcumin allows for keto–enol tautomerism. We optimized chromatographic conditions for both tautomers of THC to be resolved easily as the keto and enol forms that had a retention time of 1.4 min and 2.7 min, respectively. Similarly, the keto and enol tautomers of curcumin were easily resolved, having retention times of 1.2 min and 3.2 min, respectively (Figure 2). The enol and keto forms of each compound have the same molecular weight and fragmentation spectra, so the mass spectrometer on its own is incapable of differentiating the two tautomers of each analyte. We reconciled the retention times of each tautomer based on the previous studies which showed that curcumin is primarily in the enol form in solutions of ~50% acetonitrile, which is very similar to the conditions we used [17]. Corroborating this, other similar studies have shown that in aqueous solutions with increasing amounts of alcohol the enol tautomer predominates [18]. We defined the larger peak with the longer retention time to be the enol tautomer for curcumin, as has been observed by others under similar conditions [17], and used the same relative retention to identify the tautomers of THC (Figure 2). For THC, we found that the two tautomers were in roughly equal proportion under these chromatographic conditions, while curcumin appeared to favour the enol tautomer by a 5:1 ratio. The sum of the peak areas for both tautomers was used to calculate the concentrations in the samples. Blank plasma samples showed that there were no interfering peaks that co-eluted with THC and curcumin (data not shown).

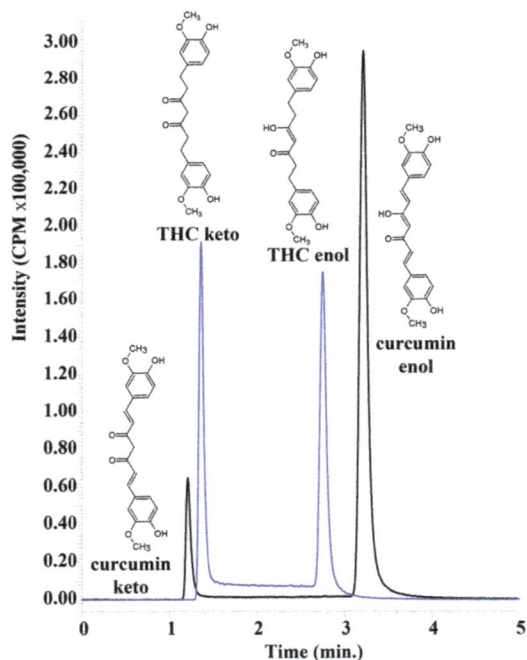

Figure 2. A representative chromatogram of curcumin and tetrahydrocurcumin (THC) Shown are the enol and keto forms of curcumin and THC using the LC–MS/MS assay. Both compounds are at a concentration of 1 µg/mL dissolved in acetonitrile.

3.2. Pharmacokinetics

The serum THC concentration versus time curve shows that more than one absorption and distribution phase was present. Initially, a rapid absorption phase with an average T_{max} of 6.8 µg/mL at 1 h was observed, followed by a short elimination phase. This was followed by two redistributions with two smaller THC maxima at 6 and 24 h (Figure 3A). Both redistribution phases had similar maxima of about 1 µg/mL (Figure 3A). The total amount of THC excreted unchanged in urine was up to 8 µg at 24 h (Figure 3B). Coinciding with the first short elimination phase, the rate of urinary excretion reached a maximum of just under 3 µg/h at 2 h. In addition, an increase in excretion rate can be observed at 12 after the second distribution. Finally, a second excretion rate maximum coincided with the final distribution phase at 24 h.

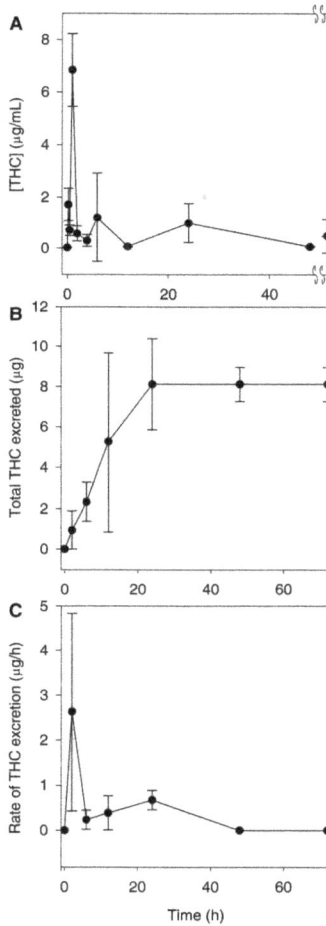

Figure 3. The pharmacokinetics of THC after a 500 mg/kg oral dose. Depicted is the serum disposition of THC in µg/mL (**A**) (the double S-marks represent a break in the Time axis from 49 to 71 h and the final time point is 72 h); the total amount of THC excreted in the urine in µg after oral administration (**B**); and the rate of urinary excretion of THC in µg/mL (**C**). All values represent a mean of 3 with standard deviation.

3.3. Cytochrome P450 Inhibition

The three curcuminoids were tested for their ability to inhibit CYP 2C9, 3A4, 1A2 and 2D6. THC, curcumin and calebin-A yielded dose-dependent inhibition of CYP2C9, and to a lesser extent, CYP3A4. All three exhibited maximum inhibition of CYP2C9 (Figure 4A) and CYP3A4 (Figure 4B) at 50 to 100 μM, compared to the positive controls sulphaphenazole and ketoconazole. Curcumin, calebin-A and THC did not show a consistent dose-response inhibition of CYP1A2 (Figure 4C) or CYP2D6 (Figure 4D) over the range of concentrations tested. In some cases, the percent inhibition exceeded 100%; this may be because percent inhibition is calculated relative to a fixed concentration of a positive control inhibitor. In those cases where percent inhibition exceeds 100%, it may be because the curcuminoid being studied is a more effective inhibitor of the CYP in question than the positive control. For Figure 4D, in some cases, curcumin appears to produce negative inhibition or increased activity, but the error associated with these values makes it difficult to determine if this is the case.

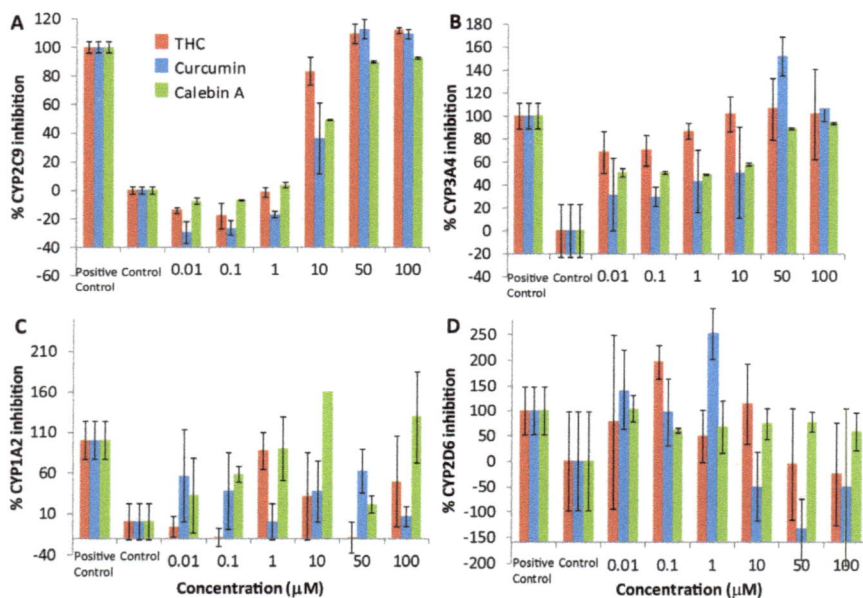

Figure 4. The inhibition of selected common drug-metabolizing enzymes by curcuminoids. Displayed are graphs showing the inhibition of CYP 2C9 (**A**); CYP3A4 (**B**); CYP1A2 (**C**); and CYP 2D6 (**D**) by THC, curcumin and calebin-A with solvent and positive controls using commercial assay kits.

3.4. Anti-Inflammatory Activity

The potential anti-inflammatory activity of HAT inhibitors, like curcumin and other curcuminoids, is thought to involve inhibition of expression of pro-inflammatory genes such as the *NF-κB* family and *COX-2*, however, it is still unclear if there is any direct inhibitory activity for curcuminoids against these pro-inflammatory proteins. Therefore, the inhibition of cyclooxygenase and lipoxygenase by THC, curcumin and calebin-A was measured using assay kits described in the methods. For the cyclooxygenase inhibition assay, we measured COX-2 and COX-1 IC_{50} and reported their COX-2/COX-1 ratios. Calebin-A and THC have similar ratios around 1, demonstrating approximately equal propensity to directly inhibit COX-2 and COX-1. Curcumin appears to show higher COX-2 inhibition with a COX-2/COX-1 ratio of 0.19 (Figure 5A). None of the curcuminoids were particularly effective inhibitors of either COX-1 or -2, with curcumin being the most effective against COX-2 with an IC$_{50}$ of ~600 µM (Table 1). We evaluated the potential lipoxygenase inhibitory activity because we found marginal COX inhibition. Calebin-A did not show any activity, but both curcumin and THC inhibited lipoxygenase as low as 1 µM (Figure 5B).

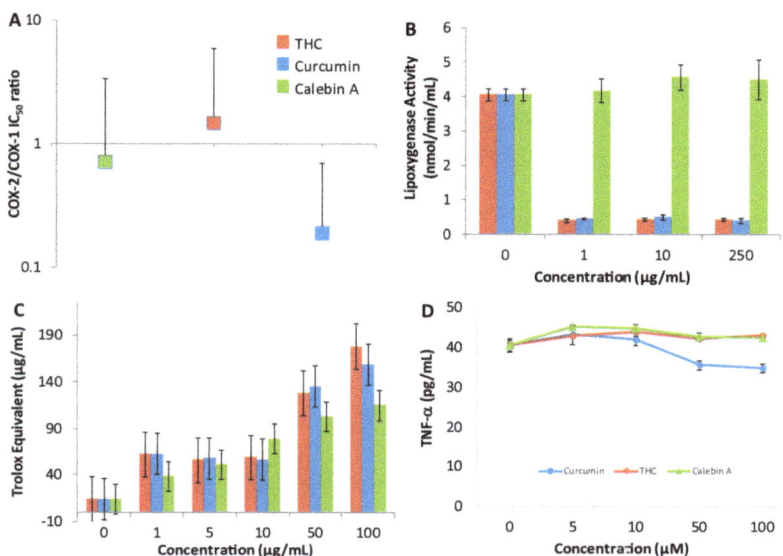

Figure 5. The anti-inflammatory and antioxidant activity of THC and other curcuminoids. The direct effects of curcuminoids on inhibition of cyclooxygenase displayed as the COX-2 to COX-1 IC$_{50}$ ratio (**A**); the inhibition of lipoxygenase by THC and other curcuminoids displayed as lipoxygenase activity in mmol/min/mL at the listed concentrations of curcuminoids (**B**); the antioxidant activity of THC and other curcuminoids as measured by the antioxidant assay kit (Cayman) (**C**); displayed are the TNF-α concentrations produced by the curcuminoids as a measure of inflammatory activity in pg/mL (**D**). Using a one-way ANOVA, the results for 50 and 100 µM levels are statistically significant $p < 0.001$. All values represent a mean of 3 with standard deviation.

Table 1. The potency of curcuminoids against cyclooxygenases.

Curcuminoid	COX-1 IC$_{50}$ (µM)	COX-2 IC$_{50}$ (µM)
THC	918 ± 1300	1348 ± 3641
Curcumin	3392 ± 8982	635 ± 367
Calebin-A	1069 ± 490	784 ± 2200

The total antioxidant activity of THC, curcumin and calebin-A was calculated with respect to Trolox as a measure of antioxidant capacity. Both THC and curcumin (and to a lesser extent calebin-A) showed their greatest antioxidant effect at 100 µM (Figure 5C).

In order to fully evaluate the anti-inflammatory activity of the curcuminoids, the concentrations of the pro-inflammatory mediators TNF-α, IFN-γ, MIG and IP-10 were measured using an ELISA assay in Sup-T1 cells treated with increasing concentrations of THC, curcumin and calebin-A. The measurements for IFN-γ, MIG and IP-10 were below detection levels for all curcuminoids. There also appeared to be no dose-response change in the concentration of TNF-α in Sup-T1 cells treated with THC and calebin-A. However, a slight decrease in TNF-α compared to no-treatment control appears to be present at the 50 and 100 µM levels for curcumin (Figure 5D).

3.5. Cell Viability

One potential therapeutic use of curcumin and THC is for the treatment of cancer [3]. It has been shown that curcumin and potentially other curcuminoids are inhibitors of HDAC and HAT. Such compounds that inhibit histone lysine acetylation and deacetylation are already being explored for their cancer treatment potential [9]. The effect of THC, curcumin and calebin-A on cancer cell viability was measured. Sup-T1 cells, T-cell lymphoblastic lymphoma cells, were treated with the curcuminoids to determine their ability to induce growth inhibition using an MTS assay, and the corresponding IC_{50} values were in the mid-to-high micromolar range (Table 2). Curcumin and calebin-A were the most potent, but THC was more than 4-fold less potent than curcumin, and at the most, resulted in a 40% growth inhibition (Figure 6A).

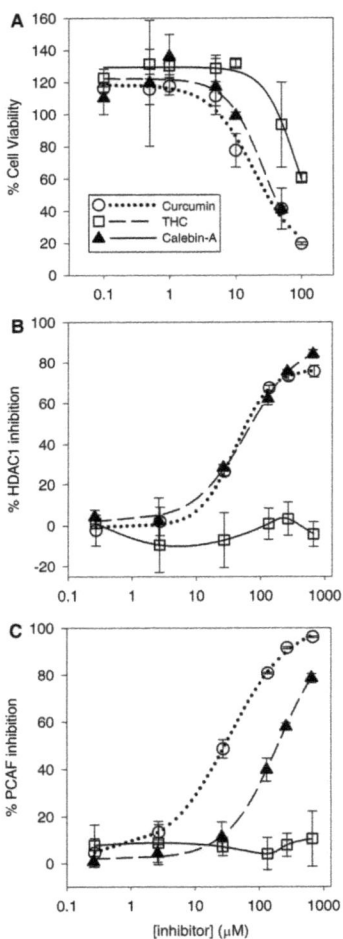

Figure 6. Cell viability and HDAC and HAT inhibition. The viability of Sup-T1 cells with increasing concentrations of the curcuminoids (**A**); the direct inhibition of the HAT PCAF by the curcuminoids as measured by an ELISA assay (**B**); the direct inhibition of the HDAC HDAC1 by the curcuminoids as measured by an ELISA assay (**C**). For each graph the points are the means of three values with an SD.

Table 2. The potency of curcuminoids on Sup-T1 growth inhibition and HDAC1/PCAF inhibition.

Curcuminoid	Viability IC$_{50}$ (µM)	HDAC1 IC$_{50}$ (µM)	PCAF IC$_{50}$ (µM)
THC	82 ± 116	NA	NA
Curcumin	19.0 ± 11	39.8 ± 3.2	33.1 ± 2.8
Calebin-A	26.2 ± 17	61.3 ± 11	200.0 ± 31

3.6. HDAC1 and HAT Inhibition

Having established the antioxidant, anti-inflammatory and cancer cell growth inhibitory properties of these curcuminoids, their activity against histone acetyltransferases (HAT) and histone deacetylases (HDAC) was evaluated, since it has been previously reported that this may be one of the many possible mechanisms for their anticancer and anti-inflammatory activities. HAT inhibitors are currently being explored as a new class of cancer treatments and have been shown to reduce expression of pro-inflammatory mediators. HDAC inhibitors are already in use alone or in combination to treat various cancers such as cutaneous T-cell lymphoma. We therefore tested the ability of the curcuminoids to inhibit HDAC1 and the HAT PCAF, using a fluorescence-based assay described in the methods. Here, we show curcumin is a potent inhibitor of the HAT PCAF (Figure 6B), an effect that has not been reported previously [4]. Calebin-A is also a PCAF inhibitor but is 6-fold less potent than curcumin (Table 2). Interestingly, THC shows no above-control inhibition of PCAF at any concentration (Figure 6C). Also as expected, curcumin and calebin-A both exhibit HDAC inhibition [5], but with similar potency, and THC shows no inhibitory activity against PCAF or HDAC1 at any concentration (Figure 6 and Table 2).

4. Discussion

A sensitive, accurate and reproducible assay was developed for the detection of tetrahydrocurcumin using UHPLC–MS/MS. It was possible to obtain baseline separation between keto and enol forms of THC and curcumin, despite the obvious similarities between the tautomers (Figure 2). Both tautomeric forms of THC and curcumin are present because of the 45% acetonitrile in the mobile phase, and they interconvert on a timescale that results in two peaks on the UHPLC chromatogram that are easily separable [17,18]. Having an alkaline mobile phase would result in only the enol form that would form an enolate, and the two peaks would converge. However, this would necessitate detection in negative MRM mode, which results in a decrease in sensitivity. The acidic mobile phase was important in obtaining the highly sensitive detection of THC and curcumin, but resulted in two separate peaks that needed to be summed in order to calculate total THC and total curcumin. We used UHPLC–MS/MS to unambiguously differentiate curcumin and THC from other serum peaks, and as expected, the plasma samples did not appear to have any other peaks that were erroneously detected as either analyte.

The choice of curcumin as an internal standard is rational in the sense that its chemical properties and structure are similar to THC. However, as mentioned above, curcumin can be metabolized to THC in the liver, and it is still possible that after plasma samples were spiked with curcumin as the internal standard, a small amount of curcumin could have been metabolized in the plasma. To mitigate this, plasma proteins in the samples were rapidly precipitated with ice-cold acetonitrile, and this would also remove any possible plasma reductases.

4.1. Disposition, Metabolism and Elimination of THC

Preliminary pharmacokinetic studies indicate that un-optimized formulations of THC have poor oral bioavailability, and it appears to only be detectable in serum and urine as glucuronides [19]. In order to detect curcumin and THC by the UHPLC–MS/MS assay, samples were treated with β-glucuronidase in order to proceed with the analysis in serum and urine. Its presence in urine indicates that THC was orally absorbed and was eliminated at least in part through the renal route.

However, it has already been long established that curcumin is excreted primarily in the bile as a glucuronide conjugate of THC [20]. More recent evidence suggests that curcumin is excreted into the bile via the active transport ABCC2 drug efflux pump [21]. Therefore, the most likely route of elimination of THC is in the bile as a glucuronide conjugate. This, together with the poor bioavailability of THC, explains why we found low concentrations of THC in the urine (Figure 3B).

4.2. THC, Curcumin and Calebin-A Inhibit CYP2C9 and CYP3A4

Curcuminoids have demonstrated inhibition of many human drug-metabolizing enzymes, especially the Phase I CYP family of oxidases in vitro [22]. We showed that THC, calebin-A and curcumin produced a consistent inhibitory dose-response relationship with CYP2C9 and 3A4, but no such dose-response relationship could be detected with CYP 1A2 and 2D6. These results suggest that THC, curcumin and calebin-A are inhibitors of CYP 2C9 and 3A4. It is not immediately obvious how these curcuminoids inhibit CYP enzymes. Curcuminoids are unlikely to be important as substrates for CYPs, as previous studies have shown that curcumin is reduced to THC by reductases and primarily converted into a THC glucuronide [19,20]. Despite this, a small proportion of each of the curcuminoids may undergo *O*-dealkylation by demethylation of the aromatic methoxy groups, and the occupancy of the enzyme may result in inhibition that is competitive. As has been observed, some curcuminoids have the potential to alkylate enzymes through the α,β-unsaturated carbonyl (Michael acceptor) [9]. This has been the mechanism proposed for curcumin and its activity against p300, however, this cannot be the mechanism of action of CYP inhibition because THC does not have such a Michael acceptor group and yet exhibits CYP inhibition. An alternative mechanism of inhibition may be nucleophilic addition at the enolic carbon (Michael donor) shared between THC and curcumin.

4.3. Curcuminoids Inhibit Some Pro-Inflammatory Mediators

None of the curcuminoids were particularly effective inhibitors of either COX-1 or -2, with curcumin being the most effective, yielding a modest IC_{50} of ~600 μM (Table 1). Nevertheless, curcumin showed a slight inhibitory preference for COX-2, suggesting it may have an effect on the activity of COX during acute inflammation. The COX ratios of calebin-A and THC were sufficiently close to 1 and the errors large enough to make it difficult to suggest that either curcuminoid exhibited a preference for either COX enzyme. Furthermore, treatment with THC and calebin-A did not reduce TNF-α release in Sup-T1 cells, and curcumin only had a moderate effect at higher doses. None of the curcuminoids tested altered the concentrations of the cytokines, IFN-γ, MIG and IP-10 in SupT1 cells. Another important group of pro-inflammatory mediators are the leukotrienes, produced by lipoxygenase. Both THC and curcumin inhibited soybean 1,5-lipoxygenase at all doses tested in comparison to a control, while calebin-A showed no such inhibitory activity. As with CYP inhibition, the inhibition of lipoxygenase activity is unclear and cannot be caused by direct Michael addition reaction because THC does not possess a Michael acceptor group, however, both THC and curcumin are very similar in structure, suggesting that this structure may be important for binding to lipoxygenase. Previous studies have used molecular docking approaches to propose potential binding sites for THC on lipoxygenase. These studies suggest that THC scavenges peroxides acting as a redox inhibitor of lipoxygenase, showing mixed inhibition [23]. Other studies confirm that curcumin and THC potently inhibit human lipoxygenase, showing that the inhibition may be clinically significant [24]. The inhibition of lipoxygenase presents the possibility that THC and curcumin may be used as a treatment for inflammatory conditions such as asthma. Lipoxygenase inhibitors such as zileuton are currently in use for treatment of asthma in children where glucocorticoids are less desirable or contraindicated.

Our data showed that THC does not inhibit HDAC or HAT; therefore, its narrower spectrum may make it a superior choice as a lipoxygenase inhibitor anti-inflammatory, because in this case, HDAC and HAT inhibitory activities would represent off-target effects. This is especially significant because we found that THC has a peak concentration of greater than 6 μg/mL (Figure 3A), with concentrations of greater than 1 µg/mL being found up to 20 h later. As we found that THC has potent lipoxygenase inhibition at 1 µg/mL (Figure 5B), this suggests that despite its poor bioavailability, THC reaches concentrations in vivo that can inhibit lipoxygenase. As far as we know, no other group has measured these activities and parameters together and made the suggestion that THC may be used as a lipoxygenase inhibitor to treat asthma and that it may be superior to curcumin. However, we acknowledge that the formulation of THC would need to be dramatically improved or an alternate route of administration chosen. In this particular case, the poor bioavailability of THC may warrant formulation into an intrapulmonary delivery system such as a metered-dose inhaler.

4.4. Curcuminoids Are Potent Antioxidants

All curcuminoids tested exhibited antioxidant capacity equivalent to the vitamin E analog antioxidant Trolox in a dose-dependent manner as measured by their free-radical-scavenging activity (ABTS) in the antioxidant assay [16]. All curcuminoids appear to be more potent than Trolox at the 50 and 100 µg/mL levels. However, the data does not suggest there is any difference in antioxidant potency among the curcuminoids. These results suggest that the curcuminoids tested have potential as potent antioxidants if their poor bioavailability can be overcome.

4.5. Curcumin and Calebin-A Potently Inhibit Sup-T1 Growth

Consistent with the previously discovered anticancer activity, curcumin induced reductions in the T-cell lymphoblastic lymphoma Sup-T1 cell line. Calebin-A also reduced viability with a similar potency to curcumin (Table 2). However, THC was at least 4-fold less cytotoxic to SupT1 cells compared to curcumin and calebin-A. This difference is likely larger as we were unable to reduce the viability of the Sup-T1 cells below the 50% level over the concentration range used. Therefore, our estimation of the IC_{50} for THC is likely higher than it would be if we were able to reduce the viability below 50%. The Sup-T1 cell line only represents one particular cell line of one type of cancer, and the different curcuminoids may have varying efficacy against different cell and cancer types. For example, THC has been shown to potently inhibit the growth of colorectal cancer cells such as SW480 and HT-29 cells, either alone or in combination [25,26]. In fact, THC has been shown to be more effective than curcumin in colon and other cancers [27,28]. Moreover, the measure of potency for reducing cell viability may not be an accurate reflection of the clinical usefulness of any drug for cancer treatment, as animal cancer models (though outside of the scope for this work) are usually more informative.

4.6. Curcumin and Calebin-A Inhibit PCAF and HDAC1

Consistent with previous findings, curcumin inhibits HDAC and HAT activity. Although previous studies have shown that curcumin binds to and inhibits the HAT activity of p300/CBP [4], as far as we know, this is the first study to show that curcumin and calebin-A inhibit PCAF. These results are not unexpected, as PCAF binds to p300/CBP and all three proteins have HAT activity, albeit with slightly different substrate specificities [29]. The suggested mechanism for inhibition of HAT activity by curcumin is alkylation of the HAT via the Michael acceptor on curcumin. This is thought to happen through HAT active-site cysteine residues [9]. Given this, it is not surprising that calebin-A also inhibits HAT, because it has a similar Michael acceptor group (Figure 1). Previous groups have identified calebin-A as having anticancer activity against a multidrug-resistant human gastric cancer line through its activity in modulating the expression of the MAP kinase family, but the mechanism of this activity was not determined directly [1]. This was recently corroborated by the finding that calebin-A inhibits phosphorylation by suppressing NF-κB signaling activation associated with osteoporosis [30]. This result is important because NF-κB is modulated through the acetylation activity of p300/CBP [31]. Here, for the first time, we can justify the activities against MAPK/NF-κB and the resulting anticancer effects of calebin-A through its direct effect inhibiting PCAF. Furthermore, calebin-A shows similar potency inhibiting HDAC1 compared to curcumin (Figure 6B), which may contribute to their anticancer activities and may be attributed to the presence of the Michael acceptor moiety on each compound. Therefore, the lack of both HDAC1 and PCAF inhibition by THC may be attributed to its lack of double bonds, which form the Michael acceptor groups present in curcumin and calebin-A (Figure 1). The observed absence of HDAC/PCAF inhibition by THC is not entirely surprising as it has long been suspected to have a different anticancer mechanism than curcumin [3]. Several studies have shown that THC is a potent antioxidant, and this study is in agreement with these findings [32–34]. Moreover, the finding that THC reduces lipoxygenase activity adds a potential anti-inflammatory mechanism that, in conjunction with its antioxidant activity, may explain the anticancer activity of THC.

Our results show that curcumin is 6-fold more potent with respect to PCAF inhibition than calebin-A, but both curcuminoids have similar IC_{50} values for inhibition of HDAC1. It is not clear why this might be the case, as both compounds are very similar. It is unlikely that enzymatic or non-enzymatic hydrolysis of the ester of calebin-A might affect its potency, as both compounds have similar potency against HDAC1 under similar conditions to the HAT assay. However, this ester is almost certainly a route of metabolism for calebin-A—that is not present in curcumin or THC—that may affect its in-vivo activity.

Acknowledgments: The authors acknowledge support from the Paul H.T. Thorlakson Foundation Fund, The Manitoba Medical Services Foundation [8-2014-03 2014], University of Manitoba Research Grants Program [UM Project # 43887, 2015], the Natural Sciences and Engineering Research Council (NSERC) Canada [RGPIN-2015-06543, 2015-2020] (to Ted M. Lakowski), the Leslie F. Buggey Graduate Scholarship, 2014 and the Research Manitoba Fellowship (to Ryan Lillico), a Canada, Brazil Science without Borders Summer Studentship (to Julia T. Novaes), and a graduate scholarship from Kuwait University, Kuwait (to Samaa Al-Rushaid). This work was also partially funded by the Sabinsa Corporation (to Neal M. Davies).

Author Contributions: Stephanie E. Martinez, Casey L. Sayre, Neal M. Davies, Kalyanam Nagabhushanam, Muhammed Majeed, Yufei Chen and Ryan Lillico conceived and designed the experiments; Julia T. Novaes, Anna P. Oliveira, Stephanie E. Martinez, Ryan Lillico, Samaa Alrushaid, performed the experiments; Julia T. Novaes, Stephanie E. Martinez, Neal M. Davies, Kalyanam Nagabhushanam, Muhammed Majeed, Ted M. Lakowski and Ryan Lillico analyzed the data; Ted M. Lakowski, Emmanuel Ho, Kalyanam Nagabhushanam, Muhammed Majeed and Neal M Davies contributed reagents/materials/analysis tools; Julia T. Novase, Ted M. Lakowski, Neal M. Davies, and Ryan Lillico wrote the paper..

Conflicts of Interest: This work was partially funded by the Sabinsa Corporation to Neal M. Davies and the authors Kalyanam Nagabushnam and Muhammed Majeed are employed with this company that supplied the tetrahydrocurcumin, curcumin and calebin-A materials for this study. All other authors declare no conflicts of interest. The authors alone are responsible for the content, writing, and interpretations in this paper.

References

1. Li, Y.; Li, S.; Han, Y.; Liu, J.; Zhang, J.; Li, F.; Wang, Y.; Liu, X.; Yao, L. Calebin-A induces apoptosis and modulates MAPK family activity in drug resistant human gastric cancer cells. *Eur. J. Pharmacol.* **2008**, *591*, 252–258. [CrossRef] [PubMed]

2. Oliveira, A.L.; Martinez, S.E.; Nagabushnam, K.; Majeed, M.; Alrushaid, S.; Sayre, C.L.; Davies, N.M. Calebin A: Analytical Development for Pharmacokinetics Study, Elucidation of Pharmacological Activities and Content Analysis of Natural Health Products. *J. Pharm. Pharm. Sci.* **2015**, *18*, 494–514. [CrossRef] [PubMed]

3. Aggarwal, B.B.; Deb, L.; Prasad, S. Curcumin differs from tetrahydrocurcumin for molecular targets, signaling pathways and cellular responses. *Molecules* **2015**, *20*, 185–205. [CrossRef] [PubMed]

4. Balasubramanyam, K.; Varier, R.A.; Altaf, M.; Swaminathan, V.; Siddappa, N.B.; Ranga, U.; Kundu, T.K. Curcumin, a novel p300/CREB-binding protein-specific inhibitor of acetyltransferase, represses the acetylation of histone/nonhistone proteins and histone acetyltransferase-dependent chromatin transcription. *J. Biol. Chem.* **2004**, *279*, 51163–51171. [CrossRef] [PubMed]

5. Reuter, S.; Gupta, S.C.; Park, B.; Goel, A.; Aggarwal, B.B. Epigenetic changes induced by curcumin and other natural compounds. *Genes Nutr.* **2011**, *6*, 93–108. [CrossRef] [PubMed]

6. Wang, S.H.; Lin, P.Y.; Chiu, Y.C.; Huang, J.S.; Kuo, Y.T.; Wu, J.C.; Chen, C.C. Curcumin-Mediated HDAC Inhibition Suppresses the DNA Damage Response and Contributes to Increased DNA Damage Sensitivity. *PLoS ONE* **2015**, *10*, e0134110. [CrossRef] [PubMed]

7. Lee, S.J.; Krauthauser, C.; Maduskuie, V.; Fawcett, P.T.; Olson, J.M.; Rajasekaran, S.A. Curcumin-induced HDAC inhibition and attenuation of medulloblastoma growth in vitro and in vivo. *BMC Cancer* **2011**, *11*, 144. [CrossRef] [PubMed]

8. Farria, A.; Li, W.; Dent, S.Y. KATs in cancer: Functions and therapies. *Oncogene* **2015**, *34*, 4901–4913. [CrossRef] [PubMed]

9. Lillico, R.; Stesco, N.; Amhad, T.K.; Cortes, C.; Namaka, M.P.; Lakowski, T.M. Inhibitors of enzymes catalyzing modifications to histone lysine residues: Structure, function and activity. *Future Med. Chem.* **2016**, *8*, 879–897. [CrossRef] [PubMed]

10. Dekker, F.J.; van den Bosch, T.; Martin, N.I. Small molecule inhibitors of histone acetyltransferases and deacetylases are potential drugs for inflammatory diseases. *Drug Discov. Today* **2014**, *19*, 654–660. [CrossRef] [PubMed]

11. Van den Bosch, T.; Boichenko, A.; Leus, N.G.; Ourailidou, M.E.; Wapenaar, H.; Rotili, D.; Mai, A.; Imhof, A.; Bischoff, R.; Haisma, H.J.; et al. The histone acetyltransferase p300 inhibitor C646 reduces pro-inflammatory gene expression and inhibits histone deacetylases. *Biochem. Pharmacol.* **2016**, *102*, 130–140. [CrossRef] [PubMed]

12. Zhu, X.Y.; Huang, C.S.; Li, Q.; Chang, R.M.; Song, Z.B.; Zou, W.Y.; Guo, Q.L. p300 exerts an epigenetic role in chronic neuropathic pain through its acetyltransferase activity in rats following chronic constriction injury (CCI). *Mol. Pain* **2012**, *8*, 84. [CrossRef] [PubMed]

13. Gerich, J. Pathogenesis and management of postprandial hyperglycemia: Role of incretin-based therapies. *Int. J. Gen. Med.* **2013**, *6*, 877–895. [CrossRef] [PubMed]

14. Pari, L.; Amali, D.R. Protective role of tetrahydrocurcumin (THC) an active principle of turmeric on chloroquine induced hepatotoxicity in rats. *J. Pharm. Pharm. Sci.* **2005**, *8*, 115–123. [PubMed]

15. Limtrakul, P.; Chearwae, W.; Shukla, S.; Phisalphong, C.; Ambudkar, S.V. Modulation of function of three ABC drug transporters, P-glycoprotein (ABCB1), mitoxantrone resistance protein (ABCG2) and multidrug resistance protein 1 (ABCC1) by tetrahydrocurcumin, a major metabolite of curcumin. *Mol. Cell. Biochem.* **2007**, *296*, 85–95. [CrossRef] [PubMed]

16. Esatbeyoglu, T.; Huebbe, P.; Ernst, I.M.; Chin, D.; Wagner, A.E.; Rimbach, G. Curcumin—From molecule to biological function. *Angew. Chem. Int. Ed. Engl.* **2012**, *51*, 5308–5332. [CrossRef] [PubMed]

17. Kawano, S.; Inohana, Y.; Hashi, Y.; Lin, J. Analysis of keto-enol tautomers of curcumin by liquid chromatography/mass spectrometry. *Chin. Chem. Lett.* **2013**, *24*, 685–687. [CrossRef]

18. Manolova, Y.; Deneva, V.; Antonov, L.; Drakalska, E.; Momekova, D.; Lambov, N. The effect of the water on the curcumin tautomerism: A quantitative approach. *Spectrochim. Acta Part A Mol. Biomol. Spectrosc.* **2014**, *132*, 815–820. [CrossRef] [PubMed]

19. Zhongfa, L.; Chiu, M.; Wang, J.; Chen, W.; Yen, W.; Fan-Havard, P.; Yee, L.D.; Chan, K.K. Enhancement of curcumin oral absorption and pharmacokinetics of curcuminoids and curcumin metabolites in mice. *Cancer Chemother. Pharmacol.* **2012**, *69*, 679–689. [CrossRef] [PubMed]

20. Holder, G.M.; Plummer, J.L.; Ryan, A.J. The metabolism and excretion of curcumin (1,7-bis-(4-hydroxy-3-methoxyphenyl)-1,6-heptadiene-3,5-dione) in the rat. *Xenobiotica* **1978**, *8*, 761–768. [CrossRef] [PubMed]

21. Lee, J.H.; Oh, J.H.; Lee, Y.J. Biliary excretion of curcumin is mediated by multidrug resistance-associated protein 2. *Biol. Pharm. Bull.* **2012**, *35*, 777–780. [CrossRef] [PubMed]

22. Volak, L.P.; Ghirmai, S.; Cashman, J.R.; Court, M.H. Curcuminoids inhibit multiple human cytochromes P450, UDP-glucuronosyltransferase, and sulfotransferase enzymes, whereas piperine is a relatively selective CYP3A4 inhibitor. *Drug Metab. Dispos.* **2008**, *36*, 1594–1605. [CrossRef] [PubMed]

23. Sneharani, A.H.; Singh, S.A.; Srinivas, P.; Rao, A.G.A. Inhibition of lipoxygenase-1 by tetrahydrocurcumin. *Eur. Food Res. Technol.* **2011**, *233*, 561. [CrossRef]

24. Hong, J.; Bose, M.; Ju, J.; Ryu, J.H.; Chen, X.; Sang, S.; Lee, M.J.; Yang, C.S. Modulation of arachidonic acid metabolism by curcumin and related beta-diketone derivatives: Effects on cytosolic phospholipase A(2), cyclooxygenases and 5-lipoxygenase. *Carcinogenesis* **2004**, *25*, 1671–1679. [CrossRef] [PubMed]

25. Chen, C.Y.; Yang, W.L.; Kuo, S.Y. Cytotoxic activity and cell cycle analysis of hexahydrocurcumin on SW 480 human colorectal cancer cells. *Nat. Prod. Commun.* **2011**, *6*, 1671–1672. [CrossRef] [PubMed]

26. Srimuangwong, K.; Tocharus, C.; Chintana, P.Y.; Suksamrarn, A.; Tocharus, J. Hexahydrocurcumin enhances inhibitory effect of 5-fluorouracil on HT-29 human colon cancer cells. *World J. Gastroenterol.* **2012**, *18*, 2383–2389. [CrossRef] [PubMed]

27. Lai, C.S.; Wu, J.C.; Yu, S.F.; Badmaev, V.; Nagabhushanam, K.; Ho, C.T.; Pan, M.H. Tetrahydrocurcumin is more effective than curcumin in preventing azoxymethane-induced colon carcinogenesis. *Mol. Nutr. Food Res.* **2011**, *55*, 1819–1828. [CrossRef] [PubMed]

28. Wu, J.C.; Tsai, M.L.; Lai, C.S.; Wang, Y.J.; Ho, C.T.; Pan, M.H. Chemopreventative effects of tetrahydrocurcumin on human diseases. *Food Funct.* **2014**, *5*, 12–17. [CrossRef] [PubMed]

29. Henry, R.A.; Kuo, Y.M.; Andrews, A.J. Differences in specificity and selectivity between CBP and p300 acetylation of histone H3 and H3/H4. *Biochemistry* **2013**, *52*, 5746–5759. [CrossRef] [PubMed]

30. Tyagi, A.K.; Prasad, S.; Majeed, M.; Aggarwal, B.B. Calebin A downregulates osteoclastogenesis through suppression of RANKL signalling. *Arch. Biochem. Biophys.* **2016**, *593*, 80–89. [CrossRef] [PubMed]

31. Greene, W.C.; Chen, L.F. Regulation of NF-kappaB action by reversible acetylation. *Novartis Found. Symp.* **2004**, *259*, 208–217. [PubMed]

32. Naito, M.; Wu, X.; Nomura, H.; Kodama, M.; Kato, Y.; Osawa, T. The protective effects of tetrahydrocurcumin on oxidative stress in cholesterol-fed rabbits. *J. Atheroscler. Thromb.* **2002**, *9*, 243–250. [CrossRef] [PubMed]

33. Somparn, P.; Phisalaphong, C.; Nakornchai, S.; Unchern, S.; Morales, N.P. Comparative antioxidant activities of curcumin and its demethoxy and hydrogenated derivatives. *Biol. Pharm. Bull.* **2007**, *30*, 74–78. [CrossRef] [PubMed]

34. Sugiyama, Y.; Kawakishi, S.; Osawa, T. Involvement of the beta-diketone moiety in the antioxidative mechanism of tetrahydrocurcumin. *Biochem. Pharmacol.* **1996**, *52*, 519–525. [CrossRef]

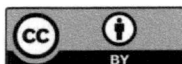

pharmaceutics

MDPI

Article

Altered Protein Expression of Cardiac CYP2J and Hepatic CYP2C, CYP4A, and CYP4F in a Mouse Model of Type II Diabetes—A Link in the Onset and Development of Cardiovascular Disease?

Benoit Drolet [1,2,*], Sylvie Pilote [2], Carolanne Gélinas [1], Alida-Douce Kamaliza [1], Audrey Blais-Boilard [1], Jessica Virgili [1,2], Dany Patoine [2] and Chantale Simard [1,2]

[1]   Faculté de Pharmacie, Université Laval, 1050 Avenue de la Médecine, Québec, QC G1V 0A6, Canada; carolanne.gelinas.1@ulaval.ca (C.G.); lovedk90@hotmail.com (A.-D.K.); audrey.blais-boilard.1@ulaval.ca (A.B.-B.); jessica.virgili.1@ulaval.ca (J.V.); chantale.simard@pha.ulaval.ca (C.S.)

[2]   Centre de Recherche, Institut Universitaire de Cardiologie et de Pneumologie de Québec, 2725 Chemin Sainte-Foy, Québec, QC G1V 4G5, Canada; sylvie.pilote@criucpq.ulaval.ca (S.P.); dany.patoine@criucpq.ulaval.ca (D.P.)

*   Correspondence: benoit.drolet@pha.ulaval.ca; Tel.: +1-418-656-8711 (ext. 5755); Fax: +1-418-656-4509

Received: 25 August 2017; Accepted: 6 October 2017; Published: 12 October 2017

Abstract: Arachidonic acid can be metabolized by cytochrome P450 (CYP450) enzymes in a tissue- and cell-specific manner to generate vasoactive products such as epoxyeicosatrienoic acids (EETs-cardioprotective) and hydroxyeicosatetraenoic acids (HETEs-cardiotoxic). Type II diabetes is a well-recognized risk factor for developing cardiovascular disease. A mouse model of Type II diabetes (C57BLKS/J-*db/db*) was used. After sacrifice, livers and hearts were collected, washed, and snap frozen. Total proteins were extracted. Western blots were performed to assess cardiac CYP2J and hepatic CYP2C, CYP4A, and CYP4F protein expression, respectively. Significant decreases in relative protein expression of cardiac CYP2J and hepatic CYP2C were observed in Type II diabetes animals compared to controls (CYP2J: 0.80 ± 0.03 vs. 1.05 ± 0.06, $n = 20$, $p < 0.001$); (CYP2C: 1.56 ± 0.17 vs. 2.21 ± 0.19, $n = 19$, $p < 0.01$). In contrast, significant increases in relative protein expression of both hepatic CYP4A and CYP4F were noted in Type II diabetes mice compared to controls (CYP4A: 1.06 ± 0.09 vs. 0.18 ± 0.01, $n = 19$, $p < 0.001$); (CYP4F: 2.53 ± 0.22 vs. 1.10 ± 0.07, $n = 19$, $p < 0.001$). These alterations induced by Type II diabetes in the endogenous pathway (CYP450) of arachidonic acid metabolism may increase the risk for cardiovascular disease by disrupting the fine equilibrium between cardioprotective (CYP2J/CYP2C-generated) and cardiotoxic (CYP4A/CYP4F-generated) metabolites of arachidonic acid.

Keywords: arachidonic acid; CYP450 enzymes; Type II diabetes; cardiovascular disease

1. Introduction

Arachidonic acid (AA) is an essential polyunsaturated fatty acid notably found in cell membrane phospholipids. It has an important role in a number of cell signaling and regulation pathways upon its cleavage from membranes via a sequence of tightly regulated events [1]. The cleavage sequence is initiated by the activation of a calcium-dependent type IV phospholipase A2 in response to a stimulus, such as ischemia [2]. The released non-esterified AA acts as a substrate for oxidation by cyclooxygenases (COX), lipoxygenases (LOX), and cytochrome P450 (CYP450) enzymes in the heart and elsewhere, thereby generating a cascade of lipid second messengers, orchestrating a broad range of critical physiological processes, including hemodynamic functions [1–3]. Both the lipoxygenase [4] and the cyclooxygenase [5] pathways have been thoroughly studied and described. Briefly, via the LOX pathway, AA is converted into a large number of lipid mediators with vasoactive and immunomodulatory effects such as lipoxins, leukotrienes, hepoxilins, eoxins, resolvins, protectins, and others [4]. On the other hand, cyclooxygenase (COX), with both its COX-1 and COX-2 isoforms, transforms AA in either prostaglandins, prostacyclins, or thromboxane; other products are known for their vasoactive, immunomodulatory, and platelet-aggregating effects [5]. In contrast, the CYP450 pathway, also known as the third pathway, was far less understood [1,6]. However, this pathway is increasingly recognized as a 'yin and yang' in relation to its potential opposing effects on the cardiac function, depending on which subfamily of the CYP enzyme is metabolizing AA. Indeed, when it is transformed by epoxidation, AA generates a number of products known as epoxyeicosatrienoic acids (EETs) that promote vasodilation, angiogenesis, and thrombolysis. It then also inhibits inflammation, smooth muscle cell migration, and apoptosis, which together lead to a preserved cardiac function [7]. In contrast, when AA is hydroxylated, it produces compounds such as hydroxyeicosatetraenoic acids (HETEs) that promote vasoconstriction, inflammation, smooth muscle cell migration, and apoptosis, all leading to cardiac dysfunction [7]. In fact, CYP450 enzymes can metabolize AA in a tissue- and cell-specific manner to generate major and highly relevant derivatives, such as cardioprotective EETs and cardiotoxic HETEs. These epoxygenated and hydroxylated lipid derivatives are known to have various biological functions, such as regulating the vascular tone and reactivity, renal and pulmonary functions, ion transport, and growth response [8]. The epoxygenases (CYP2C and CYP2J) generate EETs, while the ω-hydroxylases (CYP4A and CYP4F) generate HETEs [2,6,9]. The human CYP2C subfamily consists of four members (CYP2C8, CYP2C9, CYP2C18, and CYP2C19) and they account for approximately 20% of the P450 enzymes in the human liver. Moreover, they are expressed to variable extents in a number of tissues such as liver, kidney, gut, brain, lungs, aorta, and importantly, in the heart [10,11]. The human CYP2J subfamily has only a single gene, CYP2J2 metabolizing AA [12]. CYP2J2 was detected in tissues such as lung, intestine, liver, pancreas, and seminal vesicles, and is particularly abundant in the cardiovascular tissue [13–17]. Enzymes of the CYP4A subfamily have been identified in virtually all mammalian species. In human, CYP4A11 and CYP4A12 have been identified. The CYP4A fatty acid ω-hydroxylases are ubiquitously expressed and consistently found in strong levels in the kidney, liver, lung, intestine, skeletal muscle, and heart [18]. The mammalian CYP4F subfamily consists of seven human forms: CYP4F2 (liver and kidney), CYP4F3A (bone marrow and neutrophiles), CYP4F3B (liver and kidney), CYP4F8 (prostate), CYP4F11 (liver, kidney, heart, and skeletal muscle), CYP4F12 (gastrointestinal tract, heart, and kidney), and CYP4F22 (skin). Therefore, both CYP2 and CYP4 families are present in the heart.

CYP-derived HETEs have deleterious effects in the heart during ischemia. These include a significant pro-inflammatory effect during reperfusion and potent vasoconstriction in the coronary arteries [2]. In contrast, epoxidation of AA generates 5,6-, 8,9-, 11,12-, and 14,15-EET that have been shown to limit ischemia-reperfusion injury, to have potent anti-inflammatory effects within the vasculature, and to be potent vasodilators of the coronary arteries [2]. Once formed, EETs undergo hydrolysis by soluble epoxide hydrolase (sEH) to less biologically active dihydroeicosatrienoic acids (DHETs) [2]. Soluble epoxide hydrolase (sEH) is widely distributed in mammalian tissues. Indeed, it is present in vascular endothelia [19] and in vascular smooth muscle cells [20]. Dysregulation of lipid metabolism has frequently been associated with disorders such as inflammation, neoplasia, diabetes, and neurodegeneration, as well as cardiovascular disease [8]. In line with this, a probable link between CYP450 expression/activity and cardiovascular disease (CVD), such as high blood pressure, coronary artery disease, myocardial ischemia and infarction, congestive heart failure, stroke, dilated cardiomyopathies, and rhythm disturbances has been established [21]. It is therefore suggested that alterations in the expression and/or activity of specific CYP450 epoxygenase/hydroxylase and sEH enzymes are likely to affect the delicate balance between the cardiovascular effects of EETs, HETEs, and DHETs [2]. As a consequence, abnormalities in these pathways may contribute to and/or promote the pathogenesis of CVD [22].

Well-known to be a major contributor to the onset and development of CVD [23], Type II diabetes (T2D) is therefore thought to perturbate the fine equilibrium between cardioprotective and cardiotoxic CYP-generated metabolites of AA by contributing to the cardiotoxic side. Indeed, this modulation of AA metabolism is suggested to be associated with the onset of coronary vasoconstriction leading to endothelial dysfunction, atherosclerosis, and CVD in general [24]. Of note, while both COX- and LOX-associated cardiovascular alterations have been demonstrated in the *db/db* mouse model of T2 [25,26], such demonstration is far less clear when considering the CYP pathway.

It was therefore our objective to evaluate the T2D-induced disturbances in the CYP450 pathway of AA metabolism that may contribute to the observed increase in the risk of CVD.

2. Materials and Methods

2.1. Animal Model

Male 7-weeks old BKS.Cg-m +/+ Lepr^{db}/J mice (*db/db*: T2D) and control C57BLKS/J wild-type mice were purchased from The Jackson Laboratory (Bar Harbor, ME, USA). The animals were fed with standard chow and water ad libitum. At 12 weeks-old, blood drawns were performed by using the submandibular vein, and, thereafter, the animals were killed by cervical dislocation. Livers and hearts were quickly harvested, washed with ice-cold PBS, snap-frozen in liquid nitrogen, and further kept at −80 °C. These experiments were carried out in accordance with the Guide to the Care and Use of Experimental Animals of the Canadian Council on Animal Care. The research protocol was approved by the Comité de protection des animaux de l'Université Laval (CPAUL; Authorization # 2009140-3, on 20 December 2011).

2.2. Western Blots of Liver Proteins

Western blotting experiments were performed as previously described [27] to assess CYP2C, CYP4A, and CYP4F protein expression. Briefly, samples of frozen liver were homogenized in an ice-cold lysis buffer (in mmol/L): Tris-HCl (pH 7.4) 10, sucrose 320, EDTA 1, dithiothreitol 1, and a protease inhibitor cocktail 0.1% from Sigma-Aldrich (St. Louis, MO, USA). Total protein content was evaluated with the DC protein assay kit (Bio-Rad, Mississauga, ON, Canada). Western blot analysis of 10 μg (CYP2C), 12 μg (CYP4A), and 20 μg (CYP4F) of proteins were used to evaluate the levels of these three CYPs in the livers. The Mini-Protean TGX Stain-Free Precast Gel (Bio-Rad) or standard SDS-PAGE gel was used. The membrane was incubated overnight at 4 °C with either anti-CYP2C9 (Ab48558), anti-CYP4A (Ab3573), or anti-CYP4F12 (Ab71565) polyclonal primary antibodies (all three 1:1000; Abcam, Toronto, ON, Canada). The membrane was washed and then incubated with a goat anti-rabbit IgG HRP-linked secondary antibody (SC2004; 1:1000; Santa Cruz Biotechnology, Mississauga, ON, Canada) conjugated with horseradish peroxidase. In the specific case of CYP4F proteins, the membrane was washed, stripped in SDS/β-mercaptoethanol solution at 55 °C for 15 min to enhance the signal strength [28], and then incubated with the secondary antibody conjugated with horseradish peroxidase. Chemiluminescent immunodetection was performed by using the Luminata™ Crescendo Western HRP Substrate (EMD Millipore, Billerica, MA, USA) and the ChemiDoc™ imaging system from Bio-Rad. Expression of the proteins of interest was normalized against total lane density of loaded proteins based on Amido black staining (CYP4F) or stain-free gel technology (CYP4A and CYP2C). The linear dynamic range of sample was evaluated for each antibody to make sure that an appropriate sample loading was used.

2.3. Western Blots of Cardiac Protein

Samples of frozen ventricles were homogenized in an ice-cold lysis buffer (in mmol/L): Tris-HCl (pH 7.4) 15, NaCl 150, sodium vanadate 0.2, EGTA 1, MgCl$_2$ 1, β-mercaptoethanol 10, Triton 1%, sodium deoxycholate 0.5%, and a protease inhibitor cocktail 0.1% from Sigma-Aldrich. Total protein content was evaluated with the DC protein assay kit (Bio-Rad). Western blot analysis of 25 μg of proteins was used to assess the level of CYP2J protein in the ventricles. The membrane was incubated overnight at 4 °C with anti-CYP2J2 (Ab76176) polyclonal antibody (1:1000; Abcam). The membrane was washed and then incubated with a goat anti-rabbit IgG HRP-linked secondary antibody (SC2004; 1:1000; Santa Cruz Biotechnology) conjugated with horseradish peroxidase. Chemiluminescent immunodetection was performed using the Luminata™ Crescendo Western HRP Substrate (EMD Millipore) and the ChemiDoc™ imaging system from Bio-Rad. Expression of the proteins of interest was normalized against total protein loaded based on Amido black staining of whole lanes. Again, the linear dynamic range of the method was evaluated.

2.4. Data Analysis

Student's *t*-test followed by a Mann-Whitney rank sum test (when the test for normality failed) were used to evaluate the differences between groups (SigmaPlot 12.5, Jandel Scientific Software, San Rafael, CA, USA). All the results are expressed as mean ± SEM. Statistical significance was set at $p < 0.05$.

3. Results

Table 1 shows body weight and biochemical blood parameters of mice at sacrifice (week 12). Many clinical features of human Type II diabetes were shown to be present in the *db/db* mice (T2D) at sacrifice: severe obesity, hyperglycemia, hyperinsulinemia, hypertriglyceridemia, and hypercholesterolemia; thus confirming the validity of this T2D animal model.

Table 1. Body weight and biochemical blood parameters at sacrifice (week 12). (** $p < 0.01$, *** $p < 0.001$ vs. control).

Measures at Sacrifice (Week 12)	Control Mice ($n = 17$)	BKS.Cg-m +/+ Lepr^{db}/J Mice (*db/db*: T2D) ($n = 20$)
Weight (g)	23.5 ± 0.5	41.3 ± 0.9 ***
Glycemia (mM)	8.2 ± 0.7	31.3 ± 0.6 ***
Insulinemia (ng/mL)	0.67 ± 0.06	3.90 ± 0.50 ***
HDL-C (mM)	2.10 ± 0.05	3.18 ± 0.13 ***
Triglyceridemia (mM)	1.67 ± 0.07	2.33 ± 0.22 **
Cholesterolemia (mM)	2.32 ± 0.17	3.77 ± 0.11 ***

As shown in Figure 1 (lower panel), a significant reduction in relative expression of CYP2J proteins was observed in the cardiac ventricles of T2D mice, when compared to the control animals (0.80 ± 0.03 vs. 1.05 ± 0.06; $p < 0.001$). Upper panel shows the representative blot images of cardiac CYP2J and the total proteins loaded for both the control and T2D groups. Figure 2 (lower panel) also shows a significant reduction in relative expression of CYP2C proteins that was observed in the liver of T2D mice when compared to the control animals (1.56 ± 0.17 vs. 2.21 ± 0.19; $p < 0.01$). Upper panel shows the representative blot images of hepatic CYP2C and the total proteins loaded for both the control and T2D groups. In contrast, Figure 3 (lower panel) shows a significant increase in relative expression of CYP4A proteins that was observed in the liver of T2D mice when compared to the control animals (1.06 ± 0.09 vs. 0.18 ± 0.01; $p < 0.001$).

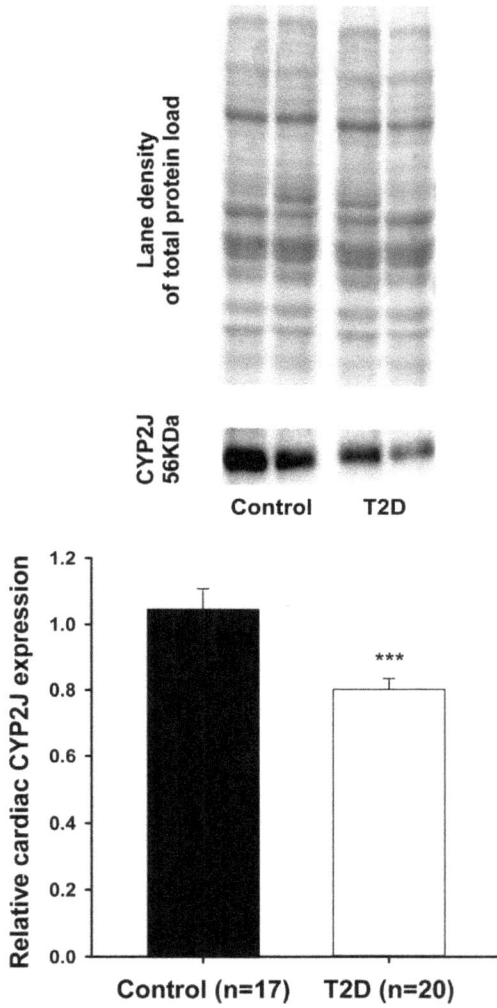

Figure 1. A significant decrease (*** $p < 0.001$) was observed in the relative protein expression of cardiac CYP2J in Type II diabetes (T2D) mice (0.80 ± 0.03) compared to controls (1.05 ± 0.06).

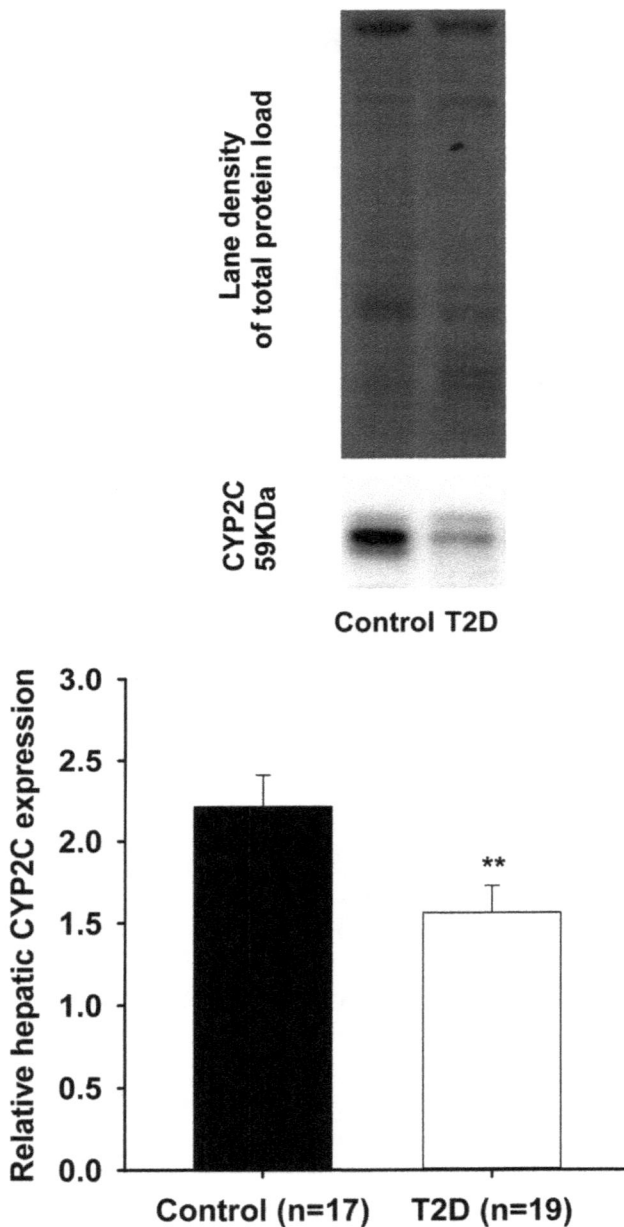

Figure 2. A significant decrease (** $p < 0.01$) was observed in the relative protein expression of hepatic CYP2C in T2D mice (1.56 ± 0.17) compared to controls (2.21 ± 0.19).

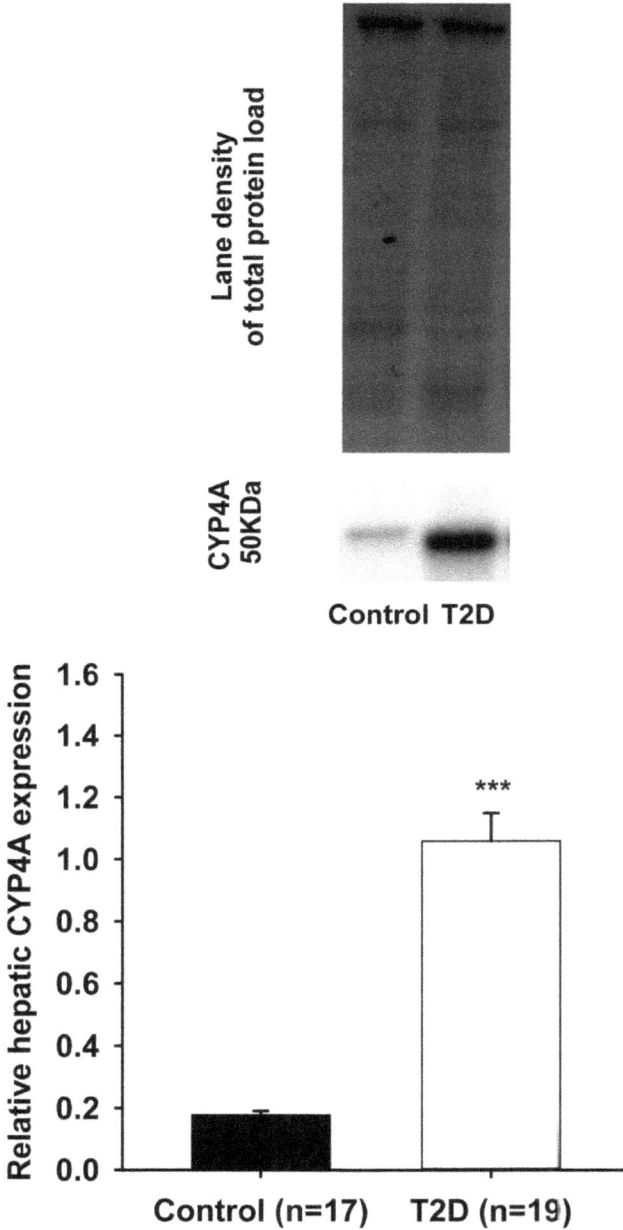

Figure 3. A significant increase (*** $p < 0.001$) was observed in the protein expression of hepatic CYP4A in T2D mice (1.06 ± 0.09) compared to controls (0.18 ± 0.01).

Upper panel shows the representative blot images of hepatic CYP4A and the total proteins loaded for both the control and T2D groups. Moreover, as seen with CYP4A, Figure 4 (lower panel) shows a significant increase in relative expression of CYP4F proteins that was observed in the liver of T2D mice when compared to the control animals (2.53 ± 0.22 vs. 1.10 ± 0.07; $p < 0.001$). Upper panel shows the representative blot images of hepatic CYP4F and the total proteins loaded for both the control and T2D groups.

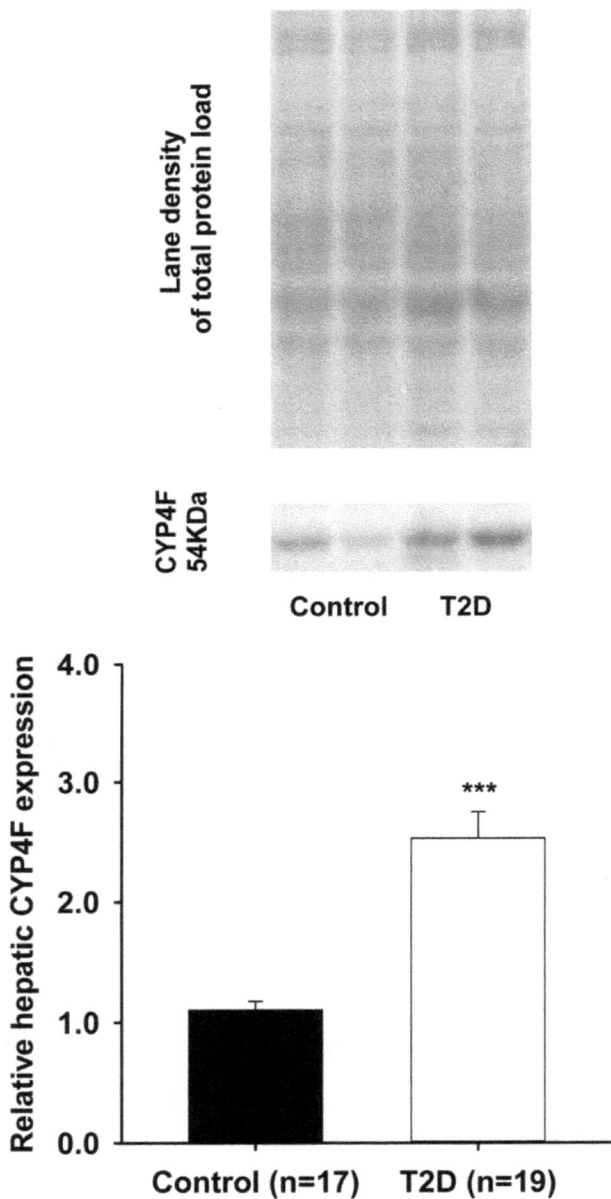

Figure 4. A significant increase (*** $p < 0.001$) was observed in the protein expression of hepatic CYP4F in T2D mice (2.53 ± 0.22) compared to controls (1.10 ± 0.07).

4. Discussion

The pathophysiology of CVD is highly complex, and a constellation of risk factors contribute to its development and progression. Consequence of the current worldwide obesity epidemic, one major risk factor of CVD that is becoming epidemic as well is Type II diabetes. Interestingly, we have already shown that CYPs expression and metabolic activity are altered in a number of conditions such as metabolic syndrome and renal insufficiency in different animal models [29,30]. Besides, Imig et al. demonstrated a decrease in renal expression of CYP2C epoxygenase enzymes in diabetic obese Zucker rats and in high fat diet-fed insulin resistant rats [31]. They concluded that eicosanoids metabolites are altered in Type II diabetes and contribute to the progression of renal injury. Moreover, Shimojo et al. reported an induction of hepatic and renal CYP4A subfamily enzymes in diabetic rats [32]. Yousif et al. demonstrated that CYP4 family expression is twice as high in the hearts of diabetic rats when compared to normal animals [33]. Enriquez et al. showed that expression of murine CYP4A10 and 4A14 in the obese mice, and 4A2 in the male fatty Zucker rat, were greatly increased [34]. Zhao et al. [35] studied the mesenteric artery protein expression in lean and obese Zucker rats. They concluded that mesenteric arterial CYP2C11 and CYP2J proteins were decreased by 38% and 43%, respectively, in obese Zucker rats. In contrast, sEH mRNA and protein expressions were significantly increased in obese Zucker rat mesenteric arteries [35]. A previous study has shown that the synthesis of renal CYP450 (CYP)-derived eicosanoids is downregulated in genetic or high-fat diet-induced obese rats [36]. These results demonstrated that the PPAR-alpha agonist fenofibrate increased renal CYP-derived eicosanoids and restored endothelial dilator function in obese Zucker rats [36]. A study from Theken et al. [37] evaluated CYP epoxygenase (EET+DHET) and ω-hydroxylase (20-HETE) metabolic activity in liver and kidney in wild-type mice fed with a high fat diet, which promoted weight gain and significantly increased insulinemia. Hepatic CYP epoxygenase metabolic activity was significantly suppressed, while renal CYP ω-hydroxylase metabolic activity was significantly induced in high fat diet-fed mice. A significantly higher 20-HETE:EET+DHET formation rate ratio was observed in both tissues [37]. They concluded that the observed changes in CYP epoxygenase and hydroxylase metabolic activity were driven by high fat diet rather than by genotype.

Interestingly, there are recent clinical studies that begin to bridge the gap between animal models of CYP-mediated arachidonic acid metabolism and cardiovascular disease in humans. Indeed, Akasaka et al. [38] examined CYP2C19 genotypes in 81 patients with microvascular angina (MVA) caused by coronary microvascular dysfunction. They found that CYP2C19 poor metabolizers had declined levels of EETs, suggesting insufficient defensive mechanism against chronic inflammation, a risk factor for MVA. Moreover, Theken et al. [39] evaluated the role of CYP-derived eicosanoids in humans with stable atherosclerotic cardiovascular disease (CVD, $n = 82$) versus healthy volunteers ($n = 36$). Among other things, they noted that obesity was significantly associated with low plasma EET levels and 14,15-EET:14,15 DHET ratios. Collectively, their findings suggest that CYP-mediated eicosanoid metabolism is dysregulated in certain subsets of CVD patients and demonstrate that biomarkers of CYP epoxygenase are altered in stable CVD patients relative to healthy individuals. Later on, the same group came up with a study [24] of 106 patients with stable coronary artery disease (CAD) in which relationships between biomarkers of CYP-mediated eicosanoid metabolism and vascular function phenotypes were evaluated. Collectively, their findings demonstrated that enhanced CYP ω-hydroxylases (generating HETEs) and sEH (degradating EETs) metabolic functions are associated with more advanced endothelial dysfunction and vascular inflammation, respectively, in patients with established atherosclerotic CVD.

In the present study, we show that Type II diabetes, a major CVD-associated pathological condition, significantly decreases the cardiac protein expression of cytochrome P450 CYP2J and of hepatic CYP2C in *db/db* mice. As CYP2J and CYP2C are the major AA epoxygenases in the cardiovascular and hepatic systems [2], where they are widely expressed respectively [40], down regulation of these two CYP epoxygenases could compromise the formation of EETs, which play many crucial roles in cardiovascular homeostasis. In fact, in addition to their potent vasodilating effect, EETs have potent anti-inflammatory properties, inhibit platelet aggregation, promote fibrinolysis, and reduce vascular smooth muscle cell proliferation [41]. In addition, our results also show increased hepatic protein expression of both cytochrome P450 CYP4A and CYP4F in *db/db* mice. CYP4F2 is known to be the key AA ω-hydroxylase in human liver and kidney with a more superior substrate specificity for AA than the already established AA ω-hydroxylase CYP4A11 [42]. The massive formation of 20-HETE, along with its potent detrimental pro-inflammatory effects during ischemia-reperfusion and vasoconstrictor effect in the coronary arteries [2], suggests that it could also serve as an intracellular second messenger underlying the regulation of vascular tone [43].

5. Conclusions

Taken together, Type II diabetes-induced combined alterations of cardiac CYP2J, and hepatic CYP2C, CYP4A, and CYP4F protein expression are likely to play a significant role in CVD. As these four CYP isoforms were shown to generate the most vasoactive eicosanoid metabolites, Type II diabetes likely generates deleterious in situ alterations in the endogenous disposition of AA. Their net effect is thought to further promote CVD by disrupting the fine equilibrium between cardioprotective (CYP2C/CYP2J-generated) and cardiotoxic (CYP4A/CYP4F-generated) AA metabolites, adding weight on the cardiotoxic side of the balance.

6. Limitation

CVD-associated pathophysiological features of the diabetic mice such as (coronary disease, vasoconstriction, endothelial dysfunction, atherosclerosis, etc.) were not compared to those of the control animals. Such further studies, beyond the scope of this article, would help to elucidate how and how much the altered CYPs in Type II diabetes may influence the onset and progression of cardiovascular disease.

Acknowledgments: This study received support from the Fondation de l'Institut universitaire de cardiologie et de pneumologie de Québec and from Diabète Québec (grants to Benoit Drolet and Chantale Simard). Carolanne Gélinas and Audrey Blais-Boilard were recipients of summer studentship awards from the Fonds d'Enseignement et de Recherche (FER) de la Faculté de pharmacie de l'Université Laval. Jessica Virgili was the recipient of a doctoral studentship award from the FER. Benoit Drolet and Chantale Simard were scholars of the Fonds de recherche du Québec-Santé (FRQ-S). The funding sponsors had no role in the design of the study; in the collection, analyses, or interpretation of data; in the writing of the manuscript; or in the decision to publish the results.

Author Contributions: Sylvie Pilote, Carolanne Gélinas, Alida-Douce Kamaliza, Audrey Blais-Boilard, Jessica Virgili, and Dany Patoine performed the experiments. Jessica Virgili, Sylvie Pilote, and Dany Patoine analysed the data. Benoit Drolet and Chantale Simard contributed reagents/materials/analysis tools. Benoit Drolet and Chantale Simard wrote the paper.

Conflicts of Interest: The authors declare no conflict of interest.

References

1. Kaspera, R.; Totah, R.A. Epoxyeicosatrienoic acids: Formation, metabolism and potential role in tissue physiology and pathophysiology. *Expert Opin. Drug Metab. Toxicol.* **2009**, *5*, 757–771. [CrossRef] [PubMed]
2. Seubert, J.M.; Zeldin, D.C.; Nithipatikom, K.; Gross, G.J. Role of epoxyeicosatrienoic acids in protecting the myocardium following ischemia/reperfusion injury. *Prostaglandins Other Lipid Mediat.* **2007**, *82*, 50–59. [CrossRef] [PubMed]
3. Jenkins, C.M.; Cedars, A.; Gross, R.W. Eicosanoid signalling pathways in the heart. *Cardiovasc. Res.* **2009**, *82*, 240–249. [CrossRef] [PubMed]
4. Kuhn, H.; Banthiya, S.; van Leyen, K. Mammalian lipoxygenases and their biological relevance. *Biochim. Biophys. Acta* **2015**, *1851*, 308–330. [CrossRef] [PubMed]
5. Luo, W.; Liu, B.; Zhou, Y. The endothelial cyclooxygenase pathway: Insights from mouse arteries. *Eur. J. Pharmacol.* **2016**, *780*, 148–158. [CrossRef] [PubMed]
6. Fleming, I. Epoxyeicosatrienoic acids, cell signaling and angiogenesis. *Prostaglandins Other Lipid Mediat.* **2007**, *82*, 60–67. [CrossRef] [PubMed]

7. Jamieson, K.L.; Endo, T.; Darwesh, A.M.; Samokhvalov, V.; Seubert, J.M. Cytochrome P450-derived eicosanoids and heart function. *Pharmacol Ther.* **2017**. [CrossRef] [PubMed]
8. Huwiler, A.; Pfeilschifter, J. Lipids as targets for novel anti-inflammatory therapies. *Pharmacol. Ther.* **2009**, *124*, 96–112. [CrossRef] [PubMed]
9. Ayajiki, K.; Okamura, T.; Fujioka, H.; Imaoka, S.; Funae, Y.; Toda, N. Involvement of CYP3A-derived arachidonic acid metabolite(s) in responses to endothelium-derived K+ channel opening substance in monkey lingual artery. *Br. J. Pharmacol.* **1999**, *128*, 802–808. [CrossRef] [PubMed]
10. Delozier, T.C.; Kissling, G.E.; Coulter, S.J.; Dai, D.; Foley, J.F.; Bradbury, J.A.; Murphy, E.; Steenbergen, C.; Zeldin, D.C.; Goldstein, J.A. Detection of human CYP2C8, CYP2C9, and CYP2J2 in cardiovascular tissues. *Drug Metab. Dispos.* **2007**, *35*, 682–688. [CrossRef] [PubMed]
11. Klose, T.S.; Blaisdell, J.A.; Goldstein, J.A. Gene structure of CYP2C8 and extrahepatic distribution of the human CYP2Cs. *J. Biochem. Mol. Toxicol.* **1999**, *13*, 289–295. [CrossRef]
12. Lee, C.A.; Neul, D.; Clouser-Roche, A.; Dalvie, D.; Wester, M.R.; Jiang, Y.; Jones, J.P.; Friewald, S.; Zientek, M.; Totah, R.A. Identification of novel substrates for human cytochrome P450 2J2. *Drug Metab. Dispos.* **2010**, *38*, 347–356. [CrossRef] [PubMed]
13. Wu, S.; Moomaw, C.R.; Tomer, K.B.; Falck, J.R.; Zeldin, D.C. Molecular cloning and expression of CYP2J2, a human cytochrome P450 arachidonic acid epoxygenase highly expressed in heart. *J. Biol. Chem.* **1996**, *271*, 3460–3468. [CrossRef] [PubMed]
14. Zeldin, D.C.; Foley, J.; Goldsworthy, S.M.; Cook, M.E.; Boyle, J.E.; Ma, J.; Moomaw, C.R.; Tomer, K.B.; Steenbergen, C.; Wu, S. CYP2J subfamily cytochrome P450s in the gastrointestinal tract: Expression, localization, and potential functional significance. *Mol. Pharmacol.* **1997**, *51*, 931–943. [CrossRef] [PubMed]
15. Zeldin, D.C.; Foley, J.; Ma, J.; Boyle, J.E.; Pascual, J.M.; Moomaw, C.R.; Tomer, K.B.; Steenbergen, C.; Wu, S. CYP2J subfamily P450s in the lung: Expression, localization, and potential functional significance. *Mol. Pharmacol.* **1996**, *50*, 1111–1117. [PubMed]
16. Zeldin, D.C.; Foley, J.; Boyle, J.E.; Moomaw, C.R.; Tomer, K.B.; Parker, C.; Steenbergen, C.; Wu, S. Predominant expression of an arachidonate epoxygenase in islets of Langerhans cells in human and rat pancreas. *Endocrinology* **1997**, *138*, 1338–1346. [CrossRef] [PubMed]
17. Borlak, J.; Walles, M.; Levsen, K.; Thum, T. Verapamil: metabolism in cultures of primary human coronary arterial endothelial cells. *Drug Metab. Dispos.* **2003**, *31*, 888–891. [CrossRef] [PubMed]
18. Graham, R.A.; Goodwin, B.; Merrihew, R.V.; Krol, W.L.; Lecluyse, E.L. Cloning, tissue expression, and regulation of beagle dog CYP4A genes. *Toxicol. Sci.* **2006**, *92*, 356–367. [CrossRef] [PubMed]
19. Zhang, D.; Xie, X.; Chen, Y.; Hammock, B.D.; Kong, W.; Zhu, Y. Homocysteine upregulates soluble epoxide hydrolase in vascular endothelium in vitro and in vivo. *Circ Res.* **2012**, *110*, 808–817. [CrossRef] [PubMed]
20. Davis, B.B.; Thompson, D.A.; Howard, L.L.; Morisseau, C.; Hammock, B.D.; Weiss, R.H. Inhibitors of soluble epoxide hydrolase attenuate vascular smooth muscle cell proliferation. *Proc. Natl. Acad. Sci. USA* **2002**, *99*, 2222–2227. [CrossRef] [PubMed]
21. Elbekai, R.H.; El-Kadi, A.O. Cytochrome P450 enzymes: Central players in cardiovascular health and disease. *Pharmacol. Ther.* **2006**, *112*, 564–587. [CrossRef] [PubMed]
22. Roman, R.J.; Maier, K.G.; Sun, C.W.; Harder, D.R.; Alonso-Galicia, M. Renal and cardiovascular actions of 20-hydroxyeicosatetraenoic acid and epoxyeicosatrienoic acids. *Clin. Exp. Pharmacol. Physiol.* **2000**, *27*, 855–865. [CrossRef] [PubMed]
23. Abdul-Ghani, M.; DeFronzo, R.A.; Del Prato, S.; Chilton, R.; Singh, R.; Ryder, R.E.J. Cardiovascular Disease and Type 2 Diabetes: Has the Dawn of a New Era Arrived? *Diabetes Care* **2017**, *40*, 813–820. [CrossRef] [PubMed]
24. Schuck, R.N.; Theken, K.N.; Edin, M.L.; Caughey, M.; Bass, A.; Ellis, K.; Tran, B.; Steele, S.; Simmons, B.P.; Lih, F.B.; et al. Cytochrome P450-derived eicosanoids and vascular dysfunction in coronary artery disease patients. *Atherosclerosis* **2013**, *227*, 442–448. [CrossRef] [PubMed]
25. Guo, Z.; Su, W.; Allen, S.; Pang, H.; Daugherty, A.; Smart, E.; Gong, M.C. COX-2 Up-regulation and vascular smooth muscle contractile hyperreactivity in spontaneous diabetic *db/db* mice. *Cardiovasc. Res.* **2005**, *67*, 723–735. [CrossRef] [PubMed]
26. Hatley, M.E.; Srinivasan, S.; Reilly, K.B.; Bolick, D.T. Increased Production of 12/15 Lipoxygenase Eicosanoids Accelerates Monocyte/Endothelial Interactions in Diabetic *db/db* Mice. *J. Biol. Chem.* **2003**, *278*, 25369–25375. [CrossRef] [PubMed]

27. Patoine, D.; Levac, X.; Pilote, S.; Drolet, B.; Simard, C. Decreased CYP3A expression and activity in guinea pig models of diet-induced metabolic syndrome: Is fatty liver infiltration involved? *Drug Metab. Dispos.* **2013**, *41*, 952–957. [CrossRef] [PubMed]

28. Pilote, S.; Virgili, J.; Patoine, D.; Drolet, B.; Simard, C. Altered hepatic protein expression of CYP4F in mouse models of Type I and Type II diabetes. In Proceedings of the 5th ICCR Congress on Chronic Societal Cardiometabolic Diseases, Quebec City, QC, Canada, 8–12 July 2015; Volume 7, p. 28.

29. Patoine, D.; Petit, M.; Pilote, S.; Picard, F.; Drolet, B.; Simard, C. Modulation of CYP3a expression and activity in mice models of Type 1 and Type 2 diabetes. *Pharmacol. Res. Perspect.* **2014**, *2*, e00082:1–8. [CrossRef] [PubMed]

30. Kingma, J.; Simard, D.; Patoine, D.; Pilote, S.; Drolet, B.; Rouleau, J.; Simard, C. Chronic kidney disease augments cardiovascular risk: Modulation of myocardial blood flow regulation and CYP450 arachidonic acid metabolites. International Academy of Cardiology Annual Scientific Sessions 2014. In Proceedings of the 19th World Congress on Heart Disease, Boston, MA, USA, 25–28 July 2014. *Cardiology* **2014**, *128* (Suppl. 1), 115.

31. Imig, J.D. Eicosanoids and renal damage in cardiometabolic syndrome. *Exp. Opin. Drug Metab. Toxicol.* **2008**, *4*, 165–174. [CrossRef] [PubMed]

32. Shimojo, N.; Ishizaki, T.; Imaoka, S.; Funae, Y.; Fujii, S.; Okuda, K. Changes in amounts of cytochrome P450 isozymes and levels of catalytic activities in hepatic and renal microsomes of rats with streptozocin-induced diabetes. *Biochem. Pharmacol.* **1993**, *46*, 621–627. [CrossRef]

33. Yousif, M.H.; Benter, I.F.; Roman, R.J. Cytochrome P450 metabolites of arachidonic acid play a role in the enhanced cardiac dysfunction in diabetic rats following ischaemic reperfusion injury. *Auton. Autacoid. Pharmacol.* **2009**, *29*, 33–41. [CrossRef] [PubMed]

34. Enriquez, A.; Leclercq, I.; Farrell, G.C.; Robertson, G. Altered expression of hepatic CYP2E1 and CYP4A in obese, diabetic ob/ob mice, and fa/fa Zucker rats. *Biochem. Biophys. Res. Commun.* **1999**, *255*, 300–306. [CrossRef] [PubMed]

35. Zhao, X.; Dey, A.; Romanko, O.P.; Stepp, D.W.; Wang, M.H.; Zhou, Y.; Jin, L.; Pollock, J.S.; Clinton Webb, R.; Imig, J.D. Decreased epoxygenase and increased epoxide hydrolase expression in the mesenteric artery of obese Zucker rats. *Am. J. Physiol. Regul. Integr. Comp. Physiol.* **2005**, *288*, R188–R196. [CrossRef] [PubMed]

36. Zhao, X.; Quigley, J.E.; Yuan, J.; Wang, M.H.; Zhou, Y.; Imig, J.D. PPAR-alpha activator fenofibrate increases renal CYP-derived eicosanoid synthesis and improves endothelial dilator function in obese Zucker rats. *Am. J. Physiol. Heart Circ. Physiol.* **2006**, *290*, H2187–H2195. [CrossRef] [PubMed]

37. Theken, K.N.; Deng, Y.; Schuck, R.N.; Oni-Orisan, A.; Miller, T.M.; Kannon, M.A.; Poloyac, S.M.; Lee, C.R. Enalapril reverses high-fat diet-induced alterations in cytochrome P450-mediated eicosanoid metabolism. *Am. J. Physiol. Endocrinol. Metab.* **2012**, *302*, E500–E509. [CrossRef] [PubMed]

38. Akasaka, T.; Sueta, D.; Arima, Y.; Tabata, N.; Takashio, S.; Izumiya, Y.; Yamamoto, E.; Tsujita, K.; Kojima, S.; Kaikita, K.; et al. CYP2C19 variants and epoxyeicosatrienoic acids in patients with microvascular angina. *IJC Heart Vasc.* **2017**, *15*, 15–20. [CrossRef] [PubMed]

39. Theken, K.N.; Schuck, R.N.; Edin, M.L.; Tran, B.; Ellis, K.; Bass, A.; Lih, F.B.; Tomer, K.B.; Poloyac, S.M.; Wu, M.C.; et al. Evaluation of cytochrome P450-derived eicosanoids in humans with stable atherosclerotic cardiovascular disease. *Atherosclerosis* **2012**, *222*, 530–536. [CrossRef] [PubMed]

40. Alsaad, A.M.; Zordoky, B.N.; Tse, M.M.; El-Kadi, A.O. Role of cytochrome P450-mediated arachidonic acid metabolites in the pathogenesis of cardiac hypertrophy. *Drug Metab. Rev.* **2013**, *45*, 173–195. [CrossRef] [PubMed]

41. Tacconelli, S.; Patrignani, P. Inside epoxyeicosatrienoic acids and cardiovascular disease. *Front Pharmacol.* **2014**, *5*, 239. [CrossRef] [PubMed]

42. Powell, P.K.; Wolf, I.; Jin, R.; Lasker, J.M. Metabolism of arachidonic acid to 20-hydroxy-5,8,11, 14-eicosatetraenoic acid by P450 enzymes in human liver: Involvement of CYP4F2 and CYP4A11. *J. Pharmacol. Exp. Ther.* **1998**, *285*, 1327–1336. [PubMed]

43. Roman, R.J. P-450 metabolites of arachidonic acid in the control of cardiovascular function. *Physiol. Rev.* **2002**, *82*, 131–185. [CrossRef] [PubMed]

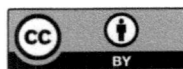

Article

Study of Statin- and Loratadine-Induced Muscle Pain Mechanisms Using Human Skeletal Muscle Cells

Yat Hei Leung [1,2], Jacques Turgeon [1] and Veronique Michaud [1,2,*]

[1] Faculty of Pharmacy, Université de Montréal, Montreal, QC H2X 0A9, Canada; yat.hei.leung@umontreal.ca (Y.H.L.); turgeoja@gmail.com (J.T.)

[2] Centre de Recherche du Centre Hospitalier de l'Université de Montréal (CRCHUM), Montreal, QC H2X 0A9, Canada

* Correspondence: v.michaud@umontreal.ca; Tel.: +1-514-890-8000 (ext. 15812)

Received: 31 August 2017; Accepted: 1 October 2017; Published: 10 October 2017

Abstract: Many drugs can cause unexpected muscle disorders, often necessitating the cessation of an effective medication. Inhibition of monocarboxylate transporters (MCTs) may potentially lead to perturbation of L-lactic acid homeostasis and muscular toxicity. Previous studies have shown that statins and loratadine have the potential to inhibit L-lactic acid efflux by MCTs (MCT1 and 4). The main objective of this study was to confirm the inhibitory potentials of atorvastatin, simvastatin (acid and lactone forms), rosuvastatin, and loratadine on L-lactic acid transport using primary human skeletal muscle cells (SkMC). Loratadine (IC_{50} 31 and 15 uM) and atorvastatin (IC_{50} ~130 and 210 μM) demonstrated the greatest potency for inhibition of L-lactic acid efflux at pH 7.0 and 7.4, respectively (~2.5-fold L-lactic acid intracellular accumulation). Simvastatin acid exhibited weak inhibitory potency on L-lactic acid efflux with an intracellular lactic acid increase of 25–35%. No L-lactic acid efflux inhibition was observed for simvastatin lactone or rosuvastatin. Pretreatment studies showed no change in inhibitory potential and did not affect lactic acid transport for all tested drugs. In conclusion, we have demonstrated that loratadine and atorvastatin can inhibit the efflux transport of L-lactic acid in SkMC. Inhibition of L-lactic acid efflux may cause an accumulation of intracellular L-lactic acid leading to the reported drug-induced myotoxicity.

Keywords: statins; loratadine; drug-transporters; MCT; monocarboxylate transporters; lactic acid; skeletal muscle cell; drug-induced muscle disorders

---

1. Introduction

Adverse drug reactions (ADRs) are an important public health problem. Death caused by ADRs has increased over the years and, since 2011, has actually surpassed motor vehicle traffic-related injuries [1]. There are many factors that can contribute to this situation, such as polypharmacy in the aging population, drug-drug interactions, and interindividual genetic variability modulating the pharmacodynamics and pharmacokinetics of drugs inside the organism [2–4]. Many common medications can induce musculoskeletal disorders, while their incidence is still unclear due to the lack of clear definitions (e.g., under drug-drug interaction conditions). However, drug-related musculoskeletal disorders have been reported more frequently since the introduction into the market of widely prescribed lipid lowering drugs, such as fibrates and statins [5]. Drug-induced myopathies can range from mild myalgias to myopathies with weakness and severe life-threatening rhabdomyolysis. While mild myalgias are more or less tolerable, chronic myopathies can affect quality of life. Therefore, an early recognition of these ADRs is really important for the patients, since most of them are partially or completely reversible when the offending drug is substituted or the dose is adjusted [6,7].

Statins, 3-hydroxy-3-methylglutaryl-coenzyme A (HMG-CoA) reductase inhibitors, form the number one class of drugs prescribed in the United States for the prevention of cardiovascular disease [8]. However, muscle pain is a known side effect associated with statin treatment. Statin therapy is usually well tolerated, but muscle symptoms can limit treatment adhesion or even lead to its discontinuation [9]. The definitive mechanism of statin-induced muscle disorders is still not known, although different hypotheses have been proposed, including alteration in cellular membrane cholesterol, alterations in protein synthesis and degradation, cell apoptosis, immune reactions, increased lysosomal activity, injuries to electrolytes homeostasis, inhibition of myogenesis, mitochondrial impairments, and oxidative stress [10–12].

Muscle is one of the largest human organs, and it is well-perfused, which means that it is also highly exposed to circulating drugs, making it quite susceptible to ADRs [13]. Since skeletal muscle is the major producer of L-lactic acid, the transport of L-lactic acid is critical for the maintenance of intracellular pH and homeostasis. We have previously hypothesized that drug-induced myotoxicities can be caused by an excess intracellular level of L-lactic acid. Indeed, we demonstrated that some statins are able to inhibit the efflux of L-lactic acid *via* MCT1 and MCT4 in breast cancer cell lines (Hs578T selectively expressing MCT1 and MDA-MB-231 selectively expressing MCT4). In those studies, atorvastatin and loratadine were associated with the greatest inhibitory potential on the efflux of L-lactic acid, leading to intracellular accumulation of lactic acid using cancer cells [14].

The main objective of our study was to corroborate our previous findings in physiologically relevant settings. Therefore, we proposed to characterize the effects of atorvastatin, loratadine, simvastatin lactone, simvastatin hydroxy acid, and rosuvastatin, on the transport of L-lactic acid using human skeletal muscle cells (SkMCs) at resting pH of 7.4 and at pH 7.0. A more acidic pH value was tested, since evidence suggests that drug-related muscle disorders can be exacerbated by exercise.

2. Materials and Methods

2.1. Materials

[^{14}C] L-lactic acid sodium salt was purchased from PerkinElmer (Walthman, MA, USA). L-lactic acid sodium salt was obtained from Sigma-Aldrich (St. Louis, MO, USA). Atorvastatin, loratadine, phloretin, rosuvastatin, simvastatin, and simvastatin hydroxyl acid ammonium salt were purchased from Toronto Research Center (Toronto, ON, Canada). Cryopreserved human primary skeletal muscle cells (from adult), Human Skeletal Muscle Cells Growth medium, Human Skeletal Muscle Cells Differentiation medium, and Subculture Reagent Kit were purchased from Cell Applications Inc. (San Diego, CA, USA).

2.2. Cell Culture

SkMCs were grown in all-in-one-ready-to-use Human Skeletal Muscle Cells Growth medium and were used within 5 passages or 15 population doublings after thawing upon arrival or from storage in liquid nitrogen. Cells were first cultured in plastic culture flasks (Sarstedt, Newton, NC, USA) at 37 °C with 5% CO_2. When they reached 60–80% confluence, they were harvested with Subculture Reagent Kit which includes HBSS, Trypsin/EDTA and Trypsin Neutralizing Solution, resuspended and seeded into new flasks. When the adequate amount of cells for the experiments was attained, they were again harvested, seeded on 35 × 10 mm tissue culture plates, and grown to reach 80–90% confluence before differentiation. After that, differentiation was initiated by changing the media from the Human Skeletal Muscle Cells Growth medium into the Human Skeletal Muscle Cells Differentiation medium for 6 days until the cells formed multinucleated syncytia, as seen in Figure 1A–D. The differentiation was confirmed by immunomicroscopy for expression of myosin (Skeletal, Slow) described in the next section.

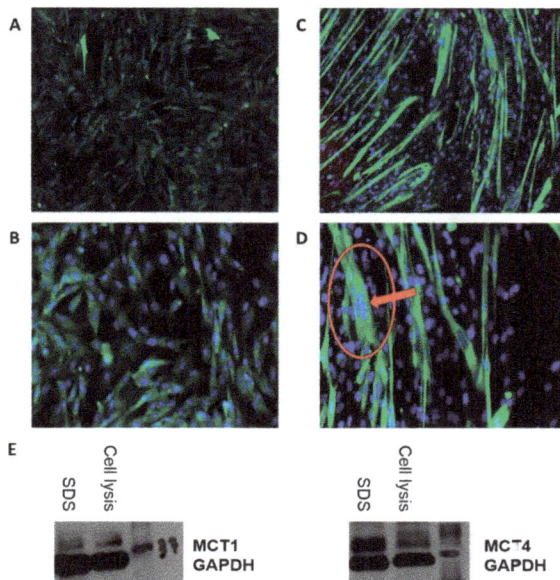

Figure 1. *SkMC*. Primary human myoblasts from Cell Applications Inc. were proliferated in 35 × 10 mm culture plates with SkMC growth medium for 25–35 days until 80–90% confluency and photographed at (**A**) 10× and (**B**) 20×. *SkMC in differentiation*. Differentiated SkMCs with multinucleated syncytia after exposition for 6 days with the SkMC differentiation medium are photographed at (**C**) 10× and (**D**) 20×. (**E**) Expression of MCT1 (**left**) and MCT4 (**right**) proteins in SkMCs was revealed by Western blotting using antibodies against MCT1, MCT4 and GAPDH (the 2 wells illustrated—SDS vs. cell lysis—represent 2 different methods tested for protein extraction).

2.3. Immunomicroscopy

The immunomiscroscopy images were obtained by having the SkMCs grown and differentiated on a glass slide cover. After removing the differentiation medium (or growth medim, if observations were made at an earlier stage), SkMCs were fixed with 3.7% formaldehyde for 15 min at room temperature and were washed twice with PBS 1× between every subsequent step. Samples were then quenched with glycine for 5 min, permeabilized with 0.2% Triton X-100 for 20 min and incubated for 3 h with BSA 3%. Cells were then incubated overnight at 4 °C with Monoclonal Anti-Myosin (Skeletal, Slow) antibody produced in mouse (Sigma-Aldrich, St. Louis, MO, USA). Cells were incubated with Alexa Fluor 488 (Invitrogen, Carlsbad, CA, USA) in BSA 3% for an hour at room temperature, followed by incubation with Hoechst for 15 min. After a final wash, images were acquired using an EE (×10 and ×20) and Zen Imaging software. The expression of MCT1 and MCT4 proteins has been assessed by Western blot during the cell culture optimization step (Figure 1E) (details of Western blotting are described in Supplementary Materials).

2.4. Transport Studies

After differentiation, and before the beginning of the transport experiments, cells were washed, and the medium replaced with HEPES (pH 7.4; 1 mL) buffer. Transport assays, including the pre-incubation period in HEPES, were performed at 37 °C. Assay conditions were previously optimized by standard incubations with L-lactic acid (e.g., incubation times). For the time-course experiments, different time points ranging from 5 s to 30 min were tested using one concentration (6 mM) of L-lactic acid.

Assessment of influx transport. At the beginning of the experiment (*t* = 0), HEPES medium was replaced by MES or HEPES (pH 7.0 or 7.4; 1 mL) buffer containing 0.03 to 30 mM [^{14}C] L-lactic acid (0.2 μCi/mL). After incubation for 2.5 min, the radioactive media was removed from the milieu. Transport assays were stopped by placing culture plates on ice, rapidly aspirating the media and cells were washed 3-times with ice-cold HEPES buffer. Cells were then solubilized using a solution of 0.2 N NaOH and 1% SDS (500 μL). The suspension was passed through $27\frac{1}{2}$ G needle 3-times. Aliquot of the cell lysate (400 μL) was transferred in a scintillation tube containing 5 mL of biodegradable scintillation counting cocktail buffer (Bio-Safe II, Research Products International Corp., Mt. Prospect, IL, USA). Radioactivity levels were quantified with a Tri-Carb liquid scintillation counter (LSC 1600TR, Packard Instrument Co., Meriden, CT, USA) to determine the intracellular [^{14}C] L-lactic acid concentrations. Protein concentrations were measured using Pierce BCA protein assay kit (Thermo Fisher Scientific, Walthman, MA, USA).

Assessment of efflux transport. A similar approach was used to measure efflux transport of L-lactic acid. For these experiments, distribution equilibrium of L-lactic acid was reached by adding MES or HEPES (pH 7.0 or 7.4; 1 mL) containing 6 mM [^{14}C] L-lactic acid (0.2 μCi/mL). After 10 min (to allow L-lactic acid to reach equilibrium), MES or HEPES buffer containing [^{14}C] L-lactic acid was replaced by L-lactic acid-free buffer for 2.5 min. Transport was stopped by placing culture plates on ice, rapidly aspirating the media and cells were washed 3-times with ice-cold HEPES buffer. Cellular radioactivity levels were determined as previously described in the Method section (Assessment of influx transport).

2.5. Inhibition Studies

In the inhibition experiments, efflux of L-lactic acid was assessed in the presence and absence of increasing concentrations of statins and loratadine. In total, 5 compounds were investigated: atorvastatin, loratadine, rosuvastatin, simvastatin hydroxy acid, and simvastatin lactone. Effects of acidic drugs on L-lactic acid transport were tested at concentrations varying from 0.25 to 300 μM. Phloretin (1 to 300 μM) was also evaluated as a known potent MCT inhibitor.

At the beginning of the experiment (*t* = 0), medium was replaced by HEPES (pH 7.4; 1 mL) buffer to wash cells. After removing the wash buffer, cells were loaded with [^{14}C] L-lactic acid (6 mM, 0.2 μCi/mL) in MES or HEPES buffer (pH 7.0 or pH 7.4). Briefly, following pre-incubation of cells in buffer containing [^{14}C] L-lactic acid for 10 min (to allow L-lactic acid to reach equilibrium), the buffer was replaced by a buffer containing [^{14}C] L-lactic acid and the potential inhibitor. This mixture was incubated for an additional 3 min in order to allow diffusion of the inhibitor in the cells without perturbing L-lactic acid equilibrium. Then, cells were washed once rapidly with buffer containing the tested inhibitors or vehicle, but without L-lactic acid. In the final step, the tested inhibitors or vehicle were added to the L-lactic acid-free buffer and incubated for 2.5 min as described previously for the assessment of the efflux transport. Culture plates were placed on ice to stop the reaction. Inhibition of L-lactic acid efflux was determined by measuring intracellular [^{14}C] L-lactic acid concentration.

2.6. Effect of Pretreatment on Lactic Acid Transport

After differentiation, the cells were put in growth media for 24 h. After stabilization, cells were exposed to atorvastatin, simvastatin acid or loratadine (added to the media in DMSO) at clinically relevant concentrations (0.033 and 0.1 μM for atorvastatin, 0.033 and 0.1 μM for simvastatin acid, and 0.023 and 0.07 μM for loratadine) for six days before conducting transport experiments. Separate experiments were thereafter carried out as described previously in the *Transport Studies* and *Inhibition Studies* sections.

2.7. Quantification of Intracellular Concentrations of Statins and Loratadine

HPLC-UV methods were used to quantify atorvastatin, loratadine, rosuvastatin, simvastatin hydroxyl acid, and simvastatin lactone in the intracellular compartment of the cells. Instruments used consisted of a SpectraSystem P4000 pump, a SpectraSystem AS3000 autosampler, a Finnigan SpectraSystem UV6000 ultraviolet detector and a SpectraSystem SN4000 System Controller from Thermo Electron Corporation (San Jose, CA, USA). An Agilent Zorbax Column, Eclipse XDB-C8, 4.6 mm × 150 mm (Agilent, Santa Clara, CA, USA) was used at a temperature of 40 °C. An isocratic mobile phase contained 10 mM ammonium formate pH 3 and acetonitrile with varying proportions, at a flow rate of 1.0 mL/min. Details for mobile phase proportions, internal standards and monitored UV wavelengths are listed in Supplementary Table S1.

The same protocol as described in the *Inhibition Studies* section was used to measure intracellular concentrations of statins and loratadine at the end of the experiments, but without radioactive product (cold L-lactic acid). After the final incubation, cells were washed twice with PBS 10% methanol and once with PBS alone. The cells were lysed with methanol containing appropriate internal standards for the compounds of interest, then transferred and centrifuged for 10 min at room temperature. The supernatant was transferred to a culture borosilicate glass tube, evaporated and reconstituted in 100 µL of 10 mM ammonium formate pH 3 and acetonitrile (50:50 *v/v*). A volume of 20 µL per sample was injected. The ChromQuest Version 4.2.34 software was used for data acquisition.

2.8. Data Analysis

For kinetic studies, the K_m (Michaelis-Menten constant) and V_{max} (maximum uptake rate) of L-lactic acid transport were estimated by non-linear least-squares regression analysis program, GraphPad Prism 5.01 (GraphPad Software Inc., La Jolla, CA, USA) using the following equation:

$$v = V_{max} \cdot [S]/(K_m + [S]) \tag{1}$$

where v and $[S]$ are uptake rate of L-lactic acid at 2.5 min and concentration of L-lactic acid, respectively. CL_{int} and IC_{50} were also estimated using the GraphPad program (Version 5.01). For the IC_{50} determination, the intracellular level of L-lactic acid measured at the end of the 10-min pre-incubation period (when equilibrium was reached, and before adding the inhibitor) was considered as the reference of the maximal intracellular concentration attained beforehand to inhibit the efflux transport.

3. Results

3.1. Kinetic Parameters of L-Lactic acid Transport in SkMC

The time-course for the uptake and efflux of L-lactic acid (6 mM) into SkMC was determined (Figure 2). The uptake and efflux of L-lactic acid were linear for the first minute while displaying a plateau thereafter. Those processes were rapid and most of the transport was completed within five minutes.

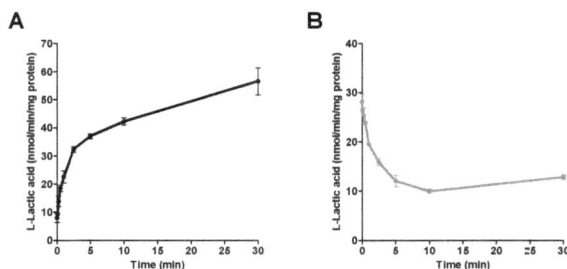

Figure 2. Intracellular concentrations of [^{14}C] L-lactic acid over time: (**A**) the uptake of L-lactic acid (6 mM), and (**B**) the efflux of L-lactic acid in SKMC at an extracellular pH of 7.4 Each point represents the mean ± S.D. of experiments performed in triplicate.

The kinetic parameters of the L-lactic acid influx transport in human skeletal muscle cells are illustrated in the Figure 3. The estimated CL_{int} value for the transport of L-lactic acid in SkMCs was higher at pH 7.0 than at pH 7.4; CL_{int} values were 5.2 $\mu L/min/mg$ protein (V_{max} 90 nmol/min/mg protein; K_m 17 mM) vs. 3.6 $\mu L/min/mg$ protein (V_{max} 82 nmol/min/mg protein; K_m 23 mM), respectively (Figure 3). The intrinsic clearance could be determined only for the influx transport.

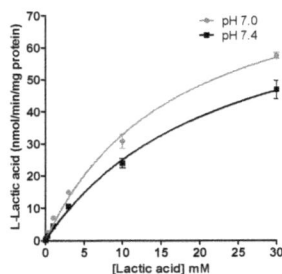

Figure 3. Kinetic parameters of L-lactic acid (0.03 to 30 mM) in SKMC determined at pH 7.0 and pH 7.4. Each point represents the mean $\pm$ S.D. of experiments performed in triplicate.

3.2. L-Lactic Acid Efflux Inhibition by Different Drugs

The inhibition of L-lactic acid efflux by statins and loratadine was tested at pH 7.0 and pH 7.4. In addition to pH 7.4, a more acidic pH value was assessed in order to determine whether an intense physical effort resulting in a lowered pH may modulate the inhibitory potential of the different compounds compared to a physiological pH. Figures 4A and 5A present the intracellular accumulation of L-lactic acid in presence of increasing concentrations of potential inhibitors, i.e., loratadine and statins, respectively. Among the drugs tested, loratadine and atorvastatin had the highest inhibitory potential on the efflux of L-lactic acid. The intracellular L-lactic acid increased 2.5-fold in the presence of 250 μM loratadine at pH 7.4 compared to the control (Figure 4A). Similarly, at the highest tested concentration of 300 μM of atorvastatin, intracellular L-lactic acid was increased by 2.5-fold (Figure 5A). For simvastatin acid (300 μM), the maximal increase of intracellular L-lactic acid was only 35%. No significant inhibitory effect on the efflux transport of L-lactic acid was observed with simvastatin lactone and rosuvastatin (Figure 5A). The IC_{50} values were estimated for the most potent inhibitors of L-lactic acid efflux observed in our study (i.e., atorvastain and loratadine) (Figure 6A,B). Our results showed that, at pH 7.4, loratadine was a more potent MCT inhibitor than atorvastatin on the L-lactic acid efllux, with IC_{50} values of 15 μM and 210 μM, respectively).

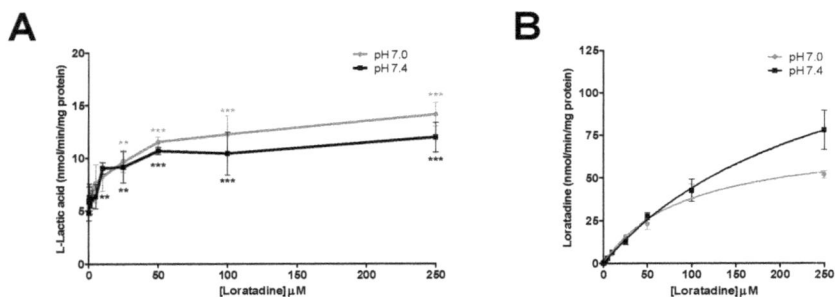

Figure 4. Drug inhibition studies with loratadine in SkMC. (**A**) Inhibitory effects of loratadine on L-lactic acid (6 mM) efflux in SkMC. The residual intracellular [^{14}C] L-lactic acid was measured after 2.5 min of efflux at pH 7.0 and pH 7.4. (**B**) Intracellular concentrations of loratadine at the end of inhibition assays in SkMC at pH 7.0 and pH 7.4. Each point represents the mean $\pm$ S.D. of experiments performed in triplicate (* $p < 0.05$, ** $p < 0.01$ and *** $p < 0.001$).

The pH value had an effect on the basal activity of lactic acid transport. The accumulation of L-lactic acid in the SkMC was higher at pH 7.0 compared to pH 7.4. However, a similar magnitude of inhibition with statin on L-lactic acid transport was observed at pH 7.0 and pH 7.4. Our results showed a 2.7-fold increase in the intracellular concentration of L-lactic acid by atorvastatin 300 μM at pH 7.0 (vs. 2.5-fold at pH 7.4). Similar observations were made with loratadine, which caused similar efflux transport inhibitions of L-lactic acid at pH 7.0 vs. 7.4 (L-lactic acid intracellular concentrations increased by 2.3- vs. 2.5-fold, respectively). Again, under these conditions, simvastatin, lactone and rosuvastatin had no significant inhibitory effect on the transport of L-lactic acid.

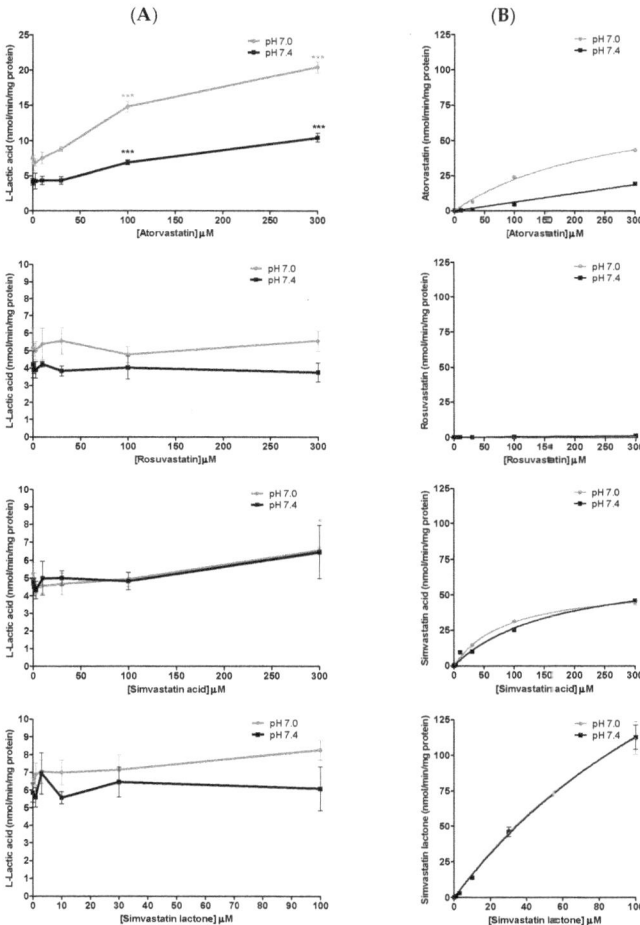

Figure 5. Drug inhibition studies with statins in SkMC. (**A**) Inhibitory effects of different statins (atorvastatin, rosuvastatin, simvastatin hydroxy acid and simvastatin lactone) on L-lactic acid (6 mM) efflux in SkMC. The residual intracellular [^{14}C] L-lactic acid was measured after 2.5 min of efflux at pH 7.0 and pH 7.4. (**B**) Intracellular concentrations of statins (atorvastatin, rosuvastatin, simvastatin hydroxy acid and simvastatin lactone) at the end of inhibition assays in SkMC at pH 7.0 and pH 7.4. Each point represents the mean ± S.D. of experiments performed in triplicate (* $p < 0.05$, ** $p < 0.01$ and *** $p < 0.001$).

A

B

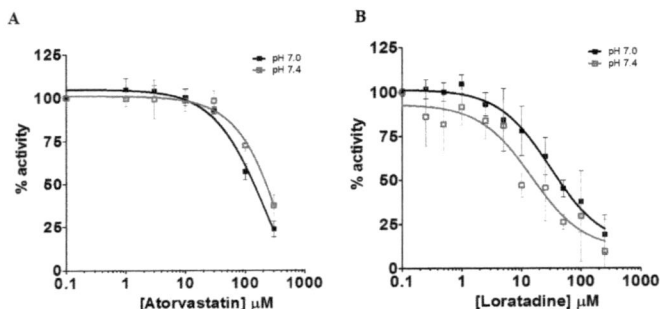

Figure 6. Inhibition of MCT-mediated efflux transport of L-lactic acid measured by the intracellular accumulation of L-lactic acid in the presence of atorvastatin (**A**) or loratadine (**B**). IC_{50} were determined at pH 7.0 and 7.4. The percentage of remaining activity was derived by substracting the maximal level of L-lactic acid after equilibrium to the residual intracellular L-lactic acid concentrations at the end of the experiment.

3.3. Uptake of Different Drugs during Lactic Acid Efflux Inhibition

Figures 4B and 5B illustrate the intracellular concentrations of the tested potential inhibitors, namely, loratadine and statins, respectively. Our results showed a higher accumulation of atorvastatin in SkMC at pH 7.0 compared to pH 7.4. Overall, pH values did not affect the intracellular penetration of simvastatin and loratadine (except at supratherapeutic concentration). Furthermore, rosuvastatin did not have a significant uptake in SkMC.

3.4. Validation of L-Lactic Acid Efflux Inhibition Using a Known Potent MCT Inhibitor

In order to compare the relative potency of the inhibition on L-lactic acid efflux via MCTs obtained with loratadine and statins, inhibition assays were also conducted with phloretin, a potent known MCT inhibitor. As shown in Figure 7, phloretin produced a maximal intracellular L-lactic acid augmentation of 2.1- and 2.2-fold at pH 7.0 and 7.4, respectively, which was similar to the observed inhibition with loratadine or atorvastatin. These results also indicated that the extent of inhibition of phloretin on MCTs was not affected by the pH tested.

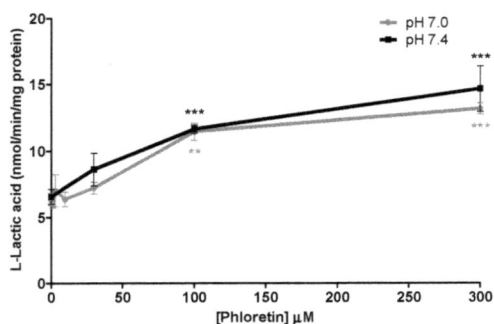

Figure 7. Inhibitory effects of phloretin, a known MCT inhibitor, on L-lactic acid efflux in SkMC. The intracellular [^{14}C] L-lactic acid was measured after 2.5 min of efflux at pH 7.0 and pH 7.4 (** $p < 0.01$ and *** $p < 0.001$).

3.5. Study of Pretreatment with Potential Inhibitors on L-Lactic Acid Transport in SkMCs

The three drugs with the highest potential inhibition (i.e., loratadine, atorvastatin and simvastatin hydroxy acid, based on prior data) of L-lactic acid efflux were selected for this study. Pretreatments with 0.033 μM and 0.1 μM of atorvastatin, 0.033 μM and 0.1 μM simvastatin acid, and 0.023 μM and 0.07 μM of loratadine were done to assess the transport capacity of L-lactic acid in SkMCs; these concentrations were selected based on clinically relevant concentrations, the highest tested concentrations were based on the maximal plasma concentrations for each substrate. Tables 1 and 2 present the effects of various pretreatments with loratadine, atorvastatin or simvastatin hydroxy acid on the basal L-lactic acid transport, both influx and efflux transport were evaluated. Our first observation was that the basal influx activity of L-lactic acid transporters did not change following a pretreatment with either of these drugs (CL_{int} at pH 7.0 vs. 7.4) as seen in Table 1. Our second observation was that pretreatment has no significant effect on the inhibition by statins and loratadine on L-lactic acid efflux transport, as shown in Table 2.

Table 1. Kinetic parameters of L-lactic acid influx following a six-day pretreatment with atorvastatin, simvastatin hydroxy acid and loratadine in SkMC at pH 7.0 and pH 7.4.

Compound	Concentration	CL_{int} (nL/min/mg Protein)	
		pH 7.0	pH 7.4
Atorvastatin	Control	5.2	3.6
	0.033 μM	4.1	3.7
	0.1 μM	4.4	2.7
Simvastatin hydroxy acid	Control	4.5	2.3
	0.033 μM	3.6	2.5
	0.1 μM	2.4	1.5
Loratadine	Control	4.5	2.3
	0.023 μM	3.4	2.4
	0.07 μM	5.3	2.4

Table 2. Intracellular L-lactic acid increase (%) during L-lactic acid efflux inhibition studies following a six-day pretreatment with atorvastatin, simvastatin hydroxy acid and loratadine in SkMC at pH 7.0 and pH 7.4.

Compound [1]	Concentrations Used for the Pretreatment	Intracellular L-Lactic Acid Increase (%)	
		pH 7.0	pH 7.4
Atorvastatin	Control	324	201
	0.033 μM	178 *	306 *
	0.1 μM	258	248
Simvastatin hydroxy acid	Control	91	65
	0.033 μM	103	51
	0.1 μM	31	35
Loratadine	Control	260	215
	0.023 μM	289	168
	0.07 μM	257	226

[1] The higest concentration of inhibitor tested during efflux experiments was used to determine the percentage of intracellular L-lactic acid increase i.e., atorvastatin 300 μM, simvastatin acid 300 μM and loratadine 250 μM and effects of pretreatment on inhibition potential were compared (* $p < 0.02$).

4. Discussion

Our previous studies demonstrated, using cell lines expressing selectively high levels of MCT1 (Hs578T) or MCT4 (MDA-MB-231), that certain acidic drugs inhibit the efflux of L-lactic acid via monocarboxylate transporters [14]. These breast cancer cell line models are great tools for rapidly screening drugs that can potentially cause an intracellular accumulation of L-lactic acid and lead to the observed muscular symptoms. However, the use of these cell lines has some limitations. First, they have a higher MCT expression due to their higher need of energy and metabolism to support their great capacity to proliferate. Second, they are not the most physiologically representative type of cells for studying muscles. To corroborate our previous findings in a more physiologically representative model, we proposed the use of primary SkMCs to confirm the effects of statins and loratadine on L-lactic acid transport.

Skeletal muscles are the major producers of L-lactic acid in the body. Therefore, it is essential that L-lactic acid transporters maintain pH homeostasis, especially during physical effort, where more L-lactic acid is formed. It was reported that physically active patients were more susceptible to experiencing drug-induced muscle disorders [15–18]. The reason and mechanisms underlying this association are not well known; although it has been postulated that coenzyme Q10 deficiency due to statin administration could lead to impaired mitochondrial energy metabolism in muscle cells, the results are still controversial [15,16]. Other hypotheses indicate that the ubiquitin proteasome pathway (UPP), involved in cell degradation and repair, or sarcoplasmic reticulum calcium cycling could be altered by statin therapy [16]. However, another proposed mechanism for drug-induced myopathies involves L-lactic acid transport. Our hypothesis and results are also supported by previous observations indicating that statins could inhibit L-lactic acid transport, causing its intracellular accumulation [19]. It could also be speculated that this effect is mediated by co-transport of statins and L-lactic acid by MCTs, leading to competitive inhibition of the transporters.

Primary SkMCs were used in our experiments as an in vitro model of the actual muscle in order to study drug-induced myopathies. Among the statins tested, only atorvastatin (IC_{50} of 130–210 μM) and simvastatin hydroxy acid (35% increases in lactic acid intracellular levels at 300 μM) were found to be significant L-lactic acid efflux inhibitors. It is important to note that the inhibitory potency of L-lactic acid transport observed for atorvastatin was similar to that of the well characterized MCT inhibitor, phloretin.

As indicated previously, our results corroborate our previous findings, as well as other studies by Kobayashi et al., which showed that some statins—mainly the lipophilic ones, such as atorvastatin and simvastatin acid—can inhibit L-lactic acid transport via MCT4 [14,19]. In their model, they reported greater inhibitory potential for L-lactic acid uptake than the one we observed for its efflux. The differences between the results can be explained by the fact that we measured efflux inhibition, whereas they measured uptake inhibition. Furthermore, they used a much lower L-lactic acid concentration (3.3 μM) than the one used for our experiments (6 mM), as well as different cell models [19–22].

Our results are also in agreement with clinical data (Primo study), in which patients experienced muscular discomfort at a higher rate for statins with greater lipophilicity, such as atorvastatin (14.9%) and simvastatin (18.9%) [23]. Clinically, the higher frequency observed with simvastatin could be due to a greater propensity for drug-drug interactions, since simvastatin has a very low oral bioavailability (<5%) and greater potential for important increases in its exposure [24,25].

Loratadine, an H1 histamine antagonist, has also been reported to cause muscle pain. It is therefore possible that this antihistaminic may cause muscular toxicity through similar mechanisms as statins. Loratadine was determined to be the most potent L-lactic acid efflux inhibitor in this study, with an average IC_{50} of 15 μM at pH 7.4. Since this drug can be obtained without prescription, it is more difficult to estimate the true frequency of loratadine-induced ADR. In the literature, it was reported that loratadine was associated with an increased risk of myopathy in some drug combinations. However, data suggests that these drug interactions do not involve inhibition of its metabolism [26]. It is hypothesized that the interaction might occur at the muscular cellular level. It has been reported that the combination of loratadine and simvastatin is associated with an increased risk for myopathy (RR = 1.69) [27].

We also investigated the effect of pH on the inhibitory potential of some drugs on L-lactic acid transporters. A pH 7.4 milieu was used as the physiological pH level and pH 7.0 was selected as a representative post-exercise physiological condition, since it is known that patients who are more physically active are generally more susceptible to these drug-induced muscular disorders. Overall, we could not demonstrate an increased potency in the blocking of L-lactic acid efflux with a more acidic pH. It could be suggested that a decrease in pH should favor intracellular accumulation of statins or loratadine due to their biophysical properties and passive diffusion. Indeed, we observed an increase in the intracellular concentrations of atorvastatin under a more acidic pH. A trend was observed between the IC_{50} values of loratadine and atorvastatin and their respective intracellular concentrations. A lower IC_{50} was estimated for loratadine at pH 7.4, where its concentrations tended to be higher. For atorvastatin, the higher intracellular concentrations were observed at pH 7.0 and associated with lower IC_{50} for the efflux of L-lactic acid.

The use of primary human skeletal muscle cells also has some limitations. First, SkMCs take an extended period of time to grow and to produce the number of cells needed for the experiment. Second, it takes about one month for each batch of cells to reach maturity, which can impose an inter-batch variability. Moreover, the proportion of differentiated cells may vary for different batches, which could lead to differences in observed basal lactic acid transport activity.

In order to study the effects of statins or loratadine on skeletal muscle during a prolonged period of time, we pretreated the SkMCs with clinical concentrations of atorvastatin, simvastatin and loratadine for 6 days. The results showed that pretreatment with these drugs did not affect L-lactic acid transport activity. Pretreatment with these drugs did not affect their inhibitory potential either. Pre-exposure periods beyond 6 days were not recommended, because of the limited amount of time for which the cells could be kept in culture after differentiation. Additionally, we performed pretreatment assays at higher concentrations to assess the effect of short-term statin treatment on mRNA transporter expression in SkMCs (Supplementary Figure S1). No difference was observed in MCT1 and MCT4 expression between the control and the pretreated batches, which could explain the absence of change in L-lactic acid transport activity levels following pre-exposition to the drug.

In conclusion, we have developed a cell model that can be used to screen for different drugs that may contribute to drug-induced myopathy by inhibiting L-lactic acid efflux. Our experiments determined the inhibitory potential of different statins and loratadine on the transport of L-lactic acid by MCTs in human skeletal cells. Our results demonstrated that loratadine and atorvastatin blocked L-lactic acid efflux transport to a significant extent, and that the magnitude of this effect was not affected by pH variation during physical activity. However, there was a higher basal accumulation of L-lactic acid at pH 7.0 vs pH 7.4. Further studies are required to relate intracellular accumulation of L-lactic acid in skeletal muscle cells and the clinical observation of drug-induced muscle pain.

Supplementary Materials: The following are available online at www.mdpi.com/1999-4923/9/4/42/s1, Figure S1: Relative mRNA expression levels of drug-transporters in SkMC following pretreatment with statins at different concentrations (0.2 and 2 µM of atorvastatin, 0.2 and 2 µM of simvastatin acid, 0.2 and 2 µM of rosuvastatin). Gene expression levels were normalized using GAPDH as an housekeeping gene and vehicle-treated SkMC were used as reference. OATP1B1 was also investigated and no expression of OATP1B1 was detected in any SkMC samples, Table S1: Summary of HPLC analytical method conditions for the quantification of statins and loratadine (flow rate of 1.0 mL/min). Details pertaining to Western blotting method are also available.

Acknowledgments: This work was supported by internal fundings from the CRCHUM, Fondation CHUM and Faculté de Pharmacie, Université de Montreal. Yat Hei Leung was a recipient of a studentship from the Fonds de la Recherche du Québec en Santé (FRQS). Veronique Michaud was the recipient of a research scholarship from FRQS in partnership with the Institut National d'Excellence en Santé et en Services Sociaux (INESSS). We are also grateful to Francois Belanger for his excellent technical assistance. We would like to thank Hasna Maachi for generating the cellular microscopy pictures.

Author Contributions: Veronique Michaud and Jacques Turgeon conceived and designed the study; Yat Hei Leung performed the experiments and the analysis; Yat Hei Leung, Veronique Michaud and Jacques Turgeon interpreted the data; Yat Hei Leung, Veronique Michaud and Jacques Turgeon wrote the paper.

Conflicts of Interest: The authors declare no conflict of interest.

References

1. Kochanek, K.D.; Murphy, S.L.; Xu, J.; Tejada-Vera, B. Deaths: Final data for 2014. *Natl. Vital Stat. Rep.* **2016**, *65*, 1–122. [PubMed]
2. Brahma, D.K.; Wahlang, J.B.; Marak, M.D.; Sangma, M.C. Adverse drug reactions in elderly. *J. Pharmacol. Pharmacother.* **2013**, *4*, 91–94. [CrossRef] [PubMed]
3. Roden, D.M.; George, A.L., Jr. The genetic basis of variability in drug responses. *Nat. Rev. Drug Discov.* **2002**, *1*, 37–44. [CrossRef] [PubMed]
4. Liu, R.; AbdulHameed, M.D.M.; Kumar, K.; Yu, X.; Wallqvist, A.; Reifman, J. Data-driven prediction of adverse drug reactions induced by drug-drug interactions. *BMC Pharmacol Toxicol.* **2017**, *18*, 44. [CrossRef] [PubMed]
5. Ghosh, B.; Sengupta, S.; Bhattacharjee, B.; Majumder, A.; Sarkar, S.B. Fenofibrate-induced myopathy. *Neurol. India* **2004**, *52*, 268–269. [PubMed]
6. Valiyil, R.; Christopher-Stine, L. Drug-related myopathies of which the clinician should be aware. *Curr. Rheumatol. Rep.* **2010**, *12*, 213–220. [CrossRef] [PubMed]
7. Mor, A.; Mitnick, H.J.; Pillinger, M.H.; Wortmann, R.L. Drug-induced myopathies. *Bull. NYU Hosp. Jt. Dis.* **2009**, *67*, 358–369. [PubMed]
8. Sathasivam, S. Statin induced myotoxicity. *Eur. J. Int. Med.* **2012**, *23*, 317–324. [CrossRef] [PubMed]
9. Rizos, C.V.; Elisaf, M.S. Statin myopathy: Navigating the maze. *Curr. Med. Res. Opin.* **2017**, *33*, 327–329. [CrossRef] [PubMed]
10. Dirks, A.J.; Jones, K.M. Statin-induced apoptosis and skeletal myopathy. *Am. J. Physiol. Cell Physiol.* **2006**, *291*, C1208–C1212. [CrossRef] [PubMed]
11. Dalakas, M.C. Toxic and drug-induced myopathies. *J. Neurol. Neurosurg. Psychiatry* **2009**, *80*, 832–838. [CrossRef] [PubMed]
12. Mastaglia, F.L.; Needham, M. Update on toxic myopathies. *Curr. Neurol. Neurosci. Rep.* **2012**, *12*, 54–61. [CrossRef] [PubMed]
13. Lee, A. *Adverse Drug Reactions*, 2nd ed.; Pharmaceutical Press: London, UK, 2006; p. 474.
14. Leung, Y.H.; Lu, J.; Papillon, M.-E.; Bélanger, F.; Turgeon, J.; Michaud, V. The role of MCT1 and MCT4 in drug-induced muscle disorders. Abstract. ASPET 2013. *FASEB J.* **2013**, *27* (Suppl. 1), 674.
15. Bosomworth, N.J. Statin Therapy as Primary Prevention in Exercising Adults: Best Evidence for Avoiding Myalgia. *J. Am. Board Fam. Med.* **2016**, *29*, 727–740. [CrossRef] [PubMed]
16. Parker, B.A.; Thompson, P.D. Effect of statins on skeletal muscle: Exercise, myopathy, and muscle outcomes. *Exerc. Sport Sci. Rev.* **2012**, *40*, 188–194. [CrossRef] [PubMed]
17. Meador, B.M.; Huey, K.A. Statin-associated myopathy and its exacerbation with exercise. *Muscle Nerve* **2010**, *42*, 469–479. [CrossRef] [PubMed]
18. Krishnan, G.M.; Thompson, P.D. The effects of statins on skeletal muscle strength and exercise performance. *Curr. Opin. Lipidol.* **2010**, *21*, 324–328. [CrossRef] [PubMed]
19. Kobayashi, M.; Otsuka, Y.; Itagaki, S.; Hirano, T.; Iseki, K. Inhibitory effects of statins on human monocarboxylate transporter 4. *Int. J. Pharm.* **2006**, *317*, 19–25. [CrossRef] [PubMed]
20. Kobayashi, M.; Kaido, F.; Kagawa, T.; Itagaki, S.; Hirano, T.; Iseki, K. Preventive effects of bicarbonate on cerivastatin-induced apoptosis. *Int. J. Pharm.* **2007**, *341*, 181–188. [CrossRef] [PubMed]
21. Kobayashi, M.; Fujita, I.; Itagaki, S.; Hirano, T.; Iseki, K. Transport Mechanism for L-Lactic Acid in Human Myocytes Using Human Prototypic Embryonal Rhabdomyosarcoma Cell Line (RD Cells). *Biol. Pharm. Bull.* **2005**, *28*, 1197–1201. [CrossRef] [PubMed]
22. Kobayashi, M.; Chisaki, I.; Narumi, K.; Hidaka, K.; Kagawa, T.; Itagaki, S.; Hirano, T.; Iseki, K. Association between risk of myopathy and cholesterol-lowering effect: A comparison of all statins. *Life Sci.* **2008**, *82*, 969–975. [CrossRef] [PubMed]
23. Bruckert, E.; Hayem, G.; Dejager, S.; Yau, C.; Begaud, B. Mild to moderate muscular symptoms with high-dosage statin therapy in hyperlipidemic patients—The PRIMO study. *Cardiovasc. Drugs Ther.* **2005**, *19*, 403–414. [CrossRef] [PubMed]
24. Merck & Co., Inc. *Zocor (Simvastatin) Tablets Prescribing Information*; West Point: New York, NY, USA, 2015.
25. McKenney, J.M. Pharmacologic characteristics of statins. *Clin. Cardiol.* **2003**, *26* (Suppl. 3), III32–III38. [CrossRef] [PubMed]

26. Han, X.; Quinney, S.K.; Wang, Z.; Zhang, P.; Duke, J.; Desta, Z.; Elmendorf, J.S.; Flockhart, D.A.; Li, L. Identification and Mechanistic Investigation of Drug-Drug Interactions Associated With Myopathy: A Translational Approach. *Clin. Pharmacol. Ther.* **2015**, *98*, 321–327. [CrossRef] [PubMed]

27. Duke, J.D.; Han, X.; Wang, Z.; Subhadarshini, A.; Karnik, S.D.; Li, X.; Hall, S.D.; Jin, Y.; Callaghan, J.T.; Overhage, M.J.; et al. Literature based drug interaction prediction with clinical assessment using electronic medical records: Novel myopathy associated drug interactions. *PLoS Comput. Biol.* **2012**, *8*, e1002614. [CrossRef] [PubMed]

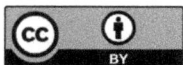

![pharmaceutics logo] *pharmaceutics*

MDPI

Article

Tissue Specific Modulation of cyp2c and cyp3a mRNA Levels and Activities by Diet-Induced Obesity in Mice: The Impact of Type 2 Diabetes on Drug Metabolizing Enzymes in Liver and Extra-Hepatic Tissues

Sarah Maximos [1,2] , Michel Chamoun [3], Sophie Gravel [1,3], Jacques Turgeon [1,2,3] and Veronique Michaud [1,2,3,*]

[1]   Centre de recherche du Centre hospitalier de l'Université de Montréal (CRCHUM),
     Montreal, QC H2X 0A9, Canada; sarah.maximos@umontreal.ca (S.M.); sophie.gravel.3@umontreal.ca (S.G.);
     turgeoja@gmail.com (J.T.)
[2]   Faculty of Medicine, Université de Montréal, Montreal, QC H3T 1J4, Canada
[3]   Faculty of Pharmacy, Université de Montréal, Montreal, QC H3T 1J4, Canada;
     michel_chamoun94@hotmail.com
*   Correspondence: v.michaud@umontreal.ca; Tel.: +1-514-890-8000 (ext. 158)

Received: 31 August 2017; Accepted: 22 September 2017; Published: 26 September 2017

Abstract: Various diseases such as type 2 diabetes (T2D) may alter drug clearance. The objective of this study was to evaluate the effects of T2D on CYP450 expressions and activities using high-fat diet (HFD) as a model of obesity-dependent diabetes in C57BL6 mice. The cyp450 mRNA expression levels for 15 different isoforms were determined in the liver and extra-hepatic tissues (kidneys, lungs and heart) of HFD-treated animals (n = 45). Modulation of cyp450 metabolic activities by HFD was assessed using eight known substrates for specific human ortholog CYP450 isoforms: in vitro incubations were conducted with liver and extra-hepatic microsomes. Expression levels of cyp3a11 and cyp3a25 mRNA were decreased in the liver (>2–14-fold) and kidneys (>2-fold) of HFD groups which correlated with a significant reduction in midazolam metabolism (by 21- and 5-fold in hepatic and kidney microsomes, respectively, $p < 0.001$). HFD was associated with decreased activities of cyp2b and cyp2c subfamilies in all organs tested except in the kidneys (for tolbutamide). Other cyp450 hepatic activities were minimally or not affected by HFD. Taken together, our data suggest that substrate-dependent and tissue-dependent modulation of cyp450 metabolic capacities by early phases of T2D are observed, which could modulate drug disposition and pharmacological effects in various tissues.

Keywords: cytochromes P450; drug metabolism; mRNA; diet induced obesity; diabetes

---

1. Introduction

Type 2 diabetes (T2D) has become a worldwide public health concern as prevalence of the disease continues to rise [1]. In 2014, the American Diabetes Association reported that 29.1 million Americans, or 9.3% of the population, had T2D [2]. In addition to anti-diabetic drugs, T2D patients commonly require multiple drug therapies to treat a wide range of comorbidities such as hypertension, stroke, dyslipidemia, atherosclerosis and coronary artery disease [3]. Clinical practice reveals that T2D patients show highly variable pharmacokinetics and responses to several drugs used to treat T2D and its related comorbidities [4–7]. For instance, variable drug dosages and effects are observed for drugs such as clopidogrel, warfarin, cyclosporine and tacrolimus, as well as for anti-hypertensive and cholesterol lowering drugs [8–14]. Hence, the treatment of co-morbidities in T2D is associated with variable drug response and unexpected toxicities [4,15–17].

Currently, information available on the underlying mechanisms responsible for this variability is uncertain. Patients with T2D have a high prevalence of metabolic syndrome (85% vs. 24% in general population), which is associated with a chronic low-grade inflammatory state [18–20]. Several reports showed that some inflammatory mediators may modulate expression levels and activities of numerous proteins including some isoenzymes of the cytochrome P450 (CYP450) superfamily [21–24]. In fact, interleukin-B (IL-1B), interleukin-6 (IL-6) and interferon-γ (INF-γ) have been associated with decreased expressions and activities of CYP450s, especially of CYP3A, in cultured human hepatocytes [25–27]. It is also known that pathophysiological changes resulting from obesity affect drug-metabolizing enzyme expressions and activities [28–30].

In humans, some studies have reported a decrease in CYP3A4 and an increase in CYP2E1 activities with obesity, while its effects on other isozymes remain uncertain [31–34]. For instance, Woolsey et al. have reported that CYP3A activity and CYP3A4 mRNA expression were reduced in humans and mice with nonalcoholic fatty liver disease [35]. However, results from animal studies are inconsistent from one study to the other [30,36–42]. These discrepancies could be explained by the type of diabetes being studied (i.e., T1D vs. T2D), and the strategy used to induce diabetes (i.e., genetically-modified animals vs. chemicals vs. diet). For instance, down-regulation of CYP1A2 and CYP3A1, and up-regulation of CYP3A2 are observed in Goto–Kakizaki rats (genetic model of non-obese T2D) [43]. Conversely, alloxan or streptozocin were associated with an increase expression of hepatic CYP1A2, CYP2B1/2, CYP3A1/23 and CYP2E1 in diabetic rats compared to controls [44–49]. No alteration in hepatic levels of cyp1a2 and cyp2e1 has been found in streptozocin-induced diabetic mice [41]. A study from Ghose et al. revealed a decrease of cyp3a activity, but unaffected cyp1a2 and cyp2e1 activities in high-fat diet (HFD) fed mice [38]. Finally, no difference was observed for cyp3a11 expression or activity in db/db mice (a genetic T2D mouse model) [37].

Several organs express various combinations of CYP450s and, thus, different patterns of CYP450 expression in tissues may be a key determinant of variability observed for drug response. Although extra-hepatic CYP450 activity is manifested to a lower magnitude compared to the liver [50], variability in tissue-specific metabolizing CYP450 enzymes may lead to variation in drug effects due to local metabolism in target organs. To date, there is a paucity of information on the influence of pathophysiological conditions such as T2D on the activity and expression of extra-hepatic CYP450s.

In this study, we sought to determine the effects of T2D on the expression and activities of hepatic and extra-hepatic CYP450 enzymes using the high fat-diet (HFD) diet-induced obesity (DIO) C57BL6 mouse as a T2D model [51]. DIO mice were stratified into two groups according to the effect of HFD on their body weight at the end of the treatment period: low-diet responders and high-diet responders. These two groups have been well characterized and correspond to the early diabetes situation observed in obese humans [51]. An extensive phenotyping characterization was conducted in many organs (liver, kidneys, lungs and heart) to assess the tissue-specific modulation of cyp450 expressions and activities.

2. Materials and Methods

2.1. Chemicals

Ebastine, hydroxyebastine, carboxyebastine, desalkylebastine, hydroxyebastine-d5, carebastine-d5, desalkylebastine-d5, bufuralol, hydroxybufuralol, hydroxybufuralol-d9, repaglinide, 2-despiperidyl-2-amino repaglinide (M1), 3′-hydroxyrepaglinide (M4), bupropion, hydroxubupropion, hydroxybupropion-d5, hydroxytolbutamide, carboxytolbutamide, 1′-hydroxytolbutaminde-d9, 4′-carboxytolbutamide-d9, 4-hydroxymidazolam, 4-hydroxymidazolam-d5, 6-hydroxychlorzoxazone and 12-hydroxydodecanoic-d20 acid were purchased from Toronto Research Chemicals (Toronto, ON, Canada). Hydroxychlorzoxazone-d2 was obtained from TLC PharmaChem (Mississauga, ON, Canada). Midazolam and 1′-hydroxymidazolam-d4 were purchased from Cerilliant (Round Road,

TX, USA). Chlorzoxazone, tolbutamide, dodecanoic acid, β-Nicotinamide-Adenine Dinucleotide Phosphate (NADP), glucose-6-phosphate (G6P), glucose-6-phosphate dehydrogenase (G6PD), dimethyl sulfoxide (DMSO), trishydroxymethylaminomethame (TRIS), and phenylmethanesulfonyl (PMSF) were purchased from Sigma-Aldrich (St. Louis, MO, USA). Ethynediaminetetraacetic acid (EDTA) and dithiothreitol were obtained from Bishop (Burlington, ON, Canada) and from Gibco®, Life Technologies Ltd. (Eugene, OR, USA), respectively. All other chemicals used were commercially available and were of analytical grade.

2.2. Animals

Five-week-old male C57BL/6 mice (n = 45) were purchased from Charles River Laboratories (Montreal, QC, Canada). Animals were housed in a temperature-, light-, and humidity-controlled environment, they were housed 2 per cage and were maintained at an ambient temperature of 21 °C on a 12-h light/dark cycle with free access to water and food ad libitum. The obese diabetic mice were developed according to the experimental protocol described previously [51]. Briefly, one week after their arrival, mice (mean weight 20.0 ± 1.0 g) were fed with a high-fat diet (HFD) (Bio-Serv Diet #F3282, Frenchtown, NJ, USA, 60% fat by energy) or the standard normal diet (ND) (Teklad Global 18% protein diet; Harlan Teklad, Madison, WI, USA, 15% fat by energy) for 8 weeks. Body weight was measured weekly while blood glucose and insulin were determined at Week 8. After 8 weeks of diet, HFD mice were stratified according to their body weight and two groups were formed as follows; low responders to HFD (LDR) (<39.9 g) and high responders to HFD (HDR) (39.9–45 g). Peyot et al. have demonstrated that the LDR are less obese, develop intermediate severity of insulin resistance and have mild impairment in glycemia, while the HDR are more obese, insulin resistant, hyperinsulinemic and hyperglycemic [51]. Animals were sacrificed by cervical dislocation, and organs including heart, lungs, kidneys and liver were quickly excised, washed with cold TRIS 100 mM buffer (pH 7.4) and immersed in liquid nitrogen (−80 °C). Experimental protocols were approved by the institutional committee of animal protection and were carried out in accordance with the Guide for the Care and Use of Experimental Animals of the Canadian Council on Animal Care.

2.3. CYP450 mRNA Levels

2.3.1. Isolation of RNA and Preparation of cDNA

For each organ tested (using a pool of 3 mice/organ), about 100 mg of tissue was homogenized in 1 mL of Trizol and incubated for 5 min at room temperature. Chloroform (200 μL) was added, the mixture shaken for 15 s and then, centrifuged at 16,000× g for 30 min at 4 °C. The aqueous supernatant (500 μL) was transferred and ethanol 70% was added (1:1 v/v). RNA was extracted using the Qiagen kit (RNeasy Mini kit; Qiagen Sciences, MD, USA) according to the manufacturer's recommendations. RNA concentration and quality was assessed by spectrometry. Total RNA (2 μg) from each sample was used for reverse transcription. RNA, random primers (6 μg) and dNTP (25 mM) were preheated for 5 min at 65 °C. Then, 5X-first strand buffer, 80 units of RNAse inhibitor, DTT (0.01 M) and 400 units of Superscript II (Invitrogen, Carlsbad, CA, USA) were added to a final volume of 40 μL. Reverse transcription was carried out for 50 min at 42 °C and stopped by heating to 70 °C for 15 min (final RNA concentration 50 ng/μL). The resulting cDNA was frozen at −80 °C until analyzed.

2.3.2. RT-qPCR Analysis

Real-time quantitative PCR was performed using TaqMan® probe and primer sets from Applied Biosystem (Foster, CA, USA). The assay IDs for selected cyp450s were: cyp2b9 (Mm00657910_m1), cyp2b10 (Mm01972453_s1), cyp2c29 (Mm00725580_s1), cyp2c37 (Mm00833845_m1), cyp2c39 (Mm04207909_g1), cyp2c40 (Mm04204172_mH), cyp2d9 (Mm00651731_m1), cyp2d10 (Mm00731648_m1), cyp2d22 (Mm00530542_m1), cyp2e1 (Mm00491127_m1), cyp2j5 (Mm00487292_m1), cyp2j6 (Mm01268197_m1), cyp3a11 (Mm00731567_m1), cyp3a13 (Mm00484110_m1), cyp3a25

(Mm01209536_m1) and cyp4a10 (Mm01622743_g1). As reference genes, gapdh (Mm99999915_g1) and b2m (Mm00437762_m1) were used as housekeeping genes. cDNA was diluted to 10 ng/reaction, mixed with TaqMan® PCR Master Mix (10 µL) and amplified using cycling conditions as follows: 45 cycles consisting of 10 s at 95 °C and 45 s at 60 °C. Reactions were run in a QuantStudio 6 Flex System (Life Technologies Inc., Burlington, ON, Canada).

The relative quantification of various gene expressions was calculated to the comparative CT method using the formula $2^{-\Delta CT}$ [52,53]. Only CT values ≤ 35 were included in the analyses. Since CT values > 35 were not reliable and considered below the detection level of the assay, a CT value of 35 to 38 was defined not quantifiable (NQ) while a value of CT > 38 as not detectable (ND). For their part, mRNA levels associated with the expression of each isoenzyme under a specific diet condition (ND, LDR, HDR) were determined using a calibrator and the following formula $2^{-\Delta\Delta CT}$ [52]. The calibrator was prepared at the same mRNA concentration using a pool of RNA obtained for each tissue (Clontech A Takara, Bio Company, Mountain View, CA, USA). Determination of mRNA levels was performed in triplicate for each sample, and three independent experiments were repeated to confirm results.

2.4. In Vitro CYP450 Metabolism in Liver and Extra-Hepatic Organs

2.4.1. Preparation of Microsomes

Microsomes from liver, kidneys, lungs and heart were prepared according to our previously described methods with slight modifications [54]. Briefly, tissue (pools of organs from 3 mice) was homogenized in an ice-cold buffer consisting of 50 mM-150 mM-1 mM TRIS-KCL-EDTA buffer (liver and kidneys) or 100 mM-150 mM-1 mM PO_4-KCL-EDTA buffer (lungs and heart) and both buffers containing protease inhibitors namely, PMFS (0.01 mM) and DTT (0.5 mM). Microsomal subcellular fraction was prepared by centrifugation (10,000 $g \times$ 20 min, at 4 °C) followed by ultra-centrifugation (100,000 $g \times$ 90 min, at 4 °C). The microsomal pellets were resuspended in the same buffer (without PMSF and DTT), and frozen at −80 °C until in vitro metabolism experiments were performed. The protein concentration of the microsomes was determined by the Bradford method using bovine serum albumin as the standard.

2.4.2. Effects of the HFD on Hepatic and Extra-Hepatic cyp450 Activities

In order to investigate the effects of the HFD as a representative model of type 2 diabetes on cyp450 activities, in vitro incubations were performed in presence of various microsomes with several probe drugs of CYP450s including bupropion, repaglinide, tolbutamide, bufuralol, chlorzoxazone, ebastine, midazolam and dodecanoic acid, which were used as markers of the functional orthologs of human CYP2B6, CYP2C8, CYP2C9, CYP2D6, CYP2J2, CYP2E1, CYP3A4/5 and CYP4A11, respectively. This study employed cocktails of probe substrates already accepted and validated to investigate the impact of diabetes on specific cyp450 activities. The production of each specific metabolite was quantified from substrate probes and variations of in vitro probes reactions can be inferred to affect all substrates metabolized by the same enzymes.

Assay conditions were previously optimized by standard incubations with probes (buffer, incubation period, protein contents and drug concentrations). All incubations were performed in triplicate. The incubation mixture containing microsomes [5 µL for liver (~20 mg proteins/mL) and 50 µL for kidney, lungs and heart microsomes (~7–14 mg proteins/mL)], NADPH-regenerating system solution (NADP 6.5 mM, G6P 16.5mM, MgCl₂ 5 mM and 0.2 U G6PD) and 100 mM phosphate buffer PO_4 (pH 7.4) or 100 mM TRIS buffer (pH 7.4, for tolbutamide and dodecanoic acid) were pre-incubated in a shaking bath for 10 min at 37 °C. Reaction was initiated by the addition of substrates (bupropion, tolbutamide, bufuralol, chlorzoxazone, midazolam, ebastine, dodecanoic acid or repaglinide) to the incubation mixture (total final volume of 500 µL). Bupropion, chlorzoxazone, ebastine and midazolam were incubated together as a cocktail as previously described whereas the other probe substrates were tested separately. The substrate concentrations used span a range from 38–620 µM for bupropion,

2.5–40 μM for bufuralol, 50–800 μM for chlorzoxazone, 0.125–2 μM for ebastine, 1.25–20 μM for dodecanoic acid, 0.25–4 μM for midazolam, 0.85–14 μM for repaglinide and 25–400 μM for tolbutamide (5 different concentrations were used with liver microsomes while one concentration (>2 km) to ensure saturation was selected to investigate cyp450 activities in extra-hepatic microsomes). After 30 min, the reaction was stopped using 1000 μL of ice-cold internal methanol containing isotope-labeled internal standard probe metabolite(s). Reaction mixtures were put on ice for 10 min, and following a centrifugation at 13,000 rpm for 10 min, and then the supernatant was transferred for analysis. For dodecanoic acid metabolite analysis, the solution was evaporated to dryness at 50 °C under a gentle stream of nitrogen, reconstituted with 200 μL of methanol and transferred to an injection vial for analysis.

2.5. High Performance Chromatography–Mass Spectrometry Analytical Methods

2.5.1. Chromatographic Conditions for the Metabolites of Bupropion, Midazolam and Ebastine

This analysis was performed on a Thermo Scientific Acclaim RSLC Polar Advantage C16 column (75 mm × 3.0 mm, 3 μm) and Phenomenex Security Guard Cartridge (C12, 4 mm × 2 mm) operating at 50 °C. The mobile phase was a gradient elution consisting of (A) 0.1% formic acid in acetonitrile and (B) 10 mM ammonium formate in water adjusted to pH 3; ratio A:B varied from 25:75 to 60:40 (v/v), at a flow rate 500 μL/min (a total run time of 10 min). A 10 μL aliquot of the extract was injected into LC-MSMS system.

A Thermo Scientific TSQ Quantiva Triple Quadrupole mass spectrometer (San Jose, CA, USA) was interfaced with a Thermo Scientific Ultimate 3000 XRS UHPLC system (San Jose, CA, USA) using a pneumatic assisted heated electrospray ion source. MS detection was performed in positive ion mode using selected reaction monitoring (SRM). Selection of optimal transitions and collision energy and tube lens voltage conditions for the metabolites and their respective internal standard are listed in Table S1.

2.5.2. Chromatographic Conditions for the Metabolites of Chlorzoxazone, Tolbutamide, Dodecanoic Acid, Bufuralol and Repaglinide

These analyses were carried out on a Phenomenex Luna PFP (2) column (150 mm × 3.0 mm I.D., 3 μm) with a Phenomenex PFP security guard cartridge operating at 40 °C. A mobile phase in isocratic mode was composed of acetonitrile and 0.01% formic acid having a fixed ratio of 40:60 (v/v) for chlorzoxazone, tolbutamide and dodecanoic acid, while a ratio of 50:50 was used for bufuralol and repaglinide. The flow rate was 0.30 mL/min (total run time 10 min). A 10 μL aliquot of the extract was injected into the LC-MSMS system.

The HPLC system consisted of a Shimadzu Prominence series UFLC pump and auto sampler (Kyoto, Japan). The tandem MS system used was a Thermo TSQ Quantum Ultra (San Jose, CA, USA). The mass spectrometer was interfaced with the HPLC system using a pneumatic assisted heated electrospray ion source. MS detection was performed in negative ion mode for chlorzoxazone, tolbutamide, and dodecanoic acid metabolites, and in positive ion mode for bufuralol and repaglinide metabolites using selected reaction monitoring (SRM). Selection of optimal transitions and collision energy and tube lens voltage conditions for the metabolites and their respective internal standard are shown in Table S2.

2.6. Statistical Analysis

Calibration curves were calculated from the equation $y = ax + b$, as determined by weighted $1/x$ and $1/x^2$ linear regressions of the calibration lines constructed from the peak-area ratios of metabolites to the internal standard (XCalibur software, Thermo Fisher, San Jose, CA, USA). Relative expression levels of CYP450s mRNAs were analyzed by one-way analysis of variance followed by the Dunnett post-hoc test. A difference with $p < 0.05$ was considered statistically significant. Enzyme kinetic parameters were determined by non-linear regression analysis using Michaelis–Menten equation and Lineweaver–Burk double reciprocal plot and data points were expressed as the mean $\pm$ S.D., K_m and V_{max} values and the 95% confidence interval for the intrinsic clearance. Data were analyzed using GraphPad Prism 5 (GraphPad Software, La Jolla, CA, USA) and SAS statistical software (Version 9.4 of the SAS System for Windows, Copyright©, SAS Institute Inc., Cary, NC, USA).

3. Results

3.1. Animal Model

Although no animal model exactly reflects human T2D, some have similar features. Human T2D is a heterogeneous disorder with a complex interplay between genetic, epigenetic and environmental factors. On one hand, diabetic animal models including chemically-induced or surgically-provoked develop hyperglycemia primarily by cytotoxic actions on beta cells rather than through insulin resistance. On the other hand, transgenic/knockout model are more useful to investigate the role of a specific candidate gene unlike heterogeneity as seen in humans. Moreover, the observed diabetes conditions are less stable; chemicals can produce toxic actions and development of digestive problems can be observed which could also affect CYP450 activities. Consequently, a validated nutritionally (high-fat diet; HFD) obese mouse model has been selected to characterize the effects of obesity-induced diabetes on CYP450 activities [51].

Weight, glycemia and insulinemia measured at week 8 were as follow; 29.2 ± 1.1 g, 9.7 ± 0.3 mmol/L and 1.37 ± 0.35 ng/mL in the chow-fed control group ($n = 12$); 36.4 ± 0.9 g, 9.4 ± 0.5 mmol/L and 2.59 ± 0.44 ng/mL for the LDR group ($n = 12$) and 43.1 ± 0.6 g, 10.5 ± 0.4 mmol/L and 6.82 ± 1.32 ng/mL, for the HDR group ($n = 16$), respectively. Weight, glycemia and insulinemia parameters were significantly higher for HFD groups compared to the control group ($p < 0.05$). Five mice were considered as extreme responders (outliers) since their weight was over 45.0 g and were excluded from our analysis.

3.2. Effects of HFD on cyp450 mRNA Expression Levels

3.2.1. General Pattern of cyp450 Expression

The relative expression of total cyp450 mRNA levels for 15 cyp450 isoforms found in hepatic and extra-hepatic tissues are illustrated for chow-fed control group (ND) and HFD groups in Figure 1 (and Table S3). Major differences were observed in the expression pattern of various cyp450s among tissues. On the other hand, the pattern of cyp450 expression was rather similar among the different diet group: hence, the HFD did not change the pattern of relative cyp450 expression levels in a specific organ. The highest relative levels of mRNAs were cyp2e1 in the liver, cyp2j5/cyp2e1 in kidneys, and cyp2d22 in both heart and lung tissues. The cyp2d, cyp2e and cyp2j subfamilies were expressed in all organs tested (i.e., liver, kidneys, heart and lungs). Moreover, high levels of cyp2b10 (representing approximately 20% of cyp450 mRNA expression) were also observed in the lungs.

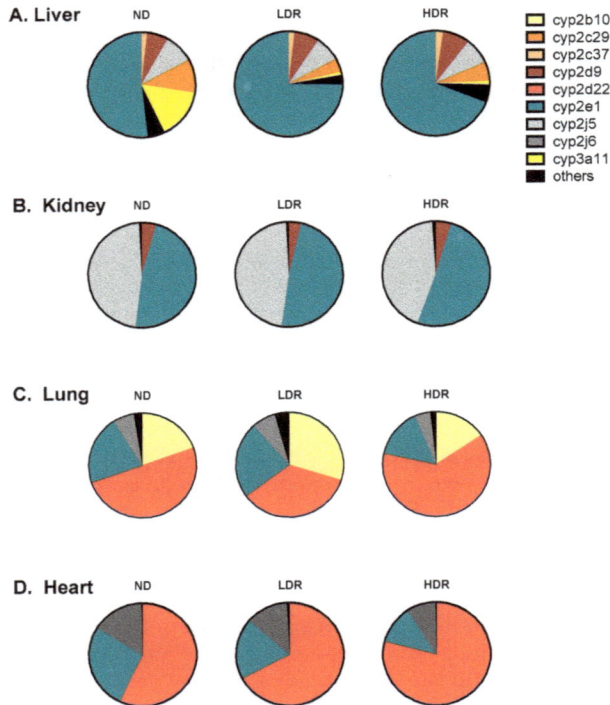

Figure 1. Cyp450 mRNA pie charts. Total mRNA transcripts for each isoenzyme are displayed as expressed in C57BL6 mouse microsomes according to diet group: (**A**) Liver; (**B**) Kidney; (**C**) Lung; and (**D**) Heart. ND, Normal diet; LDR, low-diet responders; and HDR, high-diet responders. Cyp450 mRNA transcript with a relative contribution >1% are illustrated, and "others" have a relative contribution <1%. Others include the following isoforms: Liver, cyp2b10, cyp2b29, cyp2c39, cyp2c40, cyp2d22, cyp2j6, cyp3a13, cyp3a25, and cyp4a10; Kidneys, cyp2b10, cyp2b29, cyp2c29, cyp2c37, cyp2c39, cyp2c40, cyp2d22, cyp2j6, cyp3a11, cyp3a13, cyp3a25, and cyp4a10; and Lungs, cyp2b29, cyp2c29, cyp2c37, cyp2c39, cyp2c40, cyp2d9, cyp2j5, cyp3a11, cyp3a13, cyp3a25, and cyp4a10.

3.2.2. Modulation of cyp450 mRNA Expression by HFD

Table 1 presents the relative mRNA transcripts for each cyp450 isoform found in each individual organ under HFD (LRD and HRD) vs. normal chow-diet (ND). Overall, our results showed that HFD altered the profile of mRNA expression in an isoenzyme-specific manner. Moreover, HFD altered the expression profile of cyp450 mRNAs in a tissue-specific fashion. Our major findings were: (1) mRNA levels of cyp3a11 were significantly decreased (approximately 14-fold) in the liver of both HFD groups (LRD and HRD) compared to ND ($p < 0.001$); (2) in contrast, a two-fold increase of hepatic mRNA levels of cyp2b9 ($p < 0.001$), cyp2c39 ($p < 0.01$) and cyp4a10 ($p < 0.05$) were observed in HDR compared to ND; and (3) cyp2b10 ($p < 0.01$) was also increased by two folds in the lungs.

Table 1. Relative mRNA transcripts for each cyp isoform in C57B/6 mice microsomes according to diet group.

Tissue	Diet	cyp2b9	cyp2b10	cyp2c29	cyp2c37	cyp2c39	cyp2c40	cyp2d9	cyp2d22	cyp2e1	cyp2j5	cyp2j6	cyp3a11	cyp3a13	cyp3a25	cyp4a10
Liver	ND	0.01	0.02	0.49	1.31	0.01	0.44	0.55	0.53	0.56	0.98	1.08	0.58	2.40	0.44	1.25
	LDR	4.89 *	NQ	0.25 *	1.77	0.01	0.20	0.81	0.59	1.02	1.05	0.88	0.04 †	3.07	0.17	1.22
	HDR	8.51 †	0.03	0.30	2.15	0.02 **	0.37	0.71	1.03	0.79	0.90	1.09	0.04 †	2.96	0.21	3.72
Kidney	ND	ND	0.54	2.35	ND	ND	8.62	1.65	1.32	1.28	4.89	4.56	1.41	1.37	2.00	1.42
	LDR	ND	0.46	3.08	ND	ND	3.08	1.35	1.38	1.29	4.68	4.62	0.57	2.12	1.79	1.13
	HDR	ND	0.42	1.59	ND	ND	5.92	1.65	1.50	1.29	4.18	4.03	0.72	2.41	0.95	2.43
Heart	ND	ND	1.21	0.26	ND	ND	ND	0.05	3.24	0.96	0.09	2.19	ND	NQ	ND	1.09
	LDR	ND	2.16	0.49	ND	ND	ND	0.07	3.40	0.62	0.19	1.85	ND	NQ	ND	2.15
	HDR	ND	1.68	0.30	ND	ND	ND	0.07	5.03	0.51 *	0.19	1.67	ND	NQ	NQ	1.47
Lung	ND	ND	0.73	1.11	ND	ND	ND	0.07	2.06	0.21	0.13	1.20	ND	3.26	0.06	3.28
	LDR	ND	1.66 †	2.96	ND	ND	ND	0.08	2.05	0.33 **	0.47	1.88	ND	8.15 **	0.07	9.90 *
	HDR	ND	1.17 **	1.00	ND	ND	ND	ND	5.76	0.32 *	0.83	1.69	ND	5.39	0.11	3.43

Results are expressed as mean N-fold differences in cyp gene relative to the average expression of housekeeping genes and a calibrator ($2^{-\Delta\Delta Ct\ sample}$). ND, Normal diet; LDR, low-diet responders; and HDR, high-diet responders. NQ = Not Quantifiable ($35 < Ct < 38$). ND = Not Detectable ($Ct > 38$). Each experiment was performed three times and in triplicates. One-way ANOVA was performed with Dunnett post-hoc test. LDR or HDR versus ND; * $p < 0.05$, ** $p < 0.01$, † $p < 0.001$.

3.3. Modulation of cyp450 Hepatic Activities by DIO Mouse as a Model of T2D

3.3.1. Hepatic Activities

As shown in Figure 2 (Table 2), HFD induced variations in hepatic cyp450 activities in an isoform-dependent manner. A significant decrease in midazolam metabolism, a marker of cyp3a subfamily, was observed following HFD treatment; the intrinsic clearance of 1-hydroxymidazolam was reduced in LDR and HDR (23 and 40 µL/min/mg prot) groups compared to ND (107 µL/min/mg prot) ($p < 0.001$) (Table S4). This was mostly explained by a decrease in V_{max}; formation of 1-hydroxymidazolam decreased from 0.32 (ND) to 0.06 nmol/mg protein/min (LDR and HDR, $p < 0.001$) (Table 2). HFD treatment was also associated with a diminished hepatic activity of cyp2c subfamilies compared to ND group. The intrinsic clearance of tolbutamide (used as a probe of CYP2C9 in human) was significantly reduced from 0.80 to 0.54 and 0.57 µL/min/mg prot in ND, LDR and HDR groups, respectively ($p < 0.05$) (Table S4). Similarly, HFD affected also the repaglinide hydroxylation (CL_{int} to M1-hydroxyrepaglinide) from 10.6 µL/min/mg prot in ND compared to 1.0–1.4 µL/min/mg prot in HFD groups) (Table S4). Cyp2b activity as measured by bupropion hydroxylation tended to be slightly decreased in HDR group (CL_{int} in HDR vs. ND reduced by 22%). In contrast, no significant effect was observed on the hepatic hydroxylation of bufuralol (cyp2d), dodecanoic acid (cyp4a), chlorzoxazone (cyp2e1) and ebastine (cyp2j) as demonstrated by comparable pharmacokinetics values (Table 2).

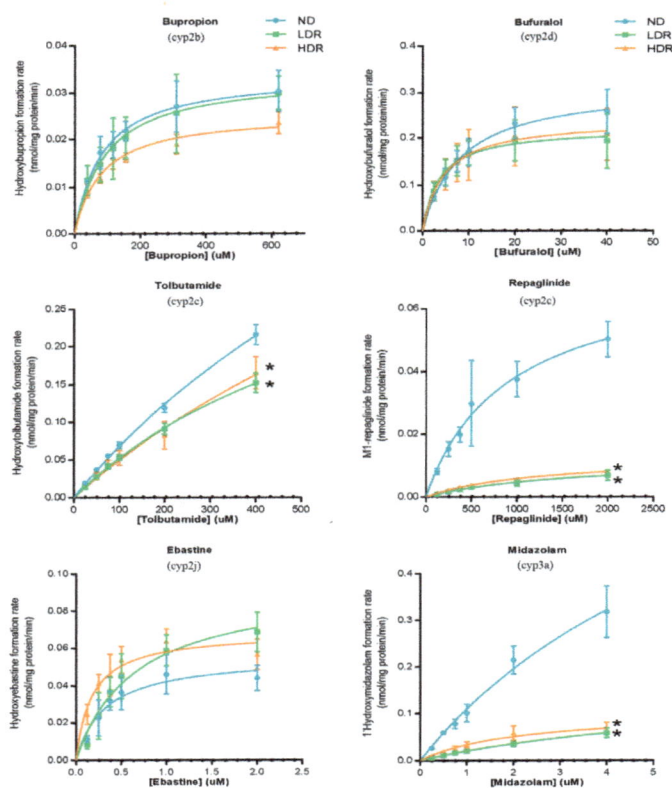

Figure 2. *Cont.*

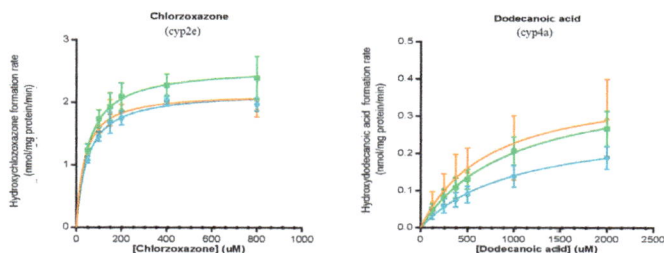

Figure 2. Hepatic cyp450 activities of cyp2b (bupropion), cyp2c (tolbutamide and repaglinide), cyp2d (bufuralol), cyp2e (chlorzoxazone), cyp2j (ebastine), cyp3a (midazolam) and cyp4a (dodecanoic acid) in C57BL6 mice fed a normal diet (ND) or a HFD (LDR, low-diet responders; and HDR, high-diet responders after an eight-week period of treatment). Data were expressed as the mean ± S.D. LDR or HDR vs. ND; * $p < 0.05$. N/F; activity not found, N/A; Not Available (in vitro incubation could not be determined) and dotted line represents the limit of quantification.

Table 2. Hepatic microsome activities for cyp2b (bupropion), cyp2c (tolbutamide and repaglinide), cyp2d (bufuralol), cyp2e (chlorzoxazone), cyp2j (ebastine), cyp3a (midazolam) and cyp4a (dodecanoic acid) in C57BL6 mice fed a normal diet (ND) or a HFD (LDR, low-diet responders; and HDR, high-diet responders after an eight-week period).

Liver	ND	LDR	HDR
	(nmol/mg protein/min)		
Bupropion → Hydroxybupropion	0.030 ± 0.004	0.030 ± 0.004	0.023 ± 0.002 **
Tolbutamide → Hydroxytolbutamide	0.22 ± 0.01	0.15 ± 0.01 ‡	0.17 ± 0.02 ‡
Repaglinide → M1-repaglinide	0.050 ± 0.006	0.007 ± 0.002 ‡	0.0081 ± 0.0003 ‡
Repaglinide → Hydroxyrepaglinide	0.0020 ± 0.0001	0.0010 ± 0.0002 ‡	0.0013 ± 0.0004 **
Bufuralol → Hydroxybufuralol	0.26 ± 0.05	0.19 ± 0.06	0.21 ± 0.06
Chlorzoxazone → Hydroxychlorzoxazone	2.0 ± 0.1	2.4 ± 0.3 **	1.9 ± 0.1
Ebastine → Hydroxyebastine and carebastine	0.044 ± 0.007	0.07 ± 0.01 ‡	0.057 ± 0.008 *
Midazolam → 1′-hydroxymidazolam	0.32 ± 0.06	0.06 ± 0.01 ‡	0.06 ± 0.01 ‡
Dodecanoic acid → 12-hydroxydecanoic acid	0.19 ± 0.03	0.27 ± 0.05	0.3 ± 0.1 *

Cyp450 activities are reported as the rate of metabolite formation in nmol/mg protein/min ± SD (* $p < 0.05$, ** $p < 0.01$, ‡ $p < 0.001$ compared to ND).

3.3.2. Extra-Hepatic Activities

Figure 3 (Table 3) illustrates the effects of diabetes induced by HFD on the formation rate of cyp450 probe metabolites measured in extra-hepatic tissues. A tissue-dependent modulation of cyp450 activities by HFD was observed. In the kidneys, HFD treatment produced a significant decrease in cyp3a activity; formation rate of 1-hydroxymidazolam was three- and five-times lower in LDR and HDR groups, respectively, compared to ND group ($p < 0.001$) (Table 3(A)). In contrast, the cyp3a activity measured in the lung was not affected by the HFD indicating a tissue-dependent modulation of cyp450 by HFD. No cyp3a activity was detectable in mouse hearts.

Our data showed that the formation of hydroxybupropion was approximately 20–50-times greater in the lungs compared to the liver and kidneys (regardless of the diet groups, $p < 0.0001$) (Table 3(B)). Renal and lung microsomes displayed a slight decrease in the hydroxylation of bupropion in HDR group vs. control diet group ($p < 0.01$) (Figure 3). Although the magnitude of activity was low, a similar observation was made for the hydroxylation of bupropion in the heart (0.150 vs. 0.037 and 0.025 pmol/mg protein/min in ND vs. LDR and HDR, respectively, $p < 0.001$) (Table 3(C)). In addition, ebastine (cyp2j) and dodecanoic acid (cyp4a) metabolisms were reduced by HFD, particularly in HDR, in renal and lung tissues. Ebastine hydroxylation in heart microsomes was not affected by HFD, whereas cyp4a activity could not be detected. In contrast, our results showed that DIO mouse were associated with an increase in tolbutamide (~20–50%) and bufuralol (~90–110%) metabolic activities in kidneys, while in lung microsomes, the hydroxylation of tolbutamide and bufuralol tended to decrease ($p < 0.01$ and $p < 0.001$, respectively, in HDR group). Overall, cyp450 activities tended to be reduced in HFD group with greater effects being observed in HDR.

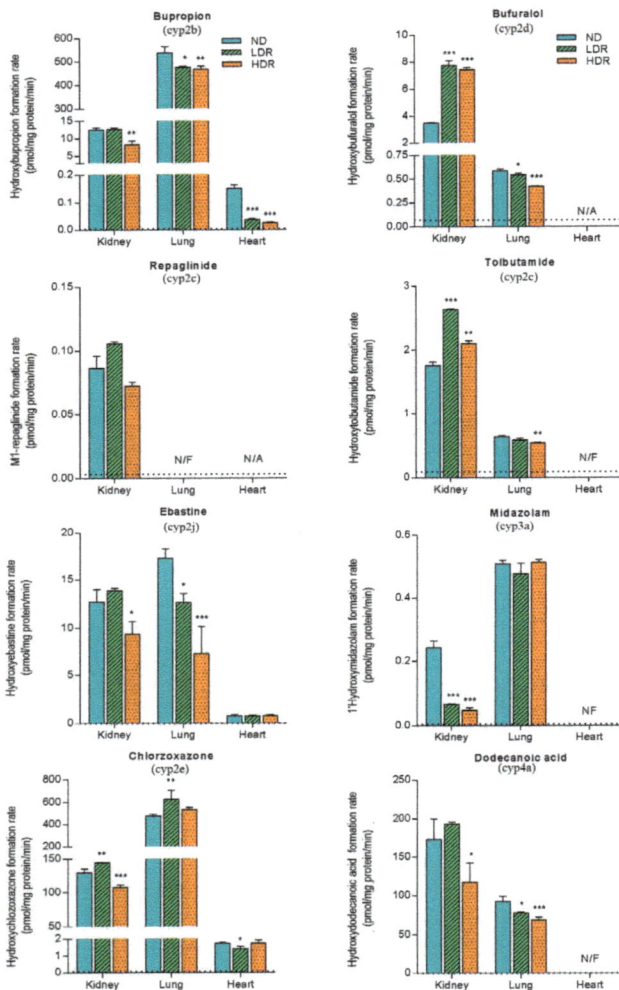

Figure 3. Extrahepatic cyp450 microsomal activities for cyp2b (bupropion), cyp2c (tolbutamide and repaglinide), cyp2d (bufuralol), cyp2e (chlorzoxazone), cyp2j (ebastine), cyp3a (midazolam) and cyp4a (dodecanoic acid) measured in the kidneys, lungs and heart in C57BL6 mice fed a normal diet (ND) or a HFD (LDR, low-diet responders; and HDR, high-diet responders after an eight-week period). Bars and error bars represent the mean ± SD, respectively. LDR or HDR vs. ND; * $p < 0.05$, ** $p < 0.01$, *** $p < 0.001$. N/F; activity not found, N/A; Not Available (in vitro incubation could not be determined) and dotted line represents the limit of quantification.

Table 3. Extra-hepatic microsome activities for cyp2b (bupropion), cyp2c (tolbutamide and repaglinide), cyp2d (bufuralol), cyp2e (chlorzoxazone), cyp2j (ebastine), cyp3a (midazolam) and cyp4a (dodecanoic acid) in C57BL6 mice fed a normal diet (ND) or a HFD (LDR, low-diet responders; and HDR, high-diet responders after an eight-week period): (**A**) renal microsomes; (**B**) lung microsomes; and (**C**) heart microsomes.

(A)			
Kidney	**ND**	**LDR**	**HDR**
	(pmol/mg protein/min)		
Bupropion → Hydroxybupropion	12.5 ± 0.6	12.6 ± 0.4	8 ± 1 **
Tolbutamide → Hydroxytolbutamide	1.76 ± 0.06	2.63 ± 0.01 ‡	2.10 ± 0.04 **
Repaglinide → M1-repaglinide	0.09 ± 0.01	0.105 ± 0.002	0.073 ± 0.003
Bufuralol → Hydroxybufuralol	3.50 ± 0.03	7.7 ± 0.4 ‡	7.4 ± 0.2 ‡
Chlorzoxazone → Hydroxychlorzoxazone	130 ± 6	144.6 ± 0.2 **	108 ± 3 **
Ebastine → Hydroxyebastine and carebastine	13 ± 1	13.9 ± 0.3	9 ± 1 *
Midazolam → 1'-hydroxymidazolam	0.24 ± 0.02	0.065 ± 0.002 ‡	0.047 ± 0.008 ‡
Dodecanoic acid → 12-hydroxydecanoic acid	173 ± 27	193 ± 3	118 ± 24 *

(B)			
Lung	**ND**	**LDR**	**HDR**
	(pmol/mg protein/min)		
Bupropion → Hydroxybupropion	538 ± 26	476 ± 4 *	467 ± 14 **
Tolbutamide → Hydroxytolbutamide	0.64 ± 0.02	0.59 ± 0.03	0.54 ± 0.01 **
Repaglinide → M1-repaglinide	N/F	N/F	N/F
Bufuralol → Hydroxybufuralol	0.59 ± 0.02	0.55 ± 0.02 *	0.425 ± 0.001 ‡
Chlorzoxazone → Hydroxychlorzoxazone	477 ± 16	629 ± 79 **	535 ± 19
Ebastine → Hydroxyebastine and carebastine	17 ± 1	12.6 ± 0.9 *	7 ± 3 ‡
Midazolam → 1'-hydroxymidazolam	0.51 ± 0.01	0.47 ± 0.04	0.51 ± 0.01
Dodecanoic acid → 12-hydroxydecanoic acid	93 ± 6	78 ± 1 *	68 ± 4 ‡

(C)			
Heart	**ND**	**LDR**	**HDR**
	(pmol/mg protein/min)		
Bupropion → Hydroxybupropion	0.15 ± 0.01	0.037 = 0.004 ‡	0.025 ± 0.003 ‡
Tolbutamide → Hydroxytolbutamide	N/F	N/F	N/F
Repaglinide → M1-repaglinide	N/A	N/A	N/A
Bufuralol → Hydroxybufuralol	N/A	N/A	N/A
Chlorzoxazone → Hydroxychlorzoxazone	1.7 ± 0.1	1.2 ± 0.1 *	1.7 ± 0.2
Ebastine → Hydroxyebastine and carebastine	0.8 ± 0.1	0.76 ± 0.06	0.78 ± 0.06
Midazolam → 1'-hydroxymidazolam	N/F	N/F	N/F
Dodecanoic acid → 12-hydroxydecanoic acid	N/F	N/F	N/F

Cyp450 activities determined at 3 km are reported as the rate of metabolite formation in pmol/mg prot/min ± SD (* $p < 0.05$, ** $p < 0.01$ and ‡ $p < 0.001$ compared to ND). N/F, activity not found; N/A, Not Available (in vitro incubation could not be determined).

4. Discussion

This study demonstrated that expression and activities of major cyp450s involved in the metabolism of drugs were modulated in DIO C57BL6 mice used as a model of T2D (Table S5). First, we demonstrated that cyp3a expression and activities were decreased by HFD. Second, cyp2c activities were reduced in all organs tested (except for tolbutamide in the kidneys). Finally, cyp2b activity, largely expressed in the lungs, was also decreased by HFD.

C57BL/6 mice were divided into three groups: ND, LDR and HDR. LDR were less obese and developed intermediate severity of insulin resistance, while HDR were more obese and developed severe insulin resistance. The extent of changes in cyp450 activities by HFD tended to be gradually decreased in LDR compared to HDR and some effects being only observed in HDR group. This observation suggests that modulation of some cyp450 activities happens at early stage of pre-diabetes and similar pathways of regulation involved in pre-diabetes development can also intervene on cyp450 activities in an isoform-dependent manner.

Obesity and diabetes have been shown to alter the expression and activity of hepatic CYP450s [14,28,29,35–38,40–42,55–57]. Clinical studies and animal experiments report mostly on hepatic CYP3A since it is the most important isoenzyme involved in the metabolism of prescribed drugs [58,59]. In humans, a significant decrease in CYP3A activity has been reported in diabetic human liver microsomes compared to healthy subjects [56], while a significant increase in CYP2E1 activity has been reported in obese T2D human liver microsomes [33]. In our study, we observed a significant decrease in hepatic cyp3a mRNA expression levels in HFD groups compared to normal diet group. Similarly, decreased levels of cyp3a11 mRNA expression have been reported in DIO mice [38,59,60]. Preliminary results from our clinical study using oral CYP450 probe cocktail demonstrate that oral clearance of midazolam was significantly reduced in subjects with T2D compared to subjects without T2D [61]. Our results on RNA transcripts are also consistent with phenotypic findings showing that cyp3a activity determined via hydroxylation of midazolam was significantly reduced in the two HFD groups compared to control group. In agreement with our finding, CYP3A activity has been reported to be also decreased in Zucker diabetic fatty (ZDF) rats using midazolam and testosterone as probes [40].

There are no or very limited data pertaining to the effects of T2D on cyp2c and cyp2b families. We observed that cyp2c and cyp2b subfamilies mRNA expression levels were not changed in the liver by HFD compared to normal group, except for cyp2b9 which was increased in HFD groups. Our results are in agreement with those reported by Yoshinari et al. and Guo et al. who demonstrated unchanged relative mRNA levels of cyp2c and cyp2b subfamilies in the liver [59,60]. In contrast, it has been reported a decrease of cyp2b10 mRNA levels in CD1 mice fed with HFD [38]. However, the relative hepatic levels of cyp2b10 mRNA measured in our study were very low or below the limit of quantification yielding a comparison analysis unreliable. In addition, our results showed that hepatic cyp2c metabolic activities, using repaglinide and tolbutamide as markers, were significantly decreased in HFD groups. Kim et al. reported that CYP2C catalytic activity determined with diclofenac was decreased in chemically induced diabetes in rats [62]. This finding, in agreement with our study, suggest that CYP2C activities are impaired, thereby lower metabolic clearance can be anticipated for drugs metabolized by CYP2Cs, particularly CYP2C8 or CYP2C9, under conditions associated with pre-diabetes or diabetes.

Our results indicate that cyp2e1 mRNA expression levels and activity remained unchanged and comparable among all groups (HFD and ND). In the same way, expression levels of cyp2e1 mRNA were reported to be unchanged in DIO mice [38,59]. In addition, activity of cyp2e1 was also unaffected in DIO and db/db mice [37,38], but increased activity was shown in ZDF [42]. No alteration in hepatic levels of cyp2e1 was found in streptozocin-induced diabetic mice [41]. These differences in cyp2e1 activity modulation could be function of the animal model of diabetes used and the stage of the disease.

Our data demonstrated a tissue-specific modulation of cyp2b activities by HFD. Indeed, no significant difference was observed for the hydroxylation of bupropion in liver microsomes. However, bupropion hydroxylation was significantly decreased in HFD groups, particularly in the lungs, the heart and kidneys (HDR group only).

To our knowledge, no study has been conducted to assess the impact of HFD induced obesity as a model of early diabetes stage in humans on CYP450s expression or activity in extrahepatic tissues. Although the magnitude of metabolic capacity and significance in total body clearance of extrahepatic CYP450s metabolism are much lower in comparison to hepatic CYP450s, extrahepatic CYP450s metabolism may affect the local exposure to xenobiotics and thus, influence their pharmacological and toxicological effects. For instance, renal cyp450 metabolites of arachidonic acid, 20-HETE and EET, play an important role in the control of blood pressure and the development of acute kidney injury [63]. In fact, arachidonic acid is metabolized by CYP4A and CYP4F families to 20-HETE (vasoconstrictor) and by CYP2C and CYP2J families to EETs (vasodilator). Our results showed a significant decrease in renal activity of cyp4a and cyp2j in the HDR group using dodecanoic acid and ebastine hydroxylation as marker, respectively. This finding indicates that diabetes could influence homeostasis by affecting local biotransformation of endogenous compounds. In high fat diet induced hypertension rats, CYP2C and CYP4A activities were found to be decreased [64]. The discrepancy observed for CYP2C activity can be explained by using different substrate markers (arachidonic acid being not specific for CYP2C but, also a CYP2J substrate).

Little is known about the effects of obesity and diabetes on CYP450 catalytic activities in the lungs, in both humans and animals. Our data showed extensive metabolic activities in lung microsomes for midazolam, bupropion, ebastine and chlorzoxazone corresponding to cyp3a, cyp2b, cyp2j and cyp2e1, respectively. In lung microsomes, HFD was associated with modulation of cyp450 catalytic activity for certain isoforms independently of patterns observed in the liver or in the kidneys. These findings support the concept that CYP450s expressed in the lungs may contribute to drug metabolism for drugs administered intravenously or locally as well as contribute to the first pass metabolism.

In conclusion, the major finding of this study was that HFD affects CYP450 expression and activities in an isoform- and tissue-dependent fashion. Our results clearly indicate that cyp3a and cyp2c metabolic activities were reduced in DIO-T2D mice (Table S5). In humans, these two CYP450 isoenzymes are involved in the metabolism of 80% of medications prescribed in clinical settings. We speculate that modulation of hepatic CYP450s by T2D diabetes may alter drug pharmacokinetics leading to intersubject variability in drug response. In addition, modulation in CYP450s expressed in extra-hepatic organs can cause variations in tissue concentrations of drugs or endogenous compounds leading to impaired pharmacological action of drugs as well as disruption of homeostasis. Therefore, variation in hepatic and extra-hepatic CYP450s makes patients with pre-diabetes and obesity more prone to adverse drug effect, toxicity or inefficacy (e.g., for prodrugs).

Supplementary Materials: Tables S1–S5 are available online at www.mdpi.com/1999-4923/9/4/40/s1.

Acknowledgments: Sarah Maximos was the recipient of a studentship from the Faculté des études supérieures et post-doctorales de l'Université de Montréal and Sophie Gravel was the recipient of a studentship from the Fonds de la Recherche du Québec en Santé (FRQS). This work was supported by Canadian Institutes of Health Research (CIHR) under the grant #299309. Veronique Michaud is the recipient of a research scholarship from FRQS in partnership with the Institut national d'excellence en santé et en services sociaux (INESSS). We thank Thierry Alquier and the CRCHUM Animal core facility for technical support and the experimental protocol for the DIO mice model. We thank Fleur Gaudette and the CRCHUM pharmacokinetics Core Facility for technical support and analytical method development. We are also grateful to Francois Belanger for his excellent technical assistance providing support in the qPCR analysis.

Author Contributions: Veronique Michaud and Jacques Turgeon conceived and designed the experiments; Sarah Maximos, Michel Chamoun (mRNA experiments) and Sophie Gravel (training for microsome and in vitro incubation protocols) performed the experiments; Sarah Maximos, Veronique Michaud and Jacques Turgeon analyzed and interpreted the data; and Sarah Maximos, Veronique Michaud and Jacques Turgeon wrote the paper.

Conflicts of Interest: The authors declare no conflict of interest.

Abbreviations

DIO	diet-induced obesity
DMSO	dimethyl sulfoxide
G6P	glucose-6-phosphate
G6PD	glucose-6-phosphate dehydrogenase
HDR	high-diet responders
HFD	high-fat diet
IFN-γ	interferon-γ
IL-1β	interleukin-1β
IL-6	interleukin-6
LC-MS/MS	liquid chromatography–tandem mass spectrometry
LDR	low-diet responders
NADP	Nicotinamide-Adenine Dinucleotide Phosphate
P450	cytochrome P450
PMSF	phenylmethanesulfonyl

RT-qPCR	real time quantitative polymerase chain reaction
T2D	type 2 diabetes
VHDR	very high-diet responders

References

1. Whiting, D.R.; Guariguata, L.; Weil, C.; Shaw, J. IDF diabetes atlas: Global estimates of the prevalence of diabetes for 2011 and 2030. *Diabetes Res. Clin. Pract.* **2011**, *94*, 311–321. [CrossRef] [PubMed]
2. Centers for Disease Control and Prevention. *National Diabetes Statistics Report: Estimates of Diabetes and Its Burden in the United States, 2014*; U.S. Department of Health and Human Services: Atlanta, GA, USA, 2014.
3. American Diabetes Association. Standards of medical care in diabetes—2015: summary of revisions. *Diabetes Care* **2015**, *38* (Suppl. 1), S4.
4. Pacanowski, M.A.; Hopley, C.W.; Aquilante, C.L. Interindividual variability in oral antidiabetic drug disposition and response: The role of drug transporter polymorphisms. *Expert Opin. Drug Metab. Toxicol.* **2008**, *4*, 529–544. [CrossRef] [PubMed]
5. Nathan, D.M.; Buse, J.B.; Davidson, M.B.; Ferrannini, E.; Holman, R.R.; Sherwin, R.; Zinman, B. Medical management of hyperglycaemia in type 2 diabetes mellitus: A consensus algorithm for the initiation and adjustment of therapy: A consensus statement from the American Diabetes Association and the European Association for the Study of Diabetes. *Diabetologia* **2009**, *52*, 17–30. [CrossRef] [PubMed]
6. Morrish, G.A.; Pai, M.P.; Green, B. The effects of obesity on drug pharmacokinetics in humans. *Expert Opin. Drug Metab. Toxicol.* **2011**, *7*, 697–706. [CrossRef] [PubMed]
7. Cheymol, G. Effects of obesity on pharmacokinetics implications for drug therapy. *Clin. Pharmacokinet.* **2000**, *39*, 215–231. [CrossRef] [PubMed]
8. Akhlaghi, F.; Dostalek, M.; Falck, P.; Mendonza, A.E.; Amundsen, R.; Gohh, R.Y.; Asberg, A. The concentration of cyclosporine metabolites is significantly lower in kidney transplant recipients with diabetes mellitus. *Ther. Drug Monit.* **2012**, *34*, 38–45. [CrossRef] [PubMed]
9. Marques, M.P.; Coelho, E.B.; Dos Santos, N.A.; Geleilete, T.J.; Lanchote, V.L. Dynamic and kinetic disposition of nisoldipine enantiomers in hypertensive patients presenting with type-2 diabetes mellitus. *Eur. J. Clin. Pharmacol.* **2002**, *58*, 607–614. [CrossRef] [PubMed]
10. Kazui, M.; Nishiya, Y.; Ishizuka, T.; Hagihara, K.; Farid, N.A.; Okazaki, O.; Ikeda, T.; Kurihara, A. Identification of the human cytochrome P450 enzymes involved in the two oxidative steps in the bioactivation of clopidogrel to its pharmacologically active metabolite. *Drug Metab. Dispos.* **2010**, *38*, 92–99. [CrossRef] [PubMed]
11. Lenzini, P.; Wadelius, M.; Kimmel, S.; Anderson, J.L.; Jorgensen, A.L.; Pirmohamed, M.; Caldwell, M.D.; Limdi, N.; Burmester, J.K.; Dowd, M.B.; et al. Integration of genetic, clinical, and INR data to refine warfarin dosing. *Clin. Pharmacol. Ther.* **2010**, *87*, 572–578. [CrossRef] [PubMed]
12. Hall, H.M.; Banerjee, S.; McGuire, D.K. Variability of clopidogrel response in patients with type 2 diabetes mellitus. *Diabetes Vasc. Dis. Res.* **2011**, *8*, 245–253. [CrossRef] [PubMed]
13. Jacobson, P.A.; Oetting, W.S.; Brearley, A.M.; Leduc, R.; Guan, W.; Schladt, D.; Matas, A.J.; Lamba, V.; Julian, B.A.; Mannon, R.B.; et al. Novel polymorphisms associated with tacrolimus trough concentrations: Results from a multicenter kidney transplant consortium. *Transplantation* **2011**, *91*, 300–308. [CrossRef] [PubMed]
14. Dostalek, M.; Sam, W.J.; Paryani, K.R.; Macwan, J.S.; Gohh, R.Y.; Akhlaghi, F. Diabetes mellitus reduces the clearance of atorvastatin lactone: Results of a population pharmacokinetic analysis in renal transplant recipients and in vitro studies using human liver microsomes. *Clin. Pharmacokinet.* **2012**, *51*, 591–606. [CrossRef] [PubMed]
15. Manolopoulos, V.G.; Ragia, G.; Tavridou, A. Pharmacogenomics of oral antidiabetic medications: Current data and pharmacoepigenomic perspective. *Pharmacogenomics* **2011**, *12*, 1161–1191. [CrossRef] [PubMed]
16. Manolopoulos, V.G. Pharmacogenomics and adverse drug reactions in diagnostic and clinical practice. *Clin. Chem. Lab. Med.* **2007**, *45*, 801–814. [CrossRef] [PubMed]
17. Holstein, A.; Beil, W. Oral antidiabetic drug metabolism: Pharmacogenomics and drug interactions. *Expert Opin. Drug Metab. Toxicol.* **2009**, *5*, 225–241. [CrossRef] [PubMed]

18. Bano, G. Glucose homeostasis, obesity and diabetes. *Best Pract. Res. Clin. Obstet. Gynaecol.* **2013**, *27*, 715–726. [CrossRef] [PubMed]

19. Paragh, G.; Seres, I.; Harangi, M.; Fulop, P. Dynamic interplay between metabolic syndrome and immunity. *Adv. Exp. Med. Biol.* **2014**, *824*, 171–190. [PubMed]

20. Dandona, P.; Aljada, A.; Bandyopadhyay, A. Inflammation: The link between insulin resistance, obesity and diabetes. *Trends Immunol.* **2004**, *25*, 4–7. [CrossRef] [PubMed]

21. Morgan, E.T. Impact of infectious and inflammatory disease on cytochrome P450-mediated drug metabolism and pharmacokinetics. *Clin. Pharmacol. Ther.* **2009**, *85*, 434–438. [CrossRef] [PubMed]

22. Rendic, S.; Guengerich, F.P. Update information on drug metabolism systems—2009, part II: Summary of information on the effects of diseases and environmental factors on human cytochrome P450 (CYP) enzymes and transporters. *Curr. Drug Metab.* **2010**, *11*, 4–84. [CrossRef] [PubMed]

23. Du Souich, P.; Fradette, C. The effect and clinical consequences of hypoxia on cytochrome P450, membrane carrier proteins activity and expression. *Expert Opin. Drug Metab. Toxicol.* **2011**, *7*, 1083–1100. [CrossRef] [PubMed]

24. Hameed, I.; Masoodi, S.R.; Mir, S.A.; Nabi, M.; Ghazanfar, K.; Ganai, B.A. Type 2 diabetes mellitus: From a metabolic disorder to an inflammatory condition. *World J. Diabetes* **2015**, *6*, 598–612. [PubMed]

25. Sunman, J.A.; Hawke, R.L.; LeCluyse, E.L.; Kashuba, A.D. Kupffer cell-mediated IL-2 suppression of CYP3A activity in human hepatocytes. *Drug Metab. Dispos.* **2004**, *32*, 359–363. [CrossRef] [PubMed]

26. Donato, M.T.; Guillen, M.I.; Jover, R.; Castell, J.V.; Gomez-Lechon, M.J. Nitric oxide-mediated inhibition of cytochrome P450 by interferon-gamma in human hepatocytes. *J. Pharmacol Exp. Ther.* **1997**, *281*, 484–490. [PubMed]

27. Jover, R.; Bort, R.; Gomez-Lechon, M.J.; Castell, J.V. Down-regulation of human CYP3A4 by the inflammatory signal interleukin-6: Molecular mechanism and transcription factors involved. *FASEB J. Off. Publ. Fed. Am. Soc. Exp. Biol.* **2002**, *16*, 1799–1801. [CrossRef] [PubMed]

28. Kotlyar, M.; Carson, S.W. Effects of obesity on the cytochrome P450 enzyme system. *Int. J. Clin. Pharmacol. Ther.* **1999**, *37*, 8–19. [PubMed]

29. Cheng, P.Y.; Morgan, E.T. Hepatic cytochrome P450 regulation in disease states. *Curr. Drug Metab.* **2001**, *2*, 165–183. [CrossRef] [PubMed]

30. Wang, M.; Tian, X.; Leung, L.; Wang, J.; Houvig, N.; Xiang, J.; Wan, Z.K.; Saiah, E.; Hahm, S.; Suri, V.; et al. Comparative pharmacokinetics and metabolism studies in lean and diet-induced obese mice: An animal efficacy model for 11beta-hydroxysteroid dehydrogenase type 1 (11beta-HSD1) inhibitors. *Drug Metab. Lett.* **2011**, *5*, 55–63. [CrossRef] [PubMed]

31. O'Shea, D.; Davis, S.N.; Kim, R.B.; Wilkinson, G.R. Effect of fasting and obesity in humans on the 6-hydroxylation of chlorzoxazone: A putative probe of CYP2E1 activity. *Clin. Pharmacol. Ther.* **1994**, *56*, 359–367. [CrossRef] [PubMed]

32. Emery, M.G.; Fisher, J.M.; Chien, J.Y.; Kharasch, E.D.; Dellinger, E.P.; Kowdley, K.V.; Thummel, K.E. CYP2E1 activity before and after weight loss in morbidly obese subjects with nonalcoholic fatty liver disease. *Hepatology* **2003**, *38*, 428–435. [CrossRef] [PubMed]

33. Wang, Z.; Hall, S.D.; Maya, J.F.; Li, L.; Asghar, A.; Gorski, J.C. Diabetes mellitus increases the in vivo activity of cytochrome P450 2E1 in humans. *Br. J. Clin. Pharmacol.* **2003**, *55*, 77–85. [CrossRef] [PubMed]

34. Fisher, C.D.; Lickteig, A.J.; Augustine, L.M.; Ranger-Moore, J.; Jackson, J.P.; Ferguson, S.S.; Cherrington, N.J. Hepatic cytochrome P450 enzyme alterations in humans with progressive stages of nonalcoholic fatty liver disease. *Drug Metab. Dispos.* **2009**, *37*, 2087–2094. [CrossRef] [PubMed]

35. Woolsey, S.J.; Mansell, S.E.; Kim, R.B.; Tirona, R.G.; Beaton, M.D. CYP3A activity and expression in nonalcoholic fatty liver disease. *Drug Metab. Dispos.* **2015**, *43*, 1484–1490. [CrossRef] [PubMed]

36. Kudo, T.; Shimada, T.; Toda, T.; Igeta, S.; Suzuki, W.; Ikarashi, N.; Ochiai, W.; Ito, K.; Aburada, M.; Sugiyama, K. Altered expression of CYP in TSOD mice: A model of type 2 diabetes and obesity. *Xenobiotica* **2009**, *39*, 889–902. [CrossRef] [PubMed]

37. Lam, J.L.; Jiang, Y.; Zhang, T.; Zhang, E.Y.; Smith, B.J. Expression and functional analysis of hepatic cytochromes P450, nuclear receptors, and membrane transporters in 10- and 25-week-old db/db mice. *Drug Metab. Dispos.* **2010**, *38*, 2252–2258. [CrossRef] [PubMed]

38. Ghose, R.; Omoluabi, O.; Gandhi, A.; Shah, P.; Strohacker, K.; Carpenter, K.C.; McFarlin, B.; Guo, T. Role of high-fat diet in regulation of gene expression of drug metabolizing enzymes and transporters. *Life Sci.* **2011**, *89*, 57–64. [CrossRef] [PubMed]

39. Patoine, D.; Petit, M.; Pilote, S.; Picard, F.; Drolet, B.; Simard, C. Modulation of CYP3a expression and activity in mice models of type 1 and type 2 diabetes. *Pharmacol. Res. Perspect.* **2014**, *2*, e00082. [CrossRef] [PubMed]

40. Zhou, X.; Rougee, L.R.; Bedwell, D.W.; Cramer, J.W.; Mohutsky, M.A.; Calvert, N.A.; Moulton, R.D.; Cassidy, K.C.; Yumibe, N.P.; Adams, L.A.; et al. Difference in the pharmacokinetics and hepatic metabolism of antidiabetic drugs in zucker diabetic fatty and sprague-dawley rats. *Drug Metab. Dispos.* **2016**, *44*, 1184–1192. [CrossRef] [PubMed]

41. Sakuma, T.; Honma, R.; Maguchi, S.; Tamaki, H.; Nemoto, N. Different expression of hepatic and renal cytochrome P450s between the streptozotocin-induced diabetic mouse and rat. *Xenobiotica* **2001**, *31*, 223–237. [CrossRef] [PubMed]

42. Khemawoot, P.; Yokogawa, K.; Shimada, T.; Miyamoto, K. Obesity-induced increase of CYP2E1 activity and its effect on disposition kinetics of chlorzoxazone in Zucker rats. *Biochem. Pharmacol.* **2007**, *73*, 155–162. [CrossRef] [PubMed]

43. Oh, S.J.; Choi, J.M.; Yun, K.U.; Oh, J.M.; Kwak, H.C.; Oh, J.G.; Lee, K.S.; Kim, B.H.; Heo, T.H.; Kim, S.K. Hepatic expression of cytochrome P450 in type 2 diabetic Goto-Kakizaki rats. *Chem. Biol. Interact.* **2012**, *195*, 173–179. [CrossRef] [PubMed]

44. Song, B.J.; Matsunaga, T.; Hardwick, J.P.; Park, S.S.; Veech, R.L.; Yang, C.S.; Gelboin, H.V.; Gonzalez, F.J. Stabilization of cytochrome P450j messenger ribonucleic acid in the diabetic rat. *Mol. Endocrinol.* **1987**, *1*, 542–547. [CrossRef] [PubMed]

45. Dong, Z.G.; Hong, J.Y.; Ma, Q.A.; Li, D.C.; Bullock, J.; Gonzalez, F.J.; Park, S.S.; Gelboin, H.V.; Yang, C.S. Mechanism of induction of cytochrome P-450ac (P-450j) in chemically induced and spontaneously diabetic rats. *Arch. Biochem. Biophys.* **1988**, *263*, 29–35. [CrossRef]

46. Yamazoe, Y.; Murayama, N.; Shimada, M.; Yamauchi, K.; Kato, R. Cytochrome P450 in livers of diabetic rats: Regulation by growth hormone and insulin. *Arch. Biochem. Biophys.* **1989**, *268*, 567–575. [CrossRef]

47. Thummel, K.E.; Schenkman, J.B. Effects of testosterone and growth hormone treatment on hepatic microsomal P450 expression in the diabetic rat. *Mol. Pharmacol.* **1990**, *37*, 119–129. [PubMed]

48. Raza, H.; Ahmed, I.; Lakhani, M.S.; Sharma, A.K.; Pallot, D.; Montague, W. Effect of bitter melon (Momordica charantia) fruit juice on the hepatic cytochrome P450-dependent monooxygenases and glutathione S-transferases in streptozotocin-induced diabetic rats. *Biochem. Pharmacol.* **1996**, *52*, 1639–1642. [CrossRef]

49. Li, L.; Zhang, Y. Changes of CYP2E1 activity in diabetic rat model. *Acta Pharm. Sin.* **1998**, *33*, 891–895.

50. Karlgren, M.; Miura, S.; Ingelman-Sundberg, M. Novel extrahepatic cytochrome P450s. *Toxicol. Appl. Pharmacol.* **2005**, *207*, 57–61. [CrossRef] [PubMed]

51. Peyot, M.L.; Pepin, E.; Lamontagne, J.; Latour, M.G.; Zarrouki, B.; Lussier, R.; Pineda, M.; Jetton, T.L.; Madiraju, S.R.; Joly, E.; et al. Beta-cell failure in diet-induced obese mice stratified according to body weight gain: Secretory dysfunction and altered islet lipid metabolism without steatosis or reduced beta-cell mass. *Diabetes* **2010**, *59*, 2178–2187. [CrossRef] [PubMed]

52. Livak, K.J.; Td, S. Analysis of relative gene expression data using real-time quantitative PCR and the 2(-Delta Delta C(T)) Method. *Methods* **2001**, *25*, 402–408. [CrossRef] [PubMed]

53. Schmittgen, T.D.; Livak, K.J. Analyzing real-time PCR data by the comparative C(T) method. *Nat. Protoc.* **2008**, *3*, 1101–1108. [CrossRef] [PubMed]

54. Michaud, V.; Frappier, M.; Dumas, M.C.; Turgeon, J. Metabolic activity and mRNA levels of human cardiac CYP450s involved in drug metabolism. *PLoS ONE* **2010**, *5*, e15666. [CrossRef] [PubMed]

55. Shayeganpour, A.; Korashy, H.; Patel, J.P.; El-Kadi, A.O.; Brocks, D.R. The impact of experimental hyperlipidemia on the distribution and metabolism of amiodarone in rat. *Int. J. Pharm.* **2008**, *361*, 78–86. [CrossRef] [PubMed]

56. Dostalek, M.; Court, M.H.; Yan, B.; Akhlaghi, F. Significantly reduced cytochrome P450 3A4 expression and activity in liver from humans with diabetes mellitus. *Br. J. Pharmacol.* **2011**, *163*, 937–947. [CrossRef] [PubMed]

57. Patoine, D.; Levac, X.; Pilote, S.; Drolet, B.; Simard, C. Decreased CYP3A expression and activity in guinea pig models of diet-induced metabolic syndrome: Is fatty liver infiltration involved? *Drug Metab. Dispos.* **2013**, *41*, 952–957. [CrossRef] [PubMed]

58. Smith, H.S. Opioid Metabolism. *Mayo Clin. Proc.* **2009**, *84*, 613–624. [CrossRef]

59. Yoshinari, K.; Takagi, S.; Yoshimasa, T.; Sugatani, J.; Miwa, M. Hepatic CYP3A expression is attenuated in obese mice fed a high-fat diet. *Pharm. Res.* **2006**, *23*, 1188–1200. [CrossRef] [PubMed]

60. Guo, Y.; Cui, J.Y.; Lu, H.; Klaassen, C.D. Effect of various diets on the expression of phase-I drug-metabolizing enzymes in livers of mice. *Xenobiotica* **2015**, *45*, 586–597. [CrossRef] [PubMed]

61. Gravel, S.; Grangeon, A.; Gaudette, F.; Chiasson, J.-L.; Dallaire, S.; Langelier, H.; Turgeon, J.; Michaud, V. Type 2 Diabetes modulates CYP450 metabolic activities; an important variability factor in drug response. In Proceedings of the ASCPT 2016, San Diego, CA, USA, 8–12 March 2016.

62. Kim, Y.C.; Oh, E.Y.; Kim, S.H.; Lee, M.G. Pharmacokinetics of diclofenac in rat model of diabetes mellitus induced by alloxan or steptozotocin. *Biopharm. Drug Dispos.* **2006**, *27*, 85–92. [CrossRef] [PubMed]

63. Fan, F.; Muroya, Y.; Roman, R.J. Cytochrome P450 eicosanoids in hypertension and renal disease. *Curr. Opin. Nephrol. Hypertens.* **2015**, *24*, 37–46. [CrossRef] [PubMed]

64. Wang, M.H.; Smith, A.; Zhou, Y.; Chang, H.H.; Lin, S.; Zhao, X.; Imig, J.D.; Dorrance, A.M. Downregulation of renal CYP-derived eicosanoid synthesis in rats with diet-induced hypertension. *Hypertension* **2003**, *42*, 594–599. [CrossRef] [PubMed]

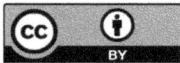

pharmaceutics

MDPI

Article

Pharmacokinetic and Toxicodynamic Characterization of a Novel Doxorubicin Derivative

Samaa Alrushaid [1], Casey L. Sayre [1,2], Jaime A. Yáñez [3], M. Laird Forrest [4],
Sanjeewa N. Senadheera [4], Frank J. Burczynski [1], Raimar Löbenberg [5] and Neal M. Davies [5,*]

[1] College of Pharmacy, Rady Faculty of Health Sciences, University of Manitoba, Winnipeg, MB R3E 0T5,
    Canada; umalrush@myumanitoba.ca (S.A.); csayre@roseman.edu (C.L.S.);
    Frank.Burczynski@umanitoba.ca (F.J.B.)
[2] College of Pharmacy, Roseman University of Health Sciences, South Jordan, UT 84096, USA
[3] YARI International Group, New Brunswick, NJ 08901 and INDETEC Corp., Lima, Peru;
    jaimeyanez@gmail.com
[4] Department of Pharmaceutical Chemistry, School of Pharmacy, University of Kansas, Lawrence, KS 66047,
    USA; mforrest@ku.edu (M.L.F.); nilendrasns@yahoo.com (S.N.S.)
[5] Faculty of Pharmacy and Pharmaceutical Sciences, University of Alberta, Edmonton, AB T6G 2R3, Canada;
    raimar@ualberta.ca
*   Correspondence: ndavies@ualberta.ca; Tel.: +1-780-492-2429

Received: 9 July 2017; Accepted: 11 September 2017; Published: 13 September 2017

Abstract: Doxorubicin (Dox) is an effective anti-cancer medication with poor oral bioavailability and systemic toxicities. DoxQ was developed by conjugating Dox to the lymphatically absorbed antioxidant quercetin to improve Dox's bioavailability and tolerability. The purpose of this study was to characterize the pharmacokinetics and safety of Dox after intravenous (IV) and oral (PO) administration of DoxQ or Dox (10 mg/kg) and investigate the intestinal lymphatic delivery of Dox after PO DoxQ administration in male Sprague–Dawley rats. Drug concentrations in serum, urine, and lymph were quantified by HPLC with fluorescence detection. DoxQ intact IV showed a 5-fold increase in the area under the curve (AUC)—18.6 ± 1.98 compared to 3.97 ± 0.71 µg * h/mL after Dox—and a significant reduction in the volume of distribution (V_{ss}): 0.138 ± 0.015 versus 6.35 ± 1.06 L/kg. The fraction excreted unchanged in urine (f_e) of IV DoxQ and Dox was ~5% and ~11%, respectively. Cumulative amounts of Dox in the mesenteric lymph fluid after oral DoxQ were twice as high as Dox in a mesenteric lymph duct cannulation rat model. Oral DoxQ increased AUC of Dox by ~1.5-fold compared to after oral Dox. Concentrations of β-N-Acetylglucosaminidase (NAG) but not cardiac troponin (cTnI) were lower after IV DoxQ than Dox. DoxQ altered the pharmacokinetic disposition of Dox, improved its renal safety and oral bioavailability, and is in part transported through intestinal lymphatics.

Keywords: doxorubicin; quercetin; pharmacokinetics; bioavailability; lymphatics transport; toxicity

1. Introduction

Doxorubicin (Dox) is an effective anti-cancer medication that has been clinically used to treat a variety of cancers including breast, ovarian, and lymphoma [1–5]. Despite the clinical effectiveness of Dox, its use is limited by off-target adverse effects, particularly dose-related cardiotoxicity and renal toxicity, which involve free radical formation and tissue damage. Dox formulations that are pegylated and in liposomes are utilized in medications, including Doxil™ and Caelyx™ [6]. Pegylated (polyethylene glycol coated) liposome-encapsulated forms of Dox result in an increased concentration of Dox in the skin and a side effect called palmar plantar erythrodysesthesia or hand–foot syndrome [7]. Non-pegylated liposomal Dox called Myocet™ does not have a polyethylene glycol coating, and therefore does not result in the same rate of hand–foot syndrome. This liposomal encapsulation of Dox limits but does not eliminate the cardiotoxic effects of the drug. This damage is caused by the generation of reactive oxidative species (ROS) such as superoxide and hydrogen peroxide upon the reduction of Dox to form electron-deficient semiquinone [8]. Various additional drug delivery approaches have been undertaken to overcome the toxicity limitations of Dox, such as utilization of micelles [9], synthetic polymer conjugates [10], and antibody targeted carriers [11], with varied degrees of success. We have previously demonstrated that hyaluronan, a biopolymeric nanocarrier, improves survival and reduces the toxicity of Dox in xenografts of human breast cancer through the localization of Dox into the lymphatics [8].

Dox is a substrate of both the P–glycoprotein (P–gp) efflux pump [12] and cytochrome P450 metabolic enzymes [13], both of which contribute to its overall disposition, poor oral absorption, and low oral bioavailability. For this reason, Dox is only currently available as a parenteral treatment administered intravenously. We have previously reported the synthesis of a Dox-quercetin derivative designed to overcome P–gp efflux and CYP inhibition [14] as quercetin is a natural flavonoid that exhibits inhibitory effects on CYP3A4 and P–gp [15] and an antioxidant that scavenges free radicals. Our in vitro investigation of DoxQ [14] revealed that both Dox and quercetin are released from the conjugate over time. Furthermore, DoxQ inhibited CYP3A4, a major metabolic enzyme involved in the first pass effect, and demonstrated higher cellular uptake by P–gp-positive (MDCK–MDR) cells compared to free Dox. The inhibitory effects of DoxQ on CYP3A4 and P–gp may improve the oral absorption and bioavailability of Dox in vivo. Additionally, DoxQ retained anti-cancer activity in a triple negative murine breast cancer cell line and was less toxic to both rat and human cardiomyocytes. The cardioprotective mechanism of DoxQ involved scavenging ROS, suppression of oxidative stress, and cardiac hypertrophy markers, and also inhibitory effects on CYP1B1, all of which contribute to Dox's induced cardiotoxicity. Taken together, the in vitro results of DoxQ showed promise at mitigating the cardiotoxicity of Dox and may also mitigate its poor oral bioavailability in vivo by inhibiting CYP3A4 and P–gp [14]. The antioxidant effects of DoxQ may also mitigate the renal toxicity induced by Dox and improve its overall tolerability in vivo.

In addition to quercetin's antioxidant activity and inhibitory effects on CYP3A4 and P–gp, it is naturally absorbed into intestinal lymphatics after gastric or intraduoderal administration [16–18]; this property may be utilized as a novel strategy to deliver Dox into lymphatics. Following oral administration, molecules and drugs are either absorbed from the intestinal mucosa into the blood stream via the hepatic portal vein or into lymphatics via the intestinal lymphatic pathway. Most small molecules and drugs administered orally enter systemic circulation via blood capillaries and become subject to hepatic metabolism before entering the vasculature. In contrast, highly lipophilic molecules and macromolecules such as proteins associate with chylomicrons in the intestinal mucosa and enter systemic circulation via the intestinal lymphatics pathway [19]. These lipophilic molecules and macromolecules are absorbed via lymphatic capillaries, which collect into the mesenteric lymph duct, followed by the thoracic lymph duct, and then drain into systemic circulation at the junction of the left subclavian and left jugular veins [19,20]. Therefore, molecules that are absorbed via the intestinal lymphatic pathway enter systemic circulation without passing through the liver. This alternative absorptive pathway may be of particular importance in drug delivery and may serve as a novel drug delivery approach to minimize the first-pass effect while increasing lymphatic exposure and ultimately improving overall systemic drug exposure [21]. Lipophilic drugs with LogP > 5 and solubility of >50 mg per g in long-chain triglyceride will likely have preferential absorption towards lymphatics owing to their ability to incorporate with intestinal lipoproteins [19]. If the drug of interest does not meet these criteria, it is also possible to alter the physicochemical properties of a small drug molecule by chemically modifying its lipophilicity, utilizing a lipid-based drug delivery system or designing a lipophilic prodrug where the parent drug is chemically conjugated to a lipophilic moiety via a linker that can be easily cleaved in vivo [19–22]. In this study, we utilized a novel Dox–quercetin conjugate where quercetin is designed to act as a lymphatically targeted carrier and may facilitate the intestinal transport of Dox into systemic circulation after oral administration and may also affect its disposition as well as overall systemic exposure after intravenous administration.

In the light of the studies discussed above and our promising DoxQ observations in vitro, this study was conducted to investigate the feasibility of utilizing the antioxidant quercetin as a lymphatically targeted carrier for Dox with the potential to improve its disposition, oral bioavailability, and tolerability in vivo. We hypothesize that the presence of quercetin in DoxQ, intact or when released from the conjugate, will act as a carrier to transport Dox into lymphatics, at least partially, thus bypassing systemic circulation and increasing the overall bioavailability of Dox. The release of quercetin from DoxQ will likely have a beneficial effect and limit the cardiotoxic and renal side effects of doxorubicin. In addition, the synthesis and change in physicochemical properties of DoxQ may alter its pharmacokinetics and metabolism; the release of quercetin from DoxQ or DoxQ intact may also have effects on CYP3A4 and P–gp, which could further augment the disposition and bioavailability of Dox in vivo. Here, the acute in vivo disposition, safety, and lymphatic uptake of DoxQ are characterized for the first time. The pharmacokinetics, toxicodynamics, and intestinal lymphatic absorption of DoxQ in comparison to free Dox are examined in a rat model. Our results demonstrate that DoxQ improves the disposition of Dox and its oral bioavailability and safety, and is partially transported via lymphatics.

2. Materials and Methods

2.1. Chemicals and Reagents

Doxorubicin, duanorubicin, cycloheximide, PEG-400, and DMSO were purchased from Sigma (St. Louis, MO, USA). Analytical grade formic acid and HPLC grade acetonitrile were purchased from Fisher Scientific (Ottawa, ON, Canada). Ultrapure water from a Milli-Q® system (Millipore, Billerica, MA, USA) was used for the mobile phase. HPLC columns, vials, inserts, and 0.2 um nylon filter membranes were purchased from Phenomenex® (Torrance, CA, USA). Silastic® laboratory tubing was purchased from the Dow Corning Corporation (Midland, MI, USA). Intramedic® polyethylene tubing was purchased from Becton Dickinson Primary Care Diagnostics, Becton Dickinson and Company (Sparks, MD, USA). Monoject® 23 gauge (0.6 × 25 mm) polypropylene hub hypodermic needles were purchased from Sherwood Medical (St. Louis, MO, USA). Synthetic absorbable surgical sutures were purchased from Wilburn Medical US (Kernesville, NC, USA). Sterile heparin/50% dextrose catheter lock solution and blunt needles were obtained from SAI Infusion Technologies, Strategic Applications (Lake Villa, IL, USA).

2.2. Synthesis of the DoxQ Conjugate

DoxQ was synthesized by conjugating Dox to quercetin via a glycine linker, as previously described [14].

2.3. Physicochemical Properties

LogP and LogS values of DoxQ were predicted using an online computer software (VCCLAB, Virtual Computational Chemistry Laboratory) [23,24]. pKa, logP, logD at pH 7.4, intrinsic solubility, and solubility at pH 7.4 were calculated using MarvinSketch v. 17.2.20.0 (ChemAxon Ltd., Cambridge, MA, USA), pKa and logP were calculated using GastroPlus v. 9.0.0007 (Simulations Plus, Inc., Lancaster, CA, USA). Portions of these results were generated by GastroPlus™ software (Version 8.0) provided by Simulations Plus, Inc. (Lancaster, CA, USA). The melting point of DoxQ was experimentally determined by MEL-TEMPII melting point apparatus from Laboratory Devices (Holliston, MA, USA).

2.4. Analytical System and Conditions

The analytical method described in [25] was adapted with some modifications. The HPLC system used was a Shimadzu LC-2010A (Kyoto, Japan) with Fluorescence RF-535 detector at 470/560 nm (excitation/emission) wavelengths. Separation was achieved using C18 Phenomenex

Kintex® (Torrance, CA, USA) column (250 µm, 250 × 4.6 mm) for serum and lymph samples or (2.6 µm, 100 × 4.60 mm) joined to (250 µm, 250 × 4.6 mm) for urine samples. The mobile phase was prepared by mixing acetonitrile with 0.1% formic acid in water (35:65, *v*/*v*), which was filtered through 0.2 µm nylon filter and degassed under reduced pressure prior to use. The separation was carried out isocratically at ambient temperature (22 ± 1 °C) with a flow rate of 0.6 mL/min. Shimadzu EZStart (Version 7.4) software was used for data collection and integration. On the day of the analysis, samples were prepared and injected into the HPLC system.

2.4.1. Preparation of Standard Solutions

Stock solutions of Dox (1 mg/mL) and the internal standard (IS) duanorubicin (1 mg/mL) were prepared in methanol, protected from light and stored at −20 °C between uses for no longer than one week. Using the stock solutions of Dox, calibration standards in serum, urine, and lymph were freshly prepared by sequential dilution with blank rat serum, urine, and lymph. A series of concentrations were obtained, particularly 0.1, 0.5, 1.0, 10.0 and 100 µg/mL.

Stock solutions of intact DoxQ (10 mg/mL) were freshly prepared in DMSO and protected from light. Calibration standards of DoxQ in serum and urine were prepared by serial dilution with blank rat serum or urine to yield concentrations of 1, 10, 20, and 100 µg/mL. The final concentration of DMSO in serum and urine spiked standards did not exceed 1%.

2.4.2. Calibration Curves

Calibration curves of Dox and DoxQ were obtained by plotting the peak area ratio of Dox or DoxQ to the internal standard (duanorubicin) versus calibration standards concentration of Dox or DoxQ through the unweighted least squares linear regression.

2.5. Animals and Surgical Procedures

Male Sprague–Dawley rats (250–300 g) were obtained from Charles River Labs (Montreal, QC, Canada) and given food (Purina Rat Chow 5001) and water ad libitum in the animal facility for at least three days before use. Rats were housed in temperature-controlled rooms with a 12 h light/dark cycle. The animal ethics protocol was revised and approved by the Bannatyne Campus Animal Care Committee at the University of Manitoba, (protocol #16-004, approved 29 March 2016).

2.6. Pharmacokinetic Study

Eight surgically modified, with exposed jugular vein catheterization (polyurethane–silastic blended catheter), adult male Sprague–Dawley rats (average weight: 250 g) were purchased from Charles River Laboratories (Saint-Constant, QC, Canada). The cannula was flushed daily with a sterile heparin/50% dextrose catheter lock solution to maintain the patency of the cannula, as advised in the technical sheet supplied with the animals from Charles River. Each animal was placed in a separate metabolic cage overnight and fasted for 12 h before dosing. On the day of experiment, the animals were dosed either intravenously or orally with Dox (10 mg/kg) or equimolar DoxQ (*n* = 4 for each treatment group). Both Dox and DoxQ were freshly reconstituted in 3% DMSO and 97% PEG-400 prior to dosing. Animals received water ad libitum pre- and post-dosing, and food (Purina Rat Chow 5001) was provided 2 h post-dosing. Doses were selected based on previous use in similar pharmacokinetic studies [13,15] and sensitivity of analytical instrumentation. Serial blood samples (0.30 mL) were collected at 0, 1 min, 15 min, and 30 min, then 1, 2, 4, 6, 12, 24, 48 and 72 h after IV administration. The same blood collection time points were applied following oral administration except for 1 min. At 72 h after administration, the animals were euthanized and exsanguinated. Immediately after all the blood collection time points (except the terminal point); the cannula was flushed with the same volume of 0.9% saline to replenish the collected blood volume. The dead volume of the cannula was filled with a small volume (~0.15 mL) of heparinized lock solution after each blood draw to maintain the patency of the cannula. The samples were collected into regular polypropylene microcentrifuge tubes, centrifuged at 15,000 rpm for 5 min (Beckman Microfuge centrifuge, Beckman Coulter Inc., Fullerton, CA, USA), and the serum collected and stored at −20 °C until further sample preparation for HPLC analysis. Urine samples were also collected at 0, 2, 6, 12, 24, 48 and 72 h following Dox or DoxQ administration. The exact urine volume of each sample was recorded then stored at −20 °C until further sample preparation for HPLC analysis.

2.7. Intestinal Lymphatic Drug Delivery

The intestinal transport of DoxQ via lymphatics was examined in vivo by two methods. In the first method, mesenteric lymph cannulated rat model was used to directly measure the concentrations of Dox in the lymph after administration of DoxQ or Dox. In the second method cycloheximide, a chylomicron blocking drug, was administered intraperitoneally prior to oral administration of DoxQ or Dox then concentrations of Dox were measured in serum to indirectly assess lymphatic transport.

2.7.1. Mesenteric Lymph Cannulation Surgery

Six male Sprague–Dawley rats (~300 g) were obtained from Charles River Labs (Montreal, QC, Canada) and given food (Purina Rat Chow 5001) and water ad libitum in the animal facility for at least three days before use. On the day of surgical operation, rats were anesthetized by isoflurane and the abdominal hair was shaved. Rats were maintained under inhaled anesthesia on a warm surgical table. A ~2.5 cm abdominal midline skin incision was made and extended through the musculature using blunt dissection beginning the incision at a point just above the xyphoid cartilage and proceeding distally. The intestine and liver were retracted using surgical retractors to locate the superior mesenteric lymph duct, which is filled with opaque white chyle. The lymph duct was isolated from the surrounding connective tissue and a small incision was made with a bent 23 G needle in the ventral wall of the lymph. A catheter was inserted through the incision and secured by placing a small cellulose patch with a drop of Vetbond™ over the point of insertion into the lymph duct. When a gradual and continuous flow of lymph was observed, an initial lymph sample was collected into a normal microtube. A single dose (10 mg/kg) of DoxQ (n = 3) or Dox (n = 3) was administered by oral gavage while the rat was under anesthesia. Thereafter, lymph samples were collected over one hour after dosing. The animals were euthanized after the last lymph sample collection.

2.7.2. Lymph Blockage by Cycloheximide

Cycloheximide (3 mg/kg) was administered intraperitoneally (IP) to jugular vein cannulated male Sprague–Dawley rats (~250 g) (n = 4) 1.5 h prior to oral administration of DoxQ to block the formation of chylomicrons in lymph [26–35]. DoxQ was then administered orally (10 mg/kg). Blood samples were collected at 0 h, 15 min, 30 min, 1 h, 2 h, 6 h, 12 h, 24 h and 48 h. The animals were euthanized after the last blood sample collection.

2.8. Treatment of Biological Samples for Analysis

2.8.1. Serum and Lymph Sample Preparation

To a 100 µL serum or lymph sample (except 0 h), 10 µM of the internal standard (duanorubicin) was added then vortexed for 30 s (Vortex Genie–2, VWR Scientific, West Chester, PA, USA). One milliliter of cold HPLC grade acetonitrile (pre-stored at −20 °C) was added to the precipitate proteins, vortexed for 2 min (Vortex Genie–2, VWR Scientific, West Chester, PA, USA), and centrifuged at 15,000 rpm for 5 min; the supernatant was transferred to new, labeled 2 mL centrifuge tubes. The samples were evaporated to dryness using a Savant SPD1010 SpeedVac Concentrator (Thermo Fisher Scientific, Inc., Asheville, NC, USA). The residue was reconstituted with 100 µL of mobile phase, vortexed for 1 min, and centrifuged at 15,000 rpm for 5 min; the supernatant was transferred to HPLC vials and 100 µL were injected into the HPLC system.

2.8.2. Urine Sample Preparation

Two hundred microliters of urine and 10 µM of the internal standard were combined and vortexed for 30 s. The proteins present in the urine samples were precipitated using 1.6 mL cold HPLC-grade acetonitrile (pre-stored at −20 °C), vortexed for 2 min, and centrifuged at 15,000 rpm for 15 min. The supernatant was transferred to new, labeled 2-mL centrifuge tubes. The samples were evaporated to dryness using SpeedVac. The residue was reconstituted with 200 µL of mobile phase, vortexed for 1 min, and centrifuged at 15,000 rpm for 15 min. The supernatant was transferred to HPLC vials and vortexed, and 100 µL was injected into the HPLC system.

2.9. Pharmacokinetic Analysis

Pharmacokinetic analysis was performed using data from individual rats, and the mean and standard error of the mean (SEM) were calculated for each group. The elimination rate constant (k_{el}) was estimated by linear regression of the serum concentrations in the log-linear terminal phase. Non-compartmental modeling of the serum concentration versus time data points was performed using Phoenix® WinNonlin® software (Version 6.3) (Pharsight Corporation. Mountain View, CA, USA) to calculate the pharmacokinetic parameters in the terminal phase, namely mean residence time (MRT), total clearance (CL_{tot}), and volume of distribution (V_{ss}). The initial maximum serum concentration (C_0) was calculated by back extrapolation using WinNonlin software. Based on the cumulative urinary excretion data, the fraction excreted in urine (f_e by dividing the total cumulative amount excreted in urine (ΣXu) by the dose), renal clearance (CL_{renal} by multiplying f_e by CL_{tot}), and hepatic clearance ($CL_{hepatic}$ by subtracting CL_{renal} from CL_{tot}, assuming that hepatic clearance is equivalent to non-renal clearance) were calculated. The fraction of a dose converted to a specific metabolite (F_m) was calculated using the following equation: $F_m = AUC_{(m,D)}/AUC_{(m)}$, where $AUC_{(m,D)}$ is the AUC of the metabolite after IV or PO administration of its precursor (Dox after DoxQ) and $AUC_{(m)}$ is the AUC of the metabolite after IV administration of an equimolar dose of the preformed metabolite (Dox after Dox) [36,37].

2.10. Assessment of Cardiac Toxicity of DoxQ and Dox

The cardiac toxicity was assessed after a single IV dose of Dox or DoxQ utilizing a rat cardiac Troponin-I (cTnI) ultra-sensitive ELISA kit from Life Diagnostics, Inc. (West Chester, PA, USA). Blood samples from pharmacokinetic studies were collected at 0, 12, 24, and 48 h from the jugular vein after a single 10 mg/kg IV dose of Dox ($n = 4$) or an equimolar dose of DoxQ ($n = 4$). Samples were centrifuged to obtain the serum and stored at −20 °C in a freezer until analysis. On the day of the analysis, cTnI concentrations were measured in serum samples following the manufacturer's instructions. The area under the effect curve (AUEC) was calculated for cTnI concentrations at 12–48 h post-dosing using the trapezoidal rule [38,39] by WinNonlin® software.

2.11. Assessment of Renal Toxicity of Dox and DoxQ

2.11.1. Urinary Output

The urinary output of rats over 24 h was monitored before and after administration of a single IV dose of Dox (10 mg/kg) or equimolar DoxQ to assess potential renal toxicity. Acute renal toxicity induced by Dox and other drugs may result in a reduction in the total urinary output [40–42]. The total urine volume excreted over 24 h post-dosing was compared to the total urine volume excreted over 24 h pre-dosing.

2.11.2. β-N-Acetylglucosaminidase (NAG)

The potential renal toxicity of Dox and DoxQ was determined by measuring β-N-acetylglucosaminidase (NAG), a marker of ongoing renal damage, in rat urine [8,43]. Urine samples from pharmacokinetics experiments were collected from metabolic cages at 0 h, 12 h, 24 h, and 48 h and stored at −20 °C until analysis. Concentrations of NAG urine samples were measured using an assay kit from ALPCO Diagnostics (Salem, NH, USA, cat. No. 73-1290050) on a Medica EasyRA automated clinical chemistry analyzer (Medica Corporation, Bedford, MA, USA) [44,45].

2.12. Statistical Analysis

Compiled data were presented as mean and standard error of the mean (mean ± SEM). Where possible, the data were analyzed for statistical significance using SigmaPlot software (v. 13.0, Systat Software, Inc., San Jose, CA, USA). Student's *t*-test was employed for unpaired samples to compare means between two groups, while one-way ANOVA was employed to compare the means of three or more groups, with subsequent *t*-tests between groups if necessary; a value of $p < 0.05$ was considered statistically significant.

3. Results

3.1. Physicochemical Properties

As DoxQ is a chemical derivative of Dox, the change in the chemical structure of Dox will likely alter the physiochemical properties of the parent drug, which may affect its disposition into biological fluids and pharmacokinetic profile. Therefore, exploring the physicochemical properties of DoxQ in comparison to Dox provides insight into the differences in their dispositions and pharmacokinetics. Computer software, namely VCCLAB [23,24], MarvinSketch, and GastroPlus, were used to predict the physicochemical properties of DoxQ and Dox (Table 1). The estimated partition coefficient (LogP) value of DoxQ (2.6–3.8) was 3–5-fold higher than Dox (logP 0.49–1.3), suggesting the higher lipophilicity of DoxQ. The distribution coefficient at pH 7.4 (LogD$_{7.4}$), which takes into account the ionizable groups at specific pH, of DoxQ was 25-fold higher than Dox (0.097) and may be a better predictor of lipophilicity. The predicted LogP and LogD$_{7.4}$ values of DoxQ are in agreement with the low predicted solubility (0.006 mg/mL) of DoxQ compared to Dox (0.243 mg/mL) at physiological pH and higher logS values of DoxQ. The predicted pKa values of DoxQ were also different than those of Dox. Furthermore, the experimentally determined melting point of DoxQ was 175 °C compared to 242 °C. The difference in the predicted pKa values of DoxQ versus Dox as well as other physicochemical properties described above indicate that DoxQ is distinct from Dox and exhibits unique physicochemical properties.

Table 1. Physicochemical properties of Dox, quercetin, and DoxQ.

Compound	Doxorubicin (Free Base)	Quercetin	DoxQ
Structure			
Molecular Weight (g/mol)	543.53	302.238	928.82
Formula	$C_{27}H_{29}NO_{11}$	$C_{15}H_{10}O_7$	$C_{45}H_{40}N_2O_{20}$
pKa (MarvinSketch)	8.00, 9.17, 9.93, 12.67, 13.49, 14.10	6.38, 7.85, 8.63, 10.29, 12.82	6.37, 7.72, 7.94, 8.97, 9.51, 10.21, 12.53, 13.10, 13.57, 14.06, 14.77
pKa (GastroPlus)	6.77, 8.43, 9.5	7.24, 8.15, 9.12, 10.25, 11.35	7.21, 8.08, 8.78, 9.38, 9.91, 10.64, 11.26
pKa (GastroPlus, after fitting solubility)	6.974, 10.08	6.582, 8.15, 10.25, 11.35	7.978, 8.08, 8.78, 9.38, 10.64, 11.26
logP (MarvinSketch)	1.30	1.75	2.60
logP (neutral, GastroPlus)	0.49	1.96	2.61
logP (VCCLAB)	1.3	1.44 ± 0.55	3.8 ± 1.5
logD$_{7.4}$ (MarvinSketch)	0.097	1.00	2.407
Intrinsic solubility (MarvinSketch)	−4.05 logS	−2.49 logS	−6.47 logS
Solubility at pH 7.4 (MarvinSketch)	−3.27 logS	−1.42 logS	−5.34 logS
Solubility at pH 7.4 (MarvinSketch)	0.243 mg/mL	15.15 mg/mL	0.006 mg/mL
logS (VCCLAB)	2.7	2.78	3.43
Melting point (experimental)	242 °C	316.5 °C *	175 °C

* PubChem [46].

3.2. HPLC Analysis of Dox

Optimal separation of Dox, DoxQ, and duanorubicin (IS) in serum, urine, and lymph was achieved with a mobile phase composed of acetonitrile with 0.1% formic acid in water 35:65, v/v and a flow rate of 0.6 mL/min on a C18 Phenomenex Kintex® (Torrance, CA, USA) column. Chromatograms were free of any interfering peaks co-eluted with peaks of interest (Figure 1). Calibration curves of Dox in serum and lymph were linear over the range of 0.05–100 µg/mL in serum and lymph and 0.1–100 µg/mL for urine, with excellent linearity ($r^2 > 0.99$) in all three matrices. Calibration curves of DoxQ in serum and urine were linear over the range of 1–100 µg/mL ($r^2 > 0.99$). The observed maximum serum concentration (C_{max}) of both Dox and DoxQ at 1 min post-dosing was within the linear range. The limit of quantification (LOQ) was 0.05 µg/mL and 1 µg/mL for Dox and DoxQ intact, respectively.

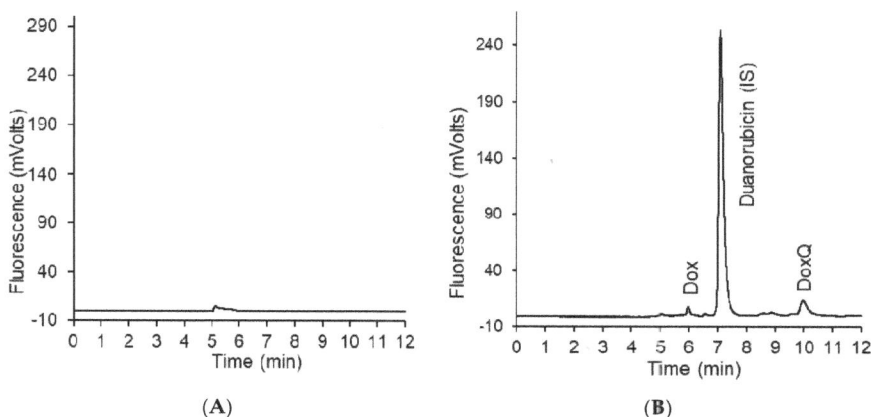

Figure 1. (**A**) Representative chromatogram of blank serum; (**B**) representative chromatogram of Dox, DoxQ, and the internal standard duanorubicin after 30 min of DoxQ IV dosing.

3.3. Pharmacokinetics of Dox and DoxQ

3.3.1. IV Administration

The disposition profiles of Dox and DoxQ intact in serum and urine following a single IV dose of Dox and an equimolar dose of DoxQ were examined (Figures 2 and 3). The serum concentration–time profile of IV DoxQ showed a rapid decline over the first 30 min and was quantifiable up to 1 h post-dosing. The concentrations of Dox after Dox were quantifiable up to 6 h post-dosing (Figure 2), with a maximum serum concentration (C_0) of Dox after Dox of ~25 µg/mL. The disposition profile of Dox after Dox, as well as its pharmacokinetic parameters, are consistent with the literature [13,15,25]. Following IV administration of DoxQ, both DoxQ intact and Dox were detected with maximum serum concentration (C_0) of intact DoxQ of ~108 µg/mL and ~1 µg/mL for free Dox (Table 2). Concentrations of intact DoxQ demonstrated a rapid decline over one hour, while concentrations of Dox after DoxQ dosing showed a slower decline and were quantifiable up to 2 h post-dosing. Notably, the maximum serum concentration (C_0) of intact DoxQ after equimolar IV DoxQ was 4–5-fold higher than C_{max} of Dox after IV Dox. The area under the concentration–time curve (AUC) of intact DoxQ (18.6 ± 1.98 µg * h/mL) was also 5-fold higher than that of Dox (3.97 ± 0.71 µg * h/mL), demonstrating higher systemic exposure to DoxQ. The volume of distribution V_{ss} of Dox was ~80-fold higher than that of DoxQ, suggesting significantly greater tissue distribution of Dox. The fraction of DoxQ metabolized into Dox was ~12%.

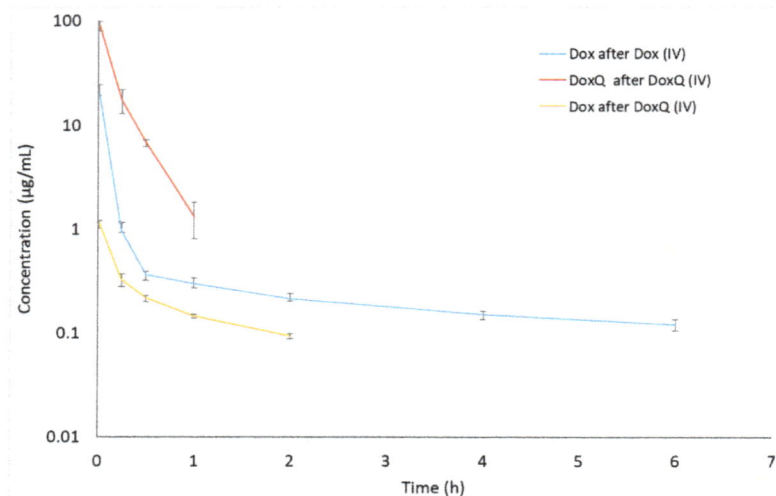

Figure 2. Concentrations of Dox and DoxQ intact after IV administration of Dox (10 mg/kg, $n = 4$ mean ± SEM) or DoxQ (equimolar dose, $n = 3$ mean ± SEM) in rat serum.

Table 2. Pharmacokinetics of Dox and DoxQ intact in rat serum after IV administration of Dox (10 mg/kg) and an equimolar dose of DoxQ (mean ± SEM, $n = 4$ unless otherwise stated).

Pharmacokinetic Parameter	Dox Administered	DoxQ Administered	
	Dox	DoxQ [1]	Dox
C_0 (µg/mL)	24.7 ± 14.2	108 ± 26.4 *	1.23 ± 0.11 [+]
k_{el} (h^{-1})	0.16 ± 0.02	4.59 ± 0.78 *	0.75 ± 0.076 [+]
$t_{1/2}$ (h)	4.69 ± 0.8 [@]	0.16 ± 0.3 *	0.87 ± 0.07
C_{last} (µg/mL)	0.12 ± 0.03	1.11 ± 0.17 *	0.09 ± 0.01 [+]
T_{last} (h) [2]	6	1	2
AUC_{last} (µg * h/mL)	3.97 ± 0.7 [@]	18.6 ± 1.98 *	0.46 ± 0.04 [+]
AUC_{inf} (µg * h/mL)	4.79 ± 1.83	NC	0.62 ± 0.03
V_{ss} (L/kg)	6.35 ± 2.11	0.08 ± 0.015	NA
CL_{renal} (L/h/kg) [1]	0.28 ± 0.84	0.02 ± 0.005	NA
$CL_{hepatic}$ (L/h/kg) [1]	2.35 ± 0.36	0.51 ± 0.06*	NA
CL_{total} (L/h/kg) [1]	2.63 ± 0.39	0.53 ± 0.01 *	NA
f_e (%)	10.73 ± 3.14	4.32 ± 1.005	NA
f_m (%)	NA	NA	11.66 ± 0.86

[1] $n = 3$; [2] Median; NC = not calculable because $r^2 < 0.8$ or AUC% extrapolated > 27%; NA = not applicable; * $p < 0.05$ Dox after Dox versus DoxQ after DoxQ, [+] $p < 0.05$ DoxQ after DoxQ versus Dox after DoxQ, [@] $p < 0.05$ Dox after Dox versus Dox after DoxQ.

In the urine, both DoxQ intact and Dox were detected after DoxQ IV dosing. Likewise, Dox was excreted unchanged after Dox IV dosing (Figure 3). The total cumulative urinary excretion plots demonstrate that DoxQ is predominantly excreted as intact DoxQ and, to a much lower extent, as free Dox after DoxQ dosing. The total cumulative amount of free Dox excreted unchanged was much higher after Dox dosing than after DoxQ. The fraction of the dose excreted unchanged in the urine (f_e) of DoxQ and Dox were 4.32 ± 1.005 and 10.73 ± 3.14, respectively, indicating that both drugs are mainly eliminated by non-renal routes.

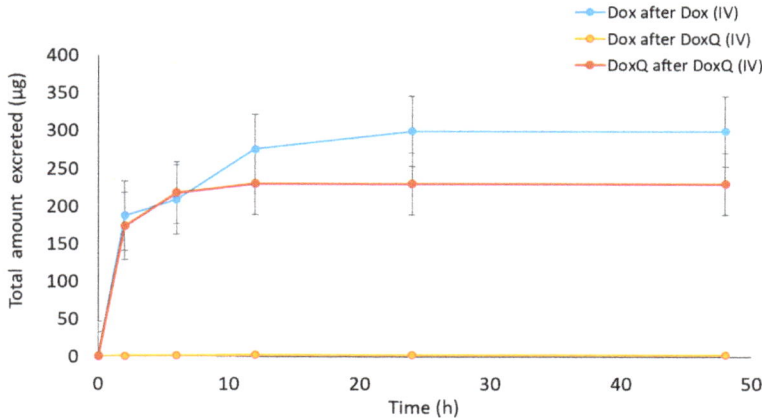

Figure 3. Cumulative amounts of Dox and DoxQ intact excreted unchanged in the urine after IV administration of Dox (10 mg/kg; $n = 3$ mean $\pm$ SEM) and equimolar DoxQ ($n = 4$ mean $\pm$ SEM) during the 48 h post-dosing.

3.3.2. Oral Administration

Following oral administration of DoxQ only the metabolite Dox was detected in serum as opposed to both DoxQ intact and Dox after IV administration (Figure 4). Following oral administration of Dox, Dox was also detected in serum. The serum concentration time plots demonstrate that concentrations of Dox after DoxQ were higher than after Dox at all time points, with resultant higher calculated AUC_{last} values of Dox after DoxQ than Dox after Dox when each was orally administered (Table 3). Bioavailability of Dox after Dox was ~8.5%, while the fraction of DoxQ metabolized into Dox was ~10.3%.

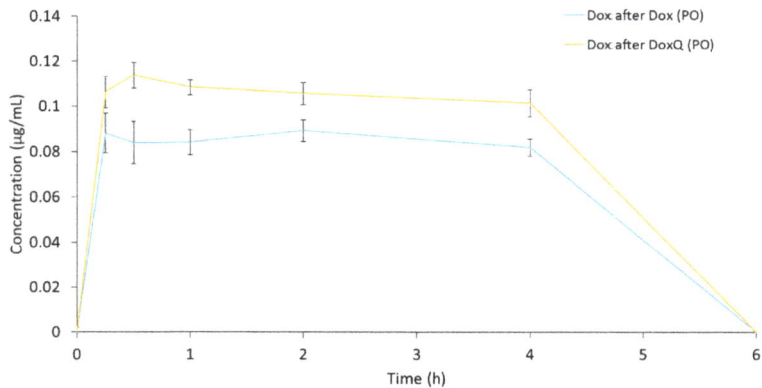

Figure 4. Concentrations of Dox after PO administration of Dox (10 mg/kg) and equimolar DoxQ in rat serum over 6 h. ($n = 3$ mean $\pm$ SEM for Dox, $n = 4$ mean $\pm$ SEM for DoxQ).

Table 3. Pharmacokinetics of Dox after oral administration of 10 mg/kg Dox and equimolar DoxQ in rat serum (mean ± SEM, *n* = 4 unless otherwise stated).

Pharmacokinetic Parameter	Dox Administered	DoxQ Administered	Cycloheximide + DoxQ Administered
	Dox [1]	Dox	Dox
C_{max} (µg/mL)	0.09 ± 0.01	0.11 ± 0.01 [+]	0.07 ± 0.001
C_{last} (µg/mL)	0.08 ± 0.01	0.10 ± 0.01	0.07 ± 0.02
T_{last} (h) [2]	4	4	4
AUC_{last} (µg * h/mL)	0.33 ± 0.04	0.41 ± 0.03 [+]	0.27 ± 0.005
F_m (%)	NA	10.32 ± 0.42 [+]	6.81 ± 0.14
F (%)	8.57 ± 0.71	NA	NA

[1] *n* = 3; [2] Median; NA = Not applicable; [+] *p* < 0.05 Dox after DoxQ versus Dox after Cycloheximide + DoxQ.

3.4. Intestinal Lymphatic Drug Delivery

3.4.1. Mesenteric Lymph Duct Cannulation

The mesenteric lymph duct cannulation rat model is commonly used as to directly examine the transport of drugs after oral administration because it enables the collection of lymphatic fluids as it flows from the intestine [20,35]. The intestinal lymphatic transport of Dox after oral administration DoxQ and Dox was investigated in a mesenteric lymph duct cannulated model to assess whether the presence of quercetin facilitates lymphatic transport of Dox. Following oral DoxQ or Dox dosing, lymph samples were collected up to one hour post-dosing and concentrations of Dox were measured by HPLC. The cumulative amount of Dox in mesenteric lymph fluid after oral DoxQ were two-fold higher than after Dox (Figure 5), suggesting that quercetin in DoxQ, intact or when released, increased the intestinal delivery of Dox into lymphatics.

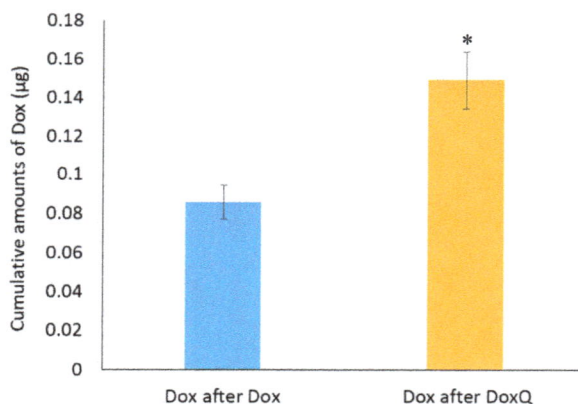

Figure 5. Cumulative amounts of Dox in mesenteric lymph fluid over one hour after oral administration of Dox (10 mg/kg) and equimolar DoxQ (*n* = 3, mean ± SEM). * *p* < 0.05 Dox after DoxQ versus Dox after Dox.

3.4.2. Lymph Blockage by Cycloheximide

Intestinal lymphatic delivery of Dox was also examined indirectly in the cycloheximide treated rat model. Lymph blockage was achieved by pre-administration of cycloheximide 1.5 h prior to oral administration of DoxQ. A 3 mg/kg intraperitoneal dose of cycloheximide was chosen based on previous studies published in the literature [26–35]. Likewise, a 1.5-h time delay prior to oral DoxQ dosing was chosen to achieve maximum lymph blockage [29].

Figure 6 demonstrates that pre-administration of cycloheximide prior to oral DoxQ reduced the systemic exposure of Dox compared to DoxQ administered alone. Given that quercetin is naturally transported via intestinal lymphatics and could act as a carrier for Dox's (Dox in DoxQ) lymphatic transport, blockage of the intestinal lymphatic pathway may reduce systemic exposure. The results suggest that quercetin in DoxQ, intact or when released from the conjugate, facilitates intestinal lymphatic transport of Dox, and that blocking the lymphatic pathway resulted in lower levels of circulating Dox.

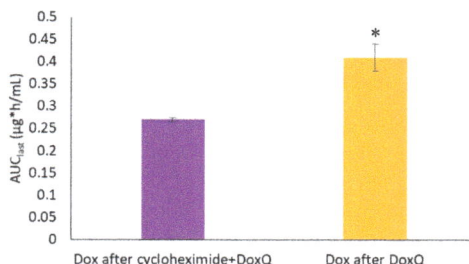

Figure 6. Systemic exposure (AUC_{last}) of Dox after PO administration of DoxQ alone or after cycloheximide IP followed by DoxQ PO in rat serum ($n = 4$ mean $\pm$ SEM). * $p < 0.05$ Dox after DoxQ versus Dox after cycloheximide + DoxQ.

3.5. Cardiotoxicity of Dox and Dox

The clinical use of Dox is limited by its dose-related cardiotoxicity, which can result in cardiac muscle injury. The extent of myocardial injury can be assessed by measuring the levels of cardiac troponins in blood. Cardiac troponins are highly sensitive and specific biomarkers of cardiac muscle damage, induced by chemotherapeutics as well as other pathological conditions [47]. cTnI is commonly used as an early marker of cardiotoxicity induced by Dox [8,48] as it is released within 2–3 h of myocardial injury and peaks at 24 h [49,50]. Based on the reported peak troponin concentrations following myocardium injury, levels of cTnI were measured in serum samples from pharmacokinetic study at 12, 24, and 48 h after a single acute IV dose (10 mg/kg) of Dox or equimolar DoxQ utilizing an ELISA kit. Figure 7 illustrates that the concentrations of cTnI at 12, 24, and 48 h post-IV-dosing of DoxQ were lower than after Dox dosing, though this did not reach statistical significance and thus the cardiac toxicity induced by DoxQ and Dox was not different using this biomarker. Although the calculated area under the effect curve (AUEC) of cTnI concentrations at 12–48 h post-DoxQ-dosing (Figure 8) was lower than the AUEC after Dox, it did not result in cardioprotective effects of DoxQ as there were no statistical differences between the treatment groups.

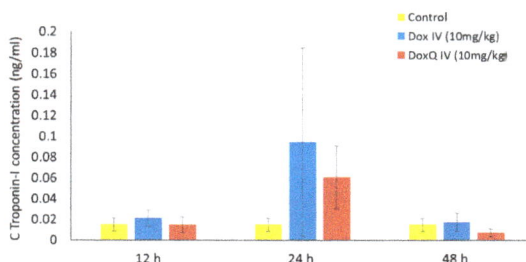

Figure 7. cTnI concentrations after IV (10 mg/kg) administration of Dox and equimolar DoxQ ($n = 4$ mean $\pm$ SEM). Data were not statistically significant.

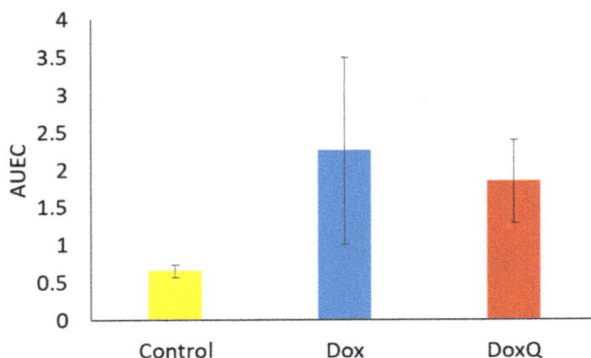

Figure 8. AUEC of cTnI concentrations 12-48 h after IV (10 mg/kg) administration of Dox and equimolar DoxQ (*n* = 4 mean ± SEM). Data were not statistically significant.

3.6. Renal Toxicity of Dox and DoxQ

3.6.1. Urinary Output over 24 h

Dox can also induce renal toxicity, which could be manifested as reduced urinary output. Thus, the effect of DoxQ on the total urinary output of rats over 24 h was examined in comparison to rats treated with Dox after a single acute IV dose. Figure 9 shows that there was no significant difference in the total urine volume over 24 h in rats treated with Dox or an equimolar dose of DoxQ.

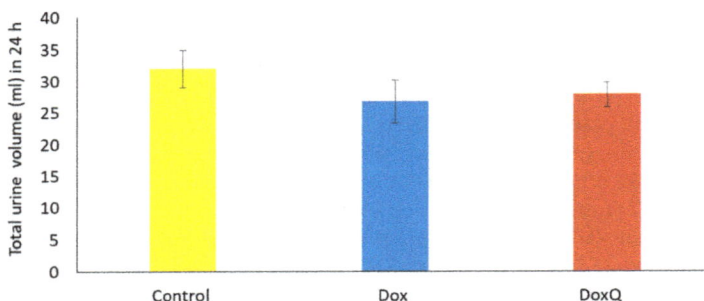

Figure 9. Average total urine volume 24 h post IV Dox (10 mg/Kg) and equimolar DoxQ compared to control untreated. Dox (*n* = 3 Mean ± SEM), DoxQ (*n* = 4 Mean ± SEM), control (*n* = 7 Mean ± SEM). Data were not statistically significant.

3.6.2. β-N-Acetylglucosaminidase (NAG)

The potential renal toxicity of Dox and DoxQ was determined by measuring β-N-acetylglucosaminidase (NAG), a lysosomal enzyme found in large concentrations in kidney tubules and a sensitive and early marker of renal damage [8,51,52]. Urine samples from pharmacokinetic studies after a single IV dose of DoxQ or Dox collected at 0, 2, 6, 12, 24 and 48 h were analyzed on a Medica easy RA analyzer for NAG concentrations. Cumulative amounts of NAG in 24 h after DoxQ dosing were lower than after Dox (Figure 10), suggesting lower renal toxicity induced after DoxQ administration compared to Dox.

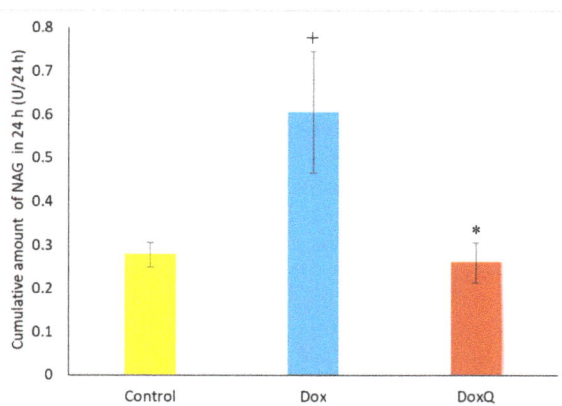

Figure 10. Total amount of NAG excreted in urine after IV administration of Dox (10 mg/kg) mean ± SEM) and equimolar DoxQ compared to control untreated ($n = 4$, mean ± SEM). + $p < 0.05$ Dox versus control ,* $p < 0.05$ DoxQ versus Dox.

4. Discussion

Dox is an anthracycline antibiotic widely used in cancer chemotherapy; however, its dose-dependent toxicity limits its clinical use. The purpose of this study was to investigate the feasibility of utilizing a Dox-bound derivative with the lymphatically absorbed antioxidant quercetin as a proof of concept linker, delivering Dox and Dox–quercetin to the systemic circulation via intestinal lymphatics after oral dosing. In addition, the flavonoid–Dox conjugate may lead to sustained release of the anti-cancer agent after IV dosing, resulting in lower peak serum concentration, which may be associated with the dose-limiting cardiotoxicity of the drug. Furthermore, the protective antioxidant effects of quercetin in DoxQ, when intact or when released, may further limit the cardiac and renal toxicity induced by Dox.

Various liposome-encapsulated formulations of Dox are currently available in human studies with the advantage of reduced acute cardiotoxicity compared to IV Dox and improved pharmacokinetics [53]. However, pegylated liposomal Dox is associated with an additional side effect of palmar plantar erythrodysesthesia [7]. In this study, we sought to examine the performance of a controlled-release Dox–quercetin conjugate with reduced side effects in vitro, which may have better tolerability compared to conventional Dox–HCl and liposomal Dox treatments.

The Dox–quercertin conjugate was synthesized using a glycine linker, resulting in a new derivative with increased lipophilicity and improved in vitro pharmacological activities. Our previous in vitro study demonstrated a controlled release of both Dox and quercetin released from DoxQ over four days [14]. Furthermore, DoxQ was less cardiotoxic than Dox to both rat and human cardiomyocytes and the mechanism of cardioprotection involved a reduction in the levels of ROS and oxidative stress markers as well as inhibitory effects on the expression and catalytic activity of CYP1B1. Additionally, DoxQ mitigated the therapeutic barriers contributing to the low oral bioavailability of Dox as it inhibited CYP3A4 and demonstrated higher cellular uptake by P–gp-positive cells (MDCK–MDR) in vitro.

In this study, our intestinal lymphatic delivery strategy was applied to the DoxQ delivery system, increasing the serum concentrations of Dox at all time points, with an overall increase in AUC_{last} of Dox after oral DoxQ administration compared to after Dox, reflecting an overall increase in the systemic exposure of Dox. In addition, only free Dox was released from oral DoxQ and detected analytically, thus it was analyzed for systemic exposure. Given that DoxQ was not detected as the intact conjugate after oral dosing of DoxQ, calculating the F of DoxQ intact was not possible; however, it was appropriate to calculate the fraction of DoxQ metabolized to Dox, as described in Section 2.9.

Therefore, the extent of systemic exposure of Dox after oral Dox and DoxQ was assessed by comparing the AUCs of Dox (Table 3).

After IV administration DoxQ was detected intact, which we have shown to be a pharmacologically active form as it retained anti-cancer activity in a triple-negative murine breast cancer cell line [14]. The actual total concentration of DoxQ intact in the serum after an equimolar dose of Dox was 5-fold higher than the concentration of Dox after Dox, allowing a greater AUC compared to the standard Dox treatment. This could result in a lower dose of DoxQ being required to achieve the same effective serum concentrations. DoxQ injections could conceivably be as effective as Dox with reduced toxicity. With regard to its pharmacokinetics, the difference in the volume of distribution between the IV Dox after Dox group and the IV DoxQ intact group was possibly due to the change in physicochemical properties and inhibition of P–gp by quercetin. Dox with a log P value of 1.3, pKa of 8.4, and a molecular weight of 543.53 g/mol rapidly crosses the lipid membrane and binds to tissues, resulting in a larger V_{ss}. On the other hand, DoxQ with a smaller V_{ss} (0.08) indicates that it is should mainly reside in the vascular compartment with much lower affinity to distribute across biological membranes compared to Dox, regardless of its higher lipophilicity (logP 2.60–3.8). This could be due to the large molecular weight of 982 g/mol and the presence of multiple potential ionization sites, which may impede its distribution across biological membranes while intact. Similar effects were observed for clozapine nano-formulation, where tissue distribution of clozapine incorporated in solid lipid nanoparticles was lower than clozapine solution because free clozapine could only be distributed after its release from nanoparticles [54]. Therefore, it is possible that DoxQ intact will distribute to a lower extent than when it is released from the conjugate or when Dox alone is administered. Examination of the total cumulative amounts of Dox and DoxQ excreted unchanged after IV dosing revealed lower cumulative amounts of DoxQ intact after DoxQ than of Dox after Dox. This could be due to the large molecular weight of DoxQ (928.8 g/mole) to be filtered at the glomerulus and also its high lipophilicity (LogP 2.6–3.8, Table 2), as opposed to Dox with a smaller size and lower lipophilicity.

With regard to intestinal lymphatic absorption of DoxQ, our results show that cumulative amounts of Dox following DoxQ oral dosing were twice as high after Dox in a mesenteric lymph cannulated rat model. This observation is likely due to the presence of quercetin in DoxQ, intact or when released, acting as a lymphatically targeted carrier to facilitate the transport of Dox into lymphatics, as quercetin has been reported to be transported via intestinal lymphatics following intragastric or intraduodenal administration [16–18]. Additionally, compounds with high lipophilicity, high logP, and large molecular size favor association with chylomicrons in the intestine, facilitating their uptake by lymphatic capillaries into the mesenteric lymph duct [19,21]. The new derivative is more lipophilic (LogP 2.6–3.8) and larger in size (molecular weight 928.8 g/mole) compared to Dox (LogP 1.3, 543.53 g/mol), both of which may in part facilitate DoxQ's lymphatic intestinal absorption. Furthermore, formulation effects of PEG-400 on the intestinal absorption and pharmacokinetics of DoxQ and even Dox are possible. PEG-400 is often utilized in dosing of rodent species [45,55] and was used as a vehicle in this study for both oral and IV administration of DoxQ and Dox because DoxQ has poor water solubility and reconstitution in 0.9% NaCl is not feasible. The diverse effects of PEG-400 on solubility, permeability, drug metabolizing enzymes, transporters, and gastrointestinal transit time may have influences on the intestinal absorption and systemic exposure of oral drugs [56–58].

In spite of the efficacy of Dox chemotherapy, its clinical use is limited due to its dose-limiting cardiac toxicity along with its renal toxicity, caused in part by the generation of oxygen species in the conversion from Dox to semiquinone, yielding very reactive hydroxyl radicals. The free radical may also cause damage to various membrane lipids and other cellular components [59]. Following a large single-dose injection of Dox (10 mg/kg IV), there was an increase in cTnI released from cardiac tissues at the 12, 24, and 48 h time points, consistent with the literature. In parallel, rats that received DoxQ (equimolar dose of Dox) also had an increase in cTnI at each time point. The significant 4–5-fold increase of circulating intact DoxQ as compared to Dox and its overall increase in systemic exposure, as well as the metabolism of DoxQ to Dox, did not result in higher cTnI compared to rats that received

Dox as no statistically significant difference in cardiac toxicity was observed between the two treatment groups (Figures 7 and 8). The in vivo cardiac effects of DoxQ in this study are different from our in vitro observations, where DoxQ formulation greatly reduced the cardiac toxicity induced by Dox in both rat and human cardiomyocytes [14]. This observation is also different from a reported study in which the combination of Dox with resveratrol and quercetin polymeric micelles was shown to mitigate Dox-induced cardiotoxicity both in vitro and in vivo [60]. The in vivo cardioprotective effects of this combination strategy were assessed by measuring levels of AST, ALT, and CK in mice and showed a significant reduction in all three biochemical markers as opposed to Dox administered alone. The observations from the later reported study [60] and our in vitro study [14] demonstrate the protective effects of quercetin on Dox-induced cardiotoxicity. The cardioprotective effects reported in [60] were attributed to the synergistic action of resveratrol and quercetin micelles when co-administered with Dox at a ratio of 10:10:1 resveratrol:quercetin:Dox, whereas our DoxQ conjugate is designed to release Dox and quercetin at a ratio of 1:1, which may have not been enough to show cardioprotection in vivo after one dose. Additionally, the use of two antioxidants, namely resveratrol and quercetin, together could have provided a greater ability to scavenge reactive oxygen species and attenuate the cardiotoxicity induced by Dox as opposed to only quercetin in the DoxQ formulation.

Urine analysis following a single acute dose of Dox showed higher cumulative amounts of β-N-acetylglucosaminidase (NAG), a lysosomal enzyme in the epithelial cells of the proximal tubules and a sensitive marker of renal damage, compared to DoxQ. This is likely due to the antioxidant protective effects of quercetin in DoxQ on Dox-induced renal toxicity and is consistent with similar studies reported in the literature [61,62].

DoxQ by injection could have greater benefits over standard dosing regimens in terms of tolerance and potential improved toxicity. Further translational efforts will focus on optimizing dose frequency, completing preclinical proof of concept in chronic studies, and examining other natural lymphatic carriers for oral delivery.

5. Conclusions

DoxQ alters the pharmacokinetic disposition of Dox both orally and intravenously and is in part transported through intestinal lymphatics. DoxQ may increase therapeutic safety compared to Dox in a rodent model and further long-term studies are warranted.

Acknowledgments: The authors would like to acknowledge Kuwait University, Faculty of Health Sciences, College of Pharmacy for the graduate scholarship awarded to Samaa Alrushaid. Sanjeewa N. Senadheera was funded by a grant from the U.S. National Cancer Institute (NCI) R01CA173292 to M. Laird Forrest.

Author Contributions: Samaa Alrushaid, Neal M. Davies, Casey L. Sayre, and M. Laird Forrest conceived and designed the experiments; Samaa Alrushaid and Sanjeewa N. Senadheera performed the experiments; Samaa Alrushaid., Neal M. Davies, Casey L. Sayre, M. Laird Forrest, Sanjeewa N. Senadheera, Jaime A. Yáñez, Frank J. Burczynski, and Raimar Löbenberg analyzed the data; Neal M. Davies, Casey L. Sayre, Jaime A. Yáñez, M. Laird Forrest, Frank J. Burczynski, and Raimar Löbenberg contributed reagents/materials/analysis tools; Samaa Alrushaid, Neal M. Davies, Casey L. Sayre, Jaime A. Yáñez, M. Laird Forrest, Sanjeewa N. Senadheera, Frank J. Burczynski, and Raimar Löbenberg wrote the paper.

Conflicts of Interest: The authors declare no conflict of interest.

References

1. Minotti, G.; Menna, P.; Salvatorelli, E.; Cairo, G.; Gianni, L. Anthracyclines: Molecular advances and pharmacologic developments in antitumor activity and cardiotoxicity. *Pharmacol. Rev.* **2004**, *56*, 185–229. [CrossRef] [PubMed]
2. Cortés-Funes, H.; Coronado, C. Role of anthracyclines in the era of targeted therapy. *Cardiovasc. Toxicol.* **2007**, *7*, 56–60. [CrossRef] [PubMed]
3. Gibbs, D.D.; Pyle, L.; Allen, M.; Vaughan, M.; Webb, A.; Johnston, S.R.; Gore, M.E. A phase I dose-finding study of a combination of pegylated liposomal doxorubicin (Doxil), carboplatin and paclitaxel in ovarian cancer. *Br. J. Cancer* **2002**, *86*, 1379–1384. [CrossRef] [PubMed]

4. Gianni, L.; Dombernowsky, P.; Sledge, G.; Martin, M.; Amadori, D.; Arbuck, S.G.; Ravdin, P.; Brown, M.; Messina, M.; Tuck, D.; et al. Cardiac function following combination therapy with paclitaxel and doxorubicin: An analysis of 657 women with advanced breast cancer. *Ann. Oncol.* **2001**, *12*, 1067–1073. [CrossRef] [PubMed]
5. McBride, N.C.; Cavenagh, J.D.; Ward, M.C.; Grant, I.; Schey, S.; Gray, A.; Hughes, A.; Mills, M.J.; Cervi, P.; Newland, A.C.; et al. Liposomal daunorubicin (DaunoXome) in combination with cyclophosphamide, vincristine and prednisolone (COP-X) as salvage therapy in poor-prognosis non-Hodgkins lymphoma. *Leuk. Lymphoma* **2001**, *42*, 89–98. [CrossRef] [PubMed]
6. Soloman, R.; Gabizon, A.A. Clinical pharmacology of liposomal anthracyclines: Focus on pegylated liposomal Doxorubicin. *Clin. Lymphoma Myeloma* **2008**, *8*, 21–32. [CrossRef] [PubMed]
7. Lorusso, D.; Stefano, A.D.; Carone, V.; Fagotti, A.; Pisconti, S.; Scambia, G. Pegylated liposomal doxorubicin-related palmar-plantar erythrodysesthesia ('hand-foot' syndrome). *Ann. Oncol.* **2007**, *18*, 1159–1164. [CrossRef] [PubMed]
8. Cai, S.; Thati, S.; Bagby, T.R.; Diab, H.M.; Davies, N.M.; Cohen, M.S.; Forrest, M.L. Localized doxorubicin chemotherapy with a biopolymeric nanocarrier improves survival and reduces toxicity in xenografts of human breast cancer. *J. Control Release* **2010**, *146*, 212–218. [CrossRef] [PubMed]
9. Matsumura, Y.; Hamaguchi, T.; Ura, T.; Muro, K.; Yamada, Y.; Shimada, Y.; Shirao, K.; Okusaka, T.; Ueno, H.; Ikeda, M.; et al. Phase I clinical trial and pharmacokinetic evaluation of NK911, a micelle-encapsulated doxorubicin. *Br. J. Cancer* **2004**, *91*, 1775–1781. [CrossRef] [PubMed]
10. Ríhová, B.; Strohalm, J.; Prausová, J.; Kubácková, K.; Jelínková, M.; Rozprimová, L.; Sírová, M.; Plocová, D.; Etrych, T.; Subr, V.; et al. Cytostatic and immunomobilizing activities of polymer-bound drugs: Experimental and first clinical data. *J. Control Release* **2003**, *91*, 1–16. [PubMed]
11. Tolcher, A.W.; Sugarman, S.; Gelmon, K.A.; Cohen, R.; Saleh, M.; Isaacs, C.; Young, L.; Healey, D.; Onetto, N.; Slichenmyer, W. Randomized phase II study of BR96-doxorubicin conjugate in patients with metastatic breast cancer. *J. Clin. Oncol.* **1999**, *17*, 478–484. [CrossRef] [PubMed]
12. Gustafson, D.L.; Merz, A.L.; Long, M.E. Pharmacokinetics of combined doxorubicin and paclitaxel in mice. *Cancer Lett.* **2005**, *220*, 161–169. [CrossRef] [PubMed]
13. Lee, H.J.; Lee, M.G. Effects of dexamethasone on the pharmacokinetics of adriamycin after intravenous administration to rats. *Res. Commun. Mol. Pathol. Pharmacol.* **1999**, *105*, 87–96. [PubMed]
14. Alrushaid, S.; Zhao, Y.; Sayre, C.L.; Maayah, Z.H.; Forrest, M.L.; Senadheera, S.N.; Chaboyer, K.; Anderson, H.D.; El-Kadi, A.; Davies, N.M. Mechanistically Elucidating the In Vitro Safety and Efficacy of a Novel Doxorubicin Derivative. *Drug Deliv. Transl. Res.* **2017**, *7*, 582–597. [CrossRef] [PubMed]
15. Choi, J.S.; Piao, Y.J.; Kang, K.W. Effects of quercetin on the bioavailability of doxorubicin in rats: Role of CYP3A4 and P-gp inhibition by quercetin. *Arch Pharm. Res.* **2011**, *34*, 607–613. [CrossRef] [PubMed]
16. Chen, I.L.; Tsai, Y.J.; Huang, C.M.; Tsai, T.H. Lymphatic absorption of quercetin and rutin in rat and their pharmacokinetics in systemic plasma. *J. Agric. Food Chem.* **2010**, *58*, 546–551. [CrossRef] [PubMed]
17. Murota, K.; Cermak, R.; Terao, J.; Wolffram, S. Influence of fatty acid patterns on the intestinal absorption pathway of quercetin in thoracic lymph duct-cannulated rats. *Br. J. Nutr.* **2013**, *109*, 2147–2153. [CrossRef] [PubMed]
18. Murota, K.; Terao, J. Quercetin appears in the lymph of unanesthetized rats as its phase II metabolites after administered into the stomach. *FEBS Lett.* **2005**, *579*, 5343–5346. [CrossRef] [PubMed]
19. Trevaskis, N.L.; Kaminskas, L.M.; Porter, C.J. From sewer to saviour—Targeting the lymphatic system to promote drug exposure and activity. *Nat. Rev. Drug Discov.* **2015**, *14*, 781–803. [CrossRef] [PubMed]
20. Trevaskis, N.L.; Hu, L.; Caliph, S.M.; Han, S.; Porter, C.J. The mesenteric lymph duct cannulated rat model: Application to the assessment of intestinal lymphatic drug transport. *J. Vis. Exp.* **2015**. [CrossRef] [PubMed]
21. Yáñez, J.A.; Wang, S.W.; Knemeyer, I.W.; Wirth, M.A.; Alton, K.B. Intestinal lymphatic transport for drug delivery. *Adv. Drug Deliv. Rev.* **2011**, *63*, 923–942. [CrossRef] [PubMed]
22. Porter, C.J.; Trevaskis, N.L.; Charman, W.N. Lipids and lipid-based formulations: Optimizing the oral delivery of lipophilic drugs. *Nat. Rev. Drug Discov.* **2007**, *6*, 231–248. [CrossRef] [PubMed]
23. Tetko, I.V.; Gasteiger, J.; Todeschini, R.; Mauri, A.; Livingstone, D.; Ertl, P.; Palyulin, V.A.; Radchenko, E.V.; Zefirov, N.S.; Makarenko, A.S.; et al. Virtual computational chemistry laboratory—Design and description. *J. Comput. Aid. Mol. Des.* **2005**, *19*, 453–463. [CrossRef] [PubMed]
24. Virtual Computational Chemistry Laboratory. Available online: http://www.vcclab.org (accessed on 24 August 2017).

25. Daeihamed, M.; Haeri, A.; Dadashzadeh, S. A Simple and Sensitive HPLC Method for Fluorescence Quantitation of Doxorubicin in Micro-volume Plasma: Applications to Pharmacokinetic Studies in Rats. *Iran J. Pharm. Res.* **2015**, *14* (Suppl. 1), 33–42. [PubMed]

26. Dahan, A.; Hoffman, A. Evaluation of a chylomicron flow blocking to investigate the intestinal lymphatic transport of lipophilic drugs. *Eur. J. Pharm. Sci.* **2005**, *24*, 381–388. [CrossRef] [PubMed]

27. Bhalekar, M.R.; Upadhaya, P.G.; Madgulkar, A.R.; Kshirsagar, S.J.; Dube, A.; Bartakke, U.S. In-Vivo bioavailability and lymphatic uptake evaluation of lipid nanoparticulates of darunavir. *Drug Deliv.* **2016**, *23*, 2581–2586. [PubMed]

28. Fu, Q.; Sun, J.; Ai, X.; Zhang, P.; Li, M.; Wang, Y.; Liu, X.; Sun, Y.; Sui, X.; Sun, L.; et al. Nimodipine nanocrystals for oral bioavailability improvement: Role of mesenteric lymph transport in the oral absorption. *Int. J. Pharm.* **2013**, *448*, 290–297. [CrossRef] [PubMed]

29. Attili-Qadri, S.; Karra, N.; Nemirovski, A.; Schwob, O.; Talmon, Y.; Nassar, T.; Benita, S. Oral delivery system prolongs blood circulation of docetaxel nanocapsules via lymphatic absorption. *Proc. Natl. Acad. Sci. USA* **2013**, *110*, 17498–17503. [CrossRef] [PubMed]

30. Sun, M.; Zhai, X.; Xue, K.; Hu, L.; Yang, X.; Li, G.; Si, L. Intestinal absorption and intestinal lymphatic transport of sirolimus from self-microemulsifying drug delivery systems assessed using the single-passintestinal perfusion (SPIP) technique and a chylomicron flow blocking approach: Linear correlation with oral bioavailabilities in rats. *Eur. J. Pharm. Sci.* **2011**, *43*, 132–140. [PubMed]

31. Lind, M.L.; Jacobsen, J.; Holm, R.; Müllertz, A. Intestinal lymphatic transport of halofantrine in rats assessed using a chylomicron flow blocking approach: The influence of polysorbate 60 and 80. *Eur. J. Pharm. Sci.* **2008**, *35*, 211–218. [CrossRef] [PubMed]

32. Gao, F.; Zhang, Z.; Bu, H.; Huang, Y.; Gao, Z.; Shen, J.; Zhao, C.; Li, Y. Nanoemulsion improves the oral absorption of candesartan cilexetil in rats:Performance and mechanism. *J. Control Release* **2011**, *149*, 168–174. [CrossRef] [PubMed]

33. Mishra, A.; Vuddanda, P.R.; Singh, S. Intestinal Lymphatic Delivery of Praziquantel by Solid Lipid Nanoparticles: Formulation Design, In Vitro and In Vivo Studies. *J. Nanotechnol. vol.* **2014**, *2014*, 1–12. [CrossRef]

34. Makwana, V.; Jain, R.; Patel, K.; Nivsarkar, M.; Joshi, A. Solid lipid nanoparticles (SLN) of Efavirenz as lymph targeting drug delivery system: Elucidation of mechanism of uptake using chylomicron flow blocking approach. *Int. J. Pharm.* **2015**, *495*, 439–446. [CrossRef] [PubMed]

35. Tsai, Y.J.; Tsai, T.H. Mesenteric lymphatic absorption and the pharmacokinetics of naringin and naringenin in the rat. *J. Agric. Food Chem.* **2012**, *60*, 12435–12442. [CrossRef] [PubMed]

36. Rowland, M.; Tozer, T.N. Metabolites and drug response. In *Clinical Pharmacokinetics and Pharmacodynamics: Concepts and applications*, 4th ed.; Tozer, R.M., Thomas, N., Eds.; Lippincott Williams & Wilkins: Baltimore, MD, USA, 2011; pp. 603–631.

37. Mehvar, R.; Jamali, F.; Watson, M.W.; Skelton, D. Pharmacokinetics of tetrabenazine and its major metabolite in man and rat. Bioavailability and dose dependency studies. *Drug Metab. Dispos.* **1987**, *15*, 250–255. [PubMed]

38. Hanafy, S.; Dagenais, N.J.; Dryden, W.F.; Jamali, F. Effects of angiotensin II blockade on inflammation-induced alterations of pharmacokinetics and pharmacodynamics of calcium channel blockers. *Br. J. Pharmacol.* **2008**, *153*, 90–99. [CrossRef] [PubMed]

39. Sattari, S.; Dryden, W.F.; Eliot, L.A.; Jamali, F. Despite increased plasma concentration, inflammation reduces potency of calcium channel antagonists due to lower binding to the rat heart. *Br. J. Pharmacol.* **2003**, *139*, 945–954. [CrossRef] [PubMed]

40. Singh, N.P.; Ganguli, A.; Prakash, A. Drug-induced kidney diseases. *J. Assoc. Physic. India* **2003**, *51*, 970–979.

41. Naughton, C.A. Drug-induced nephrotoxicity. *Am. Fam. Physic.* **2008**, *78*, 743–750.

42. Okuda, S.; Oh, Y.; Tsuruda, H.; Onoyama, K.; Fujimi, S.; Fujishima, M. Adriamycin-induced nephropathy as a model of chronic progressive glomerular disease. *Kidney Int.* **1986**, *29*, 502–510. [CrossRef] [PubMed]

43. Le, J.M.; Han, Y.H.; Choi, S.J.; Park, J.S.; Jang, J.J.; Bae, R.J.; Lee, M.J.; Kim, M.J.; Lee, Y.H.; Kim, D.; et al. Variation of nephrotoxicity biomarkers by urinary storage condition in rats. *Toxicol. Res.* **2014**, *30*, 305–309. [CrossRef] [PubMed]

44. Martinez, S.E.; Davies, N.M. Enantiospecific pharmacokinetics of isoxanthohumol and its metabolite 8-prenylnaringenin in the rat. *Mol. Nutr. Food Res.* **2015**, *59*, 1674–1689. [CrossRef] [PubMed]

45. Oliveira, A.L.; Martinez, S.E.; Nagabushnam, K.; Majeed, M.; Alrushaid, S.; Sayre, C.L.; Davies, N.M. Calebin A: Analytical Development for Pharmacokinetics Study, Elucidation of Pharmacological Activities and Content Analysis of Natural Health Products. *J. Pharm. Pharm. Sci.* **2015**, *18*, 494–514. [CrossRef] [PubMed]

46. PubChem. Available online: https://pubchem.ncbi.nlm.nih.gov/compound/5280343#section=Entrez-Crosslink (accessed on 24 August 2017).

47. Tian, S.; Hirshfield, K.M.; Jabbour, S.K.; Toppmeyer, D.; Haffty, B.G.; Khan, A.J.; Goyal, S. Serum biomarkers for the detection of cardiac toxicity after chemotherapy and radiation therapy in breast cancer patients. *Front. Oncol.* **2014**, *4*, 277. [CrossRef] [PubMed]

48. Hadi, N.; Yousif, N.G.; Al-amran, F.G.; Huntei, N.K.; Mohammad, B.I.; Ali, S.J. Vitamin E and telmisartan attenuates doxorubicin induced cardiac injury in rat through down regulation of inflammatory response. *BMC Cardiovasc. Disord.* **2012**, *12*, 63. [CrossRef] [PubMed]

49. Adamcova, M.; Sterba, M.; Simunek, T.; Potacova, A.; Popelova, O.; Mazurova, Y.; Gersl, V. Troponin as a marker of myocardiac damage in drug-induced cardiotoxicity. *Expert Opin. Drug Saf.* **2005**, *4*, 457–472. [CrossRef] [PubMed]

50. Babuin, L.; Jaffe, A.S. Troponin: The biomarker of choice for the detection of cardiac injury. *CMAJ* **2005**, *173*, 1191–1202. [CrossRef] [PubMed]

51. Teng, X.W.; Abu-Mellal, A.K.; Davies, N.M. Formulation dependent pharmacokinetics, bioavailability and renal toxicity of a selective cyclooxygenase-1 inhibitor SC-560 in the rat. *J. Pharm. Pharm. Sci.* **2003**, *6*, 205–210. [PubMed]

52. Burke, J.F.; Laucius, J.F.; Brodovsky, H.S.; Soriano, R.Z. Doxorubicin Hydrochloride-Associated Renal Failure. *Arch Int. Med.* **1977**, *137*, 385–388. [CrossRef]

53. Luo, R.; Li, Y.; He, M.; Zhang, H.; Yuan, H.; Johnson, M.; Palmisano, M.; Zhou, S.; Sun, D. Distinct biodistribution of doxorubicin and the altered dispositions mediated by different liposomal formulations. *Int. J. Pharm.* **2017**, *519*, 1–10. [CrossRef] [PubMed]

54. Manjunath, K.; Venkateswarlu, V. Pharmacokinetics, tissue distribution and bioavailability of clozapine solid nanoparticles after intravenous and intraduodenal administration. *J. Control Release* **2005**, *107*, 215–228. [CrossRef] [PubMed]

55. Martinez, S.E.; Sayre, C.L.; Davies, N.M. Pharmacometrics of 3-Methoxypterostilbene: A Component of Traditional Chinese Medicinal Plants. *Evid.-Based Complement. Altern. Med.* **2013**. [CrossRef] [PubMed]

56. Schulze, J.D.; Waddington, W.A.; Eli, P.J.; Parsons, G.E.; Coffin, M.D.; Basit, A.W. Concentration-dependent effects of polyethylene glycol 400 on gastrointestinal transit and drug absorption. *Pharm. Res.* **2003**, *20*, 1984–1988. [CrossRef] [PubMed]

57. Basit, A.W.; Newton, J.M.; Short, M.D.; Waddington, W.A.; Ell, P.J.; Lacey, L.F. The effect of polyethylene glycol 400 on gastrointestinal transit: Implications for the formulation of poorly-water soluble drugs. *Pharm. Res.* **2001**, *18*, 1146–1150. [CrossRef] [PubMed]

58. Ma, B.L.; Yang, Y.; Dai, Y.; Li, Q.; Lin, G.; Ma, Y.M. Polyethylene glycol 400 (PEG400) affects the systemic exposure of oral drugs based on multiple mechanisms: Taking berberine as an example. *RSC Adv.* **2017**, *7*, 2435–2442. [CrossRef]

59. Olson, R.D.; Mushlin, P.S. Doxorubicin cardiotoxicity: Analysis of prevailing hypotheses. *FASEB J.* **1990**, *4*, 3076–3086. [PubMed]

60. Cote, B.; Carlson, L.J.; Rao, D.A.; Alani, A.W.G. Combinatorial resveratrol and quercetin polymeric micelles mitigate doxorubicin induced cardiotoxicity in vitro and in vivo. *J. Control Release* **2015**, *213*, 128–133. [CrossRef] [PubMed]

61. Yagmurca, M.; Yasar, Z.; Bas, O. Effects of quercetin on kidney injury induced by doxorubicin. *Bratisl. Lekárske Listy* **2015**, *116*, 486–489. [CrossRef]

62. Heeba, G.H.; Mahmoud, M.E. Dual effects of quercetin in doxorubicin-induced nephrotoxicity in rats and its modulation of the cytotoxic activity of doxorubicin on human carcinoma cells. *Environ. Toxicol.* **2016**, *31*, 624–636. [CrossRef] [PubMed]

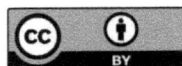

pharmaceutics

MDPI

Article

Theophylline-7β-D-Ribofuranoside (Theonosine), a New Theophylline Metabolite Generated in Human and Animal Lung Tissue

Daniel S. Sitar [1,*]**, James M. Bowen** [2] **, Juan He** [2]**, Angelo Tesoro** [2] **and Michael Spino** [2]

[1] Departments of Pharmacology and Therapeutics, Internal Medicine, and Pediatrics and Child Health, Max Rady College of Medicine, Centre on Aging, and College of Pharmacy, University of Manitoba, Winnipeg, MB R3E 0T6, Canada

[2] Leslie Dan Faculty of Pharmacy, University of Toronto, Toronto, ON M5S 3M2, Canada; bowenj@mcmaster.ca (J.M.B.); info@biopharmaservices.com (J.H.); amtesoro@rogers.com (A.T.); mspino@apopharma.com (M.S.)

* Correspondence: Daniel.Sitar@umanitoba.ca; Tel.: +1-204-789-3532

Received: 29 June 2017; Accepted: 6 August 2017; Published: 14 August 2017

Abstract: While assessing the ability of mammalian lung tissue to metabolize theophylline, a new metabolite was isolated and characterized. The metabolite was produced by the microsomal fraction of lungs from several species, including rat, rabbit, dog, pig, sheep and human tissue. Metabolite production was blocked by boiling the microsomal tissue. This new metabolite, theophylline-7β-D-ribofuranoside (theonosine), was confirmed by several spectral methods and by comparison to an authentic synthetic compound. Tissue studies from rats, rabbits, dogs, and humans for cofactor involvement demonstrated an absolute requirement for NADP and enhanced metabolite production in the presence of magnesium ion. It remains to be demonstrated whether theonosine may contribute to the known pharmacological effects of theophylline.

Keywords: theophylline; theophylline metabolism; lung; microsomes; theophylline-7β-D-ribofuranoside; theonosine

1. Introduction

The lung is known to play an important role in the metabolism of several drugs [1–3]. Most enzymes so far identified are found in lower concentrations in the lung than in the liver, but the lung receives all of the cardiac output in comparison to the liver, which receives about one quarter of it. Some drug metabolizing enzymes found in the lung are not found in the liver, suggesting the potential for lung tissue to produce unique drug metabolites [4].

More than 40 cell types have been identified in lung tissue, and drug metabolism has been detected in both endothelial and epithelial cells. Pulmonary endothelium, comprising about 70 m², is in direct contact with blood, and is active in regulating biogenic amines, prostaglandins, vasoconstrictive peptides, lipids, and nucleotides [5]. Removal of vasoconstrictive amines by the lung is more effective than by the liver [6]. Alveolar macrophages and epithelial tissue are active in drug biotransformation, particularly Clara, type I and type II cells [7]. Although it is clear that the lung can metabolize endogenous substances and drugs, its contribution to the overall metabolism of drugs remains to be better characterized [8–10].

Theophylline has been used therapeutically as a bronchodilator for more than 80 years [11]. Its metabolic disposition in humans was first reported by Brodie et al. [12]. Following a therapeutic dose, only 85% has been accounted for by measurement of known metabolites and unchanged drug excreted in urine [13] (Figure 1).

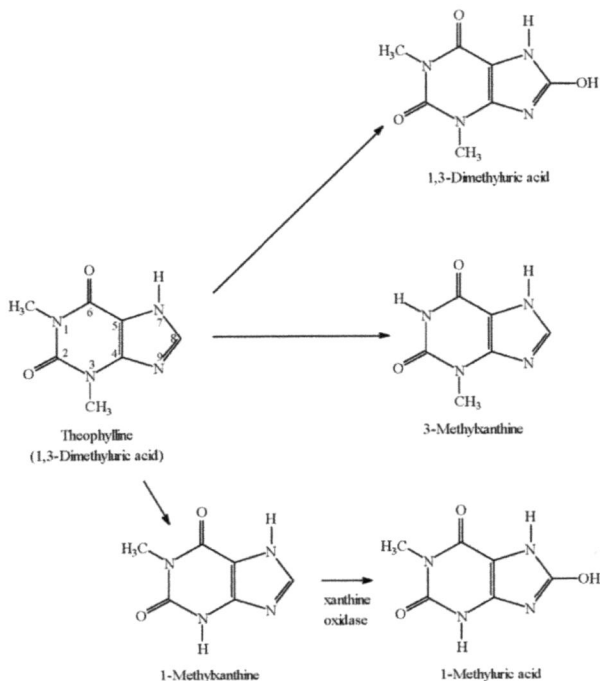

Figure 1. Summary of theophylline metabolism from urinary excretion data.

It has been observed previously that theophylline clearance is increased in patients with cystic fibrosis [14]. While testing the hypothesis that lung tissue from cystic fibrosis patients contributed to its more rapid kinetic disposition, we determined that mammalian lung microsomes from five species, including humans, biotransformed theophylline to the newly characterized metabolite, theophylline-7β-D-ribofuranoside (theonosine). This paper describes the isolation, identification, and characterization of production of this new conjugated theophylline metabolite.

2. Experimental Section

2.1. Tissue Sources and Collection

Experiments with animal lungs were completed with salvage tissue from animals killed for studies completed in accordance with protocols approved by the University of Toronto Animal Care Committee. Human lung tissue was obtained from surgical waste resulting from partial pulmonary lobectomy for carcinoma or from lung transplant recipients. Normal tissue was excised. Following resection, tissue was washed as described below for lungs from animal species and flash frozen in liquid nitrogen. Approval for use of human tissue was obtained from the Pathology Department, The Toronto Hospital (Toronto General Division), and the Review Board of the Hospital for Sick Children. Permission to conduct the study was obtained from the Human Subjects Review Committee, Hospital for Sick Children. Lungs and other tissues were removed from mongrel dogs, mixed-breed pigs, New Zealand white rabbits, and mixed-breed sheep under approved operating room conditions immediately following the death of the animals. Tissue was gently flushed with 1.15% *w/v* KCl solution to remove blood, and tissue was flash frozen in liquid nitrogen or placed on ice and transported immediately to the laboratory for preparation of microsomes.

2.2. Methods

2.2.1. Preparation of Microsomes

Frozen tissue was thawed and homogenized within one week of acquisition. Microsomes were prepared as described previously [15]. Briefly, tissue was weighed and placed in an ice-cold solution of 1.15% w/v KCl and 0.1 M sodium phosphate buffer pH 7.4. Excessive connective tissue was removed, and the remaining tissue was minced with scissors and resuspended in a fresh volume of KCL/phosphate buffer (1:4 w/v). The suspension was homogenized with a Brinkman Polytron® instrument using a PT10ST probe and centrifuged at $10,000 \times g$ at 4 °C for 20 min to remove cellular debris, nuclei, and mitochondria. The supernatant fluid was decanted into ultracentrifuge tubes and centrifuged at $105,000 \times g$ at 4 °C for 60 min (L8-80 Beckman Ultracentrifuge) to isolate the microsomal fraction. The resulting supernatant was removed and the microsomal pellet was resuspended in fresh KCl/phosphate buffer with a Teflon-glass Potter–Elvehjem homogenizer. This suspension was centrifuged again at $105,000 \times g$ at 4 °C for 60 min to isolate the microsomal fraction. The supernatant was removed, and the microsomal pellet was resuspended in fresh 0.2 M potassium phosphate buffer (pH 7.4) at a ratio of 1 g lung/mL of buffer solution. Microsomal protein was determined by the method of Lowry et al. [16].

2.2.2. In Vitro Metabolism Studies

Metabolic incubation studies for microsomal metabolism of theophylline were completed as follows. The incubation mixture, 0.50 mL, contained 40 mM pH 7.4 potassium phosphate buffer, 0.23% w/v KCl, 2 mM $MgCl_2$, 0.4 mM NADP, 4 mM glucose-6-phosphate, 0.4 U/mL glucose-6-phosphate dehydrogenase (G-6-PD), approximately 500 µg of lung microsomal protein, and varying concentrations of theophylline. All components, excepting the substrate, were preincubated for 5 min at 37 °C before the addition of theophylline substrate. The reaction was incubated in a shaking water bath at 120 rpm (Model G 86, New Brunswick Scientific Co. Inc., Edison, NJ, USA) for various time periods up to 60 min in initial studies, and for 30 min once kinetic characteristics of metabolite production were established. The reaction was stopped by the addition of 3.0 mL of acetone containing 20 µL of glacial acetic acid and β-hydroxyethyltheophylline as the internal standard. The treated incubation mixture was centrifuged at $1000 \times g$ for 10 min and the resulting supernatant removed and evaporated under a stream of nitrogen. The residue was reconstituted with 0.2 mL of distilled water and an aliquot injected for determination of theophylline metabolism by high performance liquid chromatography (HPLC) using a stepwise linear gradient elution [17]. Separation of theophylline, theonosine, and the internal standard β-hydroxyethyltheophylline was excellent with retention times of 17.0, 19.5 and 22.5 min, respectively. The limit of quantitation for theonosine was 2 ng, corresponding to a range of 0.05–1.0 pmol/mg protein/min enzyme activity. Peak height was linear to 700 pmol theonosine/reaction tube. The new metabolite was collected from the eluting solvent of the HPLC instrument and was further purified by adsorption to reversed-phase Bond Elut® columns (Varian Canada Inc., Mississauga, ON, Canada). Columns were washed with water to remove phosphate buffer. The purified metabolite was then eluted from the column by desorption with acetonitrile. The resulting compound was then subject to analyses by ultraviolet, Fourier-transformed infrared, proton nuclear magnetic resonance, and mass spectral instrumentation.

In order to determine the conditions contributing to production of the new theophylline metabolite, incubations were conducted as follows: (i) in room air; (ii) under carbon monoxide and nitrogen atmospheres to assess requirements for cytochromes P450 and oxygen; (iii) after preincubation of microsomes at 37 °C for 45 min to inactivate flavine monooxygenase [18]; (iv) with boiled microsomes to determine if the reaction was enzyme catalyzed; and (v) in the presence and absence of various cofactors described above in the standard incubation mixture. Inhibition studies were completed in the presence of varying concentrations of cimetidine, caffeine, methimazole, SKF525A, indomethacin, and antipyrine. To evaluate substrate specificity for the conjugation reaction, theonosine production was determined in the presence of added ribose, adenine, adenosine, inosine, and guanosine.

2.2.3. Synthesis of Theophylline-7β-D-Ribofuranoside

This compound was synthesized, purified, and chemically and spectrally characterized as described previously [19].

2.2.4. Chemicals

Theophylline, glucose-6-phosphate, glucose-6-phosphate dehydrogenase, β-hydroxyethylthe ophylline, caffeine, D-ribose, adenine, adenosine, inosine, guanosine, indomethacin, antipyrine, and methimazole were obtained from Sigma Chemical Co. (St. Louis, MO, USA). Cimetidine and SKF525A were gifts from Smith, Kline and French Laboratories (Toronto, ON, Canada). Other chemicals were analytical grade, excepting acetonitrile, which was HPLC grade.

2.2.5. Data Analyses

Kinetic analyses of our metabolic data were conducted using the classical assumptions of Michaelis and Menten. Data were transformed by the Lineweaver–Burk, Eadie–Hofstee, and Cornish–Bowden procedures to determine apparent K_m, V_{max}, K_i, and potential mechanisms to explain the inhibitions observed. Data are presented as mean ± SD. Statistical analyses were done with appropriate parametric tests, and a two-tailed p-value < 0.05 was the level at which a difference was accepted.

3. Results and Discussion

3.1. Microsomal Preparation

Lung microsomes prepared by the method described above resulted in the following yield of microsomal protein (mg/g lung tissue) in each of the following species: rat: 7.9 ± 2.1 ($n = 7$); rabbit: 6.0 ± 1.9 ($n = 13$); pig: 5.8 ± 0.7 ($n = 3$); sheep: 6.6 ($n = 1$); dog: 4.9 ± 1.8 ($n = 4$); human: 2.6 ± 1.3 ($n = 21$). Lung microsomal protein concentration for patients with cystic fibrosis (3.1 ± 1.3 mg/g, $n = 8$) and patients without cystic fibrosis (2.3 ± 1.2 mg/g, $n = 13$) were not different ($p < 0.21$).

3.2. Identification and Characterization of the Production of the New Theophylline Metabolite

The lung microsomal fraction among species differed both qualitatively and quantitatively in the production of theophylline metabolites. However, all species tested generated the ribosylated conjugate metabolite theonosine (Figure 2).

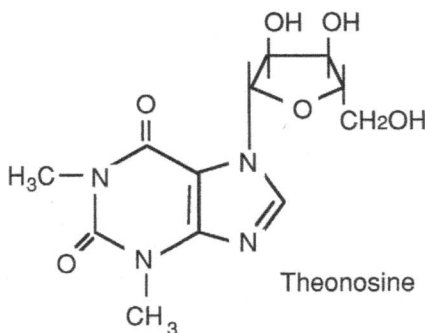

Figure 2. Theonosine structure.

There are few published data with respect to theophylline metabolism by lung tissue. Kröll et al. evaluated ^{14}C-theophylline disposition in a perfused guinea pig lung preparation, but were unable to detect any metabolites in the circulation. Uptake of the radiolabel by their lung preparation was insufficient to allow evaluation of metabolite production [20].

The wavelength maximum for theonosine's ultraviolet absorbance was 274 nm, very similar to that for theophylline, 272 nm, and much lower than that produced by oxidation of theophylline to 1,3-dimethyluric acid, 287 nm. This spectral finding confirms the initial report by Myake et al. [19]. Its elution from the HPLC column after theophylline confirms the findings of IJzerman et al. [21].

Incubation studies of theophylline with rabbit lung microsomes suggested that metabolite production was enzymatic, since it did not occur with boiled microsomes. No enzyme activity was detected in the post-microsomal supernatant, and the $10,000 \times g$ pellet produced only about 5% of the metabolite compared to lung microsomes. There was an absolute requirement for NADP, but NADP, NADPH, or an NADPH generating system were effective in supporting production of this newly isolated theophylline metabolite from lung microsomes. It was noteworthy that the reaction occurred with or without G-6-PD as long as NADP or NADPH was present (data not shown).

Studies to determine optimal conditions for production of theonosine with dog lung microsomes demonstrated that maximal activity occurred at 55 °C, with product formation being three times greater than that observed at 37 °C. The addition of Mg^{+2} up to a concentration of 6 mM increased production of the metabolite by almost two-fold, after which production plateaued.

The generation of theonosine was not inhibited by carbon monoxide, SKF525A, or antipyrine, indicating that it was not mediated by cytochromes P450. Preincubation of microsomes at 37 °C for 45 min, or coincubation with methimazole, did not affect production of the new metabolite, indicating a lack of contribution by amine oxidase. Incubation with indomethacin did not inhibit metabolite production, suggesting that cyclo-oxygenase was not involved (data not shown).

High performance liquid chromatography/mass spectral/mass spectral analysis of the metabolite gave an M + 1 ion of 313 (23% abundance) (Figure 3) with a base peak at mass 181, corresponding to that for pure theophylline when it was analyzed by the same method.

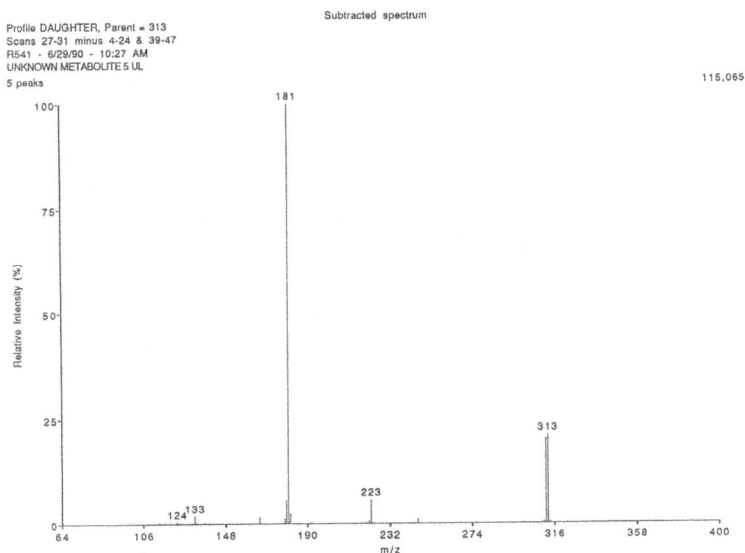

Figure 3. HPLC/MS/MS chemical ionization spectrum of theonosine.

Direct probe insertion of theonosine into the source gave an electron impact mass spectrum with a molecular ion at m/e 312 (3.4% abundance) and a base peak at m/e 180, corresponding to the molecular ion fragment of theophylline obtained by the identical technique. Fourier-transformed infrared analysis indicated the presence of a sugar conjugate. Subsequently, proton nuclear magnetic resonance analysis of a solution in deuterated water at 400 MHz suggested that the metabolite contained a 5-carbon sugar attached to nitrogen with spectral characteristics consistent with ribose.

From these data, we tentatively identified the metabolite as theophylline-7-riboside and propose the name theonosine to reflect its similarity to adenosine. Chemical synthesis and spectral analysis confirmed the identity of the metabolite as theophylline-7β-D-ribofuranoside (theonosine) [19].

Our data reveal for the first time that metabolic transformation of theophylline to a newly identified conjugate metabolite, theonosine occurs in lung tissue from several mammalian species.

Theonosine has been detected following lung microsomal incubation from all species studied to date, including human (Table 1).

Table 1. Production of theophylline-7β-D-ribofuranoside (theonosine) by lung microsomal tissue from various mammalian species incubated with 1 mM theophylline. Data are presented as mean $\pm$ SD when $n > 2$.

Species	Theonosine Production (pmol/mg protein/min)
Dog ($n = 5$)	31 ± 15
Sheep ($n = 1$)	32
Rabbit ($n = 8$)	11 ± 5
Rat ($n = 7$)	41 ± 10
Pig ($n = 3$)	40 ± 19
Human ($n = 16$)	18 ± 11

Metabolite production is linear to 1000 µg of microsomal protein per incubation tube and for 60 min. In human lung microsomes, apparent theophylline K_m for theonosine production was determined as 51 ± 24 µM with an apparent V_{max} of 63 ± 37 pmol/mg protein/min.

When incubated with dog, rabbit, pig, or human lung microsomes, 2 mM cimetidine inhibited theonosine production by about 50% with 1 mM theophylline as the substrate concentration. Studies with caffeine indicated a similar degree of inhibition of theonosine production for an equivalent molar ratio of inhibitor to substrate in the incubation medium. Inhibitory effect data from studies with representative human lung tissue are presented in Figure 4. These data suggest the potential involvement of CYP1A1/2 in the ribosylation of theophylline, since theonosine production appears to be greater in microsomal tissue from smokers [8–10]. However, lack of inhibition of theonosine production by carbon monoxide does not favour such an explanation.

Finally, we studied the effects of 0.5 mM adenine and three other nucleosides on the production of theonosine by rabbit lung microsomes. These purinergic compounds all inhibited theonosine production in the following order of decreasing potency: adenine, inosine, adenosine, and guanosine. A representative graph of these inhibitions relative to the production of 1,3-dimethyluric acid in the incubation mixture is presented in Figure 5. Studies with adenine and caffeine on the mechanism of inhibition indicated that it was not competitive, but a mixed inhibition as reflected by Dixon and Cornish–Bowden plots (data not shown). Further studies are required to more completely define the mechanisms by which inhibition of theonosine production is occurring.

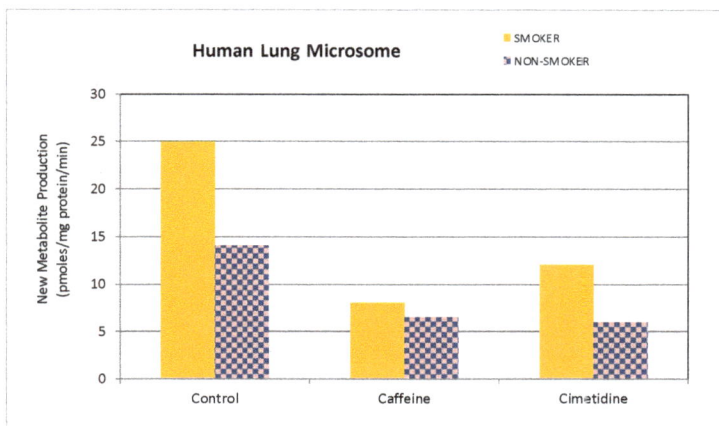

Figure 4. Inhibition of theonosine production by caffeine and cimetidine in human lung microsomes.

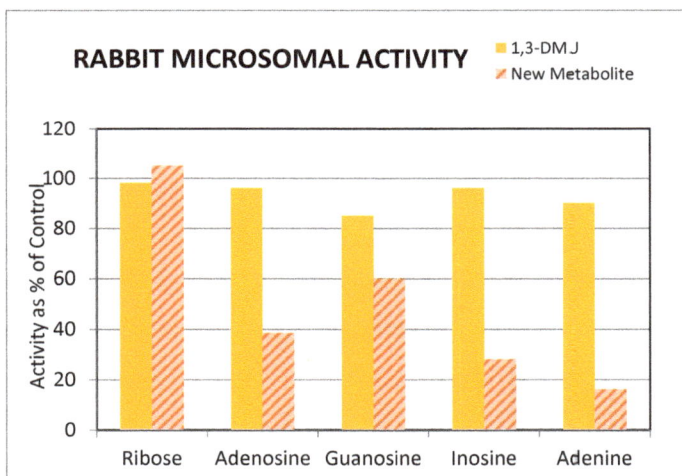

Figure 5. Inhibition of theonosine production by purinergic nucleosides in rabbit lung microsomes.

While conjugation of drugs with ribose in mammals is not common, it has been described for allopurinol [22–25]. Elion and Hitchings presented data suggesting that the liver and kidney may be the sites of production of allopurinol and oxypurinol ribosides in the rat [22]. The enzyme responsible for ribose conjugation of these drug substances has been identified as purine nucleoside phosphorylase, and its presence has been demonstrated in guinea pig small intestine and in human erythrocytes [23]. In preliminary studies in rat, dog, and rabbit tissue, in vitro, our laboratory has also demonstrated theonosine production from tissues other than the lung (unpublished observations). Further studies are required to conclusively demonstrate that this same enzyme is responsible for the conversion of theophylline to theonosine.

3.3. Potential for Pharmacological Activity of Theonosine

There is preliminary in vitro evidence that xanthine-7-ribosides bind to A_1-type adenosine receptors [26]. These conjugates have been identified as adenosine antagonists by this research group, although theophylline-7β-D-ribofuranoside is considerably less potent than theophylline in its interaction at the A_1 adenosine receptor. Subsequent to this initial report, evidence has been presented that theophylline-7-ribosides may in fact be partial agonists at the A_1 adenosine receptor [21,27]. These observations raise the possibility that theonosine may contribute to the bronchodilator effect of theophylline, since its production occurs within the lung.

4. Conclusions

Our studies have identified a new metabolite for theophylline, theophylline-7β-D-ribofuranoside (theonosine). These studies also demonstrate that theophylline serves as an additional substrate for the uncommon metabolic pathway of conjugation with ribose in mammalian species, including humans. The biological significance of this metabolic reaction warrants exploration.

Acknowledgments: The authors are grateful for the Rosenstadt Professorship from the University of Toronto provided to Daniel S. Sitar, and for funding by the Medical Research Council of Canada (MA9738) to Michael Spino. The authors also thank L. Marai of the Medical Research Council Regional GC/LC-MS facility, University of Toronto for access to the mass spectrometer. LC/MS/MS testing was done by Mann Testing Laboratories Ltd., Mississauga, ON, Canada. We thank William Reynolds of the Chemistry Department, University of Toronto for the Fourier-transformed infrared and NMR spectral analyses. We are grateful to Patterson of the Toronto Hospital Corporation for the human lung specimens. Finally, we thank V. Mas for technical assistance with the HPLC analyses.

Author Contributions: Daniel S. Sitar and Michael Spino are supervisors to James M. Bowen, Juan He, and Angelo Tesoro who conducted the experiments. All authors contributed to data analyses and manuscript preparation.

Conflicts of Interest: The authors declare no conflicts of interest.

References

1. Bend, J.R.; Serabjit-Singh, C.J.; Philpot, R.M. The pulmonary uptake, accumulation, and metabolism of xenobiotics. *Ann. Rev. Pharmacol. Toxicol.* **1985**, *25*, 97–125. [CrossRef] [PubMed]
2. Krishna, D.R.; Klotz, U. Extrahepatic metabolism of drugs in humans. *Clin. Pharmacokinet.* **1994**, *24*, 144–160. [CrossRef] [PubMed]
3. Hukkanen, J.; Pelkonen, O.; Hakkola, J.; Raunio, H. Expression and regulation of xenobiotic-metabolizing cytochrome P450 (CYP) enzymes in human lung. *Crit. Rev. Toxicol.* **2002**, *32*, 391–411. [CrossRef] [PubMed]
4. Nhamburo, P.T.; Gonzalez, F.J.; McBride, G.W.; Gelboin, H.V.; Kimura, S. Identification of a new P450 expressed in human lung: Complete cDNA sequence, cDNA-directed expression, and chromosome mapping. *Biochemistry* **1989**, *28*, 8060–8066. [CrossRef] [PubMed]
5. Upton, R.N.; Doolette, D.J. Kinetic aspects of drug disposition in the lungs. *Clin. Exp. Pharmacol. Physiol.* **1999**, *26*, 381–391. [CrossRef] [PubMed]
6. Vane, J.R. The release and fate of vaso-active hormones in the circulation. *Br. J. Pharmacol.* **1969**, *35*, 209–242. [CrossRef] [PubMed]
7. Bakhle, Y.S. Pharmacokinetic and metabolic properties of lung. *Br. J. Anaesth.* **1990**, *65*, 79–93. [CrossRef] [PubMed]
8. Hook, G.E.R.; Bend, J.R. Pulmonary metabolism of xenobiotics. *Life Sci.* **1976**, *18*, 279–290. [CrossRef]
9. Wolf, C.R.; Szutowski, M.M.; Ball, L.M.; Philpot, R.M. The rabbit pulmonary monooxygenase system: Characteristics and activities of two forms of pulmonary cytochrome P-450. *Chem. Biol. Interact.* **1978**, *21*, 29–43. [CrossRef]
10. Petruzzelli, S.; Camus, A.-M.; Carrozzi, L.; Ghelarducci, L.; Rindi, M.; Menconi, G.; Angeletti, C.A.; Ahotupa, M.; Hietanen, E.; Aitio, A.; et al. Long-lasting effects of tobacco smoking on pulmonary drug-metabolizing enzymes: A case-control study on lung cancer patients. *Cancer Res.* **1988**, *48*, 4695–4700. [PubMed]

11. Hermann, G.; Aynesworth, M.B. Successful treatment of persistent extreme dyspnea "status asthmaticus": Use of theophylline ethylene diamine (aminophylline USP) intravenously. *J. Lab. Clin. Med.* **1937**, *23*, 135–148.

12. Brodie, B.B.; Axelrod, J.; Reichenthal, A. Metabolism of theophylline (1,3-dimethylxantine) in man. *J. Biol. Chem.* **1952**, *194*, 215–222. [PubMed]

13. Tang-Liu, D.D.-S.; Williams, R.L.; Riegelman, S. Nonlinear theophylline elimination. *Clin. Pharmacol. Ther.* **1982**, *31*, 358–369. [CrossRef] [PubMed]

14. Knoppert, D.C.; Spino, M.; Beck, R.; Thiessen, J.J.; MacLeod, S.M. Cystic fibrosis: Enhanced theophylline metabolism may be linked to the disease. *Clin. Pharmacol. Ther.* **1988**, *44*, 254–264. [CrossRef] [PubMed]

15. Matsubara, T.; Prough, R.A.; Burke, M.D.; Estabrook, R.W. The preparation of microsomal fractions of rodent respiratory tract and their characterization. *Cancer Res.* **1974**, *34*, 2196–2203. [PubMed]

16. Lowry, O.H.; Rosebrough, N.J.; Farr, A.L.; Randall, R.J. Protein measurement with the Folin phenol reagent. *J. Biol. Chem.* **1951**, *193*, 265–275. [PubMed]

17. St. Pierre, M.V.; Tesoro, A.; Spino, M.; MacLeod, S.M. An HPLC method for the determination of theophylline and its metabolites in serum and urine. *J. Liquid Chromatogr.* **1984**, *7*, 1593–1608. [CrossRef]

18. Dyroff, M.C.; Neal, R.A. Studies of the mechanism of metabolism of thioacetamide S-oxide by rat liver microsomes. *Mol. Pharmacol.* **1983**, *23*, 219–227. [PubMed]

19. Miyaki, M.; Saito, A.; Shimizu, B. N→N Alkyl and glycosyl migrations of purines and pyrimidines. IV. trans-Glycosylation from pyrimidines to purines. (A novel synthetic method of purine nucleosides and nucleotides). *Chem. Pharm. Bull.* **1970**, *18*, 2459–2468. [CrossRef]

20. Kröll, F.; Karlsson, J.-A.; Nilsson, E.; Ryrfeldt, Å.; Persson, C.G.A. Rapid clearance of xanthines from airway and pulmonary tissues. *Am. Rev. Respir. Dis.* **1990**, *141*, 1167–1171. [CrossRef] [PubMed]

21. IJzerman, A.P.; Van der Wenden, R.A.A.; Mathôt, M.; Danhof, M.; Borea, P.A.; Varani, K. Partial agonism of theophylline-7-riboside on adenosine receptors. *Naunyn Schmiedebergs Arch. Pharmacol.* **1994**, *350*, 638–645. [CrossRef] [PubMed]

22. Elion, G.B.; Hitchings, G.H. Metabolic basis for the actions of analogs of purines and pyrimidines. *Adv. Chemother.* **1965**, *2*, 91–117. [PubMed]

23. Krenitsky, T.A.; Elion, G.B.; Strelitz, R.A.; Hitchings, G.H. Ribonucleosides of allopurinol and oxallopurinol. Isolation from human urine, enzymatic synthesis, and characterization. *J. Biol. Chem.* **1967**, *242*, 2675–2682. [PubMed]

24. Nelson, D.J.; Buggé, C.J.L.; Krasny, H.C.; Elion, G.B. Formation of nucleotides of [6-^{14}C] allopurinol and [6-^{14}C] oxipurinol in rat tissues and effects on uridine nucleotide pools. *Biochem. Pharmacol.* **1973**, *22*, 2003–2022. [CrossRef]

25. Reiter, S.; Simmonds, H.A.; Webster, D.R.; Watson, A.R. On the metabolism of allopurinol: Formation of allopurinol-1-riboside in purine nucleoside phosphorylase deficiency. *Biochem. Pharmacol.* **1983**, *32*, 2167–2174. [CrossRef]

26. Van Galen, P.J.M.; Uzerman, A.P. Xanthine-7-ribosides as adenosine A1 receptor antagonists: Further evidence for adenosine's anti mode of binding. *Nucleosides Nucleotides* **1990**, *9*, 275–291. [CrossRef]

27. Van der Wenden, E.M.; Hartog-Witte, H.R.; Roelen, H.C.P.F.; von Frijtag Drabbe Kunzel, J.K.; Pirovano, I.M.; Mathôt, R.A.A.; Danhof, M.; Van Aerschot, A.; Lidaks, M.J.; Ijzerman, A.P.; et al. 8-Substituted adenosine and theophylline-7-riboside analogues as potential partial agonists for the adenosine A$_1$ receptor. *Eur. J. Pharmacol.* **1995**, *290*, 189–199. [CrossRef]

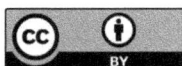

pharmaceutics

MDPI

Article

A High-Performance Liquid Chromatography Assay Method for the Determination of Lidocaine in Human Serum

Hamdah M. Al Nebaihi [1], Matthew Primrose [2], James S. Green [2] and Dion R. Brocks [1,*]

[1] Faculty of Pharmacy and Pharmaceutical Sciences, University of Alberta, Edmonton, AB T6G 2E1, Canada; alnebaih@ualberta.ca

[2] Department of Anesthesiology and Pain Medicine, Faculty of Medicine and Dentistry, University of Alberta, Edmonton, AB T6G 2B7, Canada; mprimros@ualberta.ca (M.P.); jgreen2@ualberta.ca (J.S.G.)

* Correspondence: dbrocks@ualberta.ca; Tel.: +1-780-492-2953

Received: 25 August 2017; Accepted: 15 November 2017; Published: 18 November 2017

Abstract: Here we report on the development of a selective and sensitive high-performance liquid chromatographic method for the determination of lidocaine in human serum. The extraction of lidocaine and procainamide (internal standard) from serum (0.25 mL) was achieved using diethyl ether under alkaline conditions. After liquid–liquid extraction, the separation of analytes was accomplished using reverse phase extraction. The mobile phase, a combination of acetonitrile and monobasic potassium phosphate, was pumped isocratically through a C18 analytical column. The ultraviolet (UV) wavelength was at 277 nm for the internal standard, and subsequently changed to 210 for lidocaine. The assay exhibited excellent linearity ($r^2 > 0.999$) in peak response over the concentration ranges of 50–5000 ng/mL lidocaine HCl in human serum. The mean absolute recoveries for 50 and 1000 ng/mL lidocaine HCl in serum using the present extraction procedure were 93.9 and 80.42%, respectively. The intra- and inter-day coefficients of variation in the serum were <15% at the lowest, and <12% at other concentrations, and the percent error values were less than 9%. The method displayed a high caliber of sensitivity and selectivity for monitoring therapeutic concentrations of lidocaine in human serum.

Keywords: lidocaine; pharmacokinetics; ultraviolet detection

1. Introduction

Lidocaine [also known as 2-(diethylamino)-*N*-(2,6-dimethylphenyl) acetamide] is commonly used as a local anesthetic and antiarrhythmic drug [1]. It can also be used for the management of extensive pain via either central or peripheral administration [2]. For these reasons, lidocaine is considered an essential medication for a wide array of clinical conditions [3]. Lidocaine is not a new medication, and hence many methods are available for its quantitation in biological specimens. The available methods are wide ranging, as is evident from the summary provided in Table 1. The most commonly used approach is to use reverse phase high performance liquid chromatography for separation, and ultraviolet (UV) absorbance as the detection method. This is not surprising considering that lidocaine by itself has poor fluorescence properties, and UV detectors are commonly available in laboratories.

Recently, our involvement in a clinical study necessitated that we measure lidocaine from human serum. Most of the previously available methods were based on volumes of 0.5 to 1 mL of specimen. In order to ensure that we could assay all of the samples available, we sought to develop a method that would use only 0.25 mL of specimen. Here we report on an alternative analytical method for lidocaine that was sufficiently sensitive to measure the drug in the serum using a volume of 0.25 mL.

Table 1. Comparisons of some published methods for assaying lidocaine in human matrices.

Volume of Specimen (mL)	Validated LLQ (ng/mL)	Type of Human Matrix	Sample Preparation Method	Analytical Column	Detection Method	References
0.2	50	Plasma	SPE	DB-1	GC–MS	[4]
0.5	200	Serum	LLE	C8	UV	[5]
0.1	680	Plasma	Protein ppt	C18	UV	[6]
0.5	200	Plasma	LLE	C18	UV	[7]
1	10	Serum	LLE	C18	UV	[8]
0.5	50	Plasma	LLE	C18	UV	[9]
0.1	400	Plasma	Protein ppt	C18	UV	[10]
0.5	100	Plasma	LLE	Phenyl	UV	[11]
0.5–1	25	Plasma	LLE	C18	Fluorescence of derivative	[12]
0.25	NS	Plasma	NS	C18	UV	[13]
1	1000	Plasma	LLE	C18	UV	[14]
0.01	200	Plasma	Protein ppt	C18	LC-MS/MS	[15]
1	0.2	Plasma	LLE	C18	LC-MS/MS	[16]
1	20	Serum	None	C18	UV	[17]
0.25	43	Serum	LLE	C18	UV	Current method

2. Materials and Methods

Lidocaine HCl (0.4% in 5% dextrose for injection) USP (Baxter Healthcare Corporation, Deerfield, IL, USA) was utilized as a source of lidocaine (Figure 1). Procainamide HCl was obtained from Sigma-Aldrich (St. Louis, MO, USA) (Figure 1). Ethyl ether, acetonitrile, water (all HPLC grade), triethylamine, potassium phosphate (monobasic) and sulfuric acid were purchased from Caledon Laboratories Ltd. (Georgetown, ON, Canada).

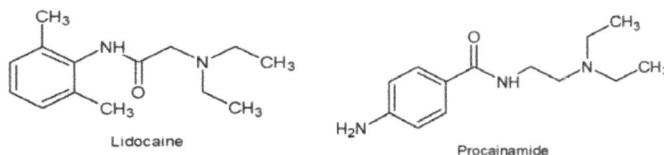

Figure 1. Chemical structure of lidocaine and procainamide, the internal standard.

2.1. Instrumentation and Chromatographic Conditions

The chromatographic system consisted of a Waters (Milford, MA, USA) 600 E multi-solvent delivery system pump, an autosampler with a variable injection valve (Waters 717), and a UV–visible tunable absorbance detector (Waters 486). The chromatograms were recorded using EZStart software (Scientific Software, Pleasanton, CA, USA) in a Windows-based computer system for data collection and processing. The chromatographic separation of lidocaine and procainamide (internal standard) were achieved using a 150 × 4.6 mm i.d., 3.5 μm particle size Alltima C18-column (Alltech, Deerfield, IL, USA) attached to a pre-guard column (Grace Alltech All-Guard™ Guard Cartridges, 7.5 mm 5 μm, Deerfield, IL, USA). The mobile phase consisted of a mixture of acetonitrile and phosphate solution (25 mM KH_2PO_4-3 mM sulfuric acid-3.6 mM triethylamine) in a ratio of 12:88 (v/v). The mobile phase was degassed prior to use by filtering it under vacuum pressure through a 0.45 μm pore size nylon filter, then pumped at a flow rate of 0.9 mL/min at room temperature.

Immediately after injection, the UV detection wavelength was set at 277 nm (the UV_{max} for procainamide). At 4 min post-injection, the UV detector was programmed to switch to a wavelength of 210 nm (the UV_{max} for lidocaine). The total analytical run time was <13 min.

2.2. Standard and Stock Solutions

The stock drug solution was 0.4% lidocaine HCl in 5% dextrose for injection. The working standard solutions were prepared daily from the stock solution by serial dilution with HPLC grade water to provide final concentrations of 40, 4 and 0.4 μg/mL lidocaine. The internal standard (IS) stock solution was prepared by dissolving 17 mg of procainamide HCl in 100 mL of water. All stock solutions were refrigerated between use. For the construction of a standard curve, samples of (0.25 mL) were prepared by adding lidocaine HCl equivalent to 50, 125, 250, 500, 1000, 2000, 2500 and 5000 ng/mL.

2.3. Extraction Procedure

A one-step liquid–liquid extraction step was used to extract lidocaine from human serum. After adding 50 μL volume of the IS stock solution and 200 μL of 1 M NaOH to 0.25 mL of human serum, 3 mL of diethyl ether was added. This was followed by vortex mixing of tubes for 30 s and centrifugation at 3000 *g* for 3 min. The organic solvent layer was pipetted to new tubes, then evaporated to dryness in vacuo. The dried residues were reconstituted using 150 μL of HPLC grade water with up to 75 μL being injected into the chromatographic system.

2.4. Recovery

Recovery was determined with lidocaine HCl concentrations of 50 and 1000 ng/mL and with an IS concentration of 0.17 mg/mL in human serum. The extraction efficiency was determined using five replicates of each concentration and comparing the extracted peak heights of analyte in the extracted samples to the peak heights of the same amounts of analyte directly injected into the HPLC without extraction.

2.5. Calibration, Accuracy and Validation

The assay was validated, generally using the guidelines published by the EMA [18]. The calibration curves were quantified by using peak height ratios of lidocaine HCl (concentration range from 50 to 5000 ng/mL) to IS versus the nominal lidocaine concentration. Intra-day validation was assessed at four different concentrations of lidocaine HCl (50, 250, 500 and 2000 ng/mL) per day in five replicates. This step was repeated on three separate days for determination of inter-day validation. For each daily run, an independent set of calibration curves samples was prepared. Accuracy and precision were assessed using the mean intra- and inter-day percentage error and percent coefficient of variation (CV%), respectively. Calibration curves were weighted by a factor of concentration^{-2} due to the wide range of concentrations (50–5000) used in the calibration curves.

Intraday, accuracy and precision of the assay were determined using a range of concentrations of lidocaine HCl. The selected concentrations were 50, 250, 500 and 2000 ng/mL of lidocaine HCl in human serum. Each concentration had five replicates. To permit the assessment of interday accuracy and precision in human serum, the assay was repeated on three separate days. For each daily run, a set of calibration samples separate from the validation samples were prepared to permit the quantification of the peak height ratios of lidocaine to IS. Precision was assessed by percentage coefficient of variation (CV%), while accuracy was represented by determining the mean intra- or inter-day percentage error.

2.6. Applicability

For the standard curve and validation samples, the serum was obtained from two healthy individuals on two separate occasions. For two of the samplings, each individual was asked to refrain from ingesting any caffeine-laden foods or drinks for 24 h before sampling.

The method was employed to determine the lidocaine concentration in human serum from one surgical patient after the injection of lidocaine as a reservoir within the rectus sheath (200 mg single dose). The patient provided written consent, and the study was approved by the University of Alberta Health Research Ethics Board. After the injection of the dose, blood samples were drawn serially into serum collection tubes until 24 h from the time of dosing. The blood samples were left for 30 min to clot, then centrifuged for 10 min. The serum was then separated and frozen at −20 °C until assayed.

3. Results

The chromatographic retention times were ~10 min for lidocaine and 2.5 min for IS (Figure 2). The chromatography displayed symmetrical peak shapes and high specificity, with a baseline resolution of IS and lidocaine. For both analytes, there was an absence of interference from endogenous components in serum (Figure 2). It was of note that the chromatograms from the serum of the healthy volunteers used in the assay development had a significant peak present that eluted at about 6.4 min, which was not seen in the patient serum sample obtained at 10 min. However, this did not interfere with the analysis of lidocaine, nor the internal standard.

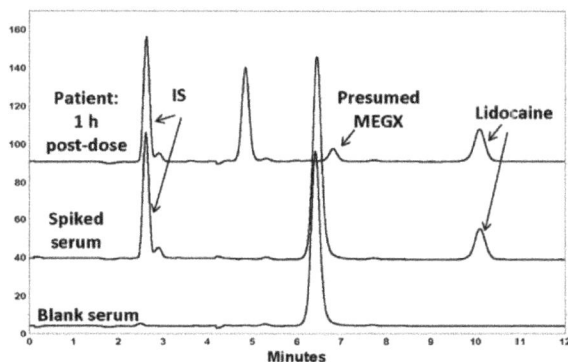

Figure 2. HPLC-UV chromatograms of blank (drug-free) serum from a healthy volunteer, volunteer serum spiked with 1000 ng/mL of lidocaine, and serum obtained 1 h after a 200 mg injection of lidocaine. The peak in the patient sample appearing at 6.8 min in the patient sample was presumed to be the lidocaine metabolite, monoethylglycinexylidide (MEGX). The peak at ~6.4 min was presumed to be from food components ingested by the volunteers who were not fasted.

The average recoveries were 97.7 ± 21% and 81.0 ± 2.4% for 50 and 1000 ng/mL lidocaine HCl in serum, respectively. The average extraction recoveries for IS at the concentration used in the assay was 55.4 ± 4.1%. There were excellent linear relationships (>0.9995) noted between the peak height ratios and lidocaine HCl concentrations over ranges of 50–5000 ng/mL serum.

From regression analysis of the concentration vs. peak height ratios of lidocaine to IS, the observed average slopes and intercepts were 0.00024 and 0.0011, respectively. The mean correlation coefficient of regression (r^2) for the serum standard curves were 0.9995. The CV of intra-and inter-day assessments were less than 15% (Table 2). The mean inter-day error in human serum was less than 9% (Table 2).

The validation assessments revealed that the assay was precise and possessed low bias. Overall, all intraday measures for mean error and CV% of the lowest concentration were less than 15%, and for the other concentrations only one fell above 10% (day three of the 216 ng/mL concentration). Except for the lowest concentration, all of the interday measures of CV% were less than 10%. All interday measures for mean error were less than 10%.

When tested for applicability in the patient samples, lidocaine serum concentrations could be measured for the full 24 h period following administration of the lidocaine dose. The observed maximal concentration was 1644 ng/mL, which occurred at 0.5 h post-dose.

The assay was reproducible and relatively fast in terms of preparation. To assay 30 samples, from the time of adding components to serum to completion of the evaporation of extracted solvent, took less than 40 min.

Table 2. Validation data for the assay of lidocaine in human serum, $n = 5$.

Nominal Concentration of Lidocaine *, ng/mL	Intraday			Interday		
	Mean ± SD ng/mL (CV%)			Mean ± SD ng/mL	CV%	Error%
43.3	45.9 ± 4.54 (9.90)	38.5 ± 5.37 (14.0)	40.8 ± 6.05 (14.8)	41.7 ± 5.32	12.9	−3.57
216	2158 ± 11.5 (5.35)	220 ± 9.60 (4.35)	226 ± 26.6 (11.8)	221 ± 15.9	7.16	1.99
433	379 ± 28.7 (7.56)	395 ± 25.6 (6.46)	407 ± 38.5 (9.47)	394 ± 30.9	7.83	−8.97
1731	1489 ± 60.5 (4.06)	1704 ± 43.3 (2.53)	1635 ± 47.1 (2.87)	1609 ± 50.3	3.16	−7.02

* To convert to lidocaine HCl salt, divide by 0.865.

4. Discussion

The HPLC method described here represents an accurate and precise avenue to determine the concentration of lidocaine in 0.25 mL volumes of human serum. The volumes of serum required are at the lower end of those volumes used by other analytical methods (Table 1). Additionally, the reported validated lower limits of quantitation are frequently greater than 50 ng/mL (Table 1). The lowest validated quantifiable concentration was found in the literature to be 10 ng/mL, though a serum volume of 1 mL was required [8]. Sintov et al. reported that the validated lower limit of quantification by using fluorescence detector was 25 ng/mL, which also required larger volumes of specimen up to 1 mL and derivatization following the extraction process [12], thereby adding elements of expense and time into sample preparation. The lower limit of quantitation (LLQ) in the current method is comparable to 50 ng/m by the GC-MS method [4].

Alkaline conditions were used to force lidocaine into its free base form, which promotes its extraction into a suitable organic solvent [12]. For the extraction of lidocaine from biological matrices, different solvents have been used in HPLC methods. These include an ethyl acetate/hexane/methanol mixture [14], dichloromethane [5], ethyl acetate [7,11], and a mixture of diethyl ether/dichloromethane [8]. Qin et al. had previously used diethyl ether as an extraction solvent for local anesthetics in human plasma, including procaine, ropivacaine, tetracaine, bupivacaine, including lidocaine [9]. The extraction of lidocaine from plasma in their hands was virtually complete, similar to what we had found. For this reason, we adopted the extraction method of Qin for use in the currently described assay method. Qin et al. had used carbamazepine as their internal standard. Due to its late elution time compared to procainamide [9], we chose to use procainamide instead. Although its recovery was less than that of lidocaine, it nevertheless extracted very consistently and provided excellent standard curves and validation indices. Procainamide would be an unlikely interfering substance in a patient as while it is chemically similar to lidocaine, it is not a popular antiarrhythmic currently, nor is it used as an anesthetic agent. The disadvantage of procainamide is that it requires that the UV detector possess the ability to program a change in wavelength after the elution of the internal standard.

In terms of mobile phase composition, acetonitrile and phosphate solution are the most common components in most of the reported studies (Table 1). Only Tam et al. and Qin et al. supplemented the mobile phase with 0.15% and 0.16% of triethylamine (TEA), respectively [7,9], while Chen et al. supplied the mobile phase with 1% diethylamine [6]. In the current method, 0.15% of triethylamine was added as it improved the peak symmetries and reduced the peak tailing of the compounds of interest, as has been noted for other compounds [19,20]. From the literature, the retention time for the compound of interest ranged from 3.6 to less than 13 min (Table 1).

The measured serum concentrations in the patient were in accordance with measures of plasma concentrations observed previously in patients administered the same dose of lidocaine HCl as depot parenteral injections [21]. The presence of a peak at 6.4 min was noticed in HPLC-UV chromatograms of blank (drug-free) human serum. Unfortunately, the appearance of this peak in the blank serum (with or without a caffeine-free period) virtually coincided with the elution of monoethylglycylxylidide (MEGX), a major metabolite of lidocaine [22]. In the first sample taken from the patient 10 min after the dose, although lidocaine was present, there was no peak observed eluting between 6 and 7 min. In later timed samples, such as 1 h after dosing (Figure 3) a peak virtually coinciding with MEGX was apparent. However, because in the volunteer serum, a large, mostly interfering peak was present, it was not possible to quantify the MEGX concentrations in the serum of the patient using the chromatographic conditions optimal for lidocaine elution. The patient differed from those subjects contributing volunteer serum in that the patients were required to fast before the surgery. Hence, it is possible that the peak in the healthy serum was from a food component, as none of the healthy volunteers had consumed any medications before contributing the blood for serum. The assay of metabolite was not a primary aim of this study, so we did not further pursue assay work as it would have meant a longer analytical run time for lidocaine, our primary analyte of interest. We did check for the elution of caffeine, and indeed it eluted at the same time as the large interfering peak in the serum of the volunteers who drank caffeine, but it was still present even after a 24 h caffeine fast. Therefore, it most likely derived from some other component of food. The patient also received other medications during surgery, and we believe that one of these may have been represented by the peak at 5.8 min (Figure 3), as it was not also seen in the volunteer serum, none of whom ingested any other drugs orally.

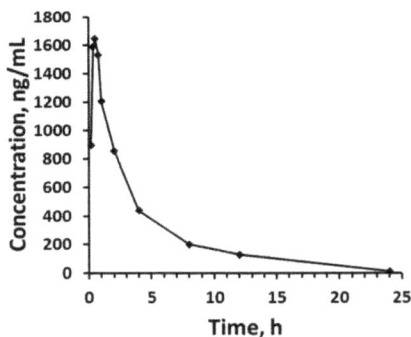

Figure 3. Serum lidocaine concentration vs. time profiles after rectus sheath injection of 200 mg lidocaine HCl to the patient volunteer.

5. Conclusions

The method demonstrated high calibers of sensitivity and selectivity for monitoring concentrations of lidocaine in human serum. The method was uncomplicated in terms of sample preparation and extraction. It was precise and accurate and was shown to have utility as a means to measure lidocaine concentration as part of a pharmacokinetic study.

Acknowledgments: Hamdah M. Al Nebaihi is the recipient of Government of Saudi Arabia scholarship.

Author Contributions: Hamdah M. Al Nebaihi performed most of the analytical method work including assay of samples and validation, and was extensively involved in data analysis and writing of the paper. Matthew Primrose and James S. Green contributed towards the concept and clinical aspect of the work. Dion R. Brocks was involved in concept, initial method workup and writing of the paper.

Conflicts of Interest: The authors declare no conflict of interest. There were no funding sponsors for the project.

Abbreviations

CV%   Coefficient of variation expressed as percent
LLQ   Lower limit of quantitation
SPE   Solid phase extraction
GC-MS   Gas chromatography-mass spectrometry
ppt   Precipitation
IS   Internal standard
LLE   Liquid-liquid extraction
UV   Ultraviolet detection
NS   Not specified or unclear

References

1. Benowitz, N.L.; Meister, W. Clinical pharmacokinetics of lignocaine. *Clin. Pharmacokinet.* **1978**, *3*, 177–201. [CrossRef] [PubMed]

2. Tremont-Lukats, I.; Teixeira, G.; Backonja, M. Systemic administration of local anesthetic agents to relieve neuropathic pain. *Anesth. Analg.* **2005**, *101*, 1736–1737.

3. World Health Organization. WHO Model List of Essential Medicines: 20th List, March 2017. Available online: http://www.who.int/medicines/publications/essentialmedicines/20th_EML2017_FINAL_amendedAug2017.png?ua=1 (accessed on 15 November 2017).

4. Ohshima, T.; Takayasu, T. Simultaneous determination of local anesthetics including ester-type anesthetics in human plasma and urine by gas chromatography-mass spectrometry with solid-phase extraction. *J. Chromatogr. B Biomed. Sci. Appl.* **1999**, *726*, 185–194. [CrossRef]

5. Piwowarska, J.; Kuczynska, J.; Pachecka, J. Liquid chromatographic method for the determination of lidocaine and monoethylglycine xylidide in human serum containing various concentrations of bilirubin for the assessment of liver function. *J. Chromatogr. B Anal. Technol. Biomed. Life Sci.* **2004**, *805*, 1–5. [CrossRef] [PubMed]

6. Chen, L.; Liao, L.; Zuo, Z.; Yan, Y.; Yang, L.; Fu, Q.; Chen, Y.; Hou, J. Simultaneous determination of nikethamide and lidocaine in human blood and cerebrospinal fluid by high performance liquid chromatography. *J. Pharm. Biomed. Anal.* **2007**, *43*, 1757–1762. [CrossRef] [PubMed]

7. Tam, Y.K.; Tawfik, S.R.; Ke, J.; Coutts, R.T.; Gray, M.R.; Wyse, D.G. High-performance liquid chromatography of lidocaine and nine of its metabolites in human plasma and urine. *J. Chromatogr.* **1987**, *423*, 199–206. [CrossRef]

8. Lotfi, H.; Debord, J.; Dreyfuss, M.F.; Marquet, P.; Ben Rhaiem, M.; Feiss, P.; Lachâtre, G. Simultaneous determination of lidocaine and bupivacaine in human plasma: Application to pharmacokinetics. *Ther. Drug Monit.* **1997**, *19*, 160–164. [CrossRef] [PubMed]

9. Qin, W.W.; Jiao, Z.; Zhong, M.K.; Shi, X.J.; Zhang, J.; Li, Z.D.; Cui, X.Y. Simultaneous determination of procaine, lidocaine, ropivacaine, tetracaine and bupivacaine in human plasma by high-performance liquid chromatography. *J. Chromatogr. B Anal. Technol. Biomed. Life Sci.* **2010**, *878*, 1185–1189. [CrossRef] [PubMed]

10. Bhusal, P.; Sharma, M.; Harrison, J.; Procter, G.; Andrews, G.; Jones, D.S.; Hill, A.G.; Svirskis, D. Development, validation and application of a stability indicating HPLC method to quantify lidocaine from polyethylene-co-vinyl acetate (EVA) matrices and biological fluids. *J. Chromatogr. Sci.* **2017**, *55*, 832–838. [CrossRef] [PubMed]

11. Nation, R.L.; Peng, G.W.; Chiou, W.L. High-performance liquid chromatographic method for the simultaneous determination of lidocaine and its N-dealkylated metabolites in plasma. *J. Chromatogr.* **1979**, *162*, 466–473. [CrossRef]

12. Sintov, A.; Siden, R.; Levy, R.J. Sensitive high-performance liquid chromatographic assay using 9-fluorenylmethylchloroformate for monitoring controlled-release lidocaine in plasma. *J. Chromatogr.* **1989**, *496*, 335–344. [CrossRef]

13. Kihara, S.; Miyabe, M.; Kakiuchi, Y.; Takahashi, S.; Fukuda, T.; Kohda, Y.; Toyooka, H. Plasma concentrations of lidocaine and its principal metabolites during continuous epidural infusion of lidocaine with or without epinephrine. *Reg. Anesth. Pain Med.* **1999**, *24*, 529–533. [CrossRef] [PubMed]

14. Dusci, L.J.; Hackett, L.P. Simultaneous determination of lidocaine, mexiletine, disopyramide, and quinidine in plasma by high performance liquid chromatography. *J. Anal. Toxicol.* **1985**, *9*, 67–70. [CrossRef] [PubMed]

15. Ter Weijden, E.; Van den Broek, M.; Ververs, F. Easy and fast LC–MS/MS determination of lidocaine and MEGX in plasma for therapeutic drug monitoring in neonates with seizures. *J. Chromatogr. B* **2012**, *881*, 111–114. [CrossRef] [PubMed]

16. Bo, L.D.; Mazzucchelli, P.; Marzo, A. Highly sensitive bioassay of lidocaine in human plasma by high-performance liquid chromatography-tandem mass spectrometry. *J. Chromatogr. A* **1999**, *854*, 3–11. [PubMed]

17. Ochoa-Aranda, E.; Esteve-Romero, J.; Rambla-Alegre, M.; Martinavarro-Domnguez, A.; Marcos-Toms, J.V.; Bose, D. Monitoring disopyramide, lidocaine, and quinidine by micellar liquic chromatography. *J. AOAC Int.* **2011**, *94*, 537–542. [PubMed]

18. Guideline on Bioanalytical Method Validation. Available online: http://www.ema.europa.eu/docs/en_GB/document_library/Scientific_guideline/2011/08/WC500109686.png (accessed on 15 November 2017).

19. Roos, R.W.; Lau-Cam, C.A. General reversed-phase high-performance liquid chromatographic method for the separation of drugs using triethylamine as a competing base. *J. Chromatogr.* **1986**, *370*, 403–418. [CrossRef]

20. Ruiz-Angel, M.; Torres-Lapasió, J.; Carda-Broch, S.; García-Alvarez-Coque, M. Improvement of peak shape and separation performance of β-blockers in conventional reversed-phase columns using solvent modifiers. *J. Chromatogr. Sci.* **2003**, *41*, 350–358. [CrossRef] [PubMed]

21. Chen, L.; Wang, Q.; Shi, K.; Liu, F.; Liu, L.; Ni, J.; Fang, X.; Xu, X. The Effects of Lidocaine Used in Sciatic Nerve on the Pharmacodynamics and Pharmacokinetics of Ropivacaine in Sciatic Nerve Combined with Lumbar Plexus Blockade: A Double-Blind, Randomized Study. *Basic Clin. Pharmacol. Toxicol.* **2013**, *112*, 203–208. [CrossRef] [PubMed]

22. Bargetzi, M.J.; Aoyama, T.; Gonzalez, F.J.; Meyer, U.A. Lidocaine metabolism in human liver microsomes by cytochrome P450IIIA4. *Clin. Pharmacol. Ther.* **1989**, *46*, 521–527. [CrossRef] [PubMed]

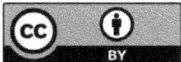

pharmaceutics

MDPI

Article

In Vitro Phase I Metabolism of CRV431, a Novel Oral Drug Candidate for Chronic Hepatitis B

Daniel J. Trepanier, Daren R. Ure and Robert T. Foster *

ContraVir Pharmaceuticals Inc., Edison, NJ 08837, USA; dtrepanier@contravir.com (D.J.T.);
dure@contravir.com (D.R.U.)
* Correspondence: rfoster@contravir.com; Tel.: +1-780-909-5041

Received: 27 August 2017; Accepted: 2 November 2017; Published: 9 November 2017

Abstract: The cytochrome P450-mediated Phase I in vitro metabolism of CRV431 was studied using selective chemical inhibition and recombinant human enzymes. Additionally, the metabolic profile of CRV431 in human, rat, and monkey liver microsomes was investigated. Liver microsomes were incubated for 0–80 min with CRV431, and the metabolite profile was assessed by electrospray ionization liquid chromatography mass spectrometry (ESI-LCMS). CRV431 was extensively metabolized through oxidation to produce various hydroxylated and demethylated species. Species identified included monohydroxylated CRV431 (two distinct products), dihydroxylated CRV431, demethylated CRV431 (two distinct products), demethylated and hydroxylated CRV431 (two distinct products), didemethylated and hydroxylated CRV431, and didemethylated and dihydroxylated CRV431. The magnitude of metabolism was greatest in monkey, followed by human, followed by rat. Importantly, all of the species identified in human microsomes were correspondingly identified in monkey and/or rat microsomes. Human liver microsome studies using selective chemical inhibition, as well as studies using recombinant human cytochrome P450 enzymes, revealed that the major enzymes involved are cytochromes P450 3A4 and 3A5. Enzymes 1A2, 2B6, 2C8, 2C9, 2C19, and 2D6 are not involved in the in vitro metabolism of CRV431. This information will be useful for the further development of CRV431 both preclinically and clinically.

Keywords: cyclophilin inhibitor; CRV431; P450; metabolism; species differences

1. Introduction

Cyclosporine A (CsA) was isolated from *Tolypocladium inflatum* in 1971, and has been used clinically since the early 1980s as an immunosuppressive drug to prevent rejection after solid organ transplantation [1]. CsA and other immunosuppressive analogues bind to cyclophilin, and the complex further binds and inhibits the activity of calcineurin, a phosphatase that activates T cells [2].

A novel investigational drug that is a non-immunosuppressive derivative of CsA, CRV431, is currently under development. The immunosuppressive property of CsA has been removed by modification of the CsA undecapeptide scaffold by introducing chemical modifications on amino acids 1 and 3. This alteration to the CsA backbone has been made to exploit the known properties of cyclophilins in normal physiology and in disease. Cyclophilins play an important role in infectious diseases, including for example, treatment of the hepatitis C virus (HCV) and hepatitis B virus (HBV). CRV431 has been shown previously to block replication of HBV, HCV, and human immunodeficiency virus type 1 (HIV-1) in vitro by inhibiting important interactions of the viruses with host cell cyclophilins [3–5]. CRV431 is currently being studied as a host-targeting investigational drug to treat chronic HBV. In in vitro [4,5] and in vivo (*unpublished data*) studies to date, CRV431 has been shown to reduce HBV and DNA, as well as target HBV proteins, including protein X (HBx) and surface antigen (HBsAg), through its ability to abrogate binding of cyclophilins to proteins. It is

Pharmaceutics **2017**, *9*, 51

anticipated that CRV431 will complement the landscape of direct acting anti-HBV drugs such as tenofovir and entecavir.

CsA undergoes extensive hepatic metabolism with elimination primarily through biliary excretion. Less than 10% of the intact drug and metabolite are excreted in urine. Cytochrome P-450 3A has been identified as the major metabolizing enzyme [6–8], which results in multiple primary hydroxylations and N-demethylations, along with secondary and tertiary products.

Here, we describe the cytochrome P450-mediated Phase I in vitro metabolism of CRV431 using selective chemical inhibition and recombinant human enzymes to gain a better understanding of the fate of the parent molecule, and understand potential routes of elimination of both parent and metabolite. Additionally, we investigate the metabolic profile of CRV431 in human, rat, and monkey liver microsomes, and identify multiple metabolites by liquid chromatography—mass spectrometry (LC-MS).

2. Materials and Methods

2.1. Drugs and Reagents

CRV431 was synthesized in-house to a purity of 97.3% by modification of cyclosporin A and stored at 5 °C. CsA was obtained from *IVAX* (Czech Republic). Human and rat liver microsomes, as well as recombinant human CYP enzymes, were obtained from Sekisui Xenotech, Kansas City, MO, USA. Monkey liver microsomes were obtained from Thermo Fisher Scientific, Waltham, MA, USA. All chemicals and reagents were purchased from Sigma-Aldrich, St. Louis. MO, USA.

2.2. Metabolic Stability of CRV431 in Human Liver Microsomes

Incubations of CRV431 (1 and 10 µM) with pooled human liver microsomes (1 mg protein/mL) were conducted for 30 min. Incubations were performed at 37 ± 1 °C in 0 2 mL incubation mixtures (final volume) containing potassium phosphate buffer (50 mM, pH 7.4), MgCl$_2$ (3 mM) and EDTA (1 mM, pH 7.4) with an NADPH-generating system as cofactor. The NADPH-generating system consisted of NADP (1 mM, pH 7.4), glucose-6-phosphate (5 mM, pH 7.4), and glucose-6-phosphate dehydrogenase (1 Unit/mL). CRV431 was added to incubations in DMSO (0.1% v/v). Additional incubations of CRV431 (1 and 10 µM) with human liver microsomes (1 mg protein/mL) were carried out at 0, 15, 30, 60, and 120 min. Reactions were initiated by the addition of the NADPH-generating system, and were stopped by the addition of 175 µL of acetonitrile. The samples were centrifuged (920× g for 10 min at 10 °C), and the supernatant fractions were analyzed by LC-MS/MS (Sciex, Redwood City, CA, USA) to quantify the amount of unchanged CRV431 based on a calibration curve (ranging from 0.01 to 15 µM). Zero-time, zero-cofactor (no NADPH), zero-substrate, and zero-protein served as blanks.

2.3. Cytochrome P450 Metabolism of CRV431 Using Recombinant Human CYP Enzymes

This experiment was carried out to determine the cytochrome P450 (CYP) enzymes capable of metabolizing CRV431. Briefly, CRV431 at two concentrations (1 and 10 µM) was incubated in duplicate with a panel of recombinant human CYP enzymes (rCYP1A2, 2B6, 2C8, 2C9, 2C19, 2D6, and 3A4 at 50 pmol CYP/mL) at 37 ± 1 °C in 0.2 mL incubation mixtures (final volume) containing potassium phosphate buffer (50 mM, pH 7.4), MgCl$_2$ (3 mM) and EDTA (1 mM, pH 7.4) with an NADPH-generating system as cofactor. The NADPH-generating system consisted of NADP (1 mM, pH 7.4), glucose-6-phosphate (5 mM, pH 7.4), and glucose-6-phosphate dehydrogenase (1 Unit/mL). CRV431 was added to the incubation mixtures in DMSO (0.1% v/v). Reactions were initiated by the addition of cofactor, and were terminated at zero and 15 min by the addition of 175 µL ice-cold methanol. After the reactions were stopped, samples were analyzed by LC-MS/MS to quantify the amount of unchanged CRV431.

2.4. Cytochrome P450 Metabolism Using Chemical Inhibition in Human Liver Microsomes

This experiment was carried out manually to verify the role of individual CYP enzymes in the metabolism of CRV431. CRV431 at 1 µM was incubated in duplicate with human liver microsomes (1 mg protein/mL) for zero and 15 min in the presence and absence of the chemical inhibitors summarized in the table below. Incubations were conducted at 37 ± 1 °C in 0.2 mL incubation mixtures (final volume) containing potassium phosphate buffer (50 mM, pH 7.4), MgCl$_2$ (3 mM) and EDTA (1 mM, pH 7.4), with an NADPH-generating system as cofactor. The NADPH-generating system consisted of NADP (1 mM, pH 7.4), glucose-6-phosphate (5 mM, pH 7.4), and glucose-6-phosphate dehydrogenase (1 Unit/mL). CRV431 was added to the incubation mixtures in DMSO (0.1% *v/v*). For incubations with direct-acting chemical inhibitors, reactions were initiated by the addition of cofactor, and stopped by the addition of an equal volume of acetonitrile stop reagent. For incubations with metabolism-dependent chemical inhibitors, 30 min pre-incubations of human liver microsomes and the inhibitor were initiated by the addition of the cofactor. CRV431 was then added to the mixture to be incubated for 15 min. Reactions were stopped by the addition of an equal volume of acetonitrile stop reagent. Samples were analyzed by LC-MS/MS to quantify the amount of unchanged CRV431. Control samples with no CYP inhibitor present were conducted in the presence of the solvent used to dissolve the CYP inhibitor ("solvent control").

2.5. LC-MS/MS Analysis of CRV431 for Cytochrome P450 Studies

Samples were analyzed by LC-MS/MS on a SCIEX 4000 QTrap mass spectrometer (Sciex, Rewood City, CA, USA). CRV431 samples were injected onto an Acquity UPLC BEH C18 analytical column (50 × 2.1 mm, 1.7 µm, Waters, Milford, MA, USA) and separated using a methanol-water gradient system (Table 1). The ammonium adducts of CRV431 (mass transition 1321.5/1304.5) were analyzed by mass spectrometry using electrospray ionization (ESI) in positive ion mode. The electrospray voltage was set at 4500 volts.

Table 1. LC-MS/MS Gradient Conditions for CRV431 Quantitation.

Time (min)	95:5 *v/v* Water: Methanol * (%)	Methanol *	Flow Rate (mL/min)
0.00	55	45	0.5
0.2	55	45	0.5
3.0	5	95	0.5
3.5	5	95	0.5
3.51	55	45	0.5
4.2	Stop	Stop	0.5

* also contains 1 mM ammonium acetate.

2.6. Microsome Incubation Procedure for Generation of CRV431 Metabolites

Human and rat liver microsomes were obtained from Xenotech (Kansas City, MO, USA) and stored at −80 °C. Monkey liver microsomes were obtained from Thermo Fisher Scientific (Waltham, MA, USA) and stored at −80 °C. Preliminary microsomal biotransformation experiments were run with 0.1, 1, and 10 µg/mL CRV431. CRV431 biotransformation was minimal at 0.1 µg/mL, while both 1 and 10 µg/mL CRV431 gave sufficient metabolite quantity and identical metabolite profiles. Additionally, preliminary experiments were conducted with human liver microsome (HLM) levels ranging for 0.125 to 1 mg. Subsequent microsomal biotransformation experiments were conducted using 0.5 mg of microsome per assay.

Thawed microsome 20 mg/mL stocks were diluted 32× into cold buffer (Phosphate pH 7.4 + MgCl2 3 mM + EDTA 1 mM) to 0.625 mg/mL, and stored on ice. For experiments with CRV431, 2 µL of 0.625 mg/mL CRV431 stocks were added to cold 1-mL microsomes (500× dilution) to generate the 1 µg/mL samples. For experiments with verapamil, 2 µL of 625 µM was added to cold 1-mL human microsomes (500× dilution). Samples were mixed by vortexing, and 160 µL was transferred into tubes containing 40 μL buffer on ice. Metabolic activity was stopped by the addition of ice-cold methanol (200 μL), followed by vortexing for an additional 10 s; these were zero-time samples. The extraction was completed by waiting 5 min, vortexing samples again for 5 s, then spinning the samples for 10 min at 3300 rpm at 4 °C in a pre-cooled microcentrifuge. The supernatant (325 μL) was transferred to new tubes and stored at −80 °C.

For time course experiments, metabolism was initiated by adding 40 μL of NADPH Regenerating System (5 mg/mL NADP, 6.5 mg/mL G6P and 5 units/mL of G6P dehydrogenase). The sample was vortexed for 2 s and placed in a 37 °C bath. For CRV431 experiments at time points 10 min, 20 min, 40 min, and 80 min, 200 μL of ice-cold methanol was added to the 200 μL microsome reactions, and extracted as described above. Samples were stored at −80 °C. For verapamil experiments at 15 min, 200 μL of ice-cold methanol was added to the 200 μL microsome reactions and extracted as described above. Samples were stored at −80 °C.

2.7. CRV431 and Metabolite Extraction from Rat, Monkey and Human Microsomes

Microsome extracts were removed from the freezer (−80 °C) and left to thaw at room temperature. Aliquots (50 μL) were removed and placed in 2 mL plastic Eppendorf microcentrifuge tubes, to which 200 μL of a 0.2 M $ZnSO_4$ solution (0.2 M $ZnSO_4$ in water, plus HPLC grade methanol, 1:4, v/v) was added as protein precipitating reagent. The tubes were capped and vortexed for 10 s, and then left on the benchtop for 10 min. Samples were then centrifuged at 3300 rpm for 10 min. The clear supernatant (≈150 μL) was transferred to an appropriately labeled LC-MS autosampler vial and capped.

2.8. LC-MS Analysis of CRV431 Metabolites

Samples were analyzed by electrospray ionization liquid chromatography mass spectrometry (ESI-LCMS) on an Agilent HP 1100 LC-MS. Samples were placed in an autosampler maintained at 5 °C. CRV431 microsomal extracts (20 μL) were injected onto a Zorbax SB-C18 reverse phase HPLC column (1.8 μm Rapid Resolution HT Cartridge, 4.6 × 30 mm (Agilent, Santa Clara, CA, USA) maintained at 75 °C, and the components were separated using an acetonitrile–water gradient system (Table 2). The sodium adducts of CRV431 (1326 m/z) and metabolites were analyzed by mass spectrometry (MS) using electrospray ionization (ESI) in positive ion mode. The ESI–MS was optimized with N_2 gas temperature set at 350 °C and drying gas at 12/L min. The fragmentor and capillary voltages were set at 260 and 4000 volts, respectively. The nebulizer pressure was set at 40 psig. For the initial analysis of the microsomal extracts, the ESI–MS was run in scan mode (1260–1460 m/z) to capture all ion signals present. Subsequently, the microsomal extracts were run in selected ion mode (SIM), with the ions identified in the scans.

Table 2. LC-MS/MS Gradient Conditions for Elution of CRV431 and Metabolites.

Time (min)	dH20 * (%)	ACN *	Flow Rate (mL/min)
0.00	55	45	1.0
16.0	25	75	1.0
16.1	0	100	1.0
18.1	0	100	1.0
18.2	55	45	1.0

* also contains 0.02% Glacial acetic acid + 20 μM Sodium Acetate.

2.9. Verapamil LC-MS Analysis for Microsome Viability

Samples were analyzed by electrospray ionization liquid chromatography mass spectrometry (ESI-LCMS) on an Agilent HP 1100 LC-MS (Agilent, Santa Clara, CA, USA). Samples were placed in an autosampler maintained at 5 °C. Verapamil microsomal extracts (2 μL) were injected onto a Zorbax SB-C18 reverse phase HPLC column (1.8 μm Rapid Resolution HT Cartridge, 4.6 × 30 mm) maintained at 75 °C, and the verapamil was separated using an acetonitrile–water gradient system

(Table 3). The sodium adduct of verapamil (455.5 m/z) was analyzed by mass spectrometry (MS) using electrospray ionization (ESI) in positive ion mode. The ESI–MS was optimized with N_2 gas temperature set at 350 °C and drying gas at 12/L min. The fragmentor and capillary voltages were set at 150 and 4500 volts, respectively. The nebulizer pressure was set at 40 psig.

Table 3. LC-MS Gradient Conditions for Elution of Verapamil.

Time (min)	dH20 * (%)	ACN *	Flow Rate (mL/min)
0.00	70	30	1.0
8.0	45	55	1.0
8.1	0	100	1.0
10.1	0	100	1.0
10.2	70	30	1.0

* also contains 0.02% Glacial acetic acid + 20 µM Sodium Acetate.

3. Results

3.1. CRV431 Metabolic Stability in Human Liver Microsomes

The biotransformation of CRV431 was nearly complete after 60 min incubation in human liver microsomes (Figure 1). In the absence of microsomal proteins and the NADPH-generating system, no biotransformation was observed over the same time period.

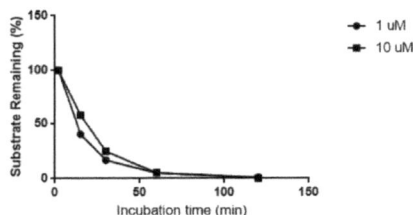

Figure 1. Biotransformation of CRV431 (1 and 10 µM) in human liver microsomes.

3.2. Cytochrome P450 Metabolism of CRV431 Using Recombinant Human CYP Enzymes

This experiment was carried out to determine the cytochrome P450 (CYP) enzymes capable of metabolizing CRV431. The disappearance of CRV431 (1 µM) was observed in incubations with recombinant human CYP1A2 (19%), CYP2C9 (27%), CYP2C19 (17%), CYP2D6 (32%), and CYP3A4 (64%), while incubations with control bactosomes resulted in 24% loss. The loss of CRV431 (10 µM) was observed in incubations with recombinant human CYP2C9 (27%) and CYP3A4 (41%). Incubations with the other recombinant human CYP enzymes evaluated resulted in less than 15% substrate loss (Figure 2).

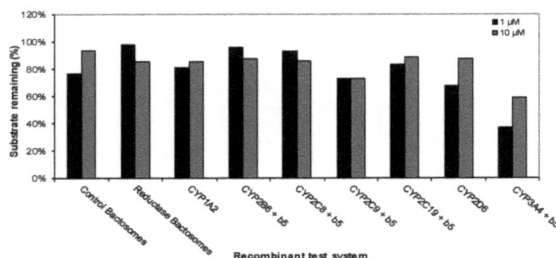

Figure 2. Metabolism of CRV431 (1 and 10 µM) by a panel of recombinant human CYP enzymes (50 pmol/mL).

3.3. Cytochrome P450 Metabolism of CRV431 Using Chemical Inhibitors

This experiment was carried out manually to verify the role of individual CYP enzymes in the metabolism of CRV431. The effect of the direct-acting inhibitors on the loss of CRV431 by human liver microsomes is shown in Figure 3. Percent inhibition was calculated by the comparison of substrate loss in samples containing chemical inhibitors to respective solvent control samples incubated for the same interval. The inhibition of CRV431 loss by direct-acting inhibitors was observed in incubations with ketoconazole (CYP3A4/5 inhibitor, 100% inhibition). Incubations with quinidine (CYP2D6 inhibitor) showed no inhibition.

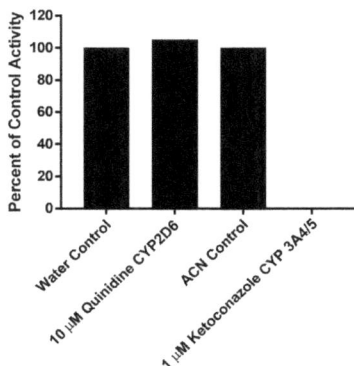

Figure 3. Effect of direct-acting chemical inhibitors on the loss of CRV431 (1 μM) by human liver microsomes.

The effect of the metabolism-dependent inhibitors on the loss of CRV431 by human liver microsomes is summarized in Figure 4. The inhibition of CRV431 loss by metabolism-dependent inhibitors was observed in incubations with tienilic acid (CYP2C9 inhibitor, 7% inhibition), esomeprazole (CYP2C19 inhibitor, 37% inhibition), and troleandomycin (CYP3A4/5 inhibitor, 100% inhibition). It is to be noted that esomeprazole is a mechanism-based inhibitor of both CYP2C19 and CYP3A4/5. Incubations with the other metabolism-dependent inhibitors evaluated resulted in no inhibition.

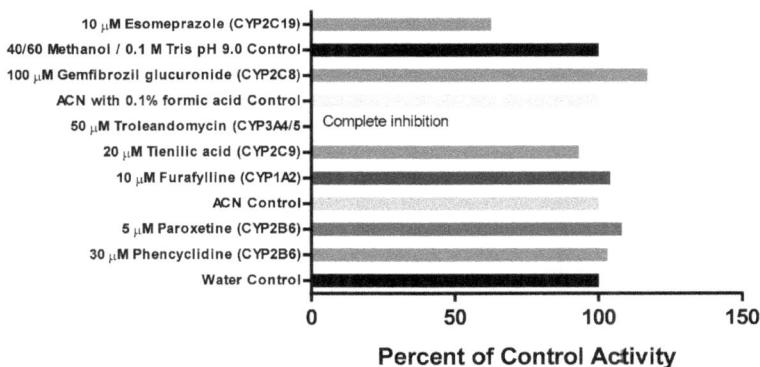

Figure 4. Effect of metabolism-dependent chemical inhibitors on the loss of CRV431 (1 μM) by human liver microsomes after 30-min preincubation.

3.4. Liver Microsome Viability for Metabolic Profiling Studies

Incubations of verapamil with human, monkey, and rat liver microsomes demonstrated rapid metabolism. The verapamil half-life in all of the microsome incubations was less than 10 min. This is in line with the metabolism rate for verapamil [9], and confirms the viability of the human, monkey, and rat liver microsomes used in this study to assess the in vitro metabolism of CRV431.

3.5. CRV431 Metabolite Identification in Human Liver Microsomes

The chemical structure of CRV431 and its potential biotransformation sites are indicated in Figure 5. The mass spectral scans for CRV431 incubated with human liver microsomes are shown in Figure 6, panels A and B. These low sensitivity scans allow for the identification of all metabolite masses. In addition to CRV431, 12 distinct masses were identified and subsequently used for more sensitive selected-ion monitoring of all CRV431 microsomal samples. The individual LC-MS metabolism profiles (0–80 min) for incubation with 1 μg/mL CRV431 are shown in Figure 7, panels A to D. The incubation of human liver microsomes with 1 μg/mL CRV431 for 0–80 min allowed for the identification of 12 distinct metabolites (M1–M12) resulting from various hydroxylation and demethylation reactions (Table 4), which are consistent with the metabolism previously reported with cyclosporine and analogues by the cytochrome P450 enzyme system [2–4]. The metabolite M4 is included for completeness, but likely arises from the demethylation of unsaturated CRV431, which is present as an impurity.

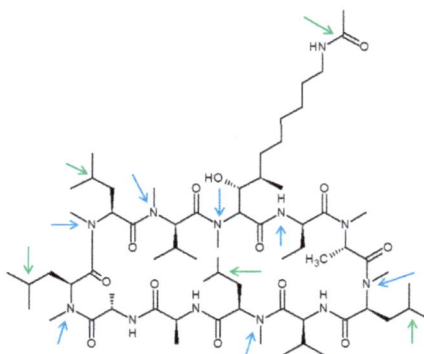

Figure 5. Chemical structure of CRV431 and proposed biotransformation sites. Potential oxidation (green arrows) and demethylation (blue arrows) sites are shown.

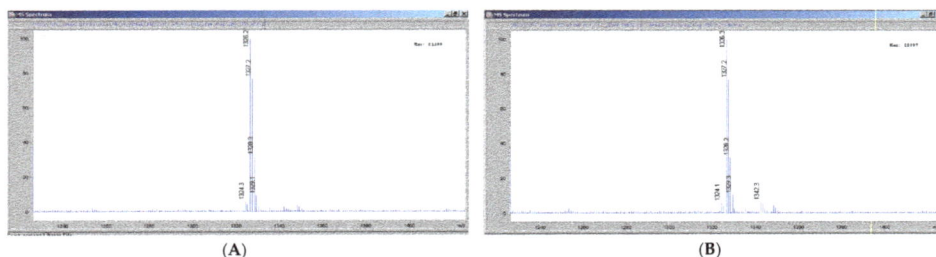

(A)   (B)

Figure 6. Mass spectral scans of human liver extracts incubated with CRV431. Human liver microsomes (1 mg/mL) were incubated with 1 μg/mL CRV431, and extracts were removed for analysis by electrospray ionization liquid chromatography mass spectrometry (ESI-LCMS) at 20 min (panel (**A**)), mass spectral scan from 1260–1460 *m/z* and 80 min (panel (**B**)), and mass spectral scan from 1260–1460 *m/z* (not shown).

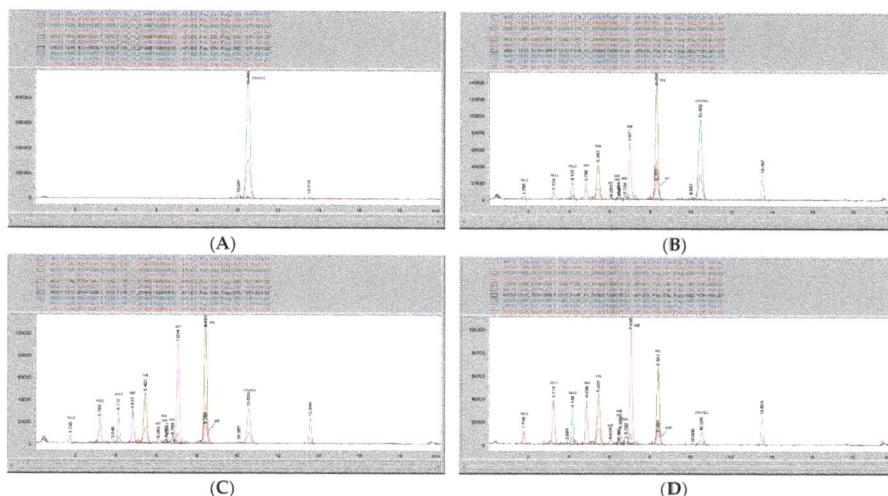

Figure 7. CRV431 metabolism in human liver microsomes. Human liver microsomes (1 mg/mL) were incubated with 1 ug/mL CRV431, and extracts were removed at 0 (panel **A**), 20 min (panel **B**), 40 min (panel **C**), and 80 min (panel **D**) for analysis by ESI-LCMS. Each liquid chromatography—mass spectrometry (LC–MS) profile displays the metabolite abundances as a function of chromatographic retention time.

Table 4. Identification of CRV431 metabolites in human liver microsomes. Human liver microsomes (1 mg/mL) were incubated with 1 ug/mL CRV431, and extracts were removed for analysis by ESI-LCMS.

Component	Proposed Biotransformation	Relative LC-MS Retention	m/z	Δ m/z	% of Total Drug-Related Mass Versus Time (minutes)				
					0 min	10 min	20 min	40 min	80 min
CRV431	NA	1.0	1326	0	96.4	57.0	27.5	10.4	4.0
CRV431 unsaturated impurity	NA	0.96	1324	NA	3.6	2.9	1.8	0.7	0.2
M1	Hydroxylation	0.8	1342	+16	0	21.2	28.3	27.4	18.3
M2	Demethylation	0.8	1312	−14	0	3.6	4.9	4.6	3.1
M3	Demethylation	0.67	1312	−14	0	5.3	13.8	21.9	27.4
M4	Demethylation of unsaturated CRV431	0.65	1310	−16	0	0.3	1.1	1.7	2.0
M5	Didemethylation	0.62	1298	−28	0	0	0.4	1.3	2.5
M6	Dihydroxylation	0.62	1358	+32	0	0	1.3	1.4	1.1
M7	Demethylation + Hydroxylation	0.58	1328	+2	0	0.1	0.6	1.2	1.7
M8	Hydroxylation	0.52	1342	+16	0	5.9	10.3	13.0	13.5
M9	Demethylation + Hydroxylation	0.47	1328	+2	0	1.1	3.2	5.6	8.6
M10	Dihydroxylation	0.39	1358	+32	0	1.2	3.3	5.3	6.6
M11	Demethylation + Hydroxylation	0.30	1328	+32	0	0.4	1.6	4.4	8.9
M12	Dihydroxylation + demethylation	0.17	1344	+18	0	0.1	0.5	1.0	1.9

3.6. CRV431 Metabolite Identification in Monkey Liver Microsomes

The mass spectral scans for CRV431 incubated with monkey liver microsomes are shown in Figure 8, panels A to C. These low sensitivity scans allow for the identification of all metabolite masses. In addition to CRV431, three distinct masses were identified and subsequently used for more sensitive selected-ion monitoring of all CRV431 microsomal samples. The individual LC-MS metabolism profiles

(0–80 min) for incubation with 1 µg/mL CRV431 are shown in Figure 9, panels A to F. The incubation of monkey liver microsomes with 1 ug/mL CRV431 for 0–80 min allowed for the identification of all 12 metabolites (M1–M12) detected in human liver microsomes. An additional 12 metabolites not observed in human liver microsomes were also seen (M13–M24) (Table 5). The rate of CRV431 metabolism in monkey liver microsomes was significantly greater (at least five-fold) than that seen in human microsomes. At 10 min incubation, the amount of CRV431 remaining in the human and monkey liver microsomes was 71.8% and 13.2%, respectively. With the exception of M15, all of the additional metabolites appeared to be a result of the further metabolism of M1–M12 (di- and tri-hydroxylations and demethylations), which was consistent with the higher metabolism rate.

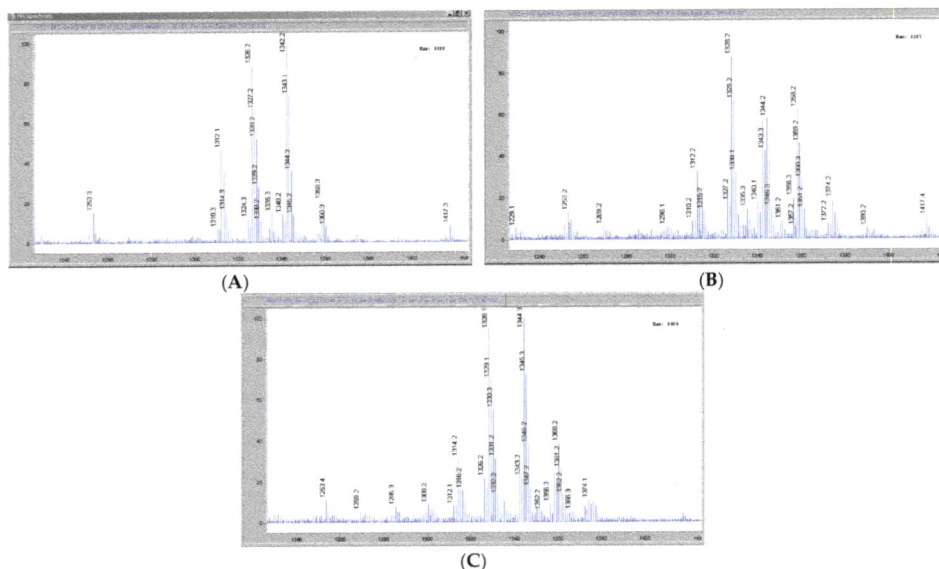

(A)   (B)

(C)

Figure 8. Mass spectral scans of monkey liver extracts incubated with CRV431. Monkey liver microsomes (1 mg/mL) were incubated with 1 µg/mL CRV431, and extracts were removed for analysis by ESI-LCMS at 5 min (panel (**A**), mass spectral scan from 1260–1460 *m/z*), 20 min (panel (**B**), mass spectral scan from 1260–1460 *m/z*) and 80 min (panel (**C**), mass spectral scan from 1260–1460 *m/z*).

(A)   (B)

Figure 9. *Cont.*

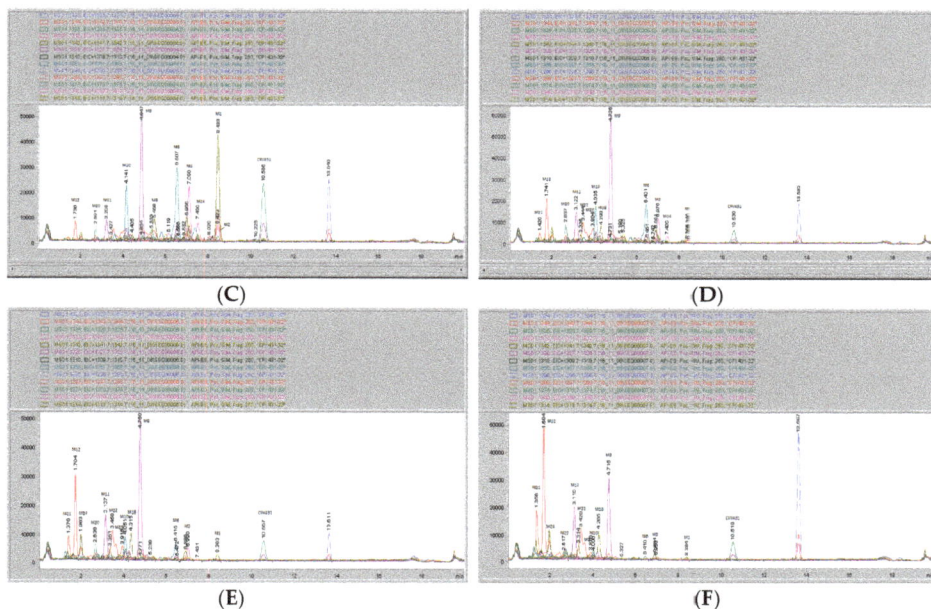

Figure 9. CRV431 metabolism in monkey liver microsomes. Monkey liver microsomes (1 mg/mL) were incubated with 1 ug/mL CRV431, and extracts were removed at 0 (panel (**A**), 5 min (panel (**B**)), 10 min (panel (**C**), 20 min (panel (**D**), 40 min (panel (**E**), and 80 min (panel (**F**) for analysis by ESI-LCMS. Each LC-MS profile displays the metabolite abundances as a function of chromatographic retention time.

Table 5. Identification of CRV431 metabolites in monkey liver microsomes. Monkey liver microsomes (1 mg/mL) were incubated with 1 ug/mL CRV431, and extracts were removed for analysis by ESI-LCMS.

Component	Proposed Biotransformation	Relative LC-MS Retention	m/z	$\Delta\ m/z$	% of Total Drug-Related Mass Versus Time (minutes)						
					0 min	2.5 min	5 min	10 min	20 min	40 min	80 min
CRV431	NA	1.0	1326	0	96.3	59.4	21.5	12.3	4.3	6.6	6.7
CRV431 unsaturated impurity	NA	0.96	1324	−2	3.7	3.8	1.7	0.8	0	0	0
M1	Hydroxylation	0.8	1342	+16	0	18.1	24.2	16.1	3.2	1.7	0.9
M2	Demethylation	0.8	1312	−14	0	3.1	6.7	2.7	0.7	0	0
M3	Demethylation	0.67	1312	−14	0	3.8	7.6	8.3	5.4	3.3	0.7
M4	Demethylation of unsaturated CRV431	0.65	1310	−16	0	0.3	0.5	0.6	0.6	0	0
M5	Didemethylation	0.62	1298	−28	0	0	0.2	0.4	0.7	0.6	0
M6	Dihydroxylation	0.62	1358	+32	0	2.4	8.2	12.6	10.9	4.8	1.3
M7	Demethylation + Hydroxylation	0.58	1328	+2	0	0	0	1.1	0	0	0
M8	Hydroxylation	0.52	1342	+16	0	1.9	3.7	3.7	2.0	0	0.4
M9	Demethylation + Hydroxylation	0.47	1328	+2	0	1.9	8.6	15.6	24.8	25.2	17.6
M10	Dihydroxylation	0.39	1358	+32	0	0.8	4.4	6.9	6.7	4.2	1.4
M11	Demethylation + Hydroxylation	0.30	1328	+32	0	0.2	1.3	2.8	6.5	8.7	11.7
M12	Dihydroxylation + demethylation	0.17	1344	+ 18	0	0.1	0.7	1.8	6.2	11.7	21.6

Table 5. *Cont.*

Component	Proposed Biotransformation	Relative LC-MS Retention	m/z	Δ m/z	% of Total Drug-Related Mass Versus Time (minutes)						
					0 min	2.5 min	5 min	10 min	20 min	40 min	80 min
Additional Metabolites Not Detected in Human Liver Microsome Experiments											
M13		0.75	1340	+14	0	1.1	1.6	1.1	0	0	0
M14		0.70	1340	+14	0	0.9	2.4	3.2	1.7	0.6	0
M15	Hydroxylation	0.65	1342	+16	0	1.6	3.3	3.9	3.3	2.4	1.7
M16	Trihydroxylation	0.50	1374	+48	0	0.4	1.8	2.6	2.2	1.4	0
M17	Trihydroxylation	0.46	1374	+48	0		0.4	0.8	0.9	1.1	0
M18	Didemethylation + hydroxylation	0.41	1314	−12	0	0	0.2	0.6	2.3	4.1	5.4
M19	Didemethylation + hydroxylation	0.31	1314	−12	0	0	0.2	0.4	1.3	1.8	2.8
M20	Trihydroxylation	0.25	1374	+48	0	0.1	0.8	1.6	3.3	2.9	1.8
M21	Dihydroxylation + demethylation	0.13	1344	+18	0	0	0	0	1.2	3.7	8.0
M22	Dihydroxylation + demethylation	0.32	1344	+18	0	0	0	0	5.6	8.4	11.1
M23	Dihydroxylation + demethylation	0.35	1344	+18	0	0	0	0	3.6	2.6	1.4
M24	Hydroxylation	0.18	1342	+16	0	0	0	0	2.3	4.0	5.7

3.7. CRV431 Metabolite Identification in Rat Liver Microsomes

The mass spectral scans for CRV431 incubated with rat liver microsomes are shown in Figure 10, panels A and B. These low-sensitivity scans allow for the identification of all of the metabolite masses present. In addition to CRV431, three distinct masses were identified and subsequently used for more sensitive selected-ion monitoring of all of the CRV431 microsomal samples. The individual LC-MS metabolism profiles (0–40 min) for incubation with 1 μg/mL CRV431 are shown in Figure 11, panels A to D. The incubation of rat liver microsomes with 1 ug/mL CRV431 for 0–80 min allowed for the identification of only four metabolites: M1, M3, M8, and M15 (Table 6). The rate of CRV431 metabolism in rat liver microsomes was significantly less (15-fold) than that seen in human microsomes. At 80 min incubation, the amount of CRV431 remaining in the human and rat liver microsomes was 5.3% and 92.3%, respectively. This slow rate of metabolism has previously been observed for cyclosporine A and other cyclosporine-based analogues in rat microsomes [personal communication].

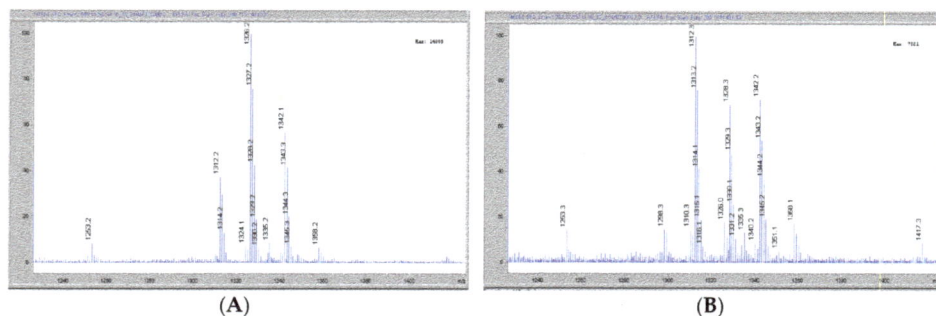

(A)   (B)

Figure 10. Mass spectral scans of rat liver extracts incubated with CRV431. Rat (Sprague-Dawley) liver microsomes (1 mg/mL) were incubated with 1 μg/mL CRV431, and extracts were removed for analysis by ESI-LCMS at 20 min (panel (**A**), mass spectral scan from 1260–1460 *m/z*) and 80 min (panel (**B**), mass spectral scan from 1260–1460 *m/z*).

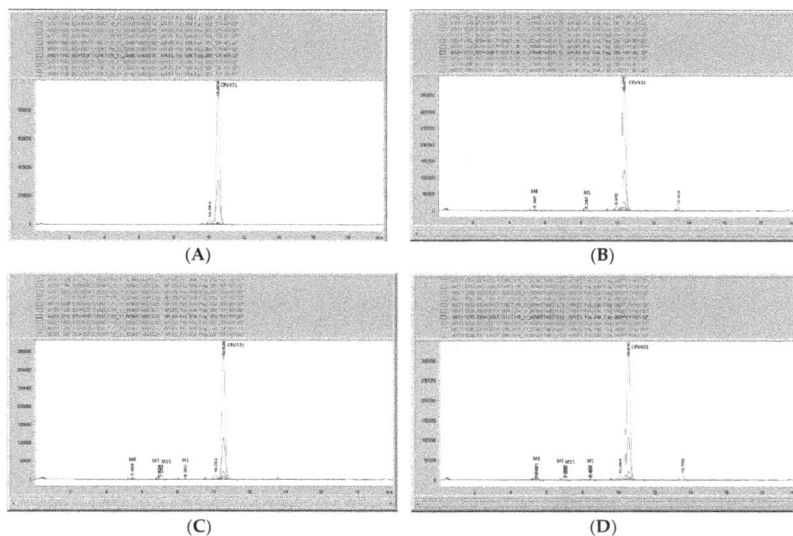

Figure 11. CRV431 metabolism in rat liver microsomes. Rat (Sprague Dawley) liver microsomes (1 mg/mL) were incubated with 1 ug/mL CRV431, and extracts were removed at 0 (panel (**A**)), 20 min (panel (**B**)), 40 min (panel (**C**)), and 80 min (panel (**D**)) for analysis by ESI-LCMS. Each LC-MS profile displays the metabolite abundances as a function of chromatographic retention time.

Table 6. Identification of CRV431 metabolites in rat liver microsomes. Rat liver microsomes (1 mg/mL) were incubated with 1 ug/mL CRV431, and extracts were removed for analysis by ESI-LCMS.

Component	Proposed Biotransformation	Relative LC-MS Retention	m/z	$\Delta\ m/z$	% of Total Drug-Related Mass Versus Time (minutes)				
					0 min	10 min	20 min	40 min	80 min
CRV431	NA	1.0	1326	0	96.2	95.4	94.6	93.6	92.3
CRV431 unsaturated impurity	NA	0.96	1324	NA	3.8	3.9	3.8	3.9	4.6
M1	Hydroxylation	0.8	1342	+16	0	0.1	0.3	0.5	0.5
M3	Demethylation	0.67	1312	−14	0	0	0.07	0.19	0.4
M8	Hydroxylation	0.52	1342	+16	0	0.4	0.8	1.3	1.7
M15	Hydroxylation	0.65	1342	+16	0	0.08	0.1	0.2	0.2

4. Conclusions and Discussion

The extensive hepatic metabolism of CsA results in three primary metabolites: the hydroxylated metabolites AMI and AM9, and the *N*-demethylated metabolite AM4n [6]. Cytochromes P450 3A4/5 are acknowledged to be predominantly responsible for the metabolism of CsA [7,8], although other cytochromes such as 3A9 may also play a role [10]. In this study, the in vitro metabolism of the CsA analogue CRV431 was shown to be NADPH-dependent in incubations with human liver microsomes. Incubations with recombinant human CYPs indicated that both CYP2D6 and CYP3A4 were able to significantly metabolize CRV431; however, in subsequent chemical inhibition (direct and metabolism-based) experiments with human liver microsomes, only CYP3A4 demonstrated significant activity. The cytochrome P450 experiments collectively indicate that CYP3A4 appears to be the predominant CYP enzyme that plays a role in the metabolism of CRV431 under the conditions evaluated.

The incubation of human liver microsomes with CRV431 allowed for the identification of 12 distinct metabolites (M1–M12) resulting from various hydroxylation and demethylation reactions (Figure 4), which is consistent with the metabolism reported for cyclosporine and analogues by the cytochrome P450 enzyme system. Monkey microsomes produced all 12 metabolites seen in human microsomes. Owing to the five-fold greater metabolism rate in monkey liver microsomes relative to human liver microsomes, an additional 12 metabolites (M13–M24) were also identified. The monkey is therefore a relevant animal species in which to study the preclinical metabolism of CRV431. Rat microsomes were very slow metabolizers of CRV431 (at least 15-fold less than human), and only M1, M3, M8, and M15 were detected.

CRV431 is being developed as a drug candidate for the treatment of certain viral infections, including hepatitis B. The current standard of care for the treatment of hepatitis B includes the use of nucleotide drugs such as tenofovir and entecavir [11]. It is anticipated that the drug–drug interaction potential between CRV431 and the nucleotide drugs used in the treatment of viral infections including hepatitis B would be minimal, as nucleotides are predominantly excreted renally, and not appreciably metabolized via cytochrome P450 enzymes.

Acknowledgments: This work was funded by ContraVir Pharmaceuticals Inc.

Author Contributions: Daniel J. Trepanier performed the experiments; Daren R. Ure contributed materials and analysis; Robert T. Foster conceived of the experiments; Daniel J. Trepanier, Daren R. Ure, and Robert T. Foster wrote the paper.

Conflicts of Interest: The authors are all employed by ContraVir Pharmaceuticals Inc.

References

1. Borel, J.F.; Kis, Z.L. The Discovery and Development of Cyclosporine (Sandimmune). *Transpl. Proc.* **1991**, *23*, 1867–1874.
2. Wiederrecht, G.; Lam, E.; Hung, S.; Martin, M.; Sigal, N. The Mechanism of Action of FK-506 and Cyclosporin A. *Ann. N. Y. Acad. Sci.* **1993**, *696*, 9–19. [CrossRef] [PubMed]
3. Gallay, P.A.; Bobardt, M.D.; Chatterji, U.; Trepanier, D.J.; Ure, D.; Ordonez, C.; Foster, R. The Novel Cyclophilin Inhibitor CRV431 Concurrently Blocks HCV and HIV-1 Infections via a Similar Mechanism of Action. *PLoS ONE* **2015**, *10*, e0134707. [CrossRef] [PubMed]
4. Ure, D.R.; Bobardt, M.D.; Chatterji, U.; Trepanier, D.J.; Gallay, P.A.; Foster, R.T. The Cyclophilin Inhibitor, CPI-431-32, is a Hepatitis B Oral Drug Candidate with Antiviral and Antifibrotic Actions. In Proceedings of the HEP DART 2015 Conference, Wailea, HI, USA, 5 October 2015.
5. Gallay, P.; Chatterji, U.; Bobardt, M.D.; Ure, D.; Trepanier, D.; Foster, R.; Ordonez, C. Novel Cyclophilin Inhibitor CPI-431-32 Shows Broad Spectrum Antiviral Action by Blocking Replication of HCV, HBV, and HIV-1. *J. Hepatol.* **2015**, *62*, S677. [CrossRef]
6. Maurer, G.; Loosli, H.R.; Schreier, E.; Keller, B. Disposition of Cyclosporine in Several Animal Species and Man. I. Structural elucidation of its metabolites. *Drug Metab. Dispos.* **1984**, *12*, 120–127. [PubMed]
7. Kronbach, T.; Fischer, V.; Meyer, U.A. Cyclosporine Metabolism in Human Liver: Identification of a Cytochrome P450 III Gene Family as the Major Cyclosporine-Metabolizing Enzyme Explains Interactions of Cyclosporine with other Drugs. *Clin. Pharmacol. Ther.* **1988**, *43*, 630–635. [CrossRef] [PubMed]
8. Combalbert, J.; Fabre, I.; Fabre, G.; Dalet, I.; Derancourt, J.; Cano, J.P.; Maurel, P. Metabolism of Cyclosporine A. IV. Purification and Identification of Rifampicin-Inducible Human Liver Cytochrome P-450 (cyclosporine A oxidase) as a Product of P-450 IIIA Gene Subfamily. *Drug Metab. Dispos.* **1989**, *17*, 197–207. [PubMed]
9. Grbac, R.T.; Stanley, F.A.; Ambo, T.; Barbara, J.E.; Haupt, L.J. High Content Automated Metabolic Stability and CYP Inhibition Cocktail Screening Assays for Early Drug Development. Personal communication, 2014.
10. Kelly, P.A.; Wang, H.; Napoli, K.L.; Kahan, B.D.; Strobel, H.W. Metabolism of Cyclosporine by Cytochromes P450 3A9 and 3A4. *Eur. J. Drug Metab. Pharm.* **1999**, *24*, 321–328. [CrossRef]
11. Kuo, A.; Gish, R. Chronic Hepatitis B Infection. *Clin. Liver Dis.* **2012**, *16*, 347–369. [CrossRef] [PubMed]

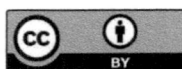

pharmaceutics

MDPI

Article

The Role of PXR Genotype and Transporter Expression in the Placental Transport of Lopinavir in Mice

Sarabjit S. Gahir [1,2] **and Micheline Piquette-Miller** [1,*]

[1] Leslie Dan Faculty of Pharmacy, University of Toronto, 144 College Street, Toronto, ON M5S 3M2, Canada; sarabjit.gahir@gmail.com

[2] Reata Pharmaceuticals, Irving, TX 75063, USA

[*] Correspondence: m.piquette.miller@utoronto.ca; Tel.: +1-416-946-3057; Fax: +1-416-978-8511

Received: 2 October 2017; Accepted: 20 October 2017; Published: 24 October 2017

Abstract: Lopinavir (LPV), an antiretroviral protease inhibitor frequently prescribed in HIV-positive pregnancies, is a substrate of Abcb1 and Abcc2. As differences in placental expression of these transporters were seen in Pregnane X Receptor (PXR) $-/-$ mice, we examined the impact of placental transporter expression and fetal PXR genotype on the fetal accumulation of LPV. PXR $+/-$ dams bearing PXR $+/+$, PXR $+/-$, and PXR $-/-$ fetuses were generated by mating PXR $+/-$ female mice with PXR $+/-$ males. On gestational day 17, dams were administered 10 mg/kg LPV (i.v.) and sacrificed 30 min post injection. Concentrations of LPV in maternal plasma and fetal tissue were measured by LC-MS/MS, and transporter expression was determined by quantitative RT-PCR. As compared to the PXR $+/+$ fetal units, placental expression of Abcb1a, Abcc2, and Abcg2 mRNA were two- to three-fold higher in PXR $-/-$ fetuses ($p < 0.05$). Two-fold higher fetal:maternal LPV concentration ratios were also seen in the PXR $+/+$ as compared to the PXR $-/-$ fetuses ($p < 0.05$), and this significantly correlated to the placental expression of Abcb1a ($r = 0.495$; $p < 0.005$). Individual differences in the expression of placental transporters due to genetic or environmental factors can impact fetal exposure to their substrates.

Keywords: antiretrovirals; transporters; P-glycoprotein; breast cancer resistance protein; multidrug resistance associated protein; gene regulation; protease inhibitor; Pregrane X Receptor; placenta; knockout mice

1. Introduction

Globally, there are over 2 million children living with HIV and, according to UNAIDS, most of these infections were caused by mother-to-child transmission (MTCT) of the virus [1]. Employing a strategy of aggressive, proactive prophylaxis when managing HIV-seropositive pregnancies by the administration of Highly Active Anti-Retroviral Therapy (HAART) has brought the rate of vertical transmission down from around 25% in the absence of these interventions to less than 2% in North America [2,3]. However, little is known about the factors controlling the transplacental trafficking of highly potent antiretrovirals.

The placenta is the principle gateway between the maternal and fetal systems, regulating the exchange of both endogenous and exogenous molecules. This barrier site also performs a critical role in limiting the access of potentially toxic xenobiotics [4,5]. The presence of several ATP Binding Cassette (ABC) drug transporters, including P-glycoprotein (PGP/ABCB1), Multidrug Resistance Associated Proteins (MRP/ABCC), and the Breast Cancer Resistance Protein (BCRP/ABCG2) at the materno-placental interface, is believed to be involved in the extrusion of a wide spectrum of drugs including antiretrovirals [6–9]. Indeed, the fetal accumulation of the protease inhibitor saquinavir has been found to be elevated in PGP-deficient mice models [10].

Lopinavir (LPV) is currently a second-line protease inhibitor (PI) that is frequently used in managing HIV-positive pregnancies [11,12]. Several in vitro and in vivo studies have established the involvement of ABCB1 and ABCC2 in the transport of LPV during the processes of absorption and disposition [13–17]. Inhibition or deficiency of PGP, which is encoded by Abcb1a and Abcb1b in rodents, has been shown to increase the oral bioavailability of LPV in addition to increasing its concentrations in the central nervous system (CNS). The placental transfer of PIs such as LPV has been shown to be highly variable in patients, in that it has been reported that the fetal cord to maternal plasma concentrations for LPV range from 0.05 to 0.34 [18–20]. Given the established role of drug transporters in LPV transport, the variability in the placental expression of these transporters may play an important part in inter- or intra-subject variability in the placental transfer of LPV into fetal tissues.

The expression of many drug transporters in the placenta has been shown to vary throughout gestation. Reports indicate that levels of PGP decline while levels of BCRP increase as gestation progresses [21–23]. The situation is further complicated by reports of disease-mediated alterations of drug transporters. In a study comparing the placental expression of PGP in HIV-infected and uninfected women, dramatically higher PGP expression was seen in placental tissue obtained from HIV-positive patients [24]. Alterations in the expression of the key drug efflux transporters in the placenta could have a serious clinical impact. In the case of drugs such as antiretrovirals, a fine balance between efficacy and safety needs to be struck, given the interplay between drug concentration, viral load suppression, and MTCT on one hand, and the potential for fetal drug toxicity on the other. Thus, it is important to be able to predict how genetic, environmental, or pathophysiological influences impact fetal drug exposure.

Nuclear receptors such as the Pregnane X Receptor (PXR) are known to be key regulators of ABC drug transporters such as Abcb1, Abcc2, Abcc3, and Abcg2 [25–28]. It is well known that PXR is activated by endogenous steroidal hormones and their metabolites, the levels of which are dramatically elevated during pregnancy. PXR is also activated by a number of dietary components, herbal remedies, and clinically important drugs [29,30]. Genetic polymorphisms of PXR are associated with decreased expression of the target genes encoding ABCB1 and CYP3A4 in patients, resulting in altered clearance of drug substrates [31,32]. While PXR activation and subsequent transporter induction at the liver and blood brain barrier has been shown to alter the bio-availability and CNS accumulation of many therapeutic agents, its role in determining fetal drug disposition is unclear and largely unexplored.

We have previously demonstrated a tissue-specific role for PXR in mice [33]. Several PXR target genes (Abcb1a, Abcc1-3, and Abcg2) were found to be elevated in the placenta in PXR null mice, with dramatically higher levels of placental transporters in the PXR $-/-$ mice as compared to the PXR $+/+$ mice. As the functional units of the placenta are almost entirely derived from fetal tissues, it is the fetal genotype that dictates the placental genotype and is therefore responsible for regulating the expression of placental transporters [34]. In this manner, alterations of fetal PXR genotype could provide us with a unique murine model with clear differences in placental transporter levels within the same dam. Therefore, by breeding PXR heterozygotes $(+/-)$, we generated a PXR $+/-$ dam bearing PXR $+/+$, PXR $+/-$, and PXR $-/-$ fetuses and placentas, allowing us to examine the impact of a range of placental transporter expression on substrate drug accumulation in the fetal units while maintaining a similar maternal physiological environment. This strategy enabled us to examine the relative contribution of placental transporters on LPV disposition without confounding maternal influences. Using this model, we explored the role of fetal PXR genotype and placental drug transporter expression on the fetal accumulation of LPV.

2. Materials and Methods

2.1. Animals and Experimental Design

All animal studies were in accordance with the guidelines of the Canadian Council of Animal Care. PXR heterozygote $(+/-)$ animals were obtained by crossing PXR $-/-$ females with PXR

+/+ males. PXR wild type (+/+) C57/BL6 mice were purchased from Charles River Canada (Montreal, QC, Canada). The PXR knockout (−/−) C57/BL6 mice were obtained with approval from Dr. Steven Kliewer (University of Texas, Southwestern Medical Center, Dallas, TX, USA) as described previously [35]. For the purpose of obtaining timed pregnancies, the PXR +/− male mice were paired overnight with PXR +/− females, and the male removed the following morning contingent to observance of a vaginal plug. On gestational day (GD) 17, pregnant PXR +/− animals were administered 10 mg/kg LPV intravenously (i.v.) via tail vein (Lopinavir; USP, Rockville, MD, USA). LPV was dissolved in ethanol:propylene glycol: 5% dextrose solution (2:4:4 ratio). Animals were sacrificed at 30 min post injection and maternal plasma and fetal tissues were collected for analysis. Previously, we found that maximal fetal accumulation occurs at 30 min after LPV i.v. administration in healthy rats [36] and pilot studies in PXR +/− mice established that this time point was optimal in detecting LPV in both maternal and fetal samples. The plasma was stored at −20 °C, while the fetal and placental tissues were snap frozen and stored at −80 °C until analysis. The fetal units were genotyped for PXR by PCR from DNA isolated from placenta and visualizing the PCR products on a 2% agarose gel. The PXR genotype did not impact fetal survival nor fetal weight (PXR +/+: 0.72 ± 0.05 g; PXR +/−: 0.69 ± 0.02 g; PXR −/−: 0.75 ± 0.06 g).

2.2. Analysis of Transporter mRNA Expression

Methods for RNA isolation, cDNA synthesis, qRT-PCR, and primer sequences have been described previously [35]. Briefly, total RNA was extracted from placental tissue using the QuickPrep RNA extraction kit (Amersham Biosciences Inc., Piscataway, NJ, USA). RNA was quantified on a NanoDrop ND-1000 spectrophotometer (Thermo Fisher Scientific, Waltham, MA, USA) and then reverse-transcribed to cDNA by use of a first-strand cDNA synthesis kit (Fermentas, Burlington, ON, Canada) according to manufacturer's protocol. qRT-PCR quantification of Abcb1a (Mdr1a), Abcc2 (Mrp2), and Abcg2 (Bcrp) mRNA were carried out by qPCR using Roche LightCycler technology with the LC FastStart DNA Master SYBR Green I Kit (Roche, Laval, QC, Canada). Oligonucleotides for previously reported primer sequences were synthesized at The Hospital for Sick Children (DNA Synthesis Centre, Toronto, ON, Canada). All transcript levels were normalized to the housekeeping gene, cyclophilin, using the efficiency-corrected ΔCq qPCR method, and the ratios are presented as the percentage of control values. Normalization to either Gapdh or 18S rRNA was found to give comparable results, and cyclophilin levels were not significantly different between genotypes. Abcb1b (Mdr1b) was very poorly expressed in the placenta of our mice, with expression in most samples being below the detectable limit. As a result, Abcb1b mRNA levels are not reported.

2.3. Lopinavir LC-MS/MS Analysis

LPV concentrations in maternal plasma and fetal tissue samples were quantified using LC-MS/MS as previously described [36]. Briefly, maternal plasma and fetal tissue samples were thawed to room temperature. Tissue samples were homogenized in glass tubes with deionized water. Then, 100 µL of plasma or fetal tissue homogenates were added into tubes containing the internal standard, ritonavir (USP, Rockville, MD, USA). Sample extraction was performed using liquid-liquid extraction. Briefly, 50 µL of 500 mM sodium carbonate was mixed with the samples followed by adding 1.2 mL of hexane/ethyl acetate (1:1 *v/v*). The mixture was then vortexed for 2 min, centrifuged at 21,000 *g* for 15 min at 4 °C, and the organic layer (700 µL) was transferred to clean vials, evaporated under nitrogen gas, and reconstituted in 200 µL of 80% methanol. The final extracts were aliquoted into autosampler vials. Unless otherwise noted, all chemical reagents were purchased from Sigma-Aldrich (Oakville, ON, Canada).

The LC-MS/MS system employed a CTC PAL autosampler unit (LEAP Technologies, Carrboro, NC, USA) with an Agilent 1100 series pump (Agilent Technologies, Santa Carla, CA, USA). Elution was achieved using a 50 mm × 4.6 mm, 5 µm Lichrosorb RP-8 column (Phenomenex, Torrance, CA, USA) with a mobile phase of 20:80 parts of 0.1% formic acid to 80% methanol (flow rate 0.700 mL/min).

MS/MS was performed with an API 4000 triple quadrupole MS equipped with a TurboIonSpray source and was set to the positive reaction monitoring mode (AB Sciex, Concord, ON, Canada). MRM transitions for LPV were m/z 629.3 to m/z 447.3 and for ritonavir, the internal standard, were m/z 721.3 to m/z 268, with the source temperature set to 500 °C. Analyst software version 1.4.2 was used (Applied Biosystems/MDS Sciex) for the analysis and quantification of LPV. The lower limit of LPV detection was <3 ng/mL and the lower limit of quantification was <10 ng/mL.

2.4. Statistical Analysis

Data were analyzed using GraphPad Prism (GraphPad Software version 5.0c, San Diego, CA, USA). Statistical significance was determined by analysis of variance (ANOVA) and significance was set to $p < 0.05$. Results are expressed as means ± standard error (SE). Pearson correlation (r) was used to analyze the strength of linear relationships between fetal LPV accumulation and transporter expression levels, and both the Pearson correlation r and absolute p-values are reported.

3. Results

3.1. Impact of Fetal PXR Genotype on Transporter Expression

As compared to the PXR +/+ fetal units, the placental mRNA expression of Abcb1a, Abcc2, and Abcg2 was approximately two- to three-fold higher in the PXR −/− fetal units (Figure 1). The expression of these transporters was significantly different in placentas obtained from PXR −/− fetal units as compared to PXR +/+ fetal units ($p < 0.05$).

Intermediate levels of these transporters were seen in fetal units with the PXR +/− genotype. While levels of Abcb1a in the PXR +/− placentae were significantly different from the PXR +/+ fetal units ($p < 0.05$), levels were not significantly different from the PXR −/− units. This provided us with an animal model with varying placental expression of transporters within the same dam.

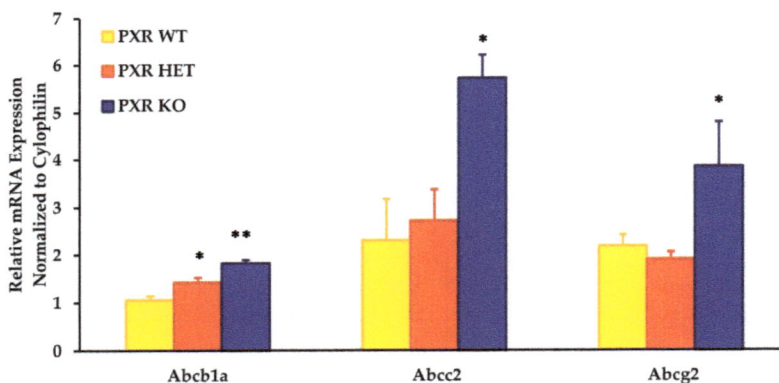

Figure 1. Effect of fetal genotype on basal mRNA expression of key placental transporters on GD 17. Fetal genotypes are PXR +/+ (PXR WT), PXR +/− (PXR HET), and PXR −/− (PXR KO). Placental mRNA expression was measured using RT-PCR and normalized to cyclophilin. Values are presented as relative expression levels ± S.E. * $p < 0.05$; ** $p < 0.01$ compared to PXR WT. $n = 10$.

3.2. Impact of Fetal PXR Genotype on Fetal Accumulation of LPV

We saw significant differences in the fetal tissue accumulation of LPV between the PXR +/+ and PXR −/− fetal units (Figure 2). The fetal tissue:maternal plasma LPV concentration was approximately 50% lower in the PXR −/− fetuses as compared to the PXR +/+ units ($p < 0.05$). There was, however, no statistically significant differences in LPV accumulation between the PXR +/+ and PXR +/− fetuses.

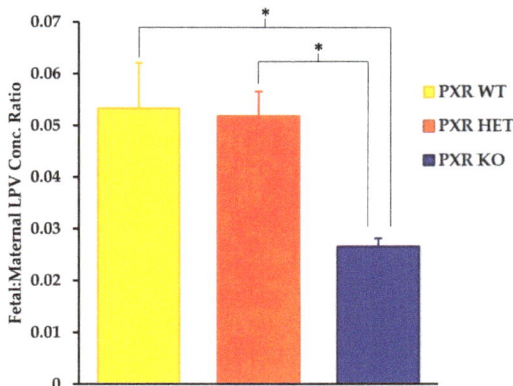

Figure 2. Effect of fetal genotype on LPV accumulation in fetal tissue. LPV concentration ratios were quantified by LC-MS/MS 30 min post-intravenous injection of LPV (10 mg/kg) as stated in the Materials and Methods section. Concentration ratios were calculated as the concentration ratio of LPV in fetal homogenate per unit weight (ng/g) to maternal plasma concentrations (ng/mL). Values are given as mean ratios ± S.E. * $p < 0.05$. $n = 10$.

3.3. Relationship of Fetal Drug Accumulation and Transporter Expression

We observed a highly significant correlation between the placental mRNA expression of Abcb1a in all fetal genotypes and the fetal accumulation of LPV (Figure 3A). There was a clear association of lower fetal tissue:maternal plasma concentration ratios with increased Abcb1a expression. A linear regression best fit the data, and the equation describing the data was $y = 15.38x + 3.3$ ($p = 0.0016$).

There was a strong trend with Abcc2 in that higher transcript levels of Abcc2 tended to be associated with lower fetal tissue:maternal plasma concentration ratios (Figure 3B). However, this association failed to reach significance ($p = 0.055$). The data were best described with a linear regression fit, with the equation of the line of best fit being $y = 1.82x + 14$. Of note, we found that the placental mRNA expression of Abcc2 was highly and significantly correlated to the expression of Abcb1a ($r = 0.54$; $p = 0.0007$). No significant correlation (linear or polynomial) between Abcg2 expression and LPV fetal accumulation was detected (Figure 3C).

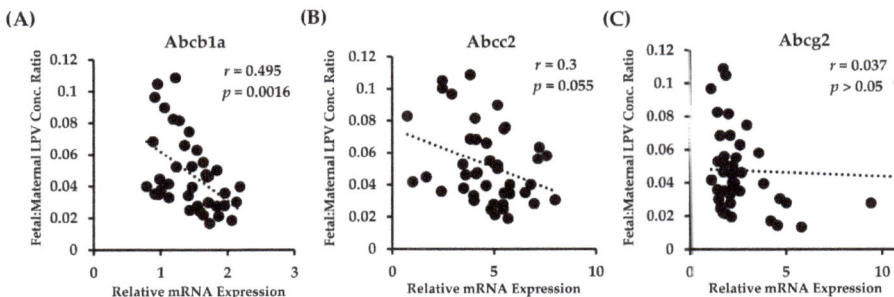

Figure 3. Relationship between fetal accumulation of LPV and placental expression of (**A**) Abcb1a; (**B**) Abcc2; and (**C**) Abcg2 in all fetal PXR genotypes. Fetal accumulation is represented as the LPV concentration of fetal homogenate (ng/g) relative to maternal plasma concentration (ng/mL). Relative placental mRNA expression was determined as described in the Materials and Methods section. $n = 39$.

4. Discussion

Many studies to date have reported low and highly variable placental transfer of protease inhibitors at delivery. While numerous in vitro and ex vivo studies have explored the role of placental transporters in drug transport, relatively little is still known about their genetic, environmental, and pathophysiological regulation, or the impact that changes in transporter expression have on fetal drug exposure. Our findings demonstrate that fetal PXR genotype affects the placental expression of drug transporters with a corresponding effect on fetal drug exposure. In this study, we found that the expression of three key ABC drug transporters, Abcb1a, Abcc2, and Abcg2, were significantly lower in fetal units with the PXR $+/+$ genotype as compared to the PXR $-/-$ genotype. Additionally, we found a corresponding change in the accumulation of LPV in that the fetal-maternal concentration ratios in fetuses with the PXR $+/+$ genotype was approximately two times higher than those seen in the PXR $-/-$ fetuses. These findings indicate that PXR genotypes that influence placental expression of transporters can also affect the fetal exposure to their substrates.

In vitro and in vivo studies have previously demonstrated that LPV is transported by PGP, which is primarily encoded by Abcb1a in murine placenta. Our model provided us with a four-fold range in the placental expression of Abcb1a between fetal units of different genotypes while maintaining a similar maternal environment. With an increase in the transcription level of placental Abcb1a, we saw a distinct decrease in the fetal accumulation of LPV. Moreover, the fetal accumulation of LPV was significantly correlated to Abcb1a expression, illustrating the important role of placental PGP on fetal exposure to LPV. These findings are in line with an ex vivo perfused human placental study that demonstrated that the inhibition of PGP increased the fetal to maternal transfer of LPV up to 10-fold [37]. Pathophysiological changes in placental Abcb1 expression were also found to significantly alter maternal-fetal transfer of LPV in rat models of infection and gestational diabetes [36,38].

We observed a very low and frequently undetectable placental expression of Abcb1b in all PXR genotypes. While PGP is encoded by Abcb1a and Abcb1b in rodents, it has been previously demonstrated that Abcb1a is the functional isoform in murine placenta. Studies in Abcb1a- and Abcb1b-deficient mice demonstrated that fetal exposure of PGP substrates such as digoxin were dependent on Abcb1a but not Abcb1b expression [39]. Moreover, only fetuses from dams with reduced Abcb1a expression (Abcb1a $-/-$ or $+/-$) were susceptible to avermectin-induced cleft palate teratogenicity, despite uniform Abcb1b placental expression [40]. This highlights Abcb1a as the vital and functional isoform of PGP in mouse placenta.

The efflux transporter ABCC2, which is localized on the apical surface of the placenta, has also been shown to mediate placental transfer of its drug substrates such as talinolol [41]. Fetal:maternal concentration ratios of LPV tended to be lower, albeit non-significant, in fetal units with higher placental levels of Abcc2, suggesting possible involvement in the placental transport of LPV. However, the contribution of ABCC2 to the in vivo disposition of LPV is not clearly known. ABCC2 has been shown to transport LPV at low concentrations in vitro in transfected cell lines [14]. However, using knockout mice models, van Waterschoot et al. (2010) demonstrated that PGP but not ABCC2 significantly influenced the oral bioavailability of LPV [17]. As we found a strong association between the expression of Abcb1a and Abcc2, it is likely that the trend between Abcc2 expression and LPV fetal accumulation was due to the fact that placentas that expressed higher levels of Abcc2 also expressed higher levels of Abcb1a as a function of the PXR genotype, rather than implicating an active role of ABCC2 in placental LPV transport. While ABCG2 is highly expressed in the placenta and plays a key role in limiting maternal-fetal transport of potentially toxic xenobiotics, LPV is not a substrate of ABCG2 [14,42]. In line with previous data, we did not observe a significant association between the fetal accumulation of LPV and Abcg2 expression. However, LPV is a potent inhibitor of ABCG2 [43]. Therefore, given the importance of ABCG2 in fetal protection and its broad range of drug substrates, the potential for drug-drug interactions should be further explored. This is particularly important when considering the clinical scenario where pregnant HIV-positive patients receive numerous antiviral agents.

Interestingly, while we found significant differences in the placental expression of transporters between the PXR +/+ and PXR −/− fetal genotypes, these differences were not as great as those seen in our previous study [33]. For instance, while we previously saw a 12-fold higher expression of Abcb1a in the placenta of PXR −/− dams as compared to PXR +/+ dams, only a two-fold difference was seen in the placental expression between the PXR +/+ and PXR −/− fetuses. This may be due to the fact that while all three genotypes were generated within a single PXR +/− mother in this study, the previous study used homozygote PXR mating pairs to generate the three PXR genotypes (i.e., PXR +/+ parents to generate PXR +/+ fetus, PXR −/− parents to generate −/− fetus, and PXR −/− and PXR +/+ mating pair to generate PXR +/− fetus). Thus, the maternal environment to which the different PXR genotypic placentas were exposed were unique and likely had an impact on the expression of PXR target genes. It is well known that progesterone is an activator of PXR and levels of this steroid hormone increase throughout pregnancy. Moreover, PXR, along with other nuclear receptors, is believed to play a role in hormonal homeostasis and may subsequently regulate transporters through hormonal changes [44,45]. Therefore, differences in genotype as well as the physiological hormone environment may influence placental transporter expression in the different dams.

In conclusion, our data demonstrates the importance of PGP expression in limiting the fetal accumulation of an important antiretroviral agent. Hence inter-individual differences in the expression of placental transporters due to genetic or environmental factors can impact fetal exposure to their substrates. The situation is further confounded by the fact that expression may be further affected by pathophysiological changes due to HIV infection or other co-morbidities. Alterations can lead to either unexpected fetal accumulation or inadequate therapeutic levels, both resulting in poor fetal outcomes. The current model can be used to study the in vivo impact of placental transporter expression on the fetal exposure to a wide array of drugs, thus helping to bridge a critical knowledge gap in the area of drug usage in pregnancy.

Acknowledgments: Funding for this study was provided by an operating grant from the Canadian Institutes of Health Research [MOP 13346]. The authors thank Ms. Eliza McColl for her assistance in the preparation of the manuscript and design of the graphical abstract.

Author Contributions: Micheline Piquette-Miller and Sarabjit S. Gahir conceived and designed the experiments; Sarabjit S. Gahir performed the experiments; Sarabjit S. Gahir analyzed the data; Micheline Piquette-Miller and Sarabjit S. Gahir wrote the paper.

Conflicts of Interest: The authors declare no conflict of interest.

Abbreviations

ABC	ATP Binding Cassette
BCRP	Brest Cancer Resistance Protein
CNS	Central Nervous System
GD	Gestational Day
HAART	Highly Active Antiretroviral Therapy
HIV	Human Immunodeficiency Virus
I.V.	Intravenously
LC-MS/MS	Liquid Chromatography-Tandem Mass Spectrometry
LPV	Lopinavir
MRP	Multidrug Resistance Associated Protein
MTCT	Mother-to-Child Transmission
PI	Protease Inhibitor
PXR	Pregnane X Receptor
qRT-PCR	Quantitative Real Time Polymerase Chain Reaction

References

1. HIV. Gov. Available online: https://www.hiv.gov/federal-response/pepfar-global-aids/global-hiv-aids-overview (accessed on 27 September 2017).
2. Sturt, A.S.; Dokubo, E.K.; Sint, T.T. Antiretroviral therapy (ART) for treating HIV infection in ART-eligible pregnant women. *Cochrane Database Sys. Rev.* **2010**, *3*, CD008440. [CrossRef]
3. Van Dyke, R.B. Mother-to-child transmission of HIV-1 in the era prior to the availability of combination antiretroviral therapy: The role of drugs of abuse. *Life Sci.* **2011**, *88*, 922–925. [CrossRef] [PubMed]
4. Prouillac, C.; Lecoeur, S. The role of the placenta in fetal exposure to xenobiotics: Importance of membrane transporters and human models for transfer studies. *Drug Metab. Dispos.* **2010**, *38*, 1623–1635. [CrossRef] [PubMed]
5. Syme, M.R.; Paxton, J.W.; Keelan, J.A. Drug transfer and metabolism by the human placenta. *Clin. Pharmacokinet.* **2004**, *43*, 487–514. [CrossRef] [PubMed]
6. Vähäkangas, K.; Myllynen, P. Drug transporters in the human blood–placental barrier. *Br. J. Pharmacol.* **2009**, *158*, 665–678. [CrossRef] [PubMed]
7. Ni, Z.; Mao, Q. ATP-binding cassette efflux transporters in human placenta. *Curr. Pharm. Biotechnol.* **2010**, *12*, 674–685. [CrossRef]
8. Tomi, M.; Nishimura, T.; Nakashima, E. Mother-to-fetus transfer of antiviral drugs and the involvement of transporters at the placental barrier. *J. Pharm. Sci.* **2011**, *100*, 3708–3718. [CrossRef] [PubMed]
9. Hutson, J.R.; Garcia-Bournissen, F.; Davis, A.; Koren, G. The human placental perfusion model: A systemic review and development of a model to predict in vivo transfer of therapeutic drugs. *Clin. Pharmacol. Ther.* **2011**, *90*, 67–76. [CrossRef] [PubMed]
10. Huisman, M.T.; Smit, J.W.; Wiltshire, H.R.; Hoetelmans, R.M.; Beijnen, J.H.; Schinkel, A.H. P-glycoprotein limits oral availability, brain, and fetal penetration of saquinavir even with high doses of ritonavir. *Mol. Pharmacol.* **2001**, *59*, 806–813. [PubMed]
11. Navér, L.; Albert, J.; Belfrage, E.; Flamholc, L.; Gisslén, M.; Gyllensten, K.; Yilmaz, A. Prophylaxis and treatment of HIV-1 infection in pregnancy: Swedish recommendations 2010. *Scand. J. Infect. Dis.* **2011**, *43*, 411–423. [CrossRef] [PubMed]
12. Baroncelli, S.; Tamburrini, E.; Ravizza, M.; Dalzero, S.; Tibaldi, C.; Ferrazzi, E.; Anzidei, G.; Fiscon, M. Italian Group on Surveillance on Antiretroviral Treatment in Pregnancy. Antiretroviral treatment in pregnancy: A six-year perspective on recent trends in prescription patters, viral load suppression, and pregnancy outcomes. *AIDS Patient Care STDS* **2009**, *23*, 513–520. [CrossRef] [PubMed]
13. Janneh, O.; Jones, E.; Chandler, B.; Owen, A.; Khoo, S.H. Inhibition of P-glycoprotein and multidrug resistance-associated proteins modulates the intracellular concentration of lopinavir in cultured CD4 T cells and primary human lymphocytes. *J. Antimicrob. Chemoth.* **2007**, *60*, 987–993. [CrossRef] [PubMed]
14. Agarwal, S.; Pal, D.; Mitra, A.K. Both P-gp and MRP2 mediate transport of lopinavir, a protease inhibitor. *Int. J. Pharm.* **2007**, *339*, 139–147. [CrossRef] [PubMed]
15. Gulati, A.; Gerk, P.M. Role of placental ABC transporters in antiretroviral therapy during pregnancy. *J. Pharm. Sci.* **2009**, *98*, 2317–2335. [CrossRef] [PubMed]
16. Kim, A.E.; Dintaman, J.M.; Waddell, D.S.; Silverman, J.A. Saquinavir, an HIV protease inhibitor, is transported by P-glycoprotein. *J. Pharmacol. Exp. Ther.* **1998**, *286*, 1439–1445. [PubMed]
17. Van Waterschoot, R.A.; ter Heine, R.; Wagenaar, E.; van der Kruijssen, C.M.; Rooswinkel, R.W.; Huitema, A.D.; Schinkel, A.H. Effects of cytochrome P450 3A (CYP3A) and the drug transporters P-glycoprotein (MDR1/ABCB1) and MRP2 (ABCC2) on the pharmacokinetics of lopinavir. *Br. J. Pharmacol.* **2010**, *160*, 1224–1233. [CrossRef] [PubMed]
18. Marzolini, C.; Rudin, C.; Decosterd, L.A.; Telenti, A.; Schreyer, A.; Biollaz, J. Swiss Mother + Child HIV Cohort Study. Transplacental passage of protease inhibitors at delivery. *AIDS* **2002**, *16*, 889–893. [CrossRef] [PubMed]
19. Mirochnick, M.; Capparelli, E. Pharmacokinetics of antiretrovirals in pregnant women. *Clin. Pharmacokinet.* **2004**, *43*, 1071–1087. [CrossRef] [PubMed]

20. Yeh, R.F.; Rezk, N.L.; Kashuba, A.D.; Dumond, J.B.; Tappouni, H.L.; Tien, H.C.; Patterson, K.B. Genital tract, cord blood, and amniotic fluid exposures of seven antiretroviral drugs during and after pregnancy in human immunodeficiency virus type 1-infected women. *Antimicrob. Agents Chemother.* **2009**, *53*, 2367–2374. [CrossRef] [PubMed]

21. Sun, M.; Kingdom, J.; Baczyk, D.; Lye, S.J.; Matthews, S.G.; Gibb, W. Expression of the multidrug resistance P-glycoprotein, (ABCB1) in the human placenta decreases with advancing gestation. *Placenta* **2006**, *27*, 602–609. [CrossRef] [PubMed]

22. Gil, S.; Saura, R.; Forestier, F.; Farinotti, R. P-glycoprotein expression of the human placenta during pregnancy. *Placenta* **2005**, *26*, 268–270. [CrossRef] [PubMed]

23. Yeboah, D.; Sun, M.; Kingdom, J.; Baczyk, D.; Lye, S.J.; Matthews, S.G.; Gibb, W. Expression of breast cancer resistance protein (BCRP/ABCG2) in human placenta throughout gestation and at term before and after labor. *Can. J. Physiol. Pharmacol.* **2006**, *84*, 1251–1258. [CrossRef] [PubMed]

24. Camus, M.; Deloménie, C.; Didier, N.; Faye, A.; Gil, S.; Dauge, M.C.; Farinotti, R. Increased expression of MDR1 mRNA and P-glycoprotein in placentas from HIV-1 infected women. *Placenta* **2006**, *27*, 699–706. [CrossRef] [PubMed]

25. Kliewer, S.A.; Goodwin, B.; Willson, T.M. The nuclear Pregnane X Receptor: A key regulator of xenobiotic metabolism. *Endocr. Rev.* **2002**, *23*, 687–702. [CrossRef] [PubMed]

26. Teng, S.; Piquette-Miller, M. Regulation of transporters by nuclear hormone receptors: Implications during inflammation. *Mol. Pharmaceut.* **2008**, *5*, 67–76. [CrossRef] [PubMed]

27. Teng, S.; Jekerle, V.; Piquette-Miller, M. Induction of ABCC3 (MRP3) by Pregnane X Receptor activators. *Drug Metab. Dispos.* **2003**, *31*, 1296–1299. [CrossRef] [PubMed]

28. Anapolsky, A.; Teng, S.; Dixit, S.; Piquette-Miller, M. The role of Pregnane X Receptor in 2-acetylaminofluorene-mediated induction of drug transport and metabolizing enzymes in mice. *Drug Metab. Dispos.* **2006**, *34*, 405–409. [CrossRef] [PubMed]

29. Chang, T.K.; Waxman, D.J. Synthetic drugs and natural products as modulators of constitutive androstane receptor (CAR) and Pregnane X Receptor (PXR). *Drug Metab. Rev.* **2006**, *38*, 51–73. [CrossRef] [PubMed]

30. Kliewer, S.A.; Moore, J.T.; Wade, L.; Staudinger, J.L.; Watson, M.A.; Jones, S.A.; Lehmann, J.M. An orphan nuclear receptor activated by pregnanes defines a novel steroid signaling pathway. *Cell* **1998**, *92*, 73–82. [CrossRef]

31. Sandanaraj, E.; Lal, S.; Selvarajan, V.; Ooi, L.L.; Wong, Z.W.; Wong, N.S.; Ang, P.C.; Lee, E.J.; Chowbay, B. PXR pharmacogenetics: Association of haplotypes with hepatic CYP3A4 and ABCB1 messenger RNA expression and doxorubicin clearance in Asian breast cancer patients. *Clin. Cancer Res.* **2008**, *14*, 7116–7126. [CrossRef] [PubMed]

32. Schipani, A.; Siccardi, M.; D'Avolio, A.; Baietto, L.; Simiele, M.; Bonora, S.; Rodríguez Novoa, S.; Cuenca, L.; Soriano, V.; Chierakul, N.; et al. Population pharmacokinetic modeling of the association between 63396C->T Pregnane X Receptor polymorphism and unboosted atazanavir clearance. *Antimicrob. Agents Chemother.* **2010**, *54*, 5242–5250. [CrossRef] [PubMed]

33. Gahir, S.S.; Piquette-Miller, M. Gestational and Pregnane X Receptor-mediated regulation of placental ATP-binding cassette drug transporters in mice. *Drug Metab. Dispos.* **2011**, *39*, 465–471. [CrossRef] [PubMed]

34. Daud, A.; Bergman, J.; Bakker, M.; Wang, H.; de Walle, H.; Plosch, T. Pharmacogenetics of drug-induced birth defects; the role of polymorphisms of placental transport proteins. *Pharmacogenomics* **2014**, *15*, 1029–1041. [CrossRef] [PubMed]

35. Teng, S.; Piquette-Miller, M. The involvement of the Pregnane X Receptor in hepatic gene regulation during inflammation in mice. *J. Pharmacol. Exp. Ther.* **2005**, *312*, 841–848. [CrossRef] [PubMed]

36. Anger, G.; Piquette-Miller, M. Mechanisms of reduced maternal and fetal lopinavir exposure in a rat model of gestational diabetes. *Drug Metab. Dispos.* **2011**, *39*, 1850–1859. [CrossRef] [PubMed]

37. Ceccaldi, P.F.; Gavard, L.; Mandelbrot, L.; Rey, E.; Farinotti, R.; Treluyer, J.M.; Gil, S. Functional role of P-glycoprotein and binding protein effect on the placental transfer of lopinavir/ritonavir in the ex vivo human perfusion model. *Obstet. Gynecol. Int.* **2009**, *2009*, 726593. [CrossRef] [PubMed]

38. Petrovic, V.; Piquette-Miller, M. Polyinosinic/Polycytidylic Acid-mediated changes in maternal and fetal disposition of lopinavir in rats. *Drug Metab. Dispos.* **2015**, *43*, 951–957. [CrossRef] [PubMed]

39. Schinkel, A.H.; Mayer, U.; Wagenaar, E.; Mol, C.A.; van Deemter, L.; Smit, J.J.; van der Valk, M.A.; Voordouw, A.C.; Spits, H.; van Tellingen, O.; et al. Normal viability and altered pharmacokinetics in mice lacking mdr1-type (drug-transporting) P-glycoproteins. *Proc. Natl. Acad. Sci. USA* **1997**, *94*, 4028–4033. [CrossRef] [PubMed]

40. Lankas, G.R.; Wise, L.D.; Cartwright, M.E.; Pippert, T.; Umbenhauer, D.R. Placental P-glycoprotein deficiency enhances susceptibility to chemically induced birth defects in mice. *Reprod. Toxicol.* **1998**, *12*, 457–463. [CrossRef]

41. May, K.; Minarikova, V.; Linnemann, K.; Zygmunt, M.; Kroemer, H.K.; Fusch, C.; Siegmund, W. Role of the multidrug transporter proteins ABCB1 and ABCC2 in the placental transport of talinolol in the term human placenta. *Drug Metab. Dispos.* **2008**, *36*, 740–744. [CrossRef] [PubMed]

42. Hahnova-Cygalova, L.; Ceckova, M.; Staud, F. Fetoprotective activity of breast cancer resistance protein (BCRP, ABCG2): Expression and function throughout pregnancy. *Drug Metab. Rev.* **2011**, *43*, 53–68. [CrossRef] [PubMed]

43. Weiss, J.; Rose, J.; Storch, C.H.; Ketabi-Kiyanvash, N.; Sauer, A.; Haefeli, W.E.; Efferth, T. Modulation of human BCRP (ABCG2) activity by anti-HIV drugs. *J. Antimicrob. Chemother.* **2007**, *59*, 238–245. [CrossRef] [PubMed]

44. Sonoda, J.; Xie, W.; Rosenfeld, J.M.; Barwick, J.L.; Guzelian, P.S.; Evans, R.M. Regulation of a xenobiotic sulfonation cascade by nuclear Pregnane X Receptor (PXR). *Prac. Natl. Acad. Sci. USA* **2002**, *99*, 13801–13806. [CrossRef] [PubMed]

45. Kliewar, S.A.; Lehmann, J.M.; Milburn, M.V.; Willson, T.M. The PPARs and PXRs: Nuclear xenobiotic receptors that define novel hormone signaling pathways. *Recent Prog. Horm. Res.* **1999**, *54*, 345–367.

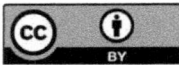

pharmaceutics

MDPI

Review

An Overview of Chitosan Nanoparticles and Its Application in Non-Parenteral Drug Delivery

Munawar A. Mohammed, Jaweria T. M. Syeda, Kishor M. Wasan and Ellen K. Wasan *

College of Pharmacy and Nutrition, University of Saskatchewan, Saskatoon, SK S7N 2Z4, Canada;
mum495@mail.usask.ca (M.A.M.); jaweria.syeda@usask.ca (J.T.M.S.); kishor.wasan@usask.ca (K.M.W.)
* Correspondence: ellen.wasan@usask.ca; Tel.: +1-(306)-966-3202

Received: 27 October 2017; Accepted: 16 November 2017; Published: 20 November 2017

Abstract: The focus of this review is to provide an overview of the chitosan based nanoparticles for various non-parenteral applications and also to put a spotlight on current research including sustained release and mucoadhesive chitosan dosage forms. Chitosan is a biodegradable, biocompatible polymer regarded as safe for human dietary use and approved for wound dressing applications. Chitosan has been used as a carrier in polymeric nanoparticles for drug delivery through various routes of administration. Chitosan has chemical functional groups that can be modified to achieve specific goals, making it a polymer with a tremendous range of potential applications. Nanoparticles (NP) prepared with chitosan and chitosan derivatives typically possess a positive surface charge and mucoadhesive properties such that can adhere to mucus membranes and release the drug payload in a sustained release manner. Chitosan-based NP have various applications in non-parenteral drug delivery for the treatment of cancer, gastrointestinal diseases, pulmonary diseases, drug delivery to the brain and ocular infections which will be exemplified in this review. Chitosan shows low toxicity both in vitro and some in vivo models. This review explores recent research on chitosan based NP for non-parenteral drug delivery, chitosan properties, modification, toxicity, pharmacokinetics and preclinical studies.

Keywords: chitosan; mucoadhesive; polymeric nanoparticles; sustained release; oral drug delivery

---

1. Introduction

The mucosal route is gaining attention for noninvasive drug delivery via the oral, nasal, pulmonary or vaginal routes [1]. At the same time, nanoparticle technology has also come to the forefront as a viable drug delivery strategy, presenting opportunities for controlled release, protection of active components from enzymatic or environmental degradation and localized retention. Nanoparticle fabrication methods are readily scalable and applicable to a broad range of drugs. Of all the nanoparticle drug delivery approaches, polymeric nanoparticles have gained significant importance as they are biodegradable, biocompatible and because formulation methods are more widely available; the range of applications has been expanding to include a variety of chemical drug classes and dosage forms [2]. Chitosan-based NP are particularly appropriate for the mucosal route, with their low toxicity, mucoadhesion and tunable physical properties. Examples will be given of chitosan-based nanoparticles used for the treatment of cancer, gastrointestinal diseases, pulmonary diseases, drug delivery to the brain and ocular infections. Recent research on chitosan-based NP for nonparenteral drug delivery is based on the field's expanding understanding of chitosan properties and methods of chemical or physical modification, which are applied to the optimization of nanoparticle drug loading and release features. We will also discuss the current understanding of in vitro and in vivo toxicity and the effect of chitosan nanoparticle formulation on drug pharmacokinetics in preclinical studies.

Chitosan

Chitosan is the most important derivative of chitin, produced by removing the acetate moiety from chitin as shown in Figure 1.

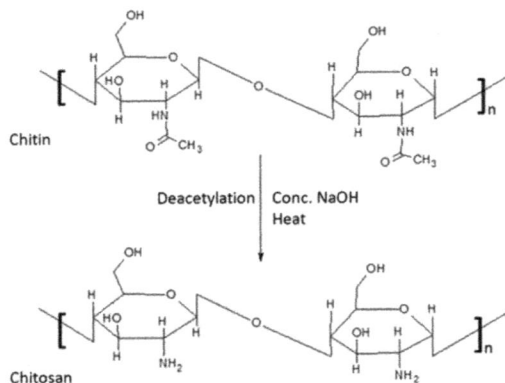

Figure 1. Deacetylation of chitin to chitosan.

It is derived from crustacean shells such as those from prawns or crabs, as well as from the cell walls of fungi. It is a naturally occurring polysaccharide, cationic, highly basic, mucoadhesive biocompatible polymer and approved by the U.S. FDA for tissue engineering and drug delivery. Chitin from natural sources is found bound to proteins and minerals, which must be removed prior to preparation of chitosan, though processes of acidification and alkalization. Purified chitin is then N-deacetylated to chitosan. This process can be modified to control the end product properties [including molecular weight and pKa (6–7.5)] [3,4] by controlling the degree of deacetylation with factors such as reaction conditions (concentration, ratios of chitin to alkali, temperature), chitin source and extent of the reaction, for example. While these chemical processes are well in hand for industrial processors, research is ongoing to more fully develop scalable biological, enzymatic or hybrid methods such as those using microorganisms [5]. It will be interesting to see how these approaches will be used to manufacture specific types of deacetylated chitosan and whether these bioprocesses will have any environmental advantage in the future.

Chitosan acts a penetration enhancer by opening the tight junctions of the epithelium. Chitosan facilitates both paracellular and transcellular transport of drugs as indicated in Figure 2. Chitosan interacts with mucus (negatively charged) to form a complex by ionic or hydrogen bonding as well as though hydrophobic interactions. The pKa of the primary amine of chitosan is ~6.5, depending on the degree of N-deacetylation. This group also contributes to the solubility of chitosan in acidic pH environments and the partial neutralization of this primary amine may also explain why chitosan has been reported to aggregate at neutral to high pH [6]. However, it should be noted that while this may be the tendency for chitosan with fraction of acetylated units <0.4 and medium/high molecular weight, chitosan with acetylation degrees in the range 40–60% are well known as being soluble even at physiological pH [4]. Thus, the nanoparticle formulator must carefully match the desired chemical and physical properties of the chitosan, as well as the anticipated biological environment, with the chitosan processing method.

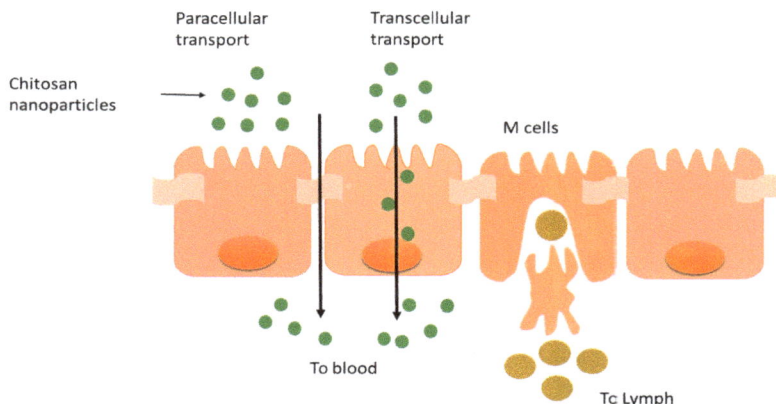

Figure 2. Schematic illustration of the presumed mechanism of transcellular and paracellular transport of chitosan NP across the epithelium.

2. Modification of Chitosan

The chitosan backbone can be modified to alter properties such as solubility, mucoadhesion and stability as discussed throughout this paper for specific applications. Both the -NH$_2$ and -OH groups of chitosan are the active sites for modification. Some of the commonly used techniques described below for preparing chitosan polymers are: blending, graft co-polymerization and curing [7]. Blending involves the simple mixing of two or more polymers. Graft co-polymerization involves the covalent bonding of polymers, while curing converts the polymers into a solidified mass by formation of three-dimensional bonds within the polymer mass by means of thermal, electrochemical or ultraviolet radiation processing methods.

2.1. Physical Modification

Physical modification is achieved by blending, which involves the physical mixing of two or more polymers. It is one of the oldest and easiest ways of modifying polymers. The quality and performance of the blend can be modified depending on the ratios of the polymers which are being mixed. Blending is the most economical technique by which the polymer properties can be tailored for specific applications [8].

Some of the common hydrophilic polymers that can be blended with chitosan to achieve oral drug delivery are poly (vinyl alcohol) (PVA), poly (vinyl pyrrolidone) (PVP) and poly (ethyl oxide) (PEO). Blending of chitosan and PVA improves the mechanical (tensile strength) and barrier properties (water vapor permeability) of chitosan films [9]. The intermolecular interactions between chitosan and PVA result in blends of PVA-chitosan that show improved mechanical properties (tensile strength) of chitosan films for controlled drug delivery [10]. An example of physical modification in controlled drug delivery is represented by amoxicillin formulated with a crosslinked chitosan/PVP blend with glutaraldehyde to form a semi-interpenetrating polymer (semi-IPN) [11]. The semi-IPN is formed because of the protonation of the amino group of chitosan, as confirmed by Fourier transform infrared spectroscopy (FTIR). Additional methods used for characterization of chitosan blends other than FTIR are: differential scanning calorimetry (DSC) [12], X-ray diffraction (XRD) [13], FTIR spectroscopy and rheology [14], enabling an understanding of the effects of processing on bonding and flow properties.

2.2. Chemical Modification

Chemical modification is achieved by altering the functional groups in a compound. Chemical modification can be done by several ways which include: chemical, radiation, photochemical, plasma-induced and enzymatic grafting methods [7]. Chemical modification of chitosan results in the formation of several derivatives such as quaternized chitosan, thiolated chitosan, carboxylated chitosan, amphiphilic chitosan, chitosan with chelating agents, PEGylated chitosan and lactose-modified chitosan. The primary amine ($-NH_2$) groups of chitosan provide a reaction site for chemical modification to achieve various pharmaceutical applications [7], reacting with sulphates, citrates and phosphates [15], which can enhance the stability and drug encapsulation efficiency [16]. For example, to improve the solubility of chitosan in intestinal media, N-trimethyl chitosan chloride (TMC), a quaternized chitosan, has been produced [17]. The two forms TMC, TMC 40 and TMC 60, enhance the intestinal permeation of hydrophilic macromolecular drugs. The mucoadhesiveness of chitosan has been further enhanced by formulating NP with thiolated chitosan [18]. Quaternization of chitosan forms several derivatives such as trimethyl (TMC), dimethylethyl (DMEC), diethylmethyl (DEMC) and triethyl chitosan (TEC). Quaternization of chitosan aids in the opening of tight junctions and improving the permeability of insulin across Caco-2 cells [19]. Chitosan-thioglycolic acid, chitosan-cysteine, chitosan-glutathione, chitosan-thioethylamidine are some of the thiolated chitosan derivatives presently in use. TMC-cysteine based NPs have shown significantly higher mucoadhesion and permeation compared to TMC NPs [20]. Grafting carboxylated chitosan with poly (methyl methacrylate) helps achieve pH-sensitive properties. The NPs made with the grafted polymer and insulin have shown very minimal drug release in simulated gastric fluid and an instant release in simulated intestinal fluid [21]. A pH sensitive polymer gel can be prepared by chemically linking D,L-lactic acid with $-NH_2$ groups of the chitosan for an application in the drug delivery to the different regions of the gastrointestinal tract (GIT) [22]. Lactose modification of the chitosan backbone (1-deoxylactit-1-yl chitosan) has been used in combination with the polyvalent ion tripolyphosphate (TPP) to form colloidal coacervates though polyionic interactions, forming highly uniform and small (200 nm diameter) nanoparticles [23,24].

3. Drug Release from Chitosan Nanoparticles

There are several mechanisms which govern drug release from chitosan nanoparticles such as: swelling of the polymer [25], diffusion of the adsorbed drug, drug diffusion through the polymeric matrix, polymer erosion or degradation and a combination of both erosion and degradation [26] as represented in Figure 3. The initial burst release from the chitosan nanoparticles is either because of swelling of the polymer, creating pores, or diffusion of the drug from the surface of the polymer [27]. Chitosan nanoparticles also exhibit a pH-dependent drug release because of the solubility of chitosan [28]. Chitosan derivatives alter the release of drug from the NP, affording tunable drug release [29] and impacting the pharmacokinetic profile of the loaded drug.

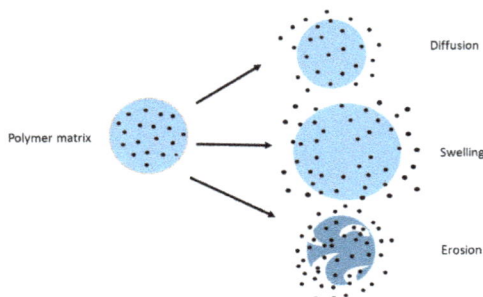

Figure 3. Diagram representing the possible mechanisms of drug release by diffusion, swelling and erosion of polymer (chitosan) matrix.

In diffusion-controlled release, the drug permeates through the interior of the polymeric matrix to the surrounding medium. Polymer chains form the diffusion barrier making it difficult for the drug to pass through and this barrier serves as the rate-limiting membrane for drug release. Diffusion may also be associated with polymer swelling or erosion. The mathematical representation of diffusion is given by Fick's law of diffusion.

$$F = -D\frac{\partial c}{\partial x} \tag{1}$$

where, F is the rate of transfer per unit area of section (flux), c is the concentration of the drug and D is the diffusion coefficient (diffusivity). To derive the parameters of Fick's law, there are few assumptions to be made such as: pseudo-steady state is maintained during drug release, the diameter of the drug particles is less than the average distance of drug diffusion through the polymeric matrix and sink conditions are always provided by the medium surrounding the nanoparticles [30].

The swelling of the polymer is characterized by the imbibition of water into the polymer until the polymer dissolves. This drug release mechanism is characterized by the solubility of the polymer in water, or the surrounding biological medium. When the polymer encounters the surrounding medium and swelling commences, the polymer chains detangle. This is followed by drug release from that region of the polymer matrix. Generally, the hydrophilicity of the polymer, the polymer swelling rate and the density of the polymer chains play a key role in the drug release profile [31]. Subsequently, this will affect the rate of drug absorption from the site of delivery in vivo, as it will affect the rate at which drug is available for membrane transport or cellular uptake.

Erosion and degradation of polymers are interrelated features. Sometimes, degradation of the polymer may cause subsequent physical erosion as bonds break. Erosion of polymers is a complex phenomenon as it involves swelling, diffusion and dissolution. Erosion occurs in two ways: homogenous and heterogeneous. Homogenous erosion is erosion of the polymer at the same rate throughout the matrix whereas heterogeneous erosion is erosion of the polymer from the surface towards the inner core. Polymer degradation may be due to the surrounding media or the presence of enzymes. The degradation of the polymer also depends on the pH of the surrounding media, the copolymer composition and water uptake by the polymer. Drug release depends on the type of polymer and internal bonding, any additives (chitosan derivatives), as well as the shape and size of the nanoparticles as this reflects surface area and free energy [32].

Generally, drug release from the chitosan nanoparticles is similar to that of PLGA (Poly(D,L-lactide-*co*-glycolide)) nanoparticles [33] but the drug release from chitosan nanoparticles is more pH-dependent [34]. As an example, exendin-4 loaded PLGA and chitosan-PLGA nanoparticles have been studied. Exendin-4 is generally used for the treatment of type-2 diabetes. The NPs were evaluated for transmembrane permeability studies in MDCK (Madin-Darby Canine Kidney) cells and in an in vivo study in male Wistar rats. The in vitro transmembrane permeability studies revealed that exendin-4 was transported across the cell layer by active transport when formulated as PLGA or chitosan-PLGA NP compared to the free drug solution. The permeability coefficient (P_{app}) with PLGA and chitosan-PLGA NP was 1.52×10^{-6} and 2.5–3.0×10^{-6}, respectively, significantly greater than exendin-4 solution alone. Some of the PLGA NPs that enter the cell are trafficked into endosomes and suffer degradation while some reach the basolateral membrane via the trans-Golgi pathway. Similar mechanisms occur with chitosan-PLGA NPs, however, due to their positive charge electrostatic interactions occur with the negatively charged cell membrane resulting in a higher P_{app}. The in vivo study revealed higher plasma drug levels and longer retention times of exendin-4 when administered as chitosan-PLGA NP compared to PLGA NP [35].

4. Chitosan in Oral Drug Delivery

Oral drug delivery certainly is the most convenient route of drug administration because of the ease of administration. But there are several challenges in achieving oral delivery such as varying pH (highly acidic stomach), the presence of enzymes, first-pass effect in the liver and the intestinal barrier to drug absorption. The above challenges limit the drug from entering the systemic circulation thereby reducing oral bioavailability [36]. Nanoparticle technology is an increasingly exploited formulation technique to overcome the limitations of oral drug delivery [7,37]. NPs have several advantages such as small particle size, large surface area and potentially a modifiable surface. Small particle size is well known to increase the dissolution rate of drugs. Besides these advantages, NPs can increase the gastrointestinal tract stability of acid-labile drugs compared to other drug delivery systems such as liposomes and lipid based systems [38]. Chitosan can be formulated as polymeric nanoparticles for various applications in oral drug delivery as explained below with several examples.

Catechin and epigallocatechin are flavonoids present in green tea and are strong antioxidants. These undergo degradation in intestinal fluid and are poorly absorbed across intestinal membranes. The intestinal absorption of catechin and epigallocatechin gallate can be improved by encapsulating them in chitosan nanoparticles [39]. Tamoxifen, an anti-cancer drug, is slightly water soluble and a good candidate for oral cancer drug delivery. Permeation of tamoxifen across the intestinal epithelium was increased by formulating tamoxifen into lecithin-chitosan nanoparticles [40]. The NPs are mucoadhesive and increase the permeation of tamoxifen by the paracellular pathway. Feng et al. have also reported a potential oral delivery strategy for anti-cancer drugs. They have prepared nanoparticles of doxorubicin hydrochloride (DOX) with chitosan and carboxymethyl chitosan. These nanostructures were found to enhance the intestinal absorption of DOX throughout the small intestine [41]. Alendronate sodium is used in the treatment of osteoporosis and suffers from low oral bioavailability and gastrointestinal side effects. High NP encapsulation efficiency of alendronate sodium was achieved by formulating chitosan nanoparticles via an ion gelation technique. Drug release was clearly pH-dependent; in 0.1N HCl, almost 80% of the drug was released within 60 min while in PBS (pH 6.8) a maximum of 40% of the drug was released over 4 h, suggesting that factors other than chitosan's pH solubility profile influenced drug release in this case and that optimization is multifactorial [28]. This highlights the importance of examining the degree of surface coverage of the nanoparticles with chitosan and of performing ongoing dissolution studies in biorelevant media during formulation development. For effective sustained delivery of sunitinib, a tyrosine kinase inhibitor, chitosan NPs were prepared by an ion crosslinking method. The encapsulation efficiency of the NPs was 98% and sustained drug release was achieved up to 72 h [42]. The harsh conditions of the GIT denature proteins such as insulin when administered orally, yet oral insulin is a highly desired goal. In one example of insulin-loaded chitosan NPs the chitosan was crosslinked with tripolyphosphate. The particle size was reduced by this crosslinking process and the stability of the NPs was increased by freeze drying. NP uptake was significant in the intestine epithelium; unfortunately, however, the NPs were unstable in gastric pH [43] and further efforts to fabricate stable oral insulin NP are still needed. Bay 41-4109, an active inhibitor of hepatitis B virus was formulated as chitosan NPs to improve drug solubility and oral bioavailability. The cytotoxicity of Bay 41-4109-chitosan NP was found to be negligible and drug uptake was higher from the NPs, which was attributed to the positive charge from the chitosan [44]. Table 1 provides detailed insight into the extensive range of applications of chitosan NP for oral drug delivery.

Table 1. Applications of chitosan nanoparticles in oral drug delivery.

Drug	Composition	Purpose	Research Findings	In Vivo	Reference
Tamoxifen citrate	Chitosan, soybean lecithin NP	Intestinal permeation of tamoxifen in lecithin/chitosan NPs through the rat intestinal wall.	Ex vivo experiment using a jejunum chamber from the small intestine of male Wistar rats. Lecithin/chitosan nanoparticles improved the non-metabolized drug passage across the rat intestinal tissue.		[40]
Sunitinib	Chitosan	Biophysical characterization	1. In vitro biodegradation was improved in the presence of lysozyme. 2. In vitro controlled release was demonstrated with 69% released within 72 h.		[42]
Hydro phobic Bay41-4109	LMW chitosan	Solubility and bioavailability enhancement.	1. In vitro drug release studies showed a sustained release profile. 2. Low cytotoxicity was demonstrated in a liver cell line.	In vivo studies were performed in rats. The absolute bioavailability of Bay41-4109 NPs was >70%, nearly 4-fold higher than other formulations	[44]
Insulin	Chitosan, TPP	Preparation, characterization and stabilization of insulin—chitosan NPs.	1. In vitro validation-Caco2 and co-culture: Caco-2 cells internalized the NPs effectively.	In vivo studies where decreased glycaemia was observed in diabetic rats after insulin NP administration.	[43]
Cyclosporin-A	Chitosan HCl, Poloxamer 188, sodium glycolate, gelatin, soya lecithin	To develop and characterize Cy-A as positive charge NPs to improve GI uptake, bioavailability	Cy-A encapsulation efficiency was very high at 88–94%.	In vivo studies in beagle dogs showed relative bioavailability of Cy-A was significantly increased by NPs.	[45]
Extra cellular products (ECPs) of *Vibrio anguillarum* (Protein carrier)	Chitosan carboxymethyl chitosan	To study the efficacy of chitosan NPs as a vehicle for oral antigen delivery in fish vaccination.	In vitro release study was performed in Tris-buffer (pH 2.0, 4.5) & PBS (pH 7.4); the highest cumulative release was 58% at pH 7.4 followed by 37% at pH 2.0.	Biodistribution showed NP uptake in spleen and kidney. Lysozyme and complement evaluation. It showed elevated specific antibody and higher concentrations of lysozyme activity and complement	[46]
Alendro-nate sodium	Chitosan LMW, sodium tripolyphosphate (TPP), fluorenyl-methyloxycarbonyl chloride (FMOC)	To study the influence of physical parameters on drug encapsulation efficiency	In vitro drug release was performed in 0.1N HCl and PBS (pH 6.8). The NPs released alendronate faster in 0.1N HCl compared to PBS. Encapsulation efficiency was ~80%.		[28]
Catechins (+) catechin (C) and (−) epigallocatechingallate (EGCg)	Chitosan LMW, sodium tripolyphos-phate, tris[(2-carboxyethyl) phosphine hydrochloride (TCEP)	To enhance the intestinal absorption by encapsulation of C, EGCg in chitosan NPs	Ex vivo study using a jejunum chamber from mice. The cumulative amounts transported after encapsulation were significantly higher for C and EGCg, respectively.		[39]

Table 1. *Cont.*

Drug	Composition	Purpose	Research Findings	In Vivo	Reference
Enoxaparin	Chitosan, STPP, sodium alginate	Alginate coated chitosan-NPs containing enoxaparin for oral controlled release	In vitro drug release showed only 2% drug release in SGF (pH 1.2) but 60% in SIF (pH 6.5).	In vivo studies were performed in albino rats: the oral bioavailability of enoxaparin in Alg-CS-NPs bioavailability was significantly higher compared to enoxaparin solution. A 60% reduction was seen in thrombus formation in rat venous thrombosis model.	[47]
Scutellarin	Chitosan, deoxycholic acid, vitamin B12	Enhancement of scutellarin oral delivery efficacy by Vit B12 modified amphiphilic chitosan derivatives to treat type II diabetes-induced retinopathy	Cytotoxicity study of Chit-DC and Chit-DC-VB12 displayed low cytotoxicity in Caco-2 cells.	In vivo studies: 1. Zebra fish embryo: development of the embryo was unaffected 2. Sprague-Dawleys rats: the AUC of scutellarin NP was 2–3 fold higher than free scutellarin and efficacy was achieved	[48]
Fucoidan	Chitosan, Tc-methylene di-phosphonate	To prepare and evaluate pH sensitivity of CS/F NPs	In vitro drug release of Tc-MDP from CS/F NPs rose as the pH levels changed from 2.5 to 7.4. CS/F NPs was stable into the stomach and decompose in the intestine.		[49]
Tolbut-amide	Chitosan, PLGA, streptozotocin	To prepare PLGA NPs modified with chitosan to form TOL-CS-PLGA NPs to improve bioavailability and reduce dose frequency.	In vitro drug release of TOL-CS-PLGA NPs showed sustained release in PBS, pH 7.4. Cytotoxicity study of TOL-CS-PLGA NPs were non-toxic in HePG2 cells.	In vivo study was performed in adult Sprague-Dawley rats: the TOL-CS-PLGA NPS showed a long-acting hypoglycemic effect over 8 h, significantly longer than metformin tablets.	[50]
Gemcita-bine	Chitosan LMW, penta sodium tripolyphos-phate	To prepare gemcitabine-loaded chitosan NPs (Gem-CS-NP) for oral bio-availability enhancement	1. In vitro drug release of Gem-CS-NPs showed controlled release by a two-phase process. 2. Absorption studies in an intestinal sac model: the absorption of Gem-CS-NPs intestinal transport increased 3–5-fold compared to free drug.		[51]
Naringenin	Sodium alginate, chitosan, streptozotocin	To prepare alginate coated chitosan core shell NPs for effective oral delivery	In vitro drug release from NPs was 15% in SGF (pH 1.2) and 90% in pH 7.4 in slow, sustained fashion.	In vivo study in rats showed lack of toxicity; and an anti-diabetic effect: naringenin NPs have better efficacy in lowering blood glucose levels compare to free drug.	[52]
Epigallocatechin gallate (EGCG)	N-carboxymethyl chitosan (MW = 61 kDa), chitosan hydrochloride	To develop EGCG-chitosan/β-Lg NPs to achieve a prolong release for oral administration in the GI tract	In vitro drug release and degradation of EGCG-chitosan/β-Lg NPs was slower in simulated stomach condition compare to control particles		[53]
Quercetin	Chitosan, sodium alginate, sodium pyruvate, L-glutamine	To develop and evaluate quercetin-chitosan/alginate NPs to preserve its antioxidant property without causing systemic toxicity.	In vitro cytotoxicity of both empty NPs and quercetin NPs exhibited nontoxic behavior in HepG2 liver cells when exposed for a period up to 72 h.	In vivo toxicity study in Wistar rats displayed no change in body weight, rat liver weight, histology, hematology and biochemical parameters after oral administration of empty NPs and quercetin loaded NPs.	[54]

Oral delivery of vaccines is critical as the antigens degrade in GIT hindering their reaching Peyer's patches, the gastrointestinal lymphoid tissue. Moreover, vaccines containing chitosan NP can only be prepared by methods that avoid organic solvents as the organic solvents may alter the immunogenicity of antigens if the peptide secondary structure is disturbed [55]. Chitosan and carboxymethyl chitosan NP were found to be excellent carriers for oral vaccine delivery of extracellular products of *V. anguillarum* (pathogenic bacteria). The NP prepared were stable in the gastric pH, had sustained release and protected the antigenic protein from entering spleen and kidney which is critical for immune response [46].

5. Chitosan in Nasal Drug Delivery

Nasal delivery is a non-invasive technique of delivering drugs to reach the respiratory system, the brain and/or systemic circulation. A significant challenge with the delivery of drugs through the nasal route is the mucociliary clearance of drugs. Moreover, hydrophilic drugs, proteins and peptides, nucleic acids and polysaccharides present difficulties because of their low permeability across the nasal epithelium. Nasal absorption is critical for the drugs to exhibit their action. The physical characteristics of drugs that govern nasal absorption include molecular weight, lipophilicity and charge. The drugs that do not cross the nasal membrane undergo mucociliary clearance. This limitation can be overcome by developing a mucoadhesive system. Chitosan is biodegradable, biocompatible, exhibits low toxicity, adheres to mucus and opens the tight junctions of nasal membrane. Owing to these properties, chitosan has applications in nasal delivery [56]. The three ways of nasal absorption is by transcellular pathway, paracellular pathway and via trigeminal nerves [57]. Several specific examples are given below.

Carbamazepine is used in the treatment of epilepsy and it is very important for the drug to cross the blood brain barrier (BBB). Carboxymethyl chitosan NPs of carbamazepine have found to enhance the bioavailability and brain targeting via the nasal route. The brain-to-plasma exposure ratio was 150% when carbamazepine was administered as chitosan NPs intranasally [25]. In Alzheimer's disease (AD), a person's sex is a risk factor and in women with AD, the levels of 17β-estradiol are found to be relatively low. Estradiol, a potent sex hormone, has been used in the prevention and treatment of AD. It is important for estradiol to achieve a sufficient tissue concentration in the brain to exhibit it effect. When estradiol is given orally, the cerebrospinal levels are very low. The cerebrospinal fluid levels of estradiol were found to be high compared to plasma levels when estradiol was administered intranasally as chitosan NPs. These results suggest that estradiol is transported to the brain directly when given through the nasal route as chitosan NPs. As another example, the bioavailability of leuprolide, used in the treatment of prostate cancer and hormone-dependent diseases, was found to be increased when formulated as thiolated-chitosan NPs [57]. Chitosan NPs and thiolated-chitosan NPs of leuprolide were prepared. There was a 2–5-fold increase in drug transport across porcine nasal mucosa when leuprolide was formulated as chitosan NPs or thiolated-chitosan NP, respectively, compared to leuprolide solution. The drug exposure, as measured by area under the plasma concentration vs. time curve AUC, increased by 6.9-fold with thiolated-chitosan NP [58].

6. Chitosan in Pulmonary Drug Delivery

Both local and systemic effects can be achieved by drug delivery to the lungs. There are several advantages to delivering drug to the lungs compared to other routes such as rapid and sustained drug delivery, high efficacy and no hepatic first-pass effect. The factors that enhance drug delivery via the lungs are the large surface area of the lungs, high tissue vascularity and the thin absorption barrier [59]. The barriers for drug delivery via the lungs include the bronchial mucus layer, the alveolar lining fluid, epithelial cells, macrophage clearance and proteolytic degradation [60]. In the recent review published by Islam and Ferro [61], drug delivery to the lungs with the help of chitosan based nanoparticles can be achieved. The authors claimed it to be beneficial that for pulmonary drug delivery, the positive charge on the surface of chitosan provides mucoadhesive properties. This adherence to the lung mucosa increases the potential for drug absorption; the positive charge on chitosan has been previously shown to open the intercellular tight junctions of the lung epithelium thereby increasing uptake. Interestingly, chitosan possesses antibacterial activity by binding to phosphoryl groups and lipopolysaccharides on bacterial cell membranes, which is an additional benefit in fighting pulmonary bacterial infections.

A NP dry powder inhalation (DPI) of rifampicin, an antitubercular drug, was formulated with chitosan as the polymer. This NP formulation has shown sustained drug release until 24 h and no toxicity at both cell and organ. An in vivo study of this formulation showed that rifampicin exhibited increased maximal plasma concentration (C_{max}), AUC and extended mean residence time (MRT) with the NP formulation [62]. Itraconazole is an anti-fungal drug which, when administered orally, suffers from low solubility. To treat pulmonary infections effectively, itraconazole has to be administered via the pulmonary route. Aerosolization would be an advantage for antifungal agents as it can provide a high drug concentration at the site of action, passive targeting and reduced systemic toxicity. The aerosolization properties of itraconazole can be significantly improved by formulating the drug in spray-dried chitosan NP with lactose, mannitol and leucine. The pulmonary deposition of itraconazole was shown to be increased when formulated as spray-dried microparticles containing itraconazole loaded chitosan NP [63]. Some of the other applications of chitosan in pulmonary drug delivery as depicted in Table 2.

Table 2. Applications of chitosan nanoparticles in pulmonary drug delivery.

Drug	Composition	Purpose	Research Findings	In Vivo	Reference
Rifampicin	TPP, lactose, Tween 80	Preparing CS-NPs dry powder to achieve local and sustained targeting of anti-tubercular drugs in order to reduce dosage and frequency	1. In vitro release showed 90% release of RFM from CS-NPs within 24 h. 2. Cell viability of J774 macrophage cells showed negligible toxicity of RFM-NPs up to 12 h exposure at concentrations up to 0.5 mg/mL.	In vivo study—male Wistar rats. A marked increase in Cmax, t1/2 and AUC was seen in RFM-NPs compared to other formulations.	[62]
Itraconazole	Hydroxypropyl-beta-cyclodextrin (HPβCD), mannitol, lactose, TPP, L-leucine	To develop chitosan NPs for pulmonary delivery of itraconazole as a dry powder formulation	1. Encapsulation efficiency of 55% was obtained in 1:3 ratio of chitosan:TPP. 2. In vitro drug release was ~80% during the first 4 h and the remaining encapsulated drug was released over 48 h.		[63]
Baclofen and siRNA	N,N,N-tri-methyl chitosan, TPP	To prepare and evaluate baclofen-trimethyl chitosan/TPP NPs (Bac-TMC/TPP NPs) in a dry powder formulation	1. Low in vitro cytotoxicity of TMC and Bac-TMC in A549 cells when treated with four different polymers for 48 h. 2. Cellular uptake of Bac-TMC3/TPP/siRNA NPs was greatly enhanced by clathrin-mediated cellular uptake pathway.		[64]
Heparin (LMWH)	Chitosan, lipoid S100, glycol chitosan	To prepare and evaluate LMWH chitosan and glycol chitosan NPs for enhancing the pulmonary absorption of LMW heparin.	In vitro drug release of lipoid S100-LMWH GCS NPs in SLF showed progressive LMWH release up to 6 h, followed by a plateau for 24 h.	In vivo studies were performed in mice: the aerosol-type administration of free LMWH and Lipoid S100-LMWH GCS NPs led to a significant elongation of the coagulation time	[65]
Theo-phylline	Chitosan thioglycolic acid, TPP	To develop and evaluate whether theophylline-thiolated chitosan NPs can enhance theophylline's capacity to alleviate allergic asthma	In vitro mucoadhesive study of TCNs exhibited a gradual increase in mucin binding and adsorption for 12 h compared to unmodified chitosan	In vivo study was performed in mice and the anti-inflammatory effects of theophylline were markedly enhanced when the drug was delivered by TCNs compared to unmodified chitosan or theophylline alone.	[66]
Leuprolide	Thiolated chitosan	To prepare and evaluate leuprolide thiolated-CS-NPs to enhance the half-life and bioavailability of leuprolide via nasal administration	In vitro drug release of leuprolide from thiolated chitosan showed slow and sustained release of drug about 43% in 2 h.	In vivo study was performed in male Sprague-Dawley rats showed improved nasal bioavailability of leuprolide thiolated NPs calculated based on AUC (0–6) was about 19.6% as compared to leuprolide solution alone 2.8%.	[60]
Estradiol (E2)	Chitosan, methylated β-cyclodextrin, TPP	To prepare estradiol-chitosan NPs for improving nasal absorption and brain targeting		In vivo study was performed in male Wister rats: The plasma concentration of E2 from E2-CS-NPs was significantly lower in intranasal administration compare to IV but CSF concentrations of E2 from E2-CS-NPs was significantly higher for intranasal administration compare to IV.	[67]
Tetanus toxoid (TT)	LMW Chitosan, TPP, trehalose	To prepare tetanus toxoid chitosan nanoparticles (TT CS NPs) as a new long-term nasal vaccine delivery vehicle	In vitro drug release of the TT from CS-NPs showed a rapid release over first 2 h followed by slow release for up to 16 days.	Intranasal immunization with two doses of TT-CS NPs in mice: The results showed the titers were significantly higher for the TT-loaded particles than for the free toxoid and at post-administration of TT-CS NPs IgA levels were significantly higher than the fluid vaccine.	[68]

7. Mucoadhesion

One of the major drawbacks of delivering proteins/peptides or macromolecules through a non-injection route is the limited absorption at mucosal sites. For local delivery in the GI tract or nasal/buccal cavity or to the vaginal, urethral or pulmonary sites, the drug delivery system should be mucoadhesive and release the drug. Mucoadhesive nanoparticles/microparticles can adhere to the mucus membrane and release the drug over time (Figure 4), with the potential to reduce dosing frequency. Uptake of drugs into the systemic circulation can be achieved by transient and reversible opening of tight junctions in between epithelial cells by certain polymers and chitosan is one such polymer [69]. Some of the other mucoadhesive polymers apart from chitosan are alginate, guar gum, pectin, carrageenan K type II, gelatin, poly (vinyl pyrrolidone), poly (vinyl amine), poly (ethylene glycol) and poly (ethylene oxide) and its copolymers and poly (acrylic acid) and poly (methacrylic acid) derivatives [70].

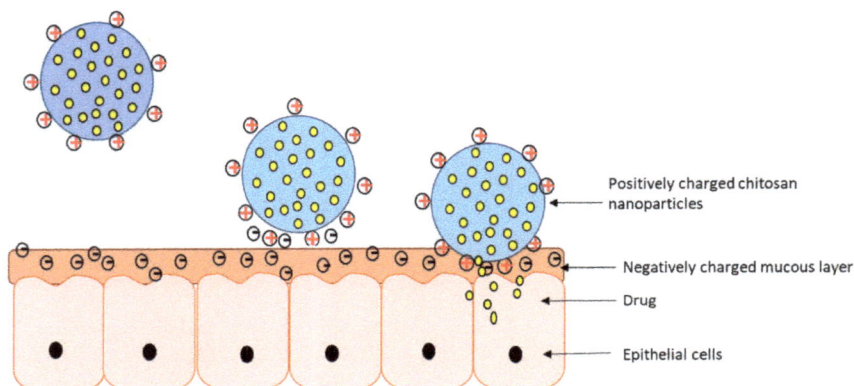

Figure 4. Schematic representation of chitosan loaded nanoparticles (CS-NP) structure and interaction with the mucus layer. From left to right: CS-NP upon reaching the mucosal layer bind to the negatively charged mucus by virtue of electrostatic attraction and release the drug over time.

As discussed earlier, the mucoadhesive property of the chitosan is attributed to its strong positive charge which helps in forming a bond with negatively charged mucus. Mucus is present in the organs of the GIT and the respiratory tract. The GIT is characterized by varying pH and an enzyme environment which makes it difficult for oral delivery of protein/peptide drugs and DNA. Chitosan is an excellent carrier for such drugs as it is mucoadhesive, permeation enhancer and forms a protective barrier for the drug [71]. Particle size also plays a role in the case of chitosan nanoparticles, as smaller particles may be more able to penetrate the mucous layer. Table 3 provides examples where the mucoadhesive property of chitosan is utilized.

Table 3. Applications of chitosan nanoparticles in mucoadhesive drug delivery.

Drug	Composition	Purpose	Research Findings	In Vivo	Reference
Doxorubicin HCL (DOX)	Chitosan (MW = 400 kDa), 4-CBS, TPP, 1-ethyl-3-(3-dimethylaminopropyl) carbodiimide HCl (EDAC)	Preparation, characterization, in vitro drug release, Topo II inhibitor activity and evaluation of DOX-loaded 4-CBS-chitosan/PLA nanoparticles.	1. In vitro drug release of DOX loaded 4-CBS-chitosan/PLA nanoparticles showed sustained release up to 26 days. 2. Cytotoxic study (MTT) of DOX loaded nanoparticles showed the lowest effect on the cell viability of HepG2 compared to SW620, KATO3 and CHAGO cell lines. 3. Over 72% inhibition of Topo II.		[72]
Alpha-mangostin (AP)	Chitosan (MW = 600 kDa), methane-sulfonic acid, oleoyl chloride, sodium bicarbonate, glycidyl-trimethyl ammonium chloride	To develop a mucoadhesive oleoyl-quaternized chitosan coated nanostructure lipid carrier (NLC) for potential oral administration with enhanced mucoadhesion	In vitro cytotoxicity of AP-NLC and CS-AP-NLC exhibited higher toxicity against Caco-2 than Hela cells.	In vivo toxicology study was performed in zebrafish embryos.	[73]
Cetirizine	Chitosan, 1-ethyl-3-(3-dimethylaminopropyl) carbodiimide hydrochloride (EDC. HCl), N-hydroxyl succinimide	Preparation and characterization of mucosal adhesion and drug release of cetirizine-chitosan NP	1. In vitro, the cumulative release of cedH from cedH:CS-NPs and cedH:CTZ-CS-1-NPs were 71% & 76% in absence of lysozyme and increased to 77% & 84% in presence of lysozyme. Burst release and lysozyme induced sustained release was achieved. 2. In vitro cytotoxicity of cedH:CTZ-CS-1 NPs showed non-toxicity in 1.929 cells and biocompatibility with RBCs.	[74]	
5-amino levulinic acid	Chitosan, lactic acid.	To develop and characterize chitosan-based 5-ALA mucoadhesive film to enhance its retention in oral mucosa	In vitro permeation and retention of 5-ALA (1.0% or 10%) were increased. However, 10% 5-ALA exhibited highest values 4 and 17 times, respectively, compared to propylene glycol vehicle.		[75]
Curcumin	Chitosan Low (CLS 50,000-190,000 Da), medium (CSM 190,000-310,00 Da), high (CSH 310,000 to >375,000 Da), polycaprolactone, glycerol	Preparation of mucoadhesive films containing curcumin-loaded NPs to prolong the residence time of the dosage form in the oral cavity and to increase drug absorption through the buccal mucosa	1. Swelling studies for mucoadhesive films containing curcumin loaded NPs showed good hydration in simulated saliva. 2. In vitro release of CSHCS-NP and CSMCS-NP exhibited high release rate approximately 3.4% and 2.8% curcumin respectively, over 24 h.		[76]
Propranolol HCl	Chitosan, TPP, Carbopol 940, poloxamer 407.	To develop a propranolol-chitosan NPs transdermal gels to improve the systemic bioavailability of the drug.	1. In vitro drug release was performed in buffer solution, only 7% and 11% of propranolol was released in 24 h from nanoparticle suspension and gel. 2. Ex vivo drug release was performed in pig ear, skin showed a slow permeation rate from nanoparticles in gel over 24 h.		[77]
C-glycosyl flavonoid enriched fractions of cecropia glaziovii (EFF-Cg)	Resomer PLGA, ploxamer 188, sorbitan monoaleate, chitosan	To develop and characterize EFF-Cg nanocomposites chitosan film containing PLGA NPs.	In vitro cytotoxicity study was performed in Vero cell line: chitosan film and nanocomposite film exhibited low toxicity.	[78]	
Alginate and pectin	Chitosan, TPP, Triton X-100	Preparation of alginate and pectin chitosan NPs for oral drug delivery	1. Cytotoxicity was performed in TR146 cells: Chit-NP showed cytocompatibility while Alg-NP, Pec-NP exhibited cytotoxicity at some concentrations. 2. Stability of NP in simulated salivary fluid: The Alg-NP were the most stable (a > 2 h), while Pec-NP and especially Chit-NP were unstable.	[79]	
Insulin	Chitosan MMW, PEG, PVP, trehalose	To develop and characterize chitosan films with insulin loaded PEG-b-PLA NPs	In vitro drug release of both insulin NPs showed pH dependent classic biphasic sustained release of protein over 5 weeks and insulin encapsulation efficiency of 30–70%.		[80]

7.1. Buccal Drug Delivery

Buccal drug delivery involves drug delivery to the buccal cavity and to the systemic circulation. The advantages by delivering drug through buccal route include; increased bioavailability, less amount of drug required and bypassing the hepatic first pass effect. Moreover, the drug need not be exposed to the harsh GI environment [81]. The high permeability of buccal mucosa is a suitable target for novel formulations [82].

Giovino and co-workers have investigated chitosan buccal films of insulin loaded poly (ethylene glycol) methyl ether-block-polylactide (PEG-b-PLA) NP [83]. The NP showed excellent mucoadhesive properties and insulin release from the NP was slow and sustained (70%). Ex vivo studies reveal 1.8-fold enhancement in insulin permeation from NP compared to pure drug. Polysaccharide-based NP of alginate, chitosan and pectin for buccal delivery were prepared and compared. Chitosan NP were not stable in the saliva compared to alginate and pectin NP. Contrary to this, chitosan NP were cytocompatible while alginate and pectin NP have shown cytotoxicity [80]. As another example of buccal delivery, curcumin prepared as polycaprolactone nanoparticles coated with chitosan. As a third example, we can consider the NP encapsulation of the enriched flavonoid fraction (EFF-Cg) obtained from *Cecropia glaziovii*. EFF-Cg is used for several purposes such as controlling blood pressure and as a diuretic, antiasthmatic and hypoglycemic agent but it suffers from low bioavailability. EFF-Cg loaded PLGA nanoparticles were prepared for buccal delivery in the form of chitosan films. The bioavailability of EFF-Cg was improved and no signs of cytotoxicity were seen [84]. Thus, addition of chitosan in this hybrid approach has enabled both a high NP encapsulation efficiency and a stronger interaction with mucus [84]. Although the above-mentioned applications of chitosan are promising, chitosan NP suffers from stability issues in oral environment.

7.2. Site Specific Delivery in the GIT

Due to its properties of mucoadhesivity, permeation enhancement, biocompatibility, biodegradability and efflux pump inhibition, chitosan is one of the most suitable polymers for oral drug delivery [81]. In the above section on oral drug delivery with chitosan formulations, there are a few examples of mucoadhesive drug delivery systems there were formulated to release drug in the small intestine [40,41]. Alternatively, Suvannasara et al. attempted to enhance the mucoadhesive property of chitosan in the acidic environment (stomach) by conjugating C2-N position of chitosan with aromatic sulfonamide, 4-carboxybenzenesulfonamide-chitosan (4-CBS-chitosan) [85]. The 4-CBS-chitosan has shown higher mucoadhesion compared to pure chitosan. Moreover, the swelling ratio was higher than the pure chitosan suggesting that the polymer can tolerate acidic stomach conditions. The authors here recommend using 4-CBS-chitosan for delivering drugs specifically to the stomach (drugs with absorption window in stomach).

For the treatment of colonic diseases such as ulcerative colitis, Chron's disease, irritable bowel disease and colon infection, colon specific drug delivery is more appropriate. Several polymers have been investigated for colon specific drug delivery [86]. Of the several natural polymers available, chitosan is best suited for colon specific delivery owing to the properties of biodegradability by enzymes in colon, chelating ability and biocompatibility [87]. Chitosan-vancomycin NPs for colon delivery were prepared by two different methods; ion gelation and spray drying. The NPs prepared by spray drying have shown high encapsulation efficiency and better drug release compared to the NPs made by ion gelation [83]. Coco et al. have compared the ability of NPs made with chitosan to other polymers for inflamed colon drug delivery [88]. Several batches of NPs were prepared by entrapping ovalbumin (OVA) into Eudragit S 100, trimethylchitosan, PLGA, PEG-PLGA and PEG-PCL, separately. Of all the NPs made, NPs with trimethyl chitosan have shown the highest permeability of OVA. However, a high permeability was also seen with PEG-PLGA NPs as they were coated with mannose for active targeting of the area of inflammation. As another example, chitosan-carboxymethyl starch nanoparticles of 5-aminosalicylic acid, another drug for inflammatory bowel disease, have been prepared which achieved high entrapment efficiency as well as controlled drug release [89].

Although chitosan has shown its ability to deliver drug to the colon, there are a few issues to be addressed such as toxicity studies in humans, the impact of the GI tract inflammation characteristic of these disorders on mucoadhesion and drug absorption, the stability of these compounds in that biological environment and achieving a manufacturing scale of fabrication [90]. Demonstration of superiority to the Eudragit polymers currently in use for colon specific drug delivery of specific drugs will also be required [91].

Some of the other drug delivery routes have been explored for mucosal delivery with chitosan are vaginal, nasal, pulmonary and ocular. Systemic absorption of insulin has been demonstrated by formulation in chitosan NPs and administration by the nasal route. Insulin loading up to 55% was achieved and nasal absorption of insulin was greater from chitosan NP [92]. Rosmarinic acid loaded chitosan NP have been prepared by an ion gelation method for ocular delivery. The NPs showed no cytotoxicity against the retinal pigment epithelium (ARPE-19) nor the human cornea cell line (HCE-T). The permeability of rosmarinic acid facilitated by the NP formulation was found to be significantly higher compared to free solution. Mucoadhesion studies reveal that the NPs interact with the ocular mucosa [93]. Imiquimod was formulated as both chitosan coated PCL nanocapsules embedded in hydroethylcellulose gel and PCL nanocapsules embedded in chitosan hydrogel for vaginal delivery to treat human papillomavirus infection [94]. The former was found to show higher mucoadhesion while the latter has shown high drug permeation. Balancing the considerations of mucoadhesion, permeation and drug retention, the latter was selected as the best delivery system [94].

8. Pharmacokinetics (PK) of Chitosan Based Formulations

The pharmacokinetics of chitosan-based NPs is similar to those of other polymeric NPs because the same principles of drug release apply as discussed above. The most important property of chitosan to be exploited is its mucoadhesion. In the following section, we explore the pharmacokinetic (PK) features of chitosan-based NP. A PK study was done in beagle dogs to assess the bioavailability of cyclosporin-A (Cy-A) encapsulated into NPs comprised of chitosan, gelatin-A or sodium glycocholate (SGC). A control group received the standard oral micro-emulsion formulation (Neoral®). The C_{max} was markedly increased in the case of both the chitosan and gelatin NP formulations while the C_{max} decreased with SGC NPs as compared to Neoral. There was a 2.6-fold increase in the AUC of Cy-A from chitosan NPs compared to SGC NPs and 1.8-fold increase in AUC from gelatin NPs compared to SGC NPs. The relative bioavailability of Cy-A from SGC NPs was decreased by 36% when compared to marketed formulation. This could be due to the negative charge of the SGC NPs which could have hindered the NPs from adhering to the intestinal mucus and thus may have reduced the drug absorption across the intestinal epithelium. This supports the idea that a positive charge on chitosan NPs can help in mucoadhesion and increase in relative bioavailability, improved by 73% in this case [45].

Chitosan based NPs of Bay 41-4109 were developed with the primary goal of prolonging circulation time of the drug in blood. A PK study in rats demonstrated a 3.3-fold increase in C_{max}, increased AUC and 4-fold increase in absolute bioavailability of chitosan NPs compared to the Bay 41-4109 suspension. The enhanced intestinal absorption of Bay 41-4109 can be attributed to either increased interaction between the positive charge of chitosan with the negative charge of cell membranes or the mucoadhesive character of chitosan NPs, enabling them to release drug over time in the small intestine [44]. Enoxaparin has little to no oral bioavailability. In order to facilitate oral bioavailability, enoxaparin-loaded alginate-coated chitosan NPs (Enx-Alg-CS-NPs) were formulated, resulting in a 3-fold increase in AUC for oral enoxaparin (50 mg/kg in rats) and representing 20% of the AUC achieved with intravenous dosing (1 mg/kg). The increased intestinal permeation of enoxaparin in rats could be due to enhanced paracellular transport of the drug across intestinal epithelium owing to the mucoadhesive property of chitosan [47]. Chitosan NPs have many applications in increasing the oral bioavailability and the in vivo efficiency, illustrated in the following schematic representation (Figure 5).

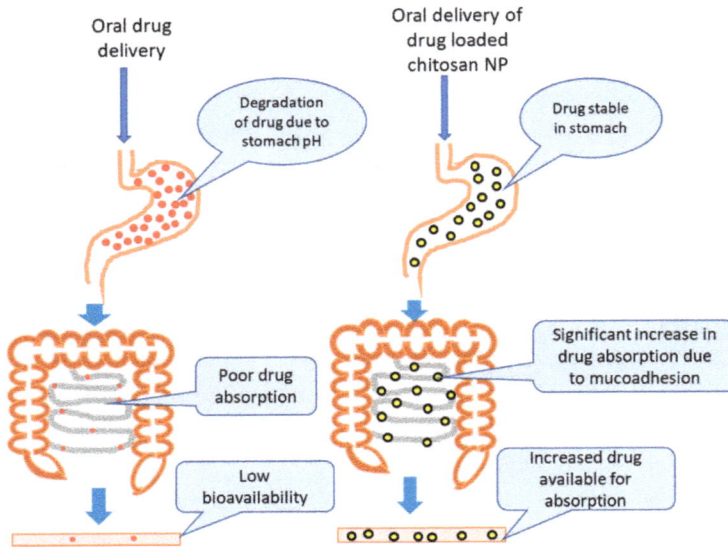

Figure 5. In vivo efficiency of drug loaded chitosan NPs in enhancing the drug absorption via the intestinal epithelium thereby increasing the drug available for absorption.

9. Toxicity and Safety of Chitosan

Chitosan is biodegradable and the process occurs either by chemical or enzyme catalysis. Degradation of chitosan is dependent on the degree of deacetylation and the availability of amino groups. Additionally, chitosan is approved as safe by US-FDA and EU for dietary use and wound dressing applications. However, the toxicity of chitosan increases by increasing charge density and degree of deacetylation [37]. As of this writing, we have not found any published data showing human toxicity of chitosan based formulations or questioning the safety of chitosan for human use. However, there are several animal toxicity studies reporting good safety in vivo and in vitro.

Aluani et al. have reported an in vivo toxicity study of two types of quercetin-loaded chitosan NPs (QR-NP1, QR-NP2) in male Wistar albino rats [56]. Briefly, the rats were divided into six groups and treated with saline, quercetin, empty NP or quercetin NPs in two related formulations. The rats were sacrificed, livers were collected, antioxidant defense marker (malondialdehyde (MDA) and glutathione (GSH)) levels were assessed. Oral administration of empty and quercetin loaded chitosan NPs indicated no change in body weight, relative rat liver weights, liver histology and hematology and biochemical parameters. There was no increase in MDA levels with both empty and quercetin loaded chitosan NP. GSH levels in animals with one of the NP formulations were slightly decreased. This data was also supported by in vitro cytotoxicity study which concludes chitosan NPs as safe carrier for quercetin in oxidative stress associated injuries.

Several airway-based cell culture models such as bronchial Calu-3 and alveolar 549 cells are in use to demonstrate the safety and toxicity of chitosan-based formulations for pulmonary drug delivery [61]. Lung toxicity of these biodegradable NPs was evaluated in mice in vivo [95]. Three NP formulations, PLGA NPs coated with chitosan, poloxamer 188 NPs and PVA NPs, were analyzed for biodistribution and inflammatory potential after a single dose administration in mice. Analysis of brancheoalveolar lavage cell population, protein secretion, cytokine release and histopathology were carried out. Chitosan-coated PLGA NPs showed better biodistribution and lower toxicity compared to non-coated NPs. Low levels of cytokine release indicate that chitosan coated PLGA NPs did not induce an inflammatory response. Chitosan-coated PLGA NPs showed a favorable biodistrbution as well [91]. Grenha et al. 2007 reported absence of toxicity in vitro with Calu-3 cells and A549 epithelial cells with NP concentrations up to 1.3 mg/mL [96].

In vitro cytotoxicity of chitosan based NP against buccal cells (TR146) was evaluated by Pistone et al. [79]. Three types of NP were prepared; alginate, Zn^{+2}—crosslinked pectin NP and chitosan NP crosslinked with TPP. An in vitro cytotoxicity test showed favorably that chitosan NPs were less cytotoxic compared to the alginate and pectin NPs. Moreover, chitosan alone was found to be more cytotoxic than the chitosan NP which could be due to the linker attached to chitosan NP or the intracellular processing response differential to free material vs NPs. The cytotoxicity of chitosan NP was shown to be further reduced either by increasing the concentration of the linker (TPP) or using chitosan with lesser degree of deacetylation.

10. Clinical Vaccine Trials of Chitosan Based Formulations

While clinical use of oral or mucoadhesive drug formulations containing chitosan remain on the horizon, there are already human vaccines in development which use chitosan as an adjuvant. CRM_{197}, a diphtheria toxoid antigen formulated as a chitosan-glutamate intranasal system, was evaluated in healthy human volunteers for the safety and immunostimulatory effects. Three groups of volunteers received intranasal diphtheria vaccine (500 µg of CRM_{197} with 9.5 mg of chitosan glutamate 213 and 2.5 mg mannitol), antigen alone (Day 0 and 28) and alum-adsorbed diphtheria toxoid vaccine via IM injection (Day 0). Serum IgG and IgA were collected on Days 27 and 42. Results suggest that chitosan was well tolerated with only minor adverse effects such as nasal discharge, blockage and discomfort. Antibody levels of the group receiving CRM_{197} and chitosan intranasally increased after the second (booster) vaccination [97].

An intranasal vaccine (NV-VLP) was formulated as spray dried powder composed of chitosan and norovirus VLP antigen with monophosphoryl lipid (MPL) as immune enhancer. This was tested in Phase 1 clinical studies, two randomized, double blinded, controlled studies with healthy volunteers. In one study, 5, 15 and 50 µg of antigen and chitosan alone were evaluated. In another trial, four groups of healthy volunteers were given MPL/chitosan (500 or 100 µg VLP per dose), chitosan only and placebo. Symptoms were recorded for a week after vaccination and safety evaluation up to 180 days. No vaccine related adverse effects were seen and significant immune response was seen with 100 µg dose. These results reveal that intranasal administration of vaccine may induce IgA secretion from intestinal mucosal tissues [98]. Similar such work has been done in healthy volunteers which provide further evidence of the efficacy of this vaccine approach [99].

11. Preparation of Chitosan Nanoparticles

Ionotropic gelation, microemulsion, emulsification solvent diffusion and emulsion based solvent evaporation are the most common methods to prepare chitosan-based nanoparticles. Usage of less organic solvent and lesser force are some of the main advantages most of these methods offer. The key characteristics that are found to affect the particle size and surface charge of chitosan NPs prepared by these methods are molecular weight and the degree of acetylation of the chitosan. Some of the mechanisms by which drugs are entrapped within the polymeric matrix are electrostatic interaction, hydrogen bonding and hydrophobic interactions. Drug loading and release are not the only key features, however. The intended use of the nanoparticles and the physiological environment at the site of administration must be taken into account, e.g. not only ionic strength, or the presence of salts, enzymes and proteins but also pH stability (consider the milieu of the eye vs the GI tract). Fortunately, we now have multiple formulation methods to choose from.

11.1. Ionotropic Gelation

This is a simple technique where the chitosan solution (positively charged) is dissolved in acetic acid or any polyanionic solution (negatively charged) with or without a stabilizing agent such as poloxamer. Nanoparticles are readily formed due to complexation between positive and negative charged species during mechanical stirring at room temperature, resulting in separation of chitosan in spherical particles of different sizes and surface charges. Generally, the reported particle size ranges from 20 to 200 and 550 to 900 nm. Chitosan-TPP/vitamin C nanoparticles were prepared via ionotropic gelation between the positively charged amino groups of chitosan-TPP and the vitamin C, with constant stirring at room temperature for just 1 h [100,101]. A few advantages of ionotropic gelation include: the processing conditions are mild and it uses an aqueous environment, low toxicity and little chance of altering the chemistry of the drug to be encapsulated. The main disadvantages of this method are its poor stability in acidic conditions and difficulty in entrapping high molecular weight drugs [2,102].

11.2. Complex Coacervation Method

Coacervation is a technique of separating spherical particles by mixing electrostatically driven liquids. DNA-chitosan nanoparticles are formed by coacervation of the positively charged amine groups of chitosan and the negatively charged DNA phosphate groups [103,104]. Entrapment efficiency and drug release are governed by the molecular weight of the two polymers [105,106]. An advantage of complex coacervation is that the process can be entirely performed in an aqueous solution at low temperature. This provides a better chance of preserving the activity of the encapsulated substances. The main disadvantages of this method are the poor stability of the NPs, low drug loading and crosslinking of the complex by a chemical reagent such as toxic glutaraldehyde is necessary [101,107,108]. In the polyelectrolyte complex (PEC) method, an anionic solution (for example, dextran sulfate DNA solution) is added to the cationic polymer (e.g., chitosan solution dissolved in acetic acid, gelatin and polyethylenimine), under mechanical stirring at room temperature followed by charge neutralization. Advantages include: the method is simple, there is an absence of harsh conditions and the nanoparticles form spontaneously [2,101]. Low molecular weight water-soluble chitosan (LMWSC) nanocarriers were developed by the PEC method for insulin, resulting in insulin-loaded chitosan NPs with a reported mean diameter of ~200 nm and sustained release profile in vitro [101].

11.3. Coprecipitation Method

The addition of a chitosan solution, prepared in low pH acetic acid solution, to a high pH 8.5–9.0 solution, such as ammonium hydroxide, results in coprecipitation and the formation of a highly monodisperse nanoparticle population. Nanoparticles of diameters as low as 10 nm can be prepared with high encapsulation efficiency [101,107]. The wide range of particle size is seen with this method which could be a disadvantage. A coprecipitation method was used to prepare lactic acid-grafted chitosan (LA-g-chitosan) nanoparticles where ammonium hydroxide was used to form coacervate drops. This method yielded spherical and uniformly distributed nanoparticles [109].

11.4. Microemulsion Method

In this method, chitosan in acetic acid solution and glutaraldehyde are added to a surfactant in an organic solvent such as hexane. This mixture is kept on continuous stirring at room temperature, allowing the nanoparticles to form overnight as the cross-linking process is completed. Organic solvent is then removed by evaporating under low pressure. The product at this point has excess surfactant which can be removed by precipitating with calcium chloride followed by centrifugation. The final nanoparticle suspension is then dialyzed and then lyophilized [110]. A very narrow size distribution is seen with this method and the size can be controlled by the concentration of glutaraldehyde in the preparation of the NPs. This method results in formation of small sized nanoparticles [111]. Some disadvantages with this method include usage of organic solvent, a lengthy process and a complex washing step [2].

11.5. Emulsification Solvent Diffusion Method

An o/w emulsion is prepared by mixing organic solvent into a solution of chitosan with stabilizer under mechanical stirring followed by high pressure homogenization [45,112]. Size range of 300–500 nm could be achieved with this method. Polymer precipitation occurs when a large amount of water is added to the emulsion, forming nanoparticles. This method is best suited for entrapment of hydrophobic drugs, for which the entrapment efficiency is found to be high. The major disadvantage of the method includes usage of high shear forces.

11.6. Emulsion Based Solvent Evaporation Method

This method is a slight modification of the above method but avoids high shear forces. Particle size of below 300 nm can be achieved with this method. An emulsion is prepared by adding organic solvent to a solution of chitosan with surfactant followed by ultrasonication. The emulsion formed is then added to a surfactant solution and allowed to stir until the organic solvent is evaporated, forming nanoparticles. The NP are then washed and centrifuged multiple times to remove excess surfactant followed, by lyophilization to achieve freeze-dried nanoparticles [113,114].

11.7. Reverse Micellar Method

The surfactant is dissolved in an organic solvent followed by the addition of chitosan, drug and crosslinking agent, under constant overnight vortex mixing. The organic solvent is evaporated results in formation of transparent dry mass, then the latter is dispersed in water and then a suitable salt is added for precipitating the surfactant [115,116]. A very narrow size range nanoparticle is seen and organic solvents are used [117]. Doxorubicin-dextran conjugate loaded chitosan nanoparticles were prepared by reverse micellar method. The surfactant used in this method was sodium bis (ethyl hexyl) sulfosuccinate (AOT) was dissolved in n-hexane. The NP are formed by adding liquid ammonia and 0.01% glutaraldehyde to AOT solution, 0.1% chitosan in acetic acid, doxorubicin–dextran conjugate upon continuous stirring at room temperature [118,119].

12. Limitations

Chitosan has low solubility in neutral and alkaline pH. For GI applications, its mucoadhesion and permeation enhancer properties are strongest in the duodenal area, which can be modulated with chitosan derivatives. The toxicological profile of chitosan derivatives is still under investigation. There are multiple preparation methods now available for chitosan nanoparticles but formulators will have to adapt methods to suit the physicochemical properties of the specific drug to be encapsulated, with a careful choice of a specific chitosan in terms of its molecular weight and degree of acetylation and consideration of chemical modification. To date, chitosan has shown little or no toxicity in animal models and there have been no reports of major adverse effects in healthy human volunteers but clinical data are lacking. Even though chitosan is approved in dietary use, wound dressing applications and cartilage formulations, as of this writing there is not yet a chitosan-based drug formulation approved for mass marketing [120]. Issues regarding scale up of fabrication methods will likely be informed by that of other polymeric formulations.

13. Conclusions and Future Work

Based on the versatility of chitosan, it has many potential applications in drug delivery via the GIT, nasal, pulmonary routes as explained in this review. Chitosan NP can effectively deliver drug at specific sites by retaining the drug locally to permit an extended time for drug absorption. Mucoadhesion and absorption enhancement of chitosan makes it possible to deliver drugs directly from the nose to the brain. Similarly, lung infections and colon diseases can be effectively targeted locally with chitosan NP. A chitosan-based nasal formulation of morphine (Rylomine^{TM}) is currently in Phase 2 clinical trials (UK and EU) and Phase 3 clinical trials in the U.S. We anticipate that when it reaches the market it will pave way for similar products in the near future as well as assist in discerning any unanticipated effects in humans [120]. And, while not specifically addressed herein, we look forward to additional advances in the use of chitosan nanoparticles in targeted cancer theranostics, dermatologic applications and targeted parenteral drug delivery systems [121–124]. With the advent of new strategies in overcoming the limitations of chitosan by improved formulation methods for a wider variety of drugs and even macromolecules, we expect to see more chitosan research work in near future, especially in nasal and pulmonary drug delivery. We hope that future work on chitosan nanoparticles prepared by chitosan or chitosan derivatives will also focus on toxicity studies in humans.

Author Contributions: Munawar A. Mohammed was the primary author of this manuscript. Jaweria T.M. Syeda prepared the tables and figures and contributed to part of the text. Kishor M. Wasan provided guidance regarding article scope and pharmacokinetics. Ellen K. Wasan conceived the design of the article, supervised its writing and had editorial responsibility.

Conflicts of Interest: The authors declare no conflict of interest.

References

1. Rampino, A.; Borgogna, M.; Blasi, P.; Bellich, B.; Cesàro, A. Chitosan nanoparticles: Preparation, size evolution and stability. *Int. J. Pharm.* **2013**, *455*, 219–228. [CrossRef] [PubMed]
2. Nagpal, K.; Singh, S.K.; Mishra, D.N. Chitosan Nanoparticles: A Promising System in Novel Drug Delivery. *Chem. Pharm. Bull.* **2010**, *58*, 1423–1430. [CrossRef] [PubMed]
3. Sorlier, P.; Denuzière, A.; Viton, C.; Domard, A. Relation between the Degree of Acetylation and the Electrostatic Properties of Chitin and Chitosan. *Biomacromolecules* **2001**, *2*, 765–772. [CrossRef] [PubMed]
4. Vårum, K.M.; Ottøy, M.H.; Smidsrød, O. Water-solubility of partially N-acetylated chitosans as a function of pH: Effect of chemical composition and depolymerisation. *Carbohydr. Polym.* **1994**, *25*, 65–70. [CrossRef]
5. Van den Broek, L.A.M.; Knoop, R.J.I.; Kappen, F.H.J.; Boeriu, C.G. Chitosan films and blends for packaging material. *Carbohydr. Polym.* **2015**, *116* (Suppl. C), 237–242. [CrossRef] [PubMed]
6. Chen, M.C.; Mi, F.L.; Liao, Z.X.; Hsiao, C.W.; Sonaje, K.; Chung, M.F.; Hsu, L.W.; Sung, H.W. Recent advances in chitosan-based nanoparticles for oral delivery of macromolecules. *Adv. Drug Deliv. Rev.* **2013**, *65*, 865–879. [CrossRef] [PubMed]
7. Shukla, S.K.; Mishra, A.K.; Arotiba, O.A.; Mamba, B.B. Chitosan-based nanomaterials: A state-of-the-art review. *Int. J. Biol. Macromol.* **2013**, *59*, 46–58. [CrossRef] [PubMed]
8. Strobl, G.R. *The Physics of Polymers*; Springer: Berlin/Heidelberg, Germany, 2007; ISBN 978-3-540-25278-8.
9. Park, S.Y.; Jun, S.T.; Marsh, K.S. Physical properties of PVOH/chitosan-blended films cast from different solvents. *Food Hydrocoll.* **2001**, *15*, 499–502. [CrossRef]
10. Mima, S.; Miya, M.; Iwamoto, R.; Yoshikawa, S. Highly deacetylated chitosan and its properties. *J. Appl. Polym. Sci.* **1983**, *28*, 1909–1917. [CrossRef]
11. Risbud, M.V.; Hardikar, A.A.; Bhat, S.V.; Bhonde, R.R. pH-sensitive freeze-dried chitosan–polyvinyl pyrrolidone hydrogels as controlled release system for antibiotic delivery. *J. Control. Release* **2000**, *68*, 23–30. [CrossRef]
12. Kolhe, P.; Kannan, R.M. Improvement in Ductility of Chitosan through Blending and Copolymerization with PEG: FTIR Investigation of Molecular Interactions. *Biomacromolecules* **2003**, *4*, 173–180. [CrossRef] [PubMed]
13. Koul, V.; Mohamed, R.; Kuckling, D.; Adler, H.-J.P.; Choudhary, V. Interpenetrating polymer network (IPN) nanogels based on gelatin and poly(acrylic acid) by inverse miniemulsion technique: Synthesis and characterization. *Colloids Surf. B Biointerfaces* **2011**, *83*, 204–213. [CrossRef] [PubMed]
14. El-Hefian, E.A.; Yahaya, A.H. Rheological study of chitosan and its blends: An overview. *Maejo Int. J. Sci. Technol.* **2010**, *4*, 210–220.
15. Dambies, L.; Vincent, T.; Domard, A.; Guibal, E. Preparation of Chitosan Gel Beads by Ionotropic Molybdate Gelation. *Biomacromolecules* **2001**, *2*, 1198–1205. [CrossRef] [PubMed]
16. Al-Qadi, S.; Grenha, A.; Carrión-Recio, D.; Seijo, B.; Remuñán-López, C. Microencapsulated chitosan nanoparticles for pulmonary protein delivery: In vivo evaluation of insulin-loaded formulations. *J. Control. Release* **2012**, *157*, 383–390. [CrossRef] [PubMed]

17. Thanou, M.M.; Kotze, A.F.; Scharringhausen, T.; Lueßen, H.L.; De Boer, A.G.; Verhoef, J.C.; Junginger, H.E. Effect of degree of quaternization of *N*-trimethyl chitosan chloride for enhanced transport of hydrophilic compounds across intestinal Caco-2 cell monolayers. *J. Control. Release* **2000**, *64*, 15–25. [CrossRef]

18. Bernkop-Schnürch, A.; Hornof, M.; Zoidl, T. Thiolated polymers—Thiomers: Synthesis and in vitro evaluation of chitosan–2-iminothiolane conjugates. *Int. J. Pharm.* **2003**, *260*, 229–237. [CrossRef]

19. Sadeghi, A.M.M.; Dorkoosh, F.A.; Avadi, M.R.; Weinhold, M.; Bayat, A.; Delie, F.; Gurny, R.; Larijani, B.; Rafiee-Tehrani, M.; Junginger, H.E. Permeation enhancer effect of chitosan and chitosan derivatives: Comparison of formulations as soluble polymers and nanoparticulate systems on insulin absorption in Caco-2 cells. *Eur. J. Pharm. Biopharm.* **2008**, *70*, 270–278. [CrossRef] [PubMed]

20. Yin, L.; Ding, J.; He, C.; Cui, L.; Tang, C.; Yin, C. Biomaterials Drug permeability and mucoadhesion properties of thiolated trimethyl chitosan nanoparticles in oral insulin delivery. *Biomaterials* **2009**, *30*, 5691–5700. [CrossRef] [PubMed]

21. Cui, F.; Qian, F.; Zhao, Z.; Yin, L.; Tang, C.; Yin, C. Preparation, Characterization and Oral Delivery of Insulin Loaded Carboxylated Chitosan Grafted Poly (methyl methacrylate) Nanoparticles. *Biomacromolecules* **2009**, *10*, 1253–1258. [CrossRef] [PubMed]

22. Kurita, K.; Hashimoto, S.; Yoshino, H.; Ishii, S.; Nishimura, S.-I. Preparation of Chitin/Polystyrene Hybrid Materials by Efficient Graft Copolymerization Based on Mercaptochitin. *Macromolecules* **1996**, *29*, 1939–1942. [CrossRef]

23. Furlani, F.; Sacco, P.; Marsich, E.; Donati, I.; Paoletti, S. Highly monodisperse colloidal coacervates based on a bioactive lactose-modified chitosan: From synthesis to characterization. *Carbohydr. Polym.* **2017**, *174* (Suppl. C), 360–368. [CrossRef] [PubMed]

24. Sacco, S.; Paoletti, M.; Cok, F.; Asaro, M.; Abrami, M.; Grassi, I. Donati Insight into the ionotropic gelation of chitosan using tripolyphosphate and pyrophosphate as cross-linkers. *Int. J. Biol. Macromol.* **2016**, *92*, 476–483. [CrossRef] [PubMed]

25. Liu, S.; Yang, S.; Ho, P.C. Intranasal administration of carbamazepine-loaded carboxymethyl chitosan nanoparticles for drug delivery to the brain. *Asian J. Pharm. Sci.* **2017**. [CrossRef]

26. Singh, R.; Lillard, J.W., Jr. Nanoparticle-based targeted drug delivery. *Exp. Mol. Pathol.* **2009**, *86*, 215–223. [CrossRef] [PubMed]

27. Yuan, Z.; Ye, Y.; Gao, F.; Yuan, H.; Lan, M.; Lou, K.; Wang, W. Chitosan-graft-β-cyclodextrin nanoparticles as a carrier for controlled drug release. *Int. J. Pharm.* **2013**, *446*, 191–198. [CrossRef] [PubMed]

28. Miladi, K.; Sfar, S.; Fessi, H.; Elaissari, A. Enhancement of alendronate encapsulation in chitosan nanoparticles. *J. Drug Deliv. Sci. Technol.* **2015**, *30*, 391–396. [CrossRef]

29. Siafaka, P.I.; Titopoulou, A.; Koukaras, E.N.; Kostoglou, M.; Koutris, E.; Karavas, E.; Bikiaris, D.N. Chitosan derivatives as effective nanocarriers for ocular release of timolol drug. *Int. J. Pharm.* **2015**, *495*, 249–264. [CrossRef] [PubMed]

30. Siepmann, J.; Siepmann, F. Modeling of diffusion controlled drug delivery. *J. Control. Release* **2012**, *161*, 351–362. [CrossRef] [PubMed]

31. Fonseca-Santos, B.; Chorilli, M. An overview of carboxymethyl derivatives of chitosan: Their use as biomaterials and drug delivery systems. *Mater. Sci. Eng. C* **2017**, *77*, 1349–1362. [CrossRef] [PubMed]

32. Göpferich, A. Mechanisms of polymer degradation and erosion. *Biomaterials* **1996**, *17*, 103–114. [CrossRef]

33. Pawar, D.; Mangal, S.; Goswami, R.; Jaganathan, K.S. Development and characterization of surface modified PLGA nanoparticles for nasal vaccine delivery: Effect of mucoadhesive coating on antigen uptake and immune adjuvant activity. *Eur. J. Pharm. Biopharm.* **2013**, *85*, 550–559. [CrossRef] [PubMed]

34. Manca, M.L.; Loy, G.; Zaru, M.; Fadda, A.M.; Antimisiaris, S.G. Release of rifampicin from chitosan, PLGA and chitosan-coated PLGA microparticles. *Colloids Surf. B Biointerfaces* **2008**, *67*, 166–170. [CrossRef] [PubMed]

35. Wang, M.; Zhang, Y.; Feng, J.; Gu, T.; Dong, Q.; Yang, X.; Sun, Y.; Wu, Y.; Chen, Y.; Kong, W. Preparation, characterization and in vitro and in vivo investigation of chitosan-coated poly (D,L-lactide-co-glycolide) nanoparticles for intestinal delivery of exendin-4. *Int. J. Nanomed.* **2013**, *8*, 1141–1154. [CrossRef]

36. Bowman, K.; Leong, K.W. Chitosan Nanoparticles for Oral Drug and Gene Delivery. *Int. J. Nanomed.* **2006**, *1*, 117–128. [CrossRef]

37. Wang, J.J.; Zeng, Z.W.; Xiao, R.Z.; Xie, T.; Zhou, G.L.; Zhan, X.R.; Wang, S.L. Recent advances of chitosan nanoparticles as drug carriers. *Int. J. Nanomed.* **2011**, *6*, 765–774. [CrossRef]

38. Palacio, J.; Agudelo, N.A.; Lopez, B.L. PEGylation of PLA nanoparticles to improve mucus-penetration and colloidal stability for oral delivery systems. *Curr. Opin. Chem. Eng.* **2016**, *11*, 14–19. [CrossRef]

39. Dube, A.; Nicolazzo, J.A.; Larson, I. Chitosan nanoparticles enhance the intestinal absorption of the green tea catechins (+)-catechin and (−)-epigallocatechin gallate. *Eur. J. Pharm. Sci.* **2010**, *41*, 219–225. [CrossRef] [PubMed]

40. Barbieri, S.; Buttini, F.; Rossi, A.; Bettini, R.; Colombo, P.; Ponchel, G.; Sonvico, F. Ex vivo permeation of tamoxifen and its 4-OH metabolite through rat intestine from lecithin/chitosan nanoparticles. *Int. J. Pharm.* **2015**, *491*, 99–104. [CrossRef] [PubMed]

41. Feng, C.; Wang, Z.; Jiang, C.; Kong, M.; Zhou, X.; Li, Y.; Cheng, X.; Chen, X. Chitosan/o-carboxymethyl chitosan nanoparticles for efficient and safe oral anticancer drug delivery: In vitro and in vivo evaluation. *Int. J. Pharm.* **2013**, *457*, 158–167. [CrossRef] [PubMed]

42. John, J.; Sangeetha, D.; Gomathi, T. Sunitinib loaded chitosan nanoparticles formulation and its evaluation. *Int. J. Biol. Macromol.* **2016**, *82*, 952–958. [CrossRef]

43. Diop, M.; Auberval, N.; Viciglio, A.; Langlois, A.; Bietiger, W.; Mura, C.; Peronet, C.; Bekel, A.; David, D.J.; Zhao, M.; et al. Design, characterisation and bioefficiency of insulin-chitosan nanoparticles after stabilisation by freeze-drying or cross-linking. *Int. J. Pharm.* **2015**, *491*, 402–408. [CrossRef] [PubMed]

44. Xue, M.; Hu, S.; Lu, Y.; Zhang, Y.; Jiang, X.; An, S.; Guo, Y.; Zhou, X.; Hou, H.; Jiang, C. Development of chitosan nanoparticles as drug delivery system for a prototype capsid inhibitor. *Int. J. Pharm.* **2015**, *495*, 771–782. [CrossRef] [PubMed]

45. El-Shabouri, M.H. Positively charged nanoparticles for improving the oral bioavailability of cyclosporin-A. *Int. J. Pharm.* **2002**, *249*, 101–108. [CrossRef]

46. Gao, P.; Xia, G.; Bao, Z.; Feng, C.; Cheng, X.; Kong, M.; Liu, Y.; Chen, X. Chitosan based nanoparticles as protein carriers for efficient oral antigen delivery. *Int. J. Biol. Macromol.* **2016**, *91*, 716–723. [CrossRef] [PubMed]

47. Bagre, A.P.; Jain, K.; Jain, N.K. Alginate coated chitosan core shell nanoparticles for oral delivery of enoxaparin: In vitro and in vivo assessment. *Int. J. Pharm.* **2013**, *456*, 31–40. [CrossRef] [PubMed]

48. Wang, J.; Tan, J.; Luo, J.; Huang, P.; Zhou, W.; Chen, L.; Long, L.; Zhang, L.; Zhu, B.; Yang, L.; et al. Enhancement of scutellarin oral delivery efficacy by vitamin B12-modified amphiphilic chitosan derivatives to treat type II diabetes induced-retinopathy. *J. Nanobiotechnol.* **2017**, *15*. [CrossRef] [PubMed]

49. Huang, Y.-C.; Chen, J.-K.; Lam, U.-I.; Chen, S.-Y. Preparing, characterizing and evaluating chitosan/fucoidan nanoparticles as oral delivery carriers. *J. Polym. Res.* **2014**, *21*, 415. [CrossRef]

50. Shi, Y.; Xue, J.; Jia, L.; Du, Q.; Niu, J.; Zhang, D. Surface-modified PLGA nanoparticles with chitosan for oral delivery of tolbutamide. *Colloids Surf. B Biointerfaces* **2018**, *161*, 67–72. [CrossRef] [PubMed]

51. Derakhshandeh, K.; Fathi, S. Role of chitosan nanoparticles in the oral absorption of Gemcitabine. *Int. J. Pharm.* **2012**, *437*, 172–177. [CrossRef] [PubMed]

52. Maity, S.; Mukhopadhyay, P.; Kundu, P.P.; Chakraborti, A.S. Alginate coated chitosan core-shell nanoparticles for efficient oral delivery of naringenin in diabetic animals—An in vitro and in vivo approach. *Carbohydr. Polym.* **2017**, *170*, 124–132. [CrossRef] [PubMed]

53. Liang, J.; Yan, H.; Yang, H.-J.; Kim, H.W.; Wan, X.; Lee, J.; Ko, S. Synthesis and controlled-release properties of chitosan/β-Lactoglobulin nanoparticles as carriers for oral administration of epigallocatechin gallate. *Food Sci. Biotechnol.* **2016**, *25*, 1583–1590. [CrossRef]

54. Aluani, D.; Tzankova, V.; Kondeva-Burdina, M.; Yordanov, Y.; Nikolova, E.; Odzhakov, F.; Apostolov, A.; Markova, T.; Yoncheva, K. Evaluation of biocompatibility and antioxidant efficiency of chitosan-alginate nanoparticles loaded with quercetin. *Int. J. Biol. Macromol.* **2017**, *103*, 771–782. [CrossRef] [PubMed]

55. Van der Lubben, I.M.; Verhoef, J.C.; Borchard, G.; Junginger, H.E. Chitosan for mucosal vaccination. *Adv. Drug Deliv. Rev.* **2001**, *52*, 139–144. [CrossRef]

56. Casettari, L.; Illum, L. Chitosan in nasal delivery systems for therapeutic drugs. *J. Control. Release* **2014**, *190*, 189–200. [CrossRef] [PubMed]

57. Lisbeth, I. Nasal drug delivery—Possibilities, problems and solutions. *J. Control. Release* **2003**, *87*, 187–198.

58. Shahnaz, G.; Vetter, A.; Barthelmes, J.; Rahmat, D.; Laffleur, F.; Iqbal, J.; Perera, G.; Schlocker, W.; Dünnhaput, S.; Augustijns, P.; et al. Thiolated chitosan nanoparticles for the nasal administration of leuprolide: Bioavailability and pharmacokinetic characterization. *Int. J. Pharm.* **2012**, *428*, 164–170. [CrossRef] [PubMed]

59. Ruge, C.A.; Kirch, J.; Lehr, C.-M. Pulmonary drug delivery: From generating aerosols to overcoming biological barriers—Therapeutic possibilities and technological challenges. *Lancet Respir. Med.* **2013**, *1*, 402–413. [CrossRef]

60. Lytting, E.; Nguyen, J.; Wang, X.; Kissel, T. Biodegradable polymeric nanocarriers for pulmonary drug delivery Biodegradable polymeric nanocarriers for pulmonary drug delivery. *Expert Opin. Drug Deliv.* **2008**, *56*, 629–639. [CrossRef] [PubMed]

61. Islam, N.; Ferro, V. Recent Advances in Chitosan-Based Nanoparticulate Pulmonary Drug Delivery. *Nanoscale* **2016**, 14341–14358. [CrossRef] [PubMed]

62. Rawal, T.; Parmar, R.; Tyagi, R.K.; Butani, S. Rifampicin loaded chitosan nanoparticle dry powder presents an improved therapeutic approach for alveolar tuberculosis. *Colloids Surf. B Biointerfaces* **2017**, *154*, 321–330. [CrossRef] [PubMed]

63. Jafarinejad, S.; Gilani, K.; Moazeni, E.; Ghazi-Khansari, M.; Najafabadi, A.R.; Mohajel, N. Development of chitosan-based nanoparticles for pulmonary delivery of itraconazole as dry powder formulation. *Powder Technol.* **2012**, *222*, 65–70. [CrossRef]

64. Ni, S.; Liu, Y.; Tang, Y.; Chen, J.; Li, S.; Pu, J.; Han, L. GABA B receptor ligand-directed trimethyl chitosan/tripolyphosphate nanoparticles and their pMDI formulation for survivin siRNA pulmonary delivery. *Carbohydr. Polym.* **2017**, *179*, 135–144. [CrossRef] [PubMed]

65. Trapani, A.; Di Gioia, S.; Ditaranto, N.; Cioffi, N.; Goycoolea, F.M.; Carbone, A.; Garcia-Fuentes, M.; Conese, M.; Alonso, M.J. Systemic heparin delivery by the pulmonary route using chitosan and glycol chitosan nanoparticles. *Int. J. Pharm.* **2013**, *447*, 115–123. [CrossRef] [PubMed]

66. Lee, D.-W.; Shirley, S.A.; Lockey, R.F.; Mohapatra, S.S. Thiolated chitosan nanoparticles enhance anti-inflammatory effects of intranasally delivered theophylline. *Respir. Res.* **2006**, *7*. [CrossRef] [PubMed]

67. Wang, X.; Chi, N.; Tang, X. Preparation of estradiol chitosan nanoparticles for improving nasal absorption and brain targeting. *Eur. J. Pharm. Biopharm.* **2008**, *70*, 735–740. [CrossRef] [PubMed]

68. Janes, K.; Behrens, I.; Kissel, T.; Vila, A.; Sa, A.; Vila, L. Low molecular weight chitosan nanoparticles as new carriers for nasal vaccine delivery in mice. *Eur. J. Pharm. Biopharm.* **2004**, *57*, 123–131. [CrossRef]

69. Van der Lubben, I.M.; Verhoef, J.C.; Borchard, G.; Junginger, H.E. Chitosan and its derivatives in mucosal drug and vaccine delivery. *Eur. J. Pharm. Sci.* **2001**, *14*, 201–207. [CrossRef]

70. Marguerite, R. Chitin and chitosan: Properties and applications. *Prog. Polym. Sci.* **2006**, *31*, 603–632. [CrossRef]

71. George, M.; Abraham, T.E. Polyionic hydrocolloids for the intestinal delivery of protein drugs: Alginate and chitosan—A review. *J. Control. Release* **2006**, *114*, 1–14. [CrossRef] [PubMed]

72. Soares, P.I.P.; Isabel, A.; Carvalho, J.; Ferreira, I.M.M.; Novo, C.M.M.; Paulo, J. Chitosan-based nanoparticles as drug delivery systems for doxorubicin: Optimization and modelling. *Carbohydr. Polym.* **2016**, *147*, 304–312. [CrossRef] [PubMed]

73. Yostawonkul, J.; Surassmo, S.; Iempridee, T.; Pimtong, W.; Suktham, K.; Sajomsang, W.; Gonil, P.; Ruktanonchai, U.R. Surface modification of nanostructure lipid carrier (NLC) by oleoyl-quaternized-chitosan as a mucoadhesive nanocarrier. *Colloids Surf. B Biointerfaces* **2017**, *149*, 301–311. [CrossRef] [PubMed]

74. Yu, X.; Mu, Y.; Xu, M.; Xia, G.; Wang, J.; Liu, Y.; Chen, X. Preparation and characterization of mucosal adhesive and two-step drug releasing cetirizine-chitosan nanoparticle. *Carbohydr. Polym.* **2017**, *173*, 600–609. [CrossRef] [PubMed]

75. Costa Idos, S.; Abranches, R.P.; Garcia, M.T.; Pierre, M.B. Chitosan-based mucoadhesive films containing 5-aminolevulinic acid for buccal cancer treatment. *J. Photochem. Photobiol. B Biol.* **2014**, *140*, 266–275. [CrossRef] [PubMed]

76. Icia-Mazzarino, L.; Borsali, R.; Lemos-senna, E. Mucoadhesive Films Containing Chitosan-Coated Nanoparticles: A New Strategy for Buccal Curcumin Release. *J. Pharm. Sci.* **2014**, *103*, 3764–3771. [CrossRef] [PubMed]

77. Al-Kassas, R.; Wen, J.; Cheng, A.E.; Kim, A.M.; Liu, S.S.M.; Yu, J. Transdermal delivery of propranolol hydrochloride through chitosan nanoparticles dispersed in mucoadhesive gel. *Carbohydr. Polym.* **2016**, *153*, 176–186. [CrossRef] [PubMed]

78. Santos, T.C.D.; Rescignano, N.; Boff, L.; Reginatto, F.H.; Simões, C.M.O.; de Campos, A.M.; Mijangos, C.U. Manufacture and characterization of chitosan/PLGA nanoparticles nanocomposite buccal films. *Carbohydr. Polym.* **2017**, *173*, 638–644. [CrossRef] [PubMed]

79. Pistone, S.; Goycoolea, F.M.; Young, A.; Smistad, G.; Hiorth, M. Formulation of polysaccharide-based nanoparticles for local administration into the oral cavity. *Eur. J. Pharm. Biopharm.* **2017**, *96*, 381–389. [CrossRef] [PubMed]

80. Giovino, C.; Ayensu, I.; Tetteh, J.; Boateng, J.S. Development and characterisation of chitosan films impregnated with insulin loaded PEG-b-PLA nanoparticles (NPs): A potential approach for buccal delivery of macromolecules. *Int. J. Pharm.* **2012**, *428*, 143–151. [CrossRef] [PubMed]

81. Kumar, A.; Vimal, A.; Kumar, A. Why Chitosan, From properties to perspective of mucosal drug delivery.pdf. *Int. J. Biol. Macromol.* **2016**, *91*, 615–622. [CrossRef] [PubMed]

82. Campisi, G.; Paderni, C.; Saccone, R.; Fede, O.; Wolff, A.; Giannola, L. Human Buccal Mucosa as an Innovative Site of Drug Delivery. *Curr. Pharm. Des.* **2010**, *16*, 641–652. [CrossRef] [PubMed]

83. Giovino, C.; Ayensu, I.; Tetteh, J.; Boateng, J.S. An integrated buccal delivery system combining chitosan films impregnated with peptide loaded PEG-b-PLA nanoparticles. *Colloids Surf. B Biointerfaces* **2013**, *112*, 9–15. [CrossRef] [PubMed]

84. Mazzarino, L.; Travelet, C.; Ortega-Murillo, S.; Otsuka, I.; Pignot-Paintrand, I.; Lemos-Senna, E.; Borsali, R. Elaboration of chitosan-coated nanoparticles loaded with curcumin for mucoadhesive applications. *J. Colloid Interface Sci.* **2012**, *370*, 58–66. [CrossRef] [PubMed]

85. Suvannasara, P.; Juntapram, K.; Praphairaksit, N.; Siralertmukul, K.; Muangsin, N. Mucoadhesive 4-carboxybenzenesulfonamide-chitosan with antibacterial properties.pdf. *Carbohydr. Polym.* **2013**, *94*, 244–252. [CrossRef] [PubMed]

86. Shukla, R.K.; Tiwari, A. Carbohydrate polymers: Applications and recent advances in delivering drugs to the colon. *Carbohydr. Polym.* **2012**, *88*, 399–416. [CrossRef]

87. Wang, Q.-S.; Wang, G.-F.; Zhou, J.; Gao, L.-N.; Cui, Y.-L. Colon targeted oral drug delivery system based on alginate-chitosan microspheres loaded with icariin in the treatment of ulcerative colitis. *Int. J. Pharm.* **2016**, *515*, 176–185. [CrossRef] [PubMed]

88. Cerchiara, T.; Abruzzo, A.; Di Cagno, M.; Bigucci, F.; Bauer-Brandl, A.; Parolin, C.; Vitali, B.; Gallucci, M.C.; Luppi, B. Chitosan based micro- and nanoparticles for colon-targeted delivery of vancomycin prepared by alternative processing methods. *Eur. J. Pharm. Biopharm.* **2015**, *92*, 112–119. [CrossRef] [PubMed]

89. Coco, R.; Plapied, L.; Pourcelle, V.; Jérôme, C.; Brayden, D.J.; Schneider, Y.-J.; Préat, V. Drug delivery to inflamed colon by nanoparticles: Comparison of different strategies. *Int. J. Pharm.* **2013**, *440*, 3–12. [CrossRef] [PubMed]

90. Saboktakin, M.R.; Tabatabaie, R.M.; Maharramov, A.; Ramazanov, M.A. Synthesis and in vitro evaluation of carboxymethyl starch chitosan nanoparticles as drug delivery system to the colon. *Int. J. Biol. Macromol.* **2010**, *48*, 381–385. [CrossRef] [PubMed]

91. Hua, S.; Marks, E.; Schneider, J.J.; Keely, S. Advances in oral nano-delivery systems for colon targeted drug delivery in inflammatory bowel disease: Selective targeting to diseased versus healthy tissue. *Nanomedicine* **2015**, *11*, 1117–1132. [CrossRef] [PubMed]

92. Fernandez-Urrusuno, R.; Calvo, P.; Remunan-Lopez, C.; Vila-Jato, J.L.; Alonso, M.J. Enhancement of nasal absorption of insulin using chitosan nanoparticles. *Pharm. Res.* **1999**, *16*, 1576–1581. [CrossRef] [PubMed]

93. Baptista da Silva, S.; Ferreira, D.; Pintado, M.; Sarmento, B. Chitosan-based nanoparticles for rosmarinic acid ocular delivery—In vitro tests. *Int. J. Biol. Macromol.* **2016**, *84*, 112–120. [CrossRef] [PubMed]

94. Frank, L.; Chaves, P.; D'Amore, C.; Contri, R.; Frank, A.; Beck, R.; Pohlman, A.; Buffon, A.; Guterres, S. The use of chitosan as cationic coating or gel vehicle for polymeric nanocapsules: Increasing penetration and adhesion of imiquimod in vaginal tissue. *Eur. J. Pharm. Biopharm.* **2017**, *114*, 202–212. [CrossRef] [PubMed]

95. Aragao-Santiago, L.; Hillaireau, H.; Grabowski, N.; Mura, S.; Nascimento, T.L.; Dufort, S.; Coll, J.-L.; Tsapis, N.; Fattal, E. Compared in vivo toxicity in mice of lung delivered biodegradable and non-biodegradable nanoparticles. *Nanotoxicology* **2016**, *10*, 292–302. [CrossRef] [PubMed]

96. Grenha, A.; Grainger, C.I.; Dailey, L.A.; Seijo, B.; Martin, G.P.; Remuñán-López, C.; Forbes, B. Chitosan nanoparticles are compatible with respiratory epithelial cells in vitro. *Eur. J. Pharm. Sci.* **2007**, *31*, 73–84. [CrossRef] [PubMed]

97. Mills, K.H.G.; Cosgrove, C.; McNeela, E.A.; Sexton, A.; Giemza, R.; Jabbal-Gill, I.; Church, A.; Lin, W.; Illum, L.; Podda, A.; et al. Protective levels of diphtheria-neutralizing antibody induced in healthy volunteers by unilateral priming-boosting intranasal immunization associated with restricted ipsilateral mucosal secretory immunoglobulin A. *Infect. Immun.* **2003**, *71*, 726–732. [CrossRef] [PubMed]

98. El-Kamary, S.S.; Pasetti, M.F.; Mendelman, P.M.; Frey, S.E.; Bernstein, D.I.; Treanor, J.J.; Ferreira, J.; Chen, W.H.; Sublett, R.; Richardson, C.; et al. Adjuvanted Intranasal Norwalk Virus-Like Particle Vaccine Elicits Antibodies and Antibody-Secreting Cells That Express Homing Receptors for Mucosal and Peripheral Lymphoid Tissues. *J. Infect. Dis.* **2010**, *202*, 1649–1658. [CrossRef] [PubMed]

99. Ramirez, K.; Wahid, R.; Richardson, C.; Bargatze, R.F.; El-Kamary, S.S.; Sztein, M.B.; Pasetti, M.F. Intranasal vaccination with an adjuvanted Norwalk virus-like particle vaccine elicits antigen-specific B memory responses in human adult volunteers. *Clin. Immunol.* **2012**, *144*, 98–108. [CrossRef] [PubMed]

100. Alishahi, A.; Mirvaghefi, A.; Tehrani, M.R.; Farahmand, H.; Koshio, S.; Dorkoosh, F.A.; Elsabee, M.Z. Chitosan nanoparticle to carry vitamin C through the gastrointestinal tract and induce the non-specific immunity system of rainbow trout (Oncorhynchus mykiss). *Carbohydr. Polym.* **2011**, *86*, 142–146. [CrossRef]

101. Hembram, K.C.; Prabha, S.; Chandra, R.; Ahmed, B.; Nimesh, S. Advances in preparation and characterization of chitosan nanoparticles for therapeutics. *Artif. Cells Nanomed. Biotechnol.* **2014**, *1401*, 1–10. [CrossRef]

102. Gonçalves, I.C.; Henriques, P.C.; Seabra, C.L.; Martins, M.C.L. The potential utility of chitosan micro/nanoparticles in the treatment of gastric infection. *Expert Rev. Anti. Infect. Ther.* **2014**, *12*, 981–992. [CrossRef] [PubMed]

103. Zhao, K.; Shi, X.; Zhao, Y.; Wei, H.; Sun, Q.; Huang, T.; Zhang, X.; Wang, Y. Preparation and immunological effectiveness of a swine influenza DNA vaccine encapsulated in chitosan nanoparticles. *Vaccine* **2011**, *29*, 8549–8556. [CrossRef] [PubMed]

104. Zhuo, Y.; Han, J.; Tang, L.; Liao, N.; Gui, G.-F.; Chai, Y.-Q.; Yuan, R. Quenching of the emission of peroxydisulfate system by ferrocene functionalized chitosan nanoparticles: A sensitive "signal off" electrochemiluminescence immunosensor. *Sens. Actuators B Chem.* **2014**, *192*, 791–795. [CrossRef]

105. Chen, Y.; Mohanraj, V.J.; Wang, F.; Benson, H.A.E. Designing Chitosan–Dextran Sulfate Nanoparticles Using Charge Ratios. *AAPS PharmSciTech* **2007**, *8*, E98. [CrossRef] [PubMed]

106. Leong, K.W.; Mao, H.-Q.; Truong-Le, V.L.; Roy, K.; Walsh, S.M.; August, J.T. DNA-polycation nanospheres as non-viral gene delivery vehicles. *J. Control. Release* **1998**, *53*, 183–193. [CrossRef]

107. Tiyaboonchai, W. Chitosan Nanoparticles: A Promising System for Drug Delivery. *Naresuan Univ. J.* **2003**, *11*, 51–66. [CrossRef]

108. Huang, M.; Fong, C.-W.; Khor, E.; Lim, L.-Y. Transfection efficiency of chitosan vectors: Effect of polymer molecular weight and degree of deacetylation. *J. Control. Release* **2005**, *106*, 391–406. [CrossRef] [PubMed]

109. Bhattarai, N.; Ramay, H.R.; Chou, S.-H.; Zhang, M. Chitosan and lactic acid-grafted chitosan nanoparticles as carriers for prolonged drug delivery. *Int. J. Nanomed.* **2006**, *1*, 181–187. [CrossRef]

110. Maitra, A.; Ghosh, P.K.; De, T.K.; Sahoo, S.K. Process for the Preparation of Highly Monodispersed Polymeric Hydrophilic Nanoparticles. US 5874111 A, 7 January 1999.

111. Wang, Y.; Wang, X.; Luo, G.; Dai, Y. Adsorption of bovin serum albumin (BSA) onto the magnetic chitosan nanoparticles prepared by a microemulsion system. *Bioresour. Technol.* **2008**, *99*, 3881–3884. [CrossRef] [PubMed]

112. Niwa, T.; Takeuchi, H.; Hino, T.; Kunou, N.; Kawashima, Y. Preparations of biodegradable nanospheres of water-soluble and insoluble drugs with D,L-lactide/glycolide copolymer by a novel spontaneous emulsification solvent diffusion method and the drug release behavior. *J. Control. Release* **1993**, *25*, 89–98. [CrossRef]

113. Vila, A.; Sanchez, A.; Tobío, M.; Calvo, P.; Alonso, M.J. Design of Biodegradable Partilces for Protein Delivery. *J. Control. Release* **2002**, *78*, 15–24. [CrossRef]

114. Zhang, L.; Zhao, Z.-L.; Wei, X.-H.; Liu, J.-H. Preparation and in vitro and in vivo characterization of cyclosporin A-loaded, PEGylated chitosan-modified, lipid-based nanoparticles. *Int. J. Nanomed.* **2013**, *8*, 601–610. [CrossRef]

115. Zeinab Sadat, S.; Hamed, S.-K.; Mohammad, I.; Mohammad, A.; Azizollah, N. Exploring the effect of formulation parameters on the particle size of carboxymethyl chitosan nanoparticles prepared via reverse micellar crosslinking. *J. Microencapsul.* **2017**, *34*, 270–279. [CrossRef]

116. Malmsten, M. *Surfactants and Polymers in Drug Delivery*; Marcel Dekker: New York, NY, USA, 2002; ISBN 9780824708047.

117. Banerjee, T.; Mitra, S.; Kumar-Singh, A.; Kumar-Sharma, R.; Maitra, A. Preparation, characterization and biodistribution of ultrafine chitosan nanoparticles. *Int. J. Pharm.* **2002**, *243*, 93–105. [CrossRef]

118. Liu, C.; Tan, Y.; Liu, C.; Chen, X.; Yu, L. Preparations, characterizations and applications of Chitosan-based nanoparticles. *J. Ocean Univ. China* **2007**, *6*, 237–243. [CrossRef]
119. Mitra, S.; Gaur, U.; Ghosh, P.C.; Maitra, A.N. Tumour targeted delivery of encapsulated dextran–doxorubicin conjugate using chitosan nanoparticles as carrier. *J. Control. Release* **2001**, *74*, 317–323. [CrossRef]
120. Bellich, B.; D'Agostino, I.; Semeraro, S.; Gamini, A.; Cesàro, A. "The good, the bad and the ugly" of chitosans. *Mar. Drugs* **2016**, *14*, 99. [CrossRef] [PubMed]
121. Key, J.; Park, K. Multicomponent, Tumor-Homing Chitosan Nanoparticles for Cancer Imaging and Therapy. *Int. J. Mol. Sci.* **2017**, *18*, E594. [CrossRef] [PubMed]
122. Zhang, X.; Yang, X.; Ji, J.; Liu, A.; Zhai, G. Tumor targeting strategies for chitosan-based nanoparticles. *Colloids Surf. B Biointerfaces* **2016**, *148*, 460–473. [CrossRef] [PubMed]
123. Ahmed, T.A.; Aljaeid, B.M. Preparation, characterization and potential application of chitosan, chitosan derivatives and chitosan metal nanoparticles in pharmaceutical drug delivery. *Drug Des. Devel. Ther.* **2016**, *10*, 483–507. [CrossRef] [PubMed]
124. Swierczewska, M.; Han, H.S.; Kim, K.; Park, J.H.; Lee, S. Polysaccharide-based nanoparticles for theranostic nanomedicine. *Adv. Drug Deliv. Rev.* **2016**, *99 Pt A*, 70–84. [CrossRef] [PubMed]

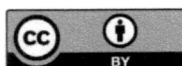

pharmaceutics

MDPI

Article

Regulation of Hepatic UGT2B15 by Methylation in Adults of Asian Descent

Steffen G. Oeser [1], Jon-Paul Bingham [1] and Abby C. Collier [2,*]

[1]   Molecular Biosciences and Bioengineering, University of Hawaii, Manoa, 1955 East-West Rd. #218, Honolulu, HI 96822, USA; steffengo@gmail.com (S.G.O.); jbingham@hawaii.edu (J.-P.B.)
[2]   Faculty of Pharmaceutical Sciences, 2405 Wesbrook Mall, University of British Columbia, Vancouver, BC V6T1Z3, Canada
*   Correspondence: abby.collier@ubc.ca; Tel.: +1-604-827-2380

Received: 12 December 2017; Accepted: 4 January 2018; Published: 7 January 2018

Abstract: The hepatic uridine 5′-diphosphate-glucuronosyl transferases (UGTs) are critical for detoxifying endo- and xenobiotics. Since UGTs are also dynamically responsive to endogenous and exogenous stimuli, we examined whether epigenetic DNA methylation can regulate hepatic UGT expression and differential effects of ethnicity, obesity, and sex. The methylation status of UGT isoforms was determined with Illumina Methylation 450 BeadChip arrays, with genotyping confirmed by sequencing and gene expression confirmed with quantitative reverse transcriptase polymerase chain reaction (q-RT-PCR). The UGT1A3 mRNA was 2-fold higher in females than males ($p < 0.05$), while UGT1A1 and UGT2B7 mRNA were significantly higher in Pacific Islanders than Caucasians (both $p < 0.05$). Differential mRNA or methylation did not occur with obesity. The methylation of the UGT2B15 locus cg09189601 in Caucasians was significantly lower than the highly methylated locus in Asians ($p < 0.001$). Three intergenic loci between UGT2B15 and 2B17 (cg07973162, cg10632656, and cg07952421) showed higher rates of methylation in Caucasians than in Asians ($p < 0.001$). Levels of UGT2B15 and UGT2B17 mRNA were significantly lower in Asians than Caucasians ($p = 0.01$ and $p < 0.001$, respectively). Genotyping and sequencing indicated that only UGT2B15 is regulated by methylation, and low UGT2B17 mRNA is due to a deletion genotype common to Asians. Epigenetic regulation of UGT2B15 may predispose Asians to altered drug and hormone metabolism and begin to explain the increased risks for adverse drug reactions and some cancers in this population.

Keywords: glucuronidation; obesity; sex; polymorphisms

1. Introduction

The uridine 5′-diphosphate-glucuronosyl transferases (UGTs, E.C. 2.4.1.17) primarily eliminate xeno- and endobiotics in humans through conjugating them with a polar sugar [1]. Alone, or in conjunction with other enzymes, the UGTs are involved in the clearance of more than 90% of clinically relevant drugs from the body [2]. Based on nucleotide sequence analysis, 22 human UGT proteins have been identified in 4 families, with the UGT1A and UGT2B subfamilies being most critical for hepatic metabolism [3–5].

The UGT enzymes are genetically polymorphic, with over 200 variant alleles described for the UGT1 and UGT2 subfamilies that can influence enzymatic function, cellular trafficking, or gene expression, modifying individual drug and endobiotic exposure [6]. Additional variants have also been identified, but have not been characterized for function. Moreover, although some of these single nucleotide polymorphisms (SNPs) are functional, changes in total glucuronidation also tend to occur when many polymorphisms are inherited together as a haplotype [6].

In addition to genetic factors, UGT enzymes are known to be regulated by environmental, xenobiotic, and endobiotic exposure, but at present there is limited information regarding epigenetic regulation, such as the effects of methylation. Methylation of UGT1A1 has been associated with colon cancer and with altered drug disposition in cancer [7,8]. More recently, a link between DNA methylation and the regulation of UGT1A1 protein expression and activity in healthy human livers has been presented [9]. This latter study implies that epigenetics are not merely a disease-state effect in UGT disposition, but may be intimately involved in modifying basal UGT enzyme expression. Therefore, examining epigenetic modifications that alter mRNA levels of UGT enzymes in common demographics, such as sex, ethnicity, and obesity, may help determine how glucuronidation varies in mixed populations. This can help determine demographic contributions to the hepatic disposition of compounds.

If glucuronidation is dysregulated or differs inherently between members of mixed populations, it is important to understand the mechanisms for these changes. These mechanisms may present druggable targets in themselves for preventing or mitigating disease and could be exploited to prevent adverse drug reactions. Moreover, epigenetic mechanisms may provide insight into the differential susceptibility of some ethnicities to diseases and syndromes, including cancer. The purpose of this study was to determine the differential methylation of all hepatic UGT isoforms in a well-characterized cohort of human livers and investigate whether hepatic methylation of UGTs is associated with sex, ethnicity, or obesity.

2. Materials and Methods

2.1. Tissue Availability and Collection

Liver samples ($n = 24$) were collected from the Hawaii Human Biorepository, which collects samples with informed consent from non-surviving organ donors' families, and with permission for future experimentation. The characteristics of this set of livers were as follows: Median age 52 ± 13 (range: 20–69), Males $n = 15$ and Females $n = 9$, Ethnicity: Caucasian $n = 9$ (38%), Asian $n = 11$ (33%), and Pacific Island (PI) $n = 4$ (16%). Three unknowns were excluded from analysis; moreover, one each of Caucasian and Asian were excluded from the methylation analysis due to poor sample quality. "Asian" in this study is reflective of Japanese, Chinese, or Korean ethnicity. The Body Mass Index (BMI) ranged from normal (20.8 kg/m^2) to morbidly obese (52.4 kg/m^2) with a median of 30.7 ± 8.5. For analysis, samples were grouped into two discrete categories, normal weight (NW) and overweight (OW), which corresponded to BMI ranges of 18.5–24.9 kg/m^2 and above 25 kg/m^2, respectively. These studies were approved by the Hawaii Institutional Review Board for Human Subjects (CHS #21144).

2.2. Liver Samples

Tissue samples (1 cm) were extracted from the anterior portion of the right lobe closest to the inferior vena cava from frozen livers. All livers were collected and archived (flash frozen) within 6 h of brain death, and these tissues were from livers that had never been thawed. None of the livers was diseased. Tissues samples were disrupted on liquid nitrogen using a mortar and pestle and stored at -80 °C until nucleic acid extraction.

2.3. DNA and RNA Extraction

DNA, RNA, and protein were extracted from 20 mg of disrupted liver sample according to the manufacturer's instructions (Qiagen AllPrep DNA/RNA/Protein Mini kit, Valencia, CA, USA). Nucleic acid purity was examined using a Nanodrop spectrophotometer (ThermoFisher Scientific, Wilmington, DE, USA), and quality was examined with a Bioanalyzer (Agilent, Palo Alto, CA, USA). To further purify DNA, ethanol precipitation was performed and the pellet re-dissolved in nuclease free water.

2.4. DNA Methylation Analysis

The Illumina Infinium Methylation Assay (Illumina Inc., San Diego, CA, USA) was performed as per the manufacturer's instructions. This assay covers 99% of RefSeq genes and 95% of Cytosine-guanine (CpG) islands in the human genome. The entire genome was interrogated and examined, but results with respect to UGT genes were the focus of this study. All CpG interrogation sites associated with all UGT genes were analyzed, but only significant results are presented. The DNA samples (1 µg) were first treated with sodium bisulfite using a Zymo Research Bisulfite conversion kit (Zymo Irvine, CA, USA) to deaminate un-methylated cytosine to produce uracil. Extraction, analysis, and visualization of the methylation data were performed using the Illumina Genome Studio software (version 2011.1) with methylation and genome viewer plug-ins (version 1.9.0, Illumina, San Diego, CA, USA). Differential methylation analysis was performed for grouped data utilizing the Illumina custom error model, resulting in a differential methylation score (diffscore) that provides directionality to the *p*-value. The diffscore was converted to an adjusted *p*-value with the formula: *p*-value = $1/((10^{|\mathrm{DiffScore}|})/10)$.

2.5. Gene Expression via Quantitative Reverse Transcriptase Polymerase Chain Reaction (q-RT-PCR)

Total RNA (1 µg) was converted to cDNA using a qScript™ cDNA synthesis kit from Quanta Biosciences (Gaithersburg, MD, USA) according to the protocol provided. After mixing, reaction was incubated using the following conditions: 5 min at 25 °C, 30 min at 42 °C, 5 min at 85 °C, and then held at 4 °C for at least 5 min. From the resulting 20 µL reaction, 4 µL of cDNA product was then combined with forward and reverse qPCR primers (Table 1) to a final concentration of 500 nM. This reaction was then combined with an equal volume of 2× Roche Power SYBR Green Master Mix containing ROX. Samples were cycled on an Applied Biosystems 7900HT qPCR machine (ABI, Foster City, CA, USA) as follows: 2 min at 50 °C, 10 min at 95 °C, then 40 cycles of 15 s at 95 °C, and 1 min at 60 °C. Additionally, a dissociation step was performed at the end of the run, utilizing a +1 °C ramp rate per second from 60 °C to 95 °C with continuous detection, to ensure that only a single product was formed. Data for q-RT-PCR were displayed utilizing Applied Biosystems SDS software version 2.1 (ABI, Foster City, CA, USA). All mRNA expression C_T values were normalized against Beta-Glucuronidase (GUSB) before relative quantitation. Resulting C_T values were analyzed and converted to fold change differences using the $\Delta\Delta C_T$ method for relative quantitation [10].

Table 1. Uridine 5′-diphosphate-glucuronosyl transferases (UGT) primer sequences used to produce quantitative polymerase chain reaction (qPCR) results for gene expression analysis. The isoform examined, forward and reverse primer sequences, as well as publication source (reference number) are listed. Primers were from references. GUSB: Beta-Glucuronidase.

UGT	Forward Primer Sequence (5′-3′)	Reverse Primer Sequence (5′-3′)
1A1	AATAAAAAAGGACTCTGCTATGCT	ACATCAAAGCTGCTTTCTGC
1A3	TGTTGAACAATATGTCTTTGGTCTA	ACCACATCAAAGGAAGTAGCA
1A4	GAACAATGTATCTTTGGCCC	ACCACATCAAAGGAAGTAGCA
1A6	CATGATTGTTATTGGCCTGTAC	TCTGTGAAAAGAGCATCAAACT
1A8	GAAAGCACAAGTACGAAGTTTG	GGGAGGGAGAAATATTTGGC
1A9	TGGAAAGCACAAGTACGAAGTATATA	GGGAGGGAGAAATATTTGGC
1A10	GAAAGCACAGGCACAAAGTATA	GGGAGGGAGAAATATTTAGCAAC
2B4	TCTTTCGATCCAACAGCC	CATCTCTTAACCGCTGCTTGATA
2B7	GGAGAATTTCTCATGCAACAGA	CAGAACTTTCTATTATGTCACCAAATATTG
2B11	AGTAACATGACAGCAGAAAGGGCCAAT	AGACCTAAGGCATCTGGTTTATTCCCG
2B15	CTTCTGAAAATCTCGATAGATGGAT	CATCTTTACAGACTTGTTACTGTAGTCAT
2B17	TTTATGAAAAGTTCGATAGATGGAC	CATCTTCACAGACTTTATATTATAGTCAG
GUSB	AGCCAGTTCCTCATCAATGG	GGTAGTGGCTGGTACGGAAA

2.6. Genotyping of the UGT2B17 Deletion

The presence or absence of the UGT2B17 gene deletion was determined. The C and J primer pairs (Table 2) were combined into a duplex reaction, generating a 316 bp fragment from within the UGT2B17 gene or an 884 bp fragment spanning the deletion breakpoint, respectively. Upon electrophoresis, individuals homozygous for the presence of UGT2B17 (Ins/Ins) show a single 316 bp product, individuals homozygous for the deletion show a single 884 bp product (Del/Del), and heterozygotes (Ins/Del) show both products with a reduction after the 316 bp fragment [11]. The PCR for the C and J primer pairs was carried out in 25 µL reactions containing 22.5 µL of Platinum Blue PCR Supermix (Invitrogen, Grand Island, NY, USA), 100 pmol each of forward and reverse primer, and 30 ng of genomic DNA. The cycle conditions were 94 °C for 3 min, 35 cycles of 94 °C for 30 s, 60 °C for 30 s, 72 °C for 3 min, and then finishing with a 4 °C hold.

Table 2. Primer sequences for PCR reactions to characterize single nucleotide polymorphisms (SNPs) and deletions. The UGT isoform being examined, region of amplification, primer name, direction, and sequence as well as the resulting amplicon size are shown. UTR: untranslated region.

UGT	Region	Primer	Orientation	Sequence (5'-3')	Amplicon (bp)
2B17	Gene	C	Forward	CCTGGAAGAGCTTGTTCAGA	316
2B17	Gene	C	Reverse	CTGCATCTTCACAGAGCTTT	316
2B17	Deletion	J	Forward	TGCACAGAGTTAAGAAATGGAGAGATGTG	884
2B17	Deletion	J	Reverse	GATCATCCTATATCCTGACAGAATTCTTTTG	884
2B15	Promoter	A	Forward	GGTCCCACTTCTTCAGATCAT	3368
2B15	Promoter	A	Reverse	GAGAGAAGGAAGAAGCCAGAAG	3368
2B15	Promoter	B	Forward	ACATAGGAAGGAGGGAACAGA	3224
2B15	Promoter	B	Reverse	TTCCTGCTGAGGGTTTGAAG	3224
2B15	UTR	D	Forward	TGGTGTGGATGTCCTTTCTG	2567
2B15	UTR	D	Reverse	GGCAGGAGAATGACTTGACTAC	2567
2B15	UTR	E	Forward	CTGCAGGTCTGTTGGAATTTG	2401
2B15	UTR	E	Reverse	GCAGTTGTAGTCCTAGCTTCTC	2401

2.7. UGT2B15 Polymerase Chain Reaction (PCR) Amplification for Promoter Region

The primers for the promoter region were designed utilizing Primer-BLAST software [12]. The A primer pair listed in Table 3 was used to amplify a 3368 bp region of the UGT2B15 promoter, and after ethanol precipitation to clean-up the PCR product, primer pair B was used to amplify that product to produce a final, specific, 3224 bp fragment for sequencing (Table 2). PCR for both reactions was carried out in a 10 µL reaction volume consisting of 9 µL of Platinum Blue PCR Supermix (Invitrogen, Grand Island, NY, USA), 1 pmol each of forward and reverse primer, and 20 ng of DNA. The cycle conditions were 94 °C for 3 min, 25 cycles of 94 °C for 30 s, 45 °C for 30 s, 72 °C for 3.5 min, and then finishing with a 4 °C hold. For SNP examination, samples were cleaned via ethanol precipitation and cycle sequenced utilizing the B forward PCR primer in addition to the sequencing primers for the promoter region listed in Table 3.

Table 3. Sequencing primers used to obtain the sequence data for the PCR reactions. The UGT isoform being examined, region of amplification, primer name, binding DNA strand, and sequence are shown.

UGT Isoform	Region	Primer #	Strand	Sequence (5'-3')
2B17	Gene	1	−	CTGGTCCCACTTCTTCAGAT
2B15	Promoter	2	+	GTTTGCAGATTTTTAATGAGGCA
2B15	Promoter	3	+	CTCCTAGGATTTGGCACCAG
2B15	Promoter	4	+	TTCTCTAATTTGACTCAGCTTCACA
2B15	Promoter	5	−	CTCAGCCCACCTGCAACC
2B15	Promoter	6	−	CCCCCTCTCCAGAATACACA
2B15	Promoter	7	−	TATCGTGGTGCAAGTAATGTCTTC
2B15	Promoter	8	−	TTATCCAATGGCTGTATTCTGTG
2B15	Promoter	9	+	ACTTTCCCACCGAAAATTCC
2B15	Promoter	10	+	TGCGTGGCAACTGTGATATT

Table 3. *Cont.*

UGT Isoform	Region	Primer #	Strand	Sequence (5′-3′)
2B15	Promoter	11	−	CAGGAAAAAGGAAATCCTCCA
2B15	Promoter	12	−	CTTTCGTGTGTAACTTTTGGATT
2B15	UTR	13	+	GAGGTTACTGCTGTCTCTTTGT
2B15	UTR	14	+	TGGTGTGGATGTCCTTTCTG
2B15	UTR	15	−	CCCTGGATCGAGCAGTCTTC
2B15	UTR	16	−	GACCAACCAATGAAGCCCCT

2.8. UGT2B15 PCR Amplification for 3′ Untranslated Regulatory Region

The primers for the untranslated regulatory region were designed utilizing the Primer-BLAST software [12]. The D primer pair listed in Table 3 was used to amplify 2567 bp of the UGT2B15 3′ untranslated regulatory region and after ethanol precipitation to clean-up the PCR product, primer pair E was used to amplify that product to produce a 2401 bp region for sequencing (Table 3). PCR for both reactions was carried out in a 10 µL reaction volume consisting of 9 µL of Platinum Blue PCR Supermix (Invitrogen, Grand Island, NY, USA), 1 pmol each of forward and reverse primer, and 20 ng of DNA. The cycle conditions were 94 °C for 3 min, 25 cycles of 94 °C for 30 s, 49 °C for 30 s, 72 °C for 3.5 min, and then finishing with a 4 °C hold. Samples were cleaned via ethanol precipitation and cycle sequenced utilizing the E forward PCR primer in addition to the listed sequencing primers for the untranslated regulatory region in Table 3. Products (300 ng) were electrophoresed on 2% (w/v) Tris-buffered EDTA (TBE) agarose gel and sized compared to a DNA ladder (Thermo Fisher, Wilmington, DE, USA) with imaging on a Typhoon Scanner 9410 (GE Healthcare, Chicago, IL, USA).

2.9. Cycle Sequencing

Each sample was sequenced in duplicate, combining 7.5 ng of PCR template with 2.5 pmol of sequencing primer in a total volume of 5 µL in a 96-well polypropylene half-skirted sequencing plate (Applied Biosystems, Foster City, CA, USA). Each 5 µL reaction was then mixed with 1.5 µL of nuclease free water, 1.5 µL of 5X Applied Biosystems Sequencing Buffer, and 2 µL of BigDye® Terminator v3.1 Ready Reaction Enzyme Mix (Life Technologies, Grand Island, NY, USA). Samples were mixed, sealed, and sequenced under the following cycling conditions: 96 °C for 1 min followed by 25 cycles of 96 °C for 10 s, 50 °C for 5 s, and 60 °C for 4 min and terminating with a 4 °C hold until samples were ready for purification.

Samples were cleaned according to the BigDye® Terminator v3.1 protocol and sequenced utilizing the Applied Biosystems DNA Analyzer 3730xl Sequencer (Foster City, CA, USA). Resulting chromatograms were examined via 4Peaks software v1.7.2 (Mek & Tosj, Amsterdam, The Netherlands), and sequences were extracted and examined for SNPs using Aliview to align and trim the sequences (Uppsala University, Uppsala, Sweden).

The resulting sequences were then entered into the BLAST program and aligned to the UGT2B15 gene (Genbank ID: NC_0000012.4). Sequences were examined and nucleotide calls recorded for each sample at each position where a known or suspected SNP exists (indicated in the BLAST program in the SNP annotation database).

2.10. Statistical Analyses

Statistical analysis was performed using the GraphPad Prism Program version 5.02 (Graph Pad, San Diego, CA, USA). Normality of the data was checked using D'Agostino–Pearson's test and variance verified using the Bartlett's test. A one-way analysis of variance (ANOVA) with Bonferroni's post-hoc comparison was used if the data were found to be normally distributed; alternatively, the Kruskal–Wallis one-way ANOVA was performed with Dunn's post hoc analysis. For binary data sets (sex), student's *t*-tests were performed with $\alpha = 0.05$.

3. Results

3.1. Summary of Methylation Beta Values for All UGT-Associated Loci

Inspection of the methylation status of all the UGT loci demonstrated that for UGT1A isoforms, most of the loci were generally moderately or hyper-methylated, but significant differential methylation was not occurring between samples. However, for UGT2B isoforms, at least four loci have differential methylation occurring with a clear splitting pattern between samples. These loci are associated with UGT2B15 (cg09189601) and both UGT2B15 and 2B17 (cg07973162, cg10632656, and cg07952421, Figure 1). No significant differences in methylation patterns were attributed to age, sex, or BMI for any of the four differentially methylated loci associated with UGT2B15 and UGT2B17.

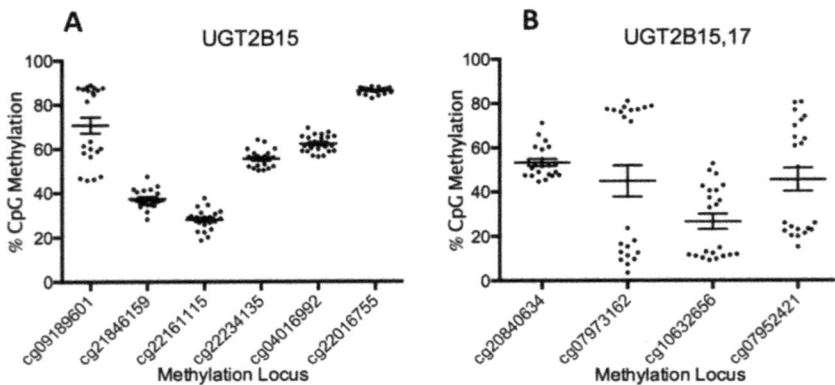

Figure 1. Grouped data showing the methylation beta values (*y*-axis) for each sample at a particular Cytosine-Guanine (CG) locus (*x*-axis) UGT2B15 (**A**) and UGT2B15/17 (**B**). Because UGT2B15/2B17 were formed by a gene duplication event, they also share common loci. Values above 70% are generally considered to be fully methylated on both strands and values below 30% are typically un-methylated on both strands with intermediate values indicating that only one of the two strands are methylated.

The only difference attributed to differential methylation was ethnicity (Figure 2). For locus cg09189601, which is associated with UGT2B15 only, we observed hyper-methylation (90%) in Asians ($n = 8$) compared to the moderate methylation (50–60%) in Caucasians ($n = 10$, $p < 0.0001$), which would imply less transcription of UGT2B15 in Asians. In contrast, at loci cg07973162, cg10632656, and cg07952421 hepatic UGT2B15 and 2B17 were hypo-methylated in Asians (<20%) compared to the more highly methylated (40–80%) Caucasian samples ($p < 0.0001$ for all loci).

The Pacific Island cohort in our study (PI, $n = 4$) displayed two samples that reflected Asian methylation patterns and two samples that reflected Caucasian patterns. Due to a limited sample size and the split nature of their methylation pattern, no significant differences in methylation patterns were determined. The ethnic makeup of our PI group was ≥50% (i.e., at least one parent PI) to define ethnicity. However, for Asian and Caucasian populations 100% (i.e., both parents of this race) defined ethnicity, hence we cannot rule out admixed genetic information in PI from other ethnic groups, and this likely explains the splitting observed. Notably, intermarriage of PI/Caucasian and PI/Asian is common in Hawaii.

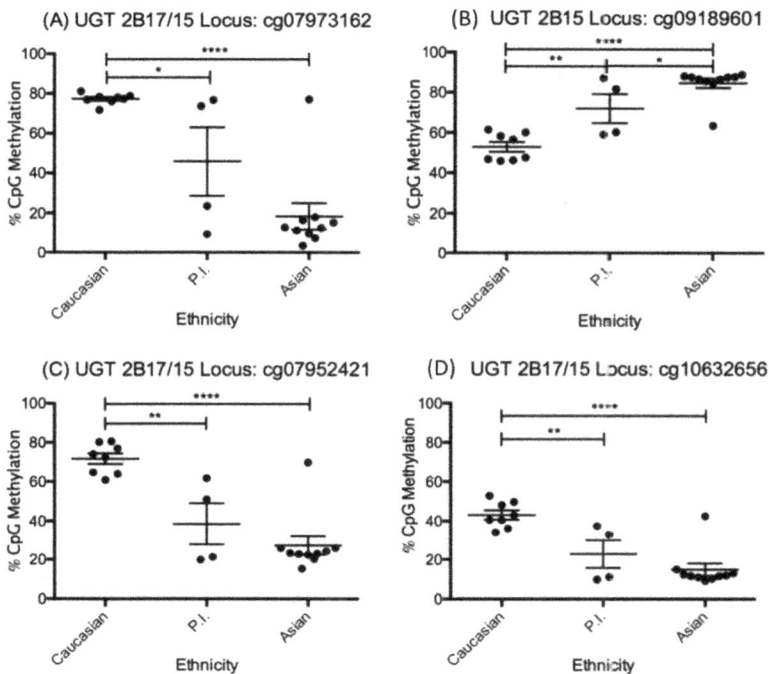

Figure 2. Graphs showing beta values (β) for differentially methylated loci associated with UGT2B15 and 2B17, grouped according to ethnicity with separate columns for Caucasians (*n* = 8), Pacific Islanders (PI, *n* = 4) and Asians (*n* = 10). The UGT isoform and the specific loci where the methylation is taking place are listed in the title for each individual graph such that loci cg07973162 (**A**), cg10632656 (**B**), cg07952421 (**C**), and cg09189601 (**D**) show different patterns of methylation between Asians, PI and Caucasians for UGT2B15 and UGT2B17. Statistical significance is listed for *p*-values ≤0.05 (*), ≤0.01 (**), and ≤0.0001 (****). As compared to PCR, two samples (one Caucasian and one Asian) were lost to analysis due to low sample quality.

3.2. The mRNA Expression of UDP-Glucuronosyl Transferase (UGT) Isoforms in This Liver Cohort

To determine differences in UGT mRNA expression and confirm methylation effects, we performed q-RT-PCR on all hepatic UGT1A and 2B isoforms. Obesity was not associated with any significant differences in mRNA levels for any UGT1A or 2B isoforms. Only UGT1A3 showed significant differences in mRNA levels with sex, where females had 2-fold higher mRNA expression than males (*p* = 0.02, data not shown).

Ethnicity was associated with significant differences in mRNA abundance for UGT1A1, where Caucasians had significantly lower mRNA levels than PI (higher ΔC_T, *p* = 0.03, Figure 3). Caution should be exercised with these data, as the number of samples in the PI group is fairly low for statistical comparison.

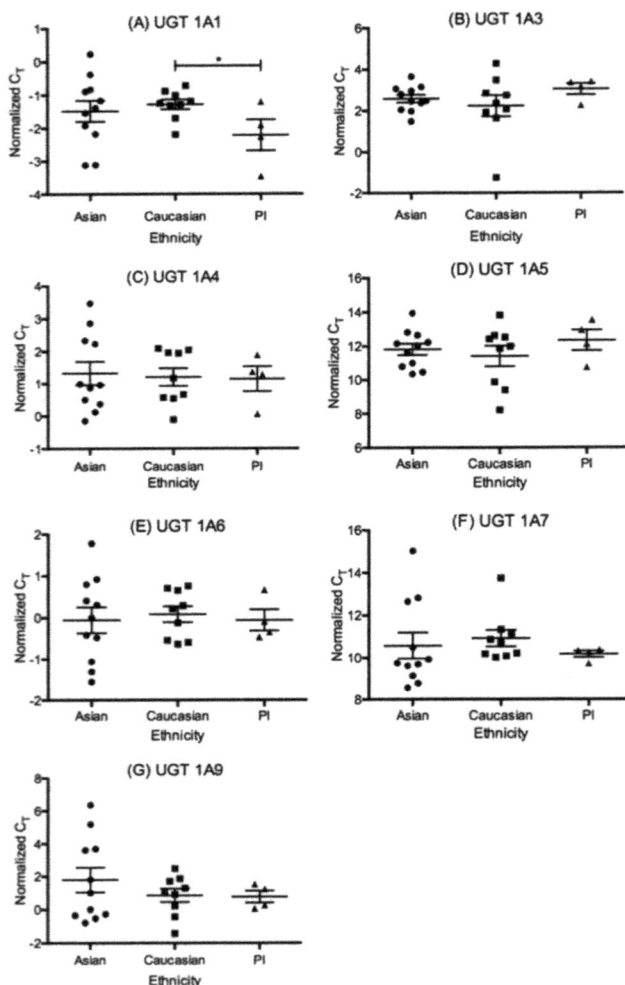

Figure 3. The quantitative PCR $\Delta\Delta C_T$ values in Asian (A, $n = 11$), Caucasian (C, $n = 9$), and Pacific Islander (PI, $n = 4$) ethnicities for all liver-specific UGT1A isoforms examined. Statistical significance is listed for p-values ≤ 0.05 (*) Note that higher $\Delta\Delta C_T$ means lower level of mRNA. (**A–G**) represent results for each individual UGT1A subfamily isoform.

Gene expression data for UGT2B samples demonstrated significantly lower UGT2B7 mRNA levels in Caucasians (higher ΔC_T) as compared to PI ($p = 0.038$, Figure 4). When mRNA expression of UGT2B15 (Figure 4) was determined across the three ethnicities, Asians show significantly lower mRNA expression than Caucasians ($p = 0.02$) and approached significance for PI ($p = 0.08$). Finally, for UGT2B17 (Figure 4), Asians exhibited significantly lower mRNA levels than Caucasians ($p = 0.001$) and approached significance as compared to PI ($p = 0.08$). These data translate to a 3-fold significant downregulation in UGT2B15 in Asians as compared to Caucasians and PI. For UGT2B17, there is no fold change between Caucasians and PI, but there is a 1500-fold downregulation between Caucasians and the three Asian samples that produced gene expression data for this isoform.

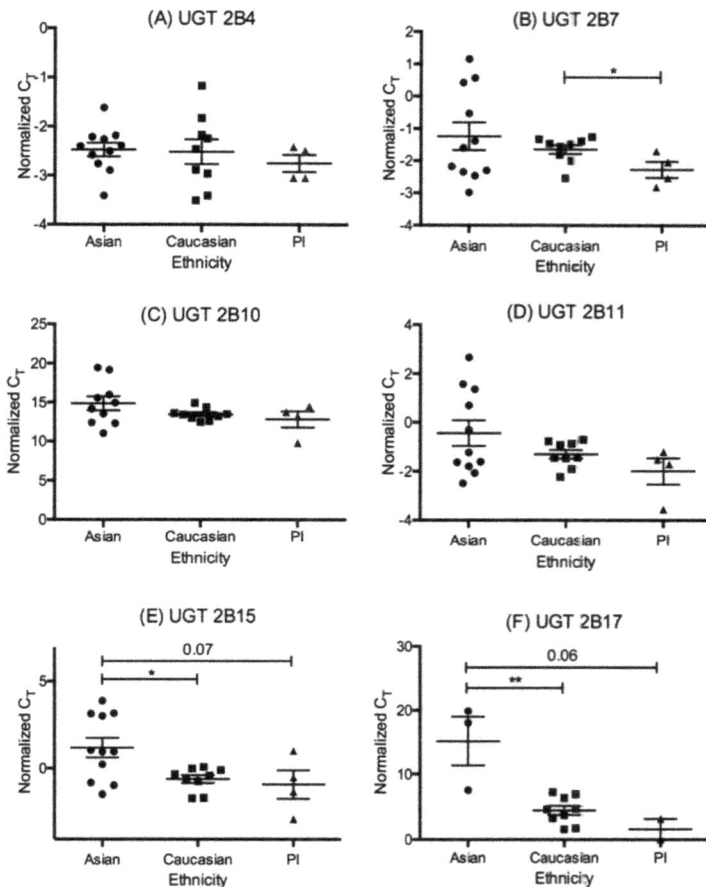

Figure 4. The quantitative PCR ΔC_T values in Asian (A, $n = 11$), Caucasian (C, $n = 9$), and Pacific Islander (PI, $n = 4$) ethnicities for all examined UGT2B isoforms in liver. Statistical significance is listed for p-values ≤ 0.05 (*), ≤ 0.01 (**), and p values approaching significance (<0.1). Note that a higher ΔC_T means a lower level of mRNA. (**A–F**) represent results for each individual UGT2B subfamily isoform.

3.3. UGT2B15 and UGT2B17 Genetic Analysis

Comparison of SNP data to mRNA levels demonstrates that the decreased expression for UGT2B15 in these samples is not caused by any of the known UGT2B15 SNPs in the areas interrogated. Deletion genotyping of UGT2B17 demonstrated that eight of nine Asian samples and two of the PI samples have the UGT2B17 Del/Del genotype. Caucasian samples had at least one copy of the UGT2B17 gene, with three Ins/Ins, four Ins/Del, and two samples that failed genotyping. The two PI samples that did not have the deletion are of Ins/Del genotype. These genotyping results are consistent with the q-RT-PCR data for UGT2B17, where Asian samples had either an absent, or an extremely low, expression of UGT2B17. The deletion polymorphism is the major cause for this low UGT2B17 gene expression for the Asian samples and also explains the hypo-methylated CpG loci in the UGT2B15/2B17 intergenic region that reside within the deletion.

4. Discussion

The critical finding of this study is that the mRNA expression of hepatic UGT2B15 is partially regulated by methylation in people of Asian descent, causing decreased mRNA expression. Moreover, while UGT2B17 showed differential methylation in Asians, lower levels of mRNA are caused by a deletion genotype and not epigenetics. The novel finding from the UGT2B17 studies is that methylation of the three loci cg07973162, cg07952421, and cg10632656 in the Illumina platform is predictive of the deletion genotype. This is because the range targeted by the Illumina methylation assay covers the deletion, as confirmed by genotyping. Other than the findings presented for individuals of Asian descent, methylation did not regulate UGT1A or UGT2B isoforms with age, ethnicity, obesity, or sex in this cohort. Finally, although not regulated by methylation, hepatic UGT1A3 mRNA levels were higher in females than males, while UGT1A1 mRNA levels were significantly higher in PI than Caucasians.

Because females showed significantly higher mRNA expression of UGT1A3 compared to males, this may have implications for sex-differences in drug and endobiotic metabolism and disposition if it is indicative of protein levels. The UGT1A3 isoform acts on some drugs and is an important metabolic pathway for bile acids [13]. Similarly, PI had higher mRNA expression of UGT1A1 than Caucasians. This is one of the most active UGTs in the liver, with wide substrate affinity. Differences in UGT expression between these two ethnic groups may begin to explain some of the differences in drug and chemical response in an admixed population. There are no reports in the literature indicating disproportionate glucuronidation in PIs, but, rather than contradicting our data, this is due to a lack of study in this ethnic population. A recent study by our laboratory has demonstrated that morbid obesity in pregnancy is associated with higher levels of unconjugated bilirubin in the blood of obese PI women and in their neonates (unpublished data). This suggests that there may be ethnic-specific effects on UGT in the PI population and is deserving of further study. While we did not find any associations with obesity in the current study, it has recently been reported that UGT2B17 can vary with obesity but only in males [14]. Given the mixed male and female cohort used, as well as the deletion of UGT2B17 in approximately one third of our samples, we would not have been empowered to confirm this finding.

For the locus associated solely with UGT2B15, Asian samples were hyper-methylated (90%) compared to the moderate methylation (50–60%) in Caucasians. This is opposite to the three common UGT2B15/2B17 loci, which are hypo-methylated in Asians (<20%) compared to the more highly methylated (40–80%) Caucasian samples. Taken together, these results imply a regulatory mechanism by which both UGT2B15 and 2B17 are methylated simultaneously at the intergenic region and UGT2B15 is modified at another site to modulate its glucuronidation separately. Because these two isoforms are the result of a gene duplication event in the recent past, this complex differential regulation is empirically sensible. The mRNA expression patterns are not concordant with methylation data that is typically observed in connection with gene promoters, which was expected because methylation occurs within intergenic areas for UGT2B15 and UGT2B17. In general, regulatory methylation occurs at hypo-methylated sites commonly located in CpG islands within 1.5 kb of the transcription start site of a gene, while hyper-methylated sites tend to be located in the distal intergenic and gene body regions [15–17]. Another potential explanation for this is that the liver is highly enriched in 5 hmC and the bisulfite technique does not discriminate between 5 mC and 5 hmC. Since these two CpG modifications have opposing effects, this may also explain why mRNA levels are not concordant with traditional methylation patterns. Finally, methylation patterns presenting with a beta value of 50% could represent an admixed cell population where half the cells are methylated and half are not. This is highly unlikely to be the case in our study, since the cells in the small 1–2 g pieces of human liver would be exposed to the same endo- and xenobiotic stimuli and concordance between a majority of the UGT-related CpG sites was high.

In addition to epigenetic mechanisms, functional and clinically relevant polymorphisms in UGT2B15 and 2B17 that affect drug and chemical disposition exist. This includes the UGT2B15*2 polymorphism, where reduced lorazepam and S-oxazepam clearance occurs [18,19], as well as the

UGT2B17*2 and UGT2B17 deletion genotypes, which both reduce MK-7246 and exemestane clearances, potentially leading to toxic accumulation [20,21]. Polymorphisms may also increase activity, such as with UGT2B15*4, which has a C > A nucleotide change in the coding region, increasing UGT2B15 catalysis [18,19]. Polymorphisms in UGT2B15 and 2B17 have been implicated in modifying the clearance of a wide range of drugs, reviewed in: [22]. Here, an analogy can be made with methylation because if Asians have differential methylation patterns compared to Caucasians for UGT2B15, they may also have altered glucuronidation capacity.

In addition to drugs and chemicals, UGT2B15 and 2B17 have been investigated in relation to risks for cancer and other endocrine diseases [23]. This is especially true with regard to the UGT2B17 deletion phenotype, which is more prevalent in the Asian population [24] and is particularly important because UGT2B17 is more active than UGT2B15 for testosterone glucuronidation [25,26]. Polymorphisms in both of these genes have been shown to alter steroid metabolism and also are predictors of fat mass in men [27]. Most studies indicate that genetic polymorphisms affecting UGT2B15 and/or 2B17 are risk factors for prostate cancer [28–31]. Although lifestyle and environmental factors account for some prostate cancer in Asians, these only account for a small proportion of the relative risk [32]. These prior research efforts have elucidated many of the biological effects of UGT2B15 and UGT2B17 polymorphisms, but the impact of epigenetic methylation has not previously been established. Our study implies that hyper-methylation of UGT2B15 in Asians may affect androgen disposition as compared to the Caucasian population and is a promising avenue for investigating some of the altered risk for androgen-related cancers in these populations.

Although this study contained only a relatively small sample size, making interactions between environment, genotype, and demographics difficult to establish, the numbers of samples for ethnicities, sex, and obesity were well-balanced. This is bolstered by our findings from the samples of PI ethnicity, where UGT genotypes showed commonality with Asians for two of the samples and for Caucasians with the other two samples. Since most of the PI participants were of mixed heritage ($\geq$50% PI, admixed with either Asian or Caucasian), these findings fit the rules of heritability. Moreover, a strong Asian linkage is not surprising, as PI are theorized to have originated in Asia and mixed extensively with Melanesians both depositing and accumulating genes into their genomes during colonization of the Pacific Islands [33], which has been further corroborated by both Y chromosome and mitochondrial DNA analyses [34]. Finally, our work is complemented by recent data demonstrating that hepatic UGT1A1 can be regulated during early human development by histone modification [35], a novel and interesting finding that supports the concept that UGTs can be regulated at the transcriptional level through genetic mechanisms. Having said this, we believe that future work in this area will need to encompass protein-level studies with Western blot of UGT2B15 and/or activity studies to confirm if these results found at the mRNA levels also follow through to the levels of enzyme proteins and their function.

A secondary finding here is that deletion of UGT2B17 is entirely predicted by methylation status, allowing for genotyping of the (Del/Del) allele via a methylation assay when all three UGT2B15/2B17 loci (cg07973162, cg07952421, and cg10632656) are hypo-methylated (<20%) due to the deletion of UGT2B17. In these samples, this occurred entirely within the Asian population of samples, which agrees with published research showing that this deletion is prevalent in Asian populations [24]. The deletion was also mirrored perfectly by the elimination of mRNA expression for UGT2B17. While it is currently very expensive to use methylation technologies, as the cost progressively reduces the validation of this finding may present an alternative avenue to sequencing or genotyping for determining the UGT2B17 deletion genotype.

5. Conclusions

In summary, methylation may be a mode of regulatory control for UGT2B15 in Asians, which likely acts in conjunction with SNP modification, reducing the enzyme's expression. Impairment of UGT2B15 is of clinical significance with respect to risks for prostate cancer [29] and renal disorders [36] as well as drug metabolism. As this is a small sample size, a larger cohort will be needed to confirm these findings, although with a signal-to-noise ratio as high as we observed we expect the findings to be reproducible. Elucidating the genetic and environmental regulation of UGT2B15 and 2B17 can be useful for predicting susceptibility to cancer and adverse drug reactions, but more work on the precise mechanisms of UGT2B15 methylation, the interplay of methylation and SNPs, as well as the effects on drug and hormone handling in vivo are needed to tease out the clinical significance of these findings.

Acknowledgments: All of the authors are grateful to Maarit Tirikainen for her assistance in running the Illumina chips at the University of Hawaii Cancer Research Center Genomics Facility. The Hawaii Biorepository is supported by the National Institutes of Health National Institute for Research Resources and the National Institute for Minority Health and Health Disparities Grant MD007601. The studies were supported in part by NSERC 17-03808.

Author Contributions: Steffen G. Oeser, Jon-Paul Bingham, and Abby C. Collier conceived and designed the experiments; Steffen G. Oeser performed the experiments; Steffen G. Oeser and Abby C. Collier analyzed the data; and Steffen G. Oeser, Jon-Paul Bingham, and Abby C. Collier wrote the paper.

Conflicts of Interest: The authors report no conflicts of interest.

References

1. Miners, J.O.; Mackenzie, P.I. Drug glucuronidation in humans. *Pharmacol. Ther.* **1991**, *51*, 347–369. [CrossRef]
2. Rowland, A.; Miners, J.O.; Mackenzie, P.I. The UDP-glucuronosyltransferases: Their role in drug metabolism and detoxification. *Int. J. Biochem. Cell Biol.* **2013**, *45*, 1121–1132. [CrossRef] [PubMed]
3. Mackenzie, P.I.; Bock, K.W.; Burchell, B.; Guillemette, C.; Ikushiro, S.; Iyanagi, T.; Miners, J.O.; Owens, I.S.; Nebert, D.W. Nomenclature update for the mammalian UDP glycosyltransferase (UGT) gene superfamily. *Pharmacogenet. Genom.* **2005**, *15*, 677–685. [CrossRef]
4. Miners, J.O.; Smith, P.A.; Sorich, M.J.; McKinnon, R.A.; Mackenzie, P.I. Predicting human drug glucuronidation parameters: Application of in vitro and in silico modeling approaches. *Ann. Rev. Pharmacol. Toxicol.* **2004**, *44*, 1–25. [CrossRef] [PubMed]
5. Izukawa, T.; Nakajima, M.; Fujiwara, R.; Yamanaka, H.; Fukami, T.; Takamiya, M.; Aoki, Y.; Ikushiro, S.; Sakaki, T.; Yokoi, T. Quantitative analysis of UDP-glucuronosyltransferase (UGT) 1A and UGT2B expression levels in human livers. *Drug Metab. Dispos.* **2009**, *37*, 1759–1768. [CrossRef] [PubMed]
6. Zhou, J.; Koszik, F.; Brunner, P.; Stingl, G. "Overrepresentation of T17 cells in the peripheral blood of psoriatic patients is not confined to the skin-homing T cell subset". *J. Dermatol. Sci.* **2014**, *75*, 190–193. [CrossRef] [PubMed]
7. Belanger, A.S.; Tojcic, J.; Harvey, M.; Guillemette, C. Regulation of UGT1A1 and HNF1 transcription factor gene expression by DNA methylation in colon cancer cells. *BMC Mol. Biol.* **2010**, *11*, 9. [CrossRef] [PubMed]
8. Gagnon, J.F.; Bernard, O.; Villeneuve, L.; Tetu, B.; Guillemette, C. Irinotecan inactivation is modulated by epigenetic silencing of UGT1A1 in colon cancer. *Clin. Cancer Res.* **2006**, *12*, 1850–1858. [CrossRef] [PubMed]
9. Yasar, U.; Greenblatt, D.J.; Guillemette, C.; Court, M.H. Evidence for regulation of UDP-glucuronosyltransferase (UGT) 1A1 protein expression and activity via DNA methylation in healthy human livers. *J. Pharm. Pharmacol.* **2013**, *65*, 874–883. [CrossRef] [PubMed]
10. Livak, K.J.; Schmittgen, T.D. Analysis of relative gene expression data using real-time quantitative PCR and the 2(-delta delta c(t)) method. *Methods* **2001**, *25*, 402–408. [CrossRef] [PubMed]
11. Wilson, W., 3rd.; Pardo-Manuel de Villena, F.; Lyn-Cook, B.D.; Chatterjee, P.K.; Bell, T.A.; Detwiler, D.A.; Gilmore, R.C.; Valladeras, I.C.; Wright, C.C.; Threadgill, D.W.; et al. Characterization of a common deletion polymorphism of the UGT2B17 gene linked to UGT2B15. *Genomics* **2004**, *84*, 707–714. [PubMed]
12. Ye, J.; Coulouris, G.; Zaretskaya, I.; Cutcutache, I.; Rozen, S.; Madden, T.L. Primer-blast: A tool to design target-specific primers for polymerase chain reaction. *BMC Bioinform.* **2012**, *13*, 134. [CrossRef] [PubMed]
13. Trottier, J.; Verreault, M.; Grepper, S.; Monte, D.; Belanger, J.; Kaeding, J.; Caron, P.; Inaba, T.T.; Barbier, O. Human UDP-glucuronosyltransferase (UGT) 1A3 enzyme conjugates chenodeoxycholic acid in the liver. *Hepatology* **2006**, *44*, 1158–1170. [CrossRef] [PubMed]
14. Zhu, A.Z.; Cox, L.S.; Ahluwalia, J.S.; Renner, C.C.; Hatsukami, D.K.; Benowitz, N.L.; Tyndale, R.F. Genetic and phenotypic variation in UGT2B17, a testosterone-metabolizing enzyme, is associated with BMI in males. *Pharmacogenet. Genom.* **2015**, *25*, 263–269. [CrossRef] [PubMed]

15. Gutknecht, N.; van Gogswaardt, D.; Conrads, G.; Apel, C.; Schubert, C.; Lampert, F. Diode laser radiation and its bactericidal effect in root canal wall dentin. *J. Clin. Laser Med. Surg.* **2000**, *18*, 57–60. [PubMed]

16. Wagner, J.R.; Busche, S.; Ge, B.; Kwan, T.; Pastinen, T.; Blanchette, M. The relationship between DNA methylation, genetic and expression inter-individual variation in untransformed human fibroblasts. *Genome Biol.* **2014**, *15*, R37. [CrossRef] [PubMed]

17. Jones, P.A. Functions of DNA methylation: Islands, start sites, gene bodies and beyond. *Nat. Rev. Genet.* **2012**, *13*, 484–492. [CrossRef] [PubMed]

18. Court, M.H.; Duan, S.X.; Guillemette, C.; Journault, K.; Krishnaswamy, S.; Von Moltke, L.L.; Greenblatt, D.J. Stereoselective conjugation of oxazepam by human UDP-glucuronosyltransferases (UGTs): S-oxazepam is glucuronidated by UGT2B15, while R-oxazepam is glucuronidated by UGT2B7 and UGT1A9. *Drug Metab. Dispos.* **2002**, *30*, 1257–1265. [CrossRef] [PubMed]

19. He, X.; Hesse, L.M.; Hazarika, S.; Masse, G.; Harmatz, J.S.; Greenblatt, D.J.; Court, M.H. Evidence for oxazepam as an in vivo probe of UGT2B15: Oxazepam clearance is reduced by UGT2B15 D85Y polymorphism but unaffected by UGT2B17 deletion. *Br. J. Clin. Pharmacol.* **2009**, *68*, 721–730. [CrossRef] [PubMed]

20. Sun, D.; Chen, G.; Dellinger, R.W.; Sharma, A.K.; Lazarus, P. Characterization of 17-dihydroexemestane glucuronidation: Potential role of the UGT2B17 deletion in exemestane pharmacogenetics. *Pharmacogenet. Genom.* **2010**, *20*, 575–585. [CrossRef] [PubMed]

21. Wang, Y.H.; Trucksis, M.; McElwee, J.J.; Wong, P.H.; Maciolek, C.; Thompson, C.D.; Prueksaritanont, T.; Garrett, G.C.; Declercq, R.; Vets, E.; et al. Ugt2b17 genetic polymorphisms dramatically affect the pharmacokinetics of MK-7246 in healthy subjects in a first-in-human study. *Clin. Pharmacol. Ther.* **2012**, *92*, 96–102. [CrossRef] [PubMed]

22. Stingl, J.C.; Bartels, H.; Viviani, R.; Lehmann, M.L.; Brockmoller, J. Relevance of UDP-glucuronosyltransferase polymorphisms for drug dosing: A quantitative systematic review. *Pharmacol. Ther.* **2014**, *141*, 92–116. [CrossRef] [PubMed]

23. Belanger, A.; Pelletier, G.; Labrie, F.; Barbier, O.; Chouinard, S. Inactivation of androgens by UDP-glucuronosyltransferase enzymes in humans. *Trends Endocrinol. Metab.* **2003**, *14*, 473–479. [CrossRef] [PubMed]

24. Nadeau, G.; Bellemare, J.; Audet-Walsh, E.; Flageole, C.; Huang, S.P.; Bao, B.Y.; Douville, P.; Caron, P.; Fradet, Y.; Lacombe, L.; et al. Deletions of the androgen-metabolizing UGT2B genes have an effect on circulating steroid levels and biochemical recurrence after radical prostatectomy in localized prostate cancer. *J. Clin. Endocrinol. Metab.* **2011**, *96*, E1550–E1557. [CrossRef] [PubMed]

25. Sten, T.; Finel, M.; Ask, B.; Rane, A.; Ekstrom, L. Non-steroidal anti-inflammatory drugs interact with testosterone glucuronidation. *Steroids* **2009**, *74*, 971–977. [CrossRef] [PubMed]

26. Sten, T.; Bichlmaier, I.; Kuuranne, T.; Leinonen, A.; Yli-Kauhaluoma, J.; Finel, M. Udp-glucuronosyltransferases (UGTs) 2B7 and UGT2B17 display converse specificity in testosterone and epitestosterone glucuronidation, whereas UGT2A1 conjugates both androgens similarly. *Drug Metab. Dispos.* **2009**, *37*, 417–423. [CrossRef] [PubMed]

27. Swanson, C.; Mellstrom, D.; Lorentzon, M.; Vandenput, L.; Jakobsson, J.; Rane, A.; Karlsson, M.; Ljunggren, O.; Smith, U.; Eriksson, A.L.; et al. The uridine diphosphate glucuronosyltransferase 2B15 D85Y and 2B17 deletion polymorphisms predict the glucuronidation pattern of androgens and fat mass in men. *J. Clin. Endocrinol. Metab.* **2007**, *92*, 4878–4882. [CrossRef] [PubMed]

28. Gauthier-Landry, L.; Belanger, A.; Barbier, O. Multiple roles for UDP-glucuronosyltransferase (UGT) 2B15 and UGT2B17 enzymes in androgen metabolism and prostate cancer evolution. *J. Steroid Biochem. Mol. Biol.* **2014**, *145*, 187–192. [CrossRef] [PubMed]

29. Kpoghomou, M.A.; Soatiana, J.E.; Kalembo, F.W.; Bishwajit, G.; Sheng, W. UGT2B17 polymorphism and risk of prostate cancer: A meta-analysis. *ISRN Oncol.* **2013**, *201*. [CrossRef] [PubMed]

30. Park, J.; Chen, L.; Shade, K.; Lazarus, P.; Seigne, J.; Patterson, S.; Helal, M.; Pow-Sang, J. Asp85tyr polymorphism in the UDP-glucuronosyltransferase (UGT) 2B15 gene and the risk of prostate cancer. *J. Urol.* **2004**, *171*, 2484–2488. [CrossRef] [PubMed]

31. MacLeod, S.L.; Nowell, S.; Plaxco, J.; Lang, N.P. An allele-specific polymerase chain reaction method for the determination of the D85Y polymorphism in the human UDP-glucuronosyltransferase 2B15 gene in a case-control study of prostate cancer. *Ann. Surg. Oncol.* **2000**, *7*, 777–782. [CrossRef] [PubMed]

32. Whittemore, A.S.; Kolonel, L.N.; Wu, A.H.; John, E.M.; Gallagher, R.P.; Howe, G.R.; Burch, J.D.; Hankin, J.; Dreon, D.M.; West, D.W.; et al. Prostate cancer in relation to diet, physical activity, and body size in blacks, whites, and Asians in the United States and Canada. *JNCI* **1995**, *87*, 652–661. [CrossRef] [PubMed]
33. Kayser, M.; Brauer, S.; Weiss, G.; Underhill, P.A.; Roewer, L.; Schiefenhovel, W.; Stoneking, M. Melanesian origin of Polynesian Y chromosomes. *Curr. Biol.* **2000**, *10*, 1237–1246. [CrossRef]
34. Kayser, M.; Brauer, S.; Cordaux, R.; Casto, A.; Lao, O.; Zhivotovsky, L.A.; Moyse-Faurie, C.; Rutledge, R.B.; Schiefenhoevel, W.; Gil, D.; et al. Melanesian and Asian origins of Polynesians: mtDNA and Y chromosome gradients across the Pacific. *Mol. Biol. Evol.* **2006**, *23*, 2234–2244. [CrossRef] [PubMed]
35. Nie, Y.; Meng, X.; Liu, J.; Yan, L.; Wang, P.; Bi, H.; Kan, Q.; Zhang, L. Histone modifications regulate the developmental expression of human hepatic UDP-glucuronosyltransferase 1A1. *Drug Metab. Dispos.* **2017**, *45*, 1372–1378. [CrossRef] [PubMed]
36. Deshmukh, N.; Petroczi, A.; Barker, J.; Szekely, A.D.; Hussain, I.; Naughton, D.P. Potentially harmful advantage to athletes: A putative connection between UGT2B17 gene deletion polymorphism and renal disorders with prolonged use of anabolic androgenic steroids. *Subst. Abuse Treat. Prev. Policy* **2010**, *5*, 7. [CrossRef] [PubMed]

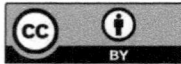

pharmaceutics

MDPI

Article

Epinephrine in Anaphylaxis: Preclinical Study of Pharmacokinetics after Sublingual Administration of Taste-Masked Tablets for Potential Pediatric Use

Ousama Rachid [1,*], Mutasem Rawas-Qalaji [2,*] and Keith J. Simons [3]

[1] College of Pharmacy, Qatar University, P.O. Box 2713 Doha, Qatar
[2] College of Pharmacy, Health Professions Division, Nova Southeastern University,
     Fort Lauderdale, FL 33328, USA
[3] College of Pharmacy, Faculty of Health Sciences, University of Manitoba, Winnipeg, MB R3E 0T5, Canada;
     Keith.Simons@umanitoba.ca
*   Correspondence: orachid@qu.edu.qa (O.R.); mr.qalaji@nova.edu (M.R.-Q.);
    Tel.: +974-4403-5631 (O.R.); +1-(954)-262-1350 (M.R.-Q.)

Received: 22 November 2017; Accepted: 12 January 2018; Published: 11 February 2018

Abstract: Epinephrine is a life-saving treatment in anaphylaxis. In community settings, a first-aid dose of epinephrine is injected from an auto-injector (EAI). Needle phobia highly contributes to EAI underuse, leading to fatalities—especially in children. A novel rapidly-disintegrating sublingual tablet (RDST) of epinephrine was developed in our laboratory as a potential alternative dosage form. The aim of this study was to evaluate the sublingual bioavailability of epinephrine 30 mg as a potential pediatric dose incorporated in our novel taste-masked RDST in comparison with intramuscular (IM) epinephrine 0.15 mg from EAI, the recommended and only available dosage form for children in community settings. We studied the rate and extent of epinephrine absorption in our validated rabbit model ($n = 5$) using a cross-over design. The positive control was IM epinephrine 0.15 mg from an EpiPen Jr®. The negative control was a placebo RDST. Tablets were placed under the tongue for 2 min. Blood samples were collected at frequent intervals and epinephrine concentrations were measured using HPLC with electrochemical detection. The mean ± SEM maximum plasma concentration (C_{max}) of 16.7 ± 1.9 ng/mL at peak time (T_{max}) of 21 min after sublingual epinephrine 30 mg did not differ significantly ($p > 0.05$) from the C_{max} of 18.8 ± 1.9 ng/mL at a T_{max} of 36 min after IM epinephrine 0.15 mg. The C_{max} of both doses was significantly higher than the C_{max} of 7.5 ± 1.7 ng/mL of endogenous epinephrine after placebo. These taste-masked RDSTs containing a 30 mg dose of epinephrine have the potential to be used as an easy-to-carry, palatable, non-invasive treatment for anaphylactic episodes for children in community settings.

Keywords: bioavailability; bioequivalence; intramuscular; auto-injector; sublingual delivery; rapidly-disintegrating; tablets; allergy; anaphylaxis; adrenaline; epinephrine

1. Introduction

Prompt injection of epinephrine in the mid-outer thigh (vastus lateralis muscle) using an auto-injector is the recommended first-aid treatment of anaphylaxis in community settings [1]. Many patients at risk of anaphylaxis in the community fail to carry their epinephrine auto-injectors consistently, due to their bulky shape and large size [2]. When anaphylaxis occurs, many patients and caregivers who have an epinephrine auto-injector available were reported to delay injecting epinephrine because of their fear of needles [3–5]. Other issues include a short shelf-life and availability of only two fixed doses (0.15 and 0.3 mg) for patients ranging in weight from <5 kg to >125 kg [2]. There is an increasingly challenging availability and affordability issue of epinephrine autoinjectors worldwide, with pharmacy acquisition costs in North America ranging from \$170 to \$430 US dollars per pack [6]. This is compounded by the need for multiple devices to be placed in various locations as part of the user's preparedness plan, such as home, work, school, and during traveling; and the need to replace expired devices almost every year. Manual techniques of removing and administering second or third epinephrine doses from used devices and filling or prefilling injections from epinephrine ampules have been suggested to overcome the high cost of autoinjectors; however, the accuracy, safety, and practicality of these techniques are questionable [7–10].

Rapidly-disintegrating sublingual tablets (RDSTs) of epinephrine have been developed as a potential non-invasive alternative epinephrine dosage form for the treatment of anaphylaxis in community settings. The highly vascular sublingual mucosa facilitates rapid drug absorption into the venous circulation through the sublingual veins [11]. Epinephrine bitartrate, a low molecular weight hydrophilic compound, is absorbed by passive diffusion driven by a concentration gradient. The high drug concentration in the sublingual space drives the drug through the mucosal epithelium into the interstitial fluid, to then be absorbed by the venous circulation [11].

In our initial preclinical studies, a dose-escalation study (10, 20, and 40 mg) was performed to determine the sublingual epinephrine dose that is bioequivalent to the intramuscular adult dose of epinephrine 0.3 mg [11]. Results showed that the administration of a first-generation RDST of epinephrine 40 mg formulation resulted in plasma epinephrine concentrations similar to those achieved after the administration of an adult dose of epinephrine 0.3 mg by intramuscular injection [11].

Later, these RDSTs were found to have a shelf-life of up to 7 years [12]. The rate of complete epinephrine dissolution was also optimized by altering excipient proportions to reach ≤60 s following fast tablet disintegration in ≤30 s [13–16]. The intrinsic bitter taste of epinephrine in the sublingual tablets was then masked by adding a taste masking excipient (citric acid), in addition to other excipients [17], since the bitter taste can be a potential barrier for patients' compliance, particularly for pediatric use. The absorption of epinephrine 40 mg from these tasted-masked sublingual tablet formulations was reevaluated again in animal model [18].

Combining the findings from the dose-escalation and taste-masking studies, we hypothesized that a taste-masked RDST formulation with a lower epinephrine dose of 30 mg would have the potential as a child dose for the treatment of anaphylaxis in a pediatric population. To our knowledge, this is the first pre-clinical study of a potential pediatric sublingual dose of epinephrine for the treatment of anaphylaxis.

The assessment of new pediatric dosage forms, new dose regimens, or new routes of administration of certain drugs and biologics was made mandatory by the FDA as per the Pediatric Research Equity Act (PREA) in 2003 [19]. According to the act, adequate pharmacokinetic data supporting dosing and administration for each pediatric subpopulation—permitting acceptable extrapolation between age groups—is a required part of the application process. The pediatric product should be a user-friendly easy-to-swallow or dissolvable dosage form with acceptable palatability. The product should also provide adequate bioavailability and be stable over a range of conditions. Taste-masking of formulations must take into consideration the effect of sweetening and/or flavoring agents on the pharmacokinetic profiles of medications being masked for their unpleasant taste.

Therefore, our objective in this preclinical study was to evaluate the pharmacokinetic profile of an epinephrine 30 mg dose from taste-masked rapidly-disintegrating sublingual tablets as a potential pediatric dose in comparison to epinephrine 0.15 mg intramuscular injection from EpiPen Jr®, the only available pediatric dose in epinephrine auto-injectors.

2. Materials and Methods

2.1. Manufacturing of Taste-Masked Rapidly-Disintegrating Sublingual Tablets (RDSTs) of Epinephrine

The composition of the formulation used to manufacture taste-masked RDSTs is shown in Table 1. Epinephrine bitartrate 54.58 mg, equivalent to 30 mg of epinephrine, was used in the preparation of epinephrine RDST (Epi 30). The ratio of total microcrystalline cellulose (both PH-301 and PH-M-06) to low-substituted hydroxypropyl cellulose was kept at 9:1 in the placebo and Epi 30 RDST formulations. This pre-determined ratio enabled optimal disintegration times, as reported previously [14,15]. Magnesium stearate was used as a lubricant and kept at 2% in a total tablet weight of 200 mg.

Table 1. The type and amounts of ingredients used in the taste-masked rapidly-disintegrating sublingual tablet formulations [1].

Ingredient (mg) [2]	Formulations	
	Placebo	Epi 30
Epinephrine bitartrate	0	54.58
Microcrystalline cellulose (Ceolus® PH-301)	123.00	80.86
Microcrystalline cellulose (Ceolus® PH-M-06)	20.50	13.48
Mannitol (Ludiflash)	34.10	34.10
Citric acid	2.50	2.50
Low-substituted hydroxypropyl cellulose (LH11)	15.90	10.48
Magnesium stearate	4.00	4.00

[1] Tablet weight was maintained at 200 mg; [2] Ratio of total microcrystalline cellulose (Ceolus® PH-301 and Ceolus® PH-M-06) to low-substituted hydroxypropyl cellulose (LH11) was kept at 9:1 in both formulations.

A 13/32 (0.4062 inch) die with flat face upper and lower punches (Natoli Engineering Company, Inc., St. Charles, MO, USA) was used to manufacture RDSTs by direct compression at a preselected range of compression forces (CFs, 18.5–23.25 kN) using a Manesty-F3 single-punch tablet press machine (Liverpool, UK) [15]. A dial caliper (Hempe Manufacturing Co., Inc., New Berlin, WI, USA) was used to measure the dimensions, diameter, and thickness of the compressed tablets.

2.2. Quality Control Testing of Taste-Masked Rapidly-Disintegrating Sublingual Tablets (RDSTs) of Epinephrine

Tablet weight variation and drug content uniformity were measured following the USP methods and criteria [20]. To determine tablet weight variation, an analytical balance (Mettler-Toledo Inc., Columbus, OH, USA) was used to individually weigh 10 out of 30 randomly selected tablets. Drug content was analyzed using a high-performance liquid chromatography (HPLC) system with ultraviolet (UV) detection at 280 nm (Waters Corp., Milford, MA, USA). An acceptance value (AV) of 15.0 was used, according to the harmonized USP method.

A hardness tester (Erweka, Heusenstamm, Germany) was used to measure the breaking force of six tablets selected randomly from each formulation batch. A friability tester (Pharma Test Apparatebau GmbH, Hainburg, Germany) was used to determine the friability according to the USP guidelines to measure the friability of compressed, uncoated tablets [21]. Briefly, the drum of the friability tester, containing a random sample of whole and dedusted tablets corresponding to 6.5 g, was rotated 100 times and tablets were removed, dedusted, and accurately reweighed. A friability value of ≤1.0% weight loss was considered acceptable.

Due to the absence of an appropriate dissolution apparatus and method that simulates the physiological conditions in the sublingual cavity, a validated novel in vitro method was followed to test the dissolution of epinephrine from RDSTs using a custom-made dissolution apparatus constructed in our laboratory [13]. The dissolution medium of 2 mL of distilled water was added into a donor glass funnel that is 15 mL in volume capacity, into which a tablet was placed to disintegrate and dissolve for 120 s without any agitation or motion. Using a vacuum pump, further drug dissolution was terminated by withdrawing the total volume of the dissolution medium into the collection tube passing through a 0.45 μm filter membrane. The dissolved drug content in the filtrate was measured by HPLC with UV detection (Waters Corp.) according to the official USP assay for Epinephrine Injection [22]. The percentage of drug dissolved (DD%) was calculated by dividing the drug content (mg) in the filtrates of six individual RDSTs by the content uniformity value of the tablet formulation batch.

2.3. Animal Study Design

A randomized three-arm cross-over placebo-controlled study was performed in New Zealand female white rabbits (*n* = 5), an epinephrine-tolerant species (mean weight ± SD = 3.6 ± 0.1 kg), using a previously reported protocol [11,18]. The studies were performed in three different study days (one treatment/arm/day) at least 4 weeks apart, as a wash-out period and to replenish blood volume. The rate and extent of epinephrine absorption from Epi 30 sublingual tablets were investigated in comparison to epinephrine absorption following 0.15 mg intramuscular injection in the mid-outer thigh using EpiPen Jr® as a positive control. In-date EpiPens Jr® 0.15 mg (Mylan Specialty L.P, Basking Ridge, NJ, USA) were purchased from the University of Manitoba pharmacy. Placebo RDSTs containing identical excipients composition and ratios of Epi 30 were used as the negative control.

The project was approved by the University of Manitoba Protocol Management and Review Committee. The guidelines published by the Canadian Council on Animal Care were followed throughout.

On each study day, an indwelling catheter was inserted into an ear artery >30 min before dosing. Blood samples of 2 mL per sample were withdrawn immediately before dosing to obtain baseline readings (endogenous epinephrine), and 5, 10, 15, 20, 30, 40, and 60 min after dosing for the measurement of plasma epinephrine concentrations.

The technique of administering sublingual tablets into the rabbit's mouth was modified from the one previously reported [11]. Briefly, the rabbit mouth was opened with the aid of a speculum, after which the tablet was placed carefully under the tongue with the aid of forceps and was kept undisturbed for 2 min [18]. Then, the tablet residues were removed from the rabbit mouth by washing with 40–50 mL distilled water to terminate any further epinephrine absorption.

2.4. Measurement of Plasma Epinephrine Concentrations

Blood samples were collected in a BD Vacutainer® PPTM Plasma Preparation Tubes, refrigerated within 1 h of sampling, and centrifuged at 4 °C. Plasma samples were frozen at −20 °C. Before analysis, plasma samples were thawed at room temperature, and epinephrine was extracted by a solid-phase extraction (SPE) process, with an efficiency of 70–80% [11], which was improved to 80–90% by optimizing the SPE conditions [23]. An aqueous solution containing 0.1 M perchloric acid (Fisher, Fair Lawn, NJ, USA) and 0.1 mM sodium metabisulfite (Sigma, St. Louis, MO, USA) to maintain the stability of epinephrine, was used for the preparation of all epinephrine stock solutions and subsequent dilutions, and for the desorption of epinephrine from alumina during epinephrine extraction from plasma samples.

A 0.5 mL volume of plasma was added to alumina, along with 50 μL of 0.1 mM sodium metabisulfite (Sigma, St. Louis, MO, USA), 400 μL of tris buffer, and precalculated concentrations of dihydroxybenzylamine (DHBA) (Sigma, St. Louis, MO, USA) as an internal standard, corresponding to the concentrations used in the calibration curve. The mixture was vortexed for 15 min to extract epinephrine and DHBA from the plasma samples, and then washed two times with distilled water to remove any plasma components and buffer. A 100 μL volume of 0.1 M perchloric acid and 0.1 mM sodium metabisulfite (1:1) solution was added, and then vortexed for 5 min to elute epinephrine and DHBA from alumina. After centrifugation, the supernatant solution was transferred into vials for injection into the HPLC system.

Epinephrine was measured using reverse-phase high performance liquid chromatography (Waters Corp.) with electrochemical detection. The potential of the glassy carbon working electrode was set at +600 mV versus ISAAC reference electrode and the detector sensitivity was set at 10 nA. All chromatography was performed on a reversed-phase Nova-Pak® C18 column, 3.9 mm × 150 mm, 60 nominal pore size, 4 μm spherical particles (Waters Corp., Milford, MA, USA). The injection volume was 20 μL.

The mobile phase was composed of buffer:methanol at a ratio of 95:5 (by volume), according to recommendations from Waters®. The buffer used was 50 mM sodium acetate (Fisher, Fair Lawn, NJ, USA), 20 mM citric acid (Fisher, Fair Lawn, NJ, USA), mixed with 3.75 mM 1-heptanesulfonic acid sodium salt (Sigma, St. Louis, MO, USA), 0.134 mM EDTA disodium salt dihydrate (Sigma, St. Louis, MO, USA), and 1 mM dibutylamine (Fisher, Fair Lawn, NJ, USA), and filtered using 22 μm nylon membrane filters (Whatman, Whatman International Ltd., Maidstone, UK). The flow rate was set at 1.0 mL/min. Under these conditions, epinephrine and DHBA eluted at 1.9 and 2.5 min, respectively.

Two stock solutions of epinephrine (25 and 250 ng/mL) were prepared using (−)-epinephrine (+) bitartrate (Sigma, St. Louis, MO, USA) and then used to prepare two sets of epinephrine standards ranging from 0.1 to 1.0 ng/mL and from 1.0 to 10.0 ng/mL spiked in anticoagulated rabbit plasma. A 40 μL volume of DHBA 5 ng/mL (0.2 ng) and a 50 μL volume of DHBA 50 ng/mL (2.5 ng) were used with the low and high range calibration curves, respectively. The low-range calibration curve was linear (R^2 of >0.95) over the range 0.1–1 ng/mL (CV%, 0.4–0.1%). The high-range calibration curve was linear (R^2 of >0.99) over the range of 1–10 ng/mL (CV%, 0.1%).

The extraction recovery from plasma was 80–90%. The CV% of the system reproducibility in solution at 1.0 ng/mL ($n = 5$) was 0.25%. The detection limit was 5 pg with a CV% of 28.8% ($n = 2$).

2.5. Data Analysis

Mean ± SEM maximum plasma epinephrine concentration (C_{max}), the time at which C_{max} was achieved (T_{max}), and the area under the plasma epinephrine concentration versus time curve ($AUC_{0-1 h}$) were calculated from the epinephrine versus time plots of each individual rabbit using WinNonlin 5.3 (Pharsight, Mountain View, CA, USA). Values were compared using ANOVA and Tukey–Kramer tests (NCSS Statistical Analysis Software). Differences were considered significant at $p < 0.05$.

3. Results

The manufactured taste-masked RDSTs resulted in acceptable tablet weight variation, drug content uniformity, breaking force, and friability. Epinephrine from the manufactured RDSTs was dissolved completely within 2 min. Table 2 summarizes the results of the quality control tests of taste-masked RDSTs.

Table 2. Mean ± SD diameter, weight variation (WV), content uniformity (CU), breaking force (BF), friability (F), and drug dissolution (DD) for the taste-masked rapidly-disintegrating sublingual tablet formulations.

Characteristics	Formulations	
	Placebo	Epi 30
Diameter (mm)	9.98 ± 0.01	9.98 ± 0.01
WV (mg), (AV) [a]	202 ± 2.58 (3.1)	211 ± 2.85 (6.47)
CU (%), (AV) [a]	N/A	102 ± 4.77 (10.94)
BF (kgf)	2.53 ± 0.02	2.50 ± 0.01
F (%)	0.1	0.7
DD (%) [b]	N/A	102.97 ± 8.28

[a] AV, USP acceptance value (values ≤15.00 were considered acceptable according to USP L1 limit);
[b] DD (%), Percentage of drug dissolved in the first 120 s.

The plasma concentration of epinephrine versus time profiles following the administration of placebo and epinephrine 30 mg sublingual tablets, and epinephrine 0.15 mg by intramuscular injection are presented in Figure 1 as means ± SEM. $C_{baseline}$, T_{max}, C_{max}, and $AUC_{0-1 h}$ values are presented in Table 3 as means ± SEM. The $C_{baseline}$ obtained following catheterization of rabbits and just before dosage forms' administration were not significantly different between the three different treatment arms ($p \geq 0.05$). The C_{max} and T_{max} values did not differ significantly after the administration of epinephrine 30 mg by sublingual tablets or epinephrine 0.15 mg by intramuscular injection ($p \geq 0.05$). However, the $AUC_{0-1 h}$ obtained after the sublingual administration of epinephrine 30 mg was significantly lower than those obtained after the intramuscular injection of epinephrine 0.15 mg ($p \leq 0.05$). The C_{max} and $AUC_{0-1 h}$ following the administration of epinephrine 30 mg sublingual tablets or epinephrine 0.15 mg by intramuscular injection were significantly higher ($p < 0.05$) than the C_{max} and $AUC_{0-1\,h}$ following the administration of placebo sublingual tablets reflecting the endogenous epinephrine levels.

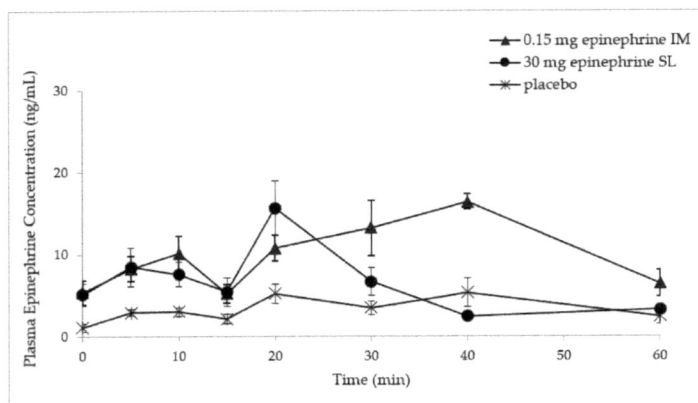

Figure 1. Plasma epinephrine concentration (mean ± SEM) versus time plots following the administration of epinephrine 0.15 mg by intramuscular injection, epinephrine 30 mg sublingually, and placebo sublingually.

Table 3. The pharmacokinetic parameters of epinephrine following the sublingual administration of epinephrine 30 mg and placebo tablets and epinephrine 0.15 mg by intramuscular injection in the thigh.

Mean ± SEM *	Placebo Sublingual Tablets (Endogenous Epinephrine)	Epinephrine Sublingual Tablets (Epi 30)	EpiPens Jr®
Epinephrine dose (mg)	0	30	0.15
$C_{baseline}$ (ng/mL)	1.1 ± 0.5	5.1 ± 1.4	5.4 ± 1.5
C_{max} (ng/mL)	7.5 ± 1.7 [†]	16.7 ± 1.9	18.8 ± 1.9
T_{max} (min) [††]	33.3 ± 7.2	21.0 ± 2.5	36.0 ± 2.5
$AUC_{0-1\,h}$ (ng/mL/min)	220.1 ± 31.8 [†]	372.3 ± 21.7 [†]	654.2 ± 39.6

$C_{baseline}$: baseline plasma concentration reflecting endogenous epinephrine; C_{max}: maximum plasma concentration (mean ± SEM of individual C_{max} values from each rabbit, regardless of the time at which C_{max} was achieved); T_{max}: time at which maximum plasma epinephrine concentration was achieved (mean ± SEM of individual T_{max} values in each rabbit); $AUC_{0-1\,h}$: area under the plasma concentration versus time curve (mean ± SEM of individual AUC values from each rabbit). * $n = 5$; [†] $p < 0.05$; [††] T_{max} is the time at which the highest peak epinephrine concentration occurred in each individual rabbit, regardless of the time since dosing. T_{max} is limited by experimental design because it is a discrete variable based on defined times of blood sampling.

4. Discussion

Visits to emergency departments due to anaphylaxis have been increasing over the years, with the highest number of visits being among children [24]. The management of anaphylaxis includes the administration of epinephrine as the drug of choice. For the first-aid treatment of anaphylaxis, autoinjectors delivering 0.15 mg of epinephrine are prescribed for children, but they are underused for a number of reasons—one of which is needle phobia. Physical injuries resulting from inadvertent and incorrect administration leading to lacerations and embedded needles caused by epinephrine autoinjector use in children have been reported [6].

Potential alternative routes to epinephrine intramuscular administration have been proposed, including inhalational route, in an effort to provide a user-friendly dosage form of epinephrine [25,26]. However, inhalers for asthma as well as autoinjectors for anaphylaxis were associated with misuse, which indicates the need for the extensive training of all caregivers [27]. In our laboratory, a rapidly-disintegrating tablet formulation of epinephrine for sublingual administration has been extensively studied [11–18,28,29]. A rabbit model was utilized for the evaluation of sublingual absorption and pharmacokinetic modeling, which has been shown to be used for many other drugs [30–33]. The challenges associated with the intramuscular administration of epinephrine have been effectively considered and overcome through the development of a rapidly-disintegrating sublingual tablet formulation of epinephrine. Compared to the intramuscular route, the sublingual route is accessible, convenient for self-administration, and has long been used for self-treatment in other medical emergencies, such as the initial treatment of angina using user-friendly sublingual nitroglycerine tablets. The design and development of taste-masked RDSTs of epinephrine enabled the application of human factor analysis, taking real-life scenarios of human use into consideration. The RDSTs are small in size, and can be easily and conveniently carried anytime and anywhere. These taste-masked RDSTs may be formulated to contain several dose ranges to accommodate the general population on a mg/kg basis.

There is a growing demand for pediatric regulatory requirement to ensure the safety and efficacy of medications in the pediatric population [34–36]. Masking the bitter taste of medications is becoming one of the major considerations in the development of a pediatric formulation to enhance administration acceptability by children. The sour taste, provided by the flavoring agent citric acid, is one of the recognized and well-accepted tastes by children and is commonly used in children's drinks, food, and medications [34]. Epinephrine's inherent bitter taste in the manufactured tablets was effectively masked by the addition of citric acid as we showed previously in our taste-masking studies using an electronic tongue [17]. However, taste-masking should not compromise the pharmacokinetics of the active pharmaceutical ingredient in the developed pediatric formulation.

In this study, it has been shown that the addition of citric acid as a taste-masking and flavoring agent did not affect the dissolution, absorption, or pharmacokinetics of a potential epinephrine pediatric dose from these developed taste-masked RDSTs, and were similar to the dissolution of our previously published data of non-taste-masked RDSTs [11,14]. Epinephrine 30 mg was completely released from the taste-masked sublingual tablets and dissolved in 2 min, which shows that the addition of citric acid to the tablet formulation did not slow down epinephrine dissolution—a critical and limiting step for epinephrine absorption.

In comparison to the intramuscularly administered pediatric dose of EpiPen Jr® 0.15 mg, the sublingually-administered epinephrine 30 mg was rapidly absorbed following its complete dissolution through sublingual mucosa, resulting in a similar maximum concentration (C_{max}) at a similar T_{max}, which are clinically significant parameters for the treatment of anaphylaxis, demonstrating that the addition of citric acid to the tablet formulation did not affect the extent and rate of epinephrine absorption, respectively (Table 3). Despite of the lack of a significant difference in the T_{max} due to the small sample size and sublingual variability, the shorter T_{max} after sublingual administration of epinephrine compared to T_{max} after intramuscular administration is in agreement with results from our previous work [11,18,29]. This can be attributed to the thin mucosa and the abundant blood supply in the sublingual area, facilitating the rapid absorption of epinephrine by passive diffusion across the epithelium into the interstitial fluid.

The administration of epinephrine resulted in two peaks at 5 min and 20 min after the administration of epinephrine 30 mg taste-masked RDSTs compared to two peaks at 10 min and 40 min after IM injection of EpiPen Jr® 0.15 mg (Figure 1).

Similar to what we have reported previously in both animal model and humans [11,18], epinephrine administration through all studied routes of administration resulted in an intermittent pattern of absorption as reflected in two or more peaks of epinephrine in the collected plasma over the duration of the study. Initially, the rapid absorption of epinephrine resulted in the first peak, which led to vasoconstriction at the administration site (i.e., sublingual mucosa or skeletal muscle). The first absorbed portion of epinephrine, consequently leading to vasoconstriction, resulted in a reduction of epinephrine absorption that was temporary due to blood circulation sink condition. However, the remaining higher portion of epinephrine dose continued to accumulate at the site of absorption and interstitial space. Therefore, the subsequent vasodilation due to the elimination of epinephrine resulted in a second phase of epinephrine absorption from the site of absorption, leading to a second, often higher, peak in the systemic circulation due to the accumulation of a larger amount of epinephrine compared to the one resulted in the first peak.

Achieving high epinephrine plasma peaks as rapidly as possible is a clinical necessity to reverse the life-threatening signs and symptoms of anaphylaxis. Epinephrine administered sublingually in a relatively high dose compared with the doses administered intramuscularly was found necessary to create the high concentration gradient that drives its diffusion through the sublingual mucosa according to Fick's law. Despite the similar magnitude of C_{max} resulting after the administration of Epi 30 and EpiPen Jr® 0.15 mg, their $AUC_{0-1 h}$ were significantly different. Paradoxically and despite its half dose, EpiPen Jr® 0.15 mg resulted in similar, but slightly higher $AUC_{0-1 h}$ (654 ng/mL/min) than that achieved after EpiPen® 0.3 mg (592 ng/mL/min) reported previously [18]. It has been shown that further epinephrine absorption from EpiPen Jr® beyond 1 h might occur [37], but it would be clinically insignificant during anaphylaxis episodes when the initial epinephrine peaks in the first hour are critical for life-saving. The $AUC_{0-1 h}$ achieved after the sublingual administration of epinephrine 30 mg in this study is about half the $AUC_{0-1 h}$ achieved after the intramuscular administration of epinephrine 0.3 mg using EpiPens® from previously reported data [18]. The ratio *F.Dose/AUC*$_{0-1 h}$ after sublingual administration of epinephrine 30 mg was 81 F L/min and the ratio calculated after sublingual administration of epinephrine 40 mg from data reported previously [18] was 59 F L/min. Assuming similar clearances, the bioavailability, F, of the 40 mg dose is higher than that of the 30 mg dose, reflecting a higher driving force of sublingual absorption with higher epinephrine doses.

A narrower dose-ranging study of epinephrine in RDSTs should be performed to determine the equivalent sublingual dose to the 0.15 mg intramuscular dose. Epinephrine microcrystals were developed in our laboratory, enhancing epinephrine absorption from RDSTs, which facilitated dose reduction [29]. Tablet dosage form and size suitability for pediatric population have been reviewed, showing positive acceptability of tablet dosage form by age groups ranging from 1 month to 18 years; and mini tablets by age groups ranging from newborns to 5 years [38–40]. A range of tablet and mini-tablet sizes can be manufactured that would enable proper administration to meet the needs of different pediatric age groups. In these pediatric age groups, sublingual administration techniques are yet to be evaluated for innovative approaches that are user-friendly, misuse resistant, and economical.

5. Conclusions

Taste-masked rapidly-disintegrating sublingual tablets containing epinephrine 30 mg resulted in comparable pharmacokinetic profiles with similar maximum concentrations, but different area under the curve, compared to intramuscular epinephrine 0.15 mg from EpiPen Jr®. Further pharmacokinetic studies are needed to determine dose equivalency in preclinical animal models. RDSTs of epinephrine might eventually be useful as an easy-to-carry, palatable, non-invasive treatment for anaphylactic episodes in community settings.

Author Contributions: All authors conceived and designed the experiments; Ousama Rachid and Keith J. Simons performed the animal experiments; Ousama Rachid and Mutasem Rawas-Qalaji analyzed the data, withdraw conclusions; and contributed to the writing of the paper.

Conflicts of Interest: The authors declare no conflict of interest.

References

1. Simons, F.E.R.; Ardusso, L.R.F.; Bilo, M.B.; El-Gamal, Y.M.; Ledford, D.K.; Ring, J.; Sanchez-Borges, M.; Senna, G.E.; Sheikh, A.; Thong, B.Y.; et al. World Allergy Organization guidelines for the assessment and management of anaphylaxis. *J. Allergy Clin. Immunol.* **2011**, *127*, 587–593.e1–e22. [CrossRef] [PubMed]
2. Simons, K.J.; Simons, F.E.R. Epinephrine and its use in anaphylaxis: Current issues. *Curr. Opin. Allergy Clin. Immunol.* **2010**, *10*, 354–361. [CrossRef] [PubMed]
3. Simons, F.E.R.; Clark, S.; Camargo, C.A. Anaphylaxis in the community: Learning from the survivors. *J. Allergy Clin. Immunol.* **2009**, *124*, 301–306. [CrossRef] [PubMed]

4. Noimark, L.; Wales, J.; Du Toit, G.; Pastacaldi, C.; Haddad, D.; Gardner, J.; Hyer, W.; Vance, G.; Townshend, C.; Alfaham, M.; et al. The use of adrenaline autoinjectors by children and teenagers. *Clin. Exp. Allergy* **2012**, *42*, 284–292. [CrossRef] [PubMed]

5. Chad, L.; Ben-Shoshan, M.; Asai, Y.; Cherkaoui, S.; Alizadehfar, R.; St-Pierre, Y.; Harada, L.; Allen, M.; Clarke, A. A majority of parents of children with peanut allergy fear using the epinephrine auto-injector. *Allergy* **2013**, *68*, 1605–1609. [CrossRef] [PubMed]

6. Brown, J.C.; Tuuri, R.E.; Akhter, S.; Guerra, L.D.; Goodman, I.S.; Myers, S.R.; Nozicka, C.; Manzi, S.; Long, K.; Turner, T.; et al. Lacerations and embedded needles caused by epinephrine autoinjector use in children. *Ann. Emerg. Med.* **2016**, *67*, 307–315. [CrossRef] [PubMed]

7. Robinson, P.E.; Lareau, S.A. Novel technique for epinephrine removal in new generation autoinjectors. *Wilderness Environ. Med.* **2016**, *27*, 252–255. [CrossRef] [PubMed]

8. Hawkins, S.C.; Weil, C.; Baty, F.; Fitzpatrick, D.; Powell, B. Retrieval of additional epinephrine from auto-injectors. *Wilderness Environ. Med.* **2013**, *24*, 434–444. [CrossRef] [PubMed]

9. Rawas-Qalaji, M.; Simons, F.E.; Collins, D.; Simons, K.J. Long-term stability of epinephrine dispensed in unsealed syringes for the first-aid treatment of anaphylaxis. *Ann. Allergy Asthma Immunol* **2009**, *102*, 500–503. [CrossRef]

10. Simons, F.E.; Chan, E.S.; Gu, X.; Simons, K.J. Epinephrine for the out-of-hospital (first-aid) treatment of anaphylaxis in infants: Is the ampule/syringe/needle method practical? *J. Allergy Clin. Immunol.* **2001**, *108*, 1040–1044. [CrossRef] [PubMed]

11. Rawas-Qalaji, M.M.; Simons, F.E.R.; Simons, K.J. Sublingual epinephrine tablets versus intramuscular injection of epinephrine: Dose-equivalence for potential treatment of anaphylaxis. *J. Allergy Clin. Immunol.* **2006**, *117*, 398–403. [CrossRef] [PubMed]

12. Rawas-Qalaji, M.; Rachid, O.; Simons, F.E.R.; Simons, K.J. Long-term stability of epinephrine sublingual tablets for the potential first-aid treatment of anaphylaxis. *Ann. Allergy Asthma Immunol.* **2013**, *111*, 568–570. [CrossRef] [PubMed]

13. Rachid, O.; Rawas-Qalaji, M.M.; Simons, F.E.R.; Simons, K.J. Dissolution testing of sublingual tablets: A novel in vitro method. *AAPS PhamSciTech* **2011**, *12*, 544–552. [CrossRef] [PubMed]

14. Rachid, O.; Rawas-Qalaji, M.; Simons, F.E.R.; Simons, K.J. Rapidly-disintegrating sublingual tablets of epinephrine: Role of non-medicinal ingredients in formulation development. *Eur. J. Pharm. Biopharm.* **2012**, *82*, 598–604. [CrossRef] [PubMed]

15. Rawas-Qalaji, M.M.; Simons, F.E.; Simons, K.J. Fast-disintegrating sublingual tablets: Effect of epinephrine load on tablet characteristics. *AAPS PharmSciTech* **2006**, *7*, E72–E78. [CrossRef] [PubMed]

16. Rawas-Qalaji, M.M.; Simons, F.E.; Simons, K.J. Fast-disintegrating sublingual epinephrine tablets: Effect of tablet dimensions on tablet characteristics. *Drug Dev. Ind. Pharm* **2007**, *33*, 523–530. [CrossRef] [PubMed]

17. Rachid, O.; Simons, F.E.R.; Rawas-Qalaji, M.; Simons, K.J. An electronic tongue: Evaluation of the masking efficacy of sweetening and/or flavouring agents on the bitter taste of epinephrine. *AAPS PharmSciTech* **2010**, *11*, 550–557. [CrossRef] [PubMed]

18. Rachid, O.; Rawas-Qalaji, M.M.; Simons, F.E.; Simons, K.J. Epinephrine (adrenaline) absorption from new-generation, taste-masked sublingual tablets: A preclinical study. *J. Allergy Clin. Immunol.* **2013**, *131*, 236–238. [CrossRef] [PubMed]

19. Food and Drug Administration. Pediatric Research Equity Act. 2003. Available online: http://www.fda.gov/downloads/Drugs/DevelopmentApprovalProcess/DevelopmentResources/UCM077853.pdf (accessed on 16 July 2017).

20. Physical tests: Uniformity of dosage Units h905i. In *USP/NF*, 26th/21st ed.; United States Pharmacopeial Convention Inc.: Rockville, MD, USA, 2003.

21. Physical tests: Tablet friability h1216i. In *USP/NF*, 26th/21st ed.; United States Pharmacopeial Convention Inc.: Rockville, MD, USA, 2003.

22. Official monograph: Epinephrine injection. In *USP/NF*, 32nd/27th ed.; United States Pharmacopeial Convention Inc.: Rockville, MD, USA, 2009; p. 2261.

23. Zahrah, F.; Shosha'a, K.; Alzahabi, K.; Khalil, A.; Rawas-Qalaji, M.; Rachid, O. A simple solid phase extraction method for optimizing the recovery of catecholamines and their metabolites from biological sample. In Proceedings of the American Association of Pharmaceutical Scientists, San Diego, CA, USA, 12–15 November 2017.

24. Motosue, M.S.; Bellolio, M.F.; Van Houten, H.K.; Shah, N.D.; Campbell, R.L. Increasing emergency department visits for anaphylaxis, 2005–2014. *J. Allergy Clin. Immunol. Pract.* **2016**, *5*, 171–175.e3. [CrossRef] [PubMed]
25. Frechen, S.; Suleiman, A.A.; Mohammad Nejad Sigaroudi, A.; Wachall, B.; Fuhr, U. Population pharmacokinetic and pharmacodynamic modeling of epinephrine administered using a mobile inhaler. *Drug Metab. Pharmacokinet.* **2015**, *30*, 391–399. [CrossRef] [PubMed]
26. Gu, X.; Simons, F.E.; Simons, K.J. Epinephrine absorption after different routes of administration in an animal model. *Biopharm. Drug Dispos.* **1999**, *20*, 401–405. [CrossRef]
27. Bonds, R.S.; Asawa, A.; Ghazi, AI. Misuse of medical devices: A persistent problem in self-management of asthma and allergic disease. *Ann. Allergy Asthma Immunol.* **2015**, *114*, 74–76. [CrossRef] [PubMed]
28. Rawas-Qalaji, M.M.; Werdy, S.; Rachid, O.; Simons, F.E.; Simons, K.J. Sublingual diffusion of epinephrine microcrystals from rapidly disintegrating tablets for the potential first-aid treatment of anaphylaxis: In vitro and ex vivo study. *AAPS PharmSciTech* **2015**, *16*, 1203–1212. [CrossRef] [PubMed]
29. Rawas-Qalaji, M.; Rachid, O.; Mendez, B.A.; Losada, A.; Simons, F.E.; Simons, K.J. Adrenaline (epinephrine) microcrystal sublingual tablet formulation: Enhanced absorption in a preclinical model. *J. Pharm. Pharmacol.* **2015**, *67*, 20–25. [CrossRef] [PubMed]
30. Kaartama, R.; Turunen, E.; Toljamo, K.; Kokki, H.; Lehtonen, M.; Ranta, V.P.; Savolainen, J.; Järvinen, K.; Jarho, P. The effect of hydroxypropyl beta-cyclodextrin and sucrose on the sublingual absorption of midazolam in rabbits. *Eur. J. Pharm. Biopharm.* **2012**, *81*, 178–183. [CrossRef] [PubMed]
31. Sheu, M.T.; Hsieh, C.M.; Chen, R.N.; Chou, P.Y.; Ho, H.O. Rapid-onset sildenafil sublingual drug delivery systems: In vitro evaluation and in vivo pharmacokinetic studies in rabbits. *J. Pharm. Sci.* **2016**, *105*, 2774–2781. [CrossRef] [PubMed]
32. Turunen, E.; Mannila, J.; Laitinen, R.; Riikonen, J.; Lehto, V.P.; Järvinen, T.; Ketolainen, J.; Järvinen, K.; Jarho, P. Fast-dissolving sublingual solid dispersion and cyclodextrin complex increase the absorption of perphenazine in rabbits. *J. Pharm. Pharmacol.* **2011**, *63*, 19–25. [CrossRef] [PubMed]
33. Hedaya, M.A.; Thomas, T.; Abdel-Hamid, M.E.; Kehinde, E.O.; Phillips, O.A. Comparative pharmacokinetic study for linezolid and two novel antibacterial oxazolidinone derivatives in rabbits: Can differences in the pharmacokinetic properties explain the discrepancies between their in vivo and in vitro antibacterial activities? *Pharmaceutics* **2017**, *9*, 34. [CrossRef] [PubMed]
34. Committee for Medicinal Products for Human Use (CHMP) of European Medicines Agency. Reflection Paper: Formulations of Choice for the Paediatric Population. EMEA/CHMP/PEG/194810/2005. Available online: http://www.ema.europa.eu/docs/en_GB/document_library/Scientific_guideline/2009/09/WC500003782.pdf (accessed on 11 March 2017).
35. Committee for Human Medicinal Products of European Medicines Agency. ICH E11(R1) Guideline on Clinical Investigation of Medicinal Products in the Pediatric Population Step 5. EMA/CPMP/ICH/2711/1999. Available online: http://www.ema.europa.eu/docs/en_GB/document_library/Scientific_guideline/2017/10/WC500236218.pdf (accessed on 20 November 2017).
36. Zisowsky, J.; Krause, A.; Dingemanse, J. Drug development for pediatric populations: Regulatory aspects. *Pharmaceutics* **2010**, *2*, 364–388. [CrossRef] [PubMed]
37. Simons, F.E.; Gu, X.; Silver, N.A.; Simons, K.J. EpiPen Jr versus EpiPen in young children weighing 15 to 30 kg at risk for anaphylaxis. *J. Allergy Clin. Immunol.* **2002**, *109*, 171–175. [CrossRef] [PubMed]
38. Mitra, B.; Chang, J.; Wu, S.J.; Wolfe, C.N.; Ternik, R.L.; Gunter, T.Z.; Victor, M.C. Feasibility of mini-tablets as a flexible drug delivery tool. *Int. J. Pharm.* **2017**, *525*, 149–159. [CrossRef] [PubMed]
39. Ranmal, S.R.; Cram, A.; Tuleu, C. Age-appropriate and acceptable paediatric dosage forms: Insights into end user perceptions, preferences and practices from the Children's Acceptability of Oral Formulations (CALF) Study. *Int. J. Pharm.* **2016**, *514*, 296–307. [CrossRef] [PubMed]
40. Walsh, J.; Ranmal, S.R.; Ernest, T.B.; Liu, F. Patient acceptability, safety and access: A balancing act for selecting age-appropriate oral dosage forms for paediatric and geriatric populations. *Int. J. Pharm.* **2017**. [CrossRef] [PubMed]

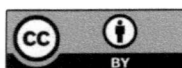

MDPI AG

St. Alban-Anlage 66

4052 Basel, Switzerland

Tel. +41 61 683 77 34

Fax +41 61 302 89 18

http://www.mdpi.com

Pharmaceutics Editorial Office

E-mail: pharmaceutics@mdpi.com

http://www.mdpi.com/journal/pharmaceutics